Pain-Relieving Procedures

The Illustrated Guide

P. Prithvi Raj MBBS, FFARCS (Eng), FIPP

Professor Emeritus
Departments of Anesthesiology and Pain Medicine
Texas Tech University Health Sciences Center
Lubbock, Texas, USA

Serdar Erdine MD, Specialist in Algology (Turkey), FIPP

Professor of Anesthesiology and Algology
Istanbul Pain Center
Istanbul, Turkey

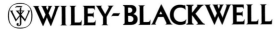

WILEY-BLACKWELL

A John Wiley & Sons, Ltd., Publication

Library of Congress Cataloging-in-Publication Data
Raj, P. Prithvi.
   Pain-relieving procedures : the illustrated guide / P. Prithvi Raj, Serdar Erdine.
       p. ; cm.
   Includes bibliographical references and index.
   ISBN 978-0-470-67038-5 (hardcover : alk. paper)
   I. Erdine, S.   II. Title.
   [DNLM: 1. Pain Management–methods–Handbooks. WL 39]

   616'.0472–dc23
                                                          2011048894

A catalogue record for this book is available from the British Library.

Cover images supplied by authors
Cover design by Steve Thompson

Wiley also publishes its books in a variety of electronic formats. Some content that appears in print may not be available in electronic books.

Set in 9/12 pt Meridien by Toppan Best-set Premedia Limited, Hong Kong
Printed and bound in Singapore by Markono Print Media Pte Ltd

1   2012

Contents

Contents

Foreword

Interventional pain medicine is a relative new specialty, with neurosurgeons and anesthesiologists as "founding fathers". Dr Sam Lipton, Dr Norman Shealy, Dr Menno Sluijter, and Dr Prithvi Raj were, with many others, pioneers of interventional pain medicine at the beginning of the 1980s. After a short period of empirical use of interventional pain techniques, the procedures have been improved and are now more target specific. Nowadays, interventional pain management techniques have become accepted and integrated into the treatment of patients with chronic pain problems. In many treatment plans of patients with chronic benign pain problems such as chronic cervical or lumbar low back pain, interventional pain procedures are now an accepted solution. The same is true for problems caused by for cancer pain such as that due to pancreas carcinoma or to lung cancer.

Since the beginning of the 2000s we have been entering the second phase of interventional pain medicine: "the episode of further professionalization." The public expect something from an interventional pain doctor nowadays: optimal medical knowledge, optimal patient care, technical skills, continuous practical-based learning, and professionalism. Pain physicians have to apply diagnostic and therapeutic interventions in the correct and safe way for the right clinical diagnosis. The clinical diagnoses in which these procedures can be applied were published in the evidence-based medicine series in *Pain Practice* in 2009/2011.

This book has been produced by the pioneer of interventional pain management Professor Dr Prithvi Raj and the key opinion leader of interventional pain at this moment Professor Dr Sedar Erdine. It covers all the relevant specific techniques of interventional pain medicine in an explicit way. More than 40 interventional procedures in and around the head, neck, thoracic, thoraco-abdominal, lumbar, and sacral regions are described.

Moreover, all the chapters are accompanied by detailed anatomical observations and the background to these procedures. This book is an important step in the further evaluation of interventional pain as a tool in the optimal treatment of patients with acute and chronic pain. It will also further improve the technical skills and the knowledge of all pain physicians.

Professor Dr Maarten van Kleef
Head, Department of Anesthesiology and Pain Management
Maastricht University Medical Centre
The Netherlands

Foreword

Pain science and pain medicine are relatively new specialties. The British Pain Society first met in 1971 and the International Association for the Study of Pain (IASP) organized its first international symposium on pain in 1973. Professor John Bonica and his colleagues established this large, multidisciplinary world society and developed the *Journal of Pain*. There have been meetings every 3 years until recently, when the frequency was changed to every 2 years.

Since the early 1970s many other groups have evolved, including the World Society of Pain Clinicians, the World Institute of Pain, and the European Federation of IASP Chapters (EFIC).

Before and during the past 40 years many specialists and general practioners have treated pain, but not in any particularly organized manner. Acute pain was generally managed reasonably well, but there were clearly difficulties in understanding the causes of, and comprehensively treating, chronic pain. Physicians used drugs whereas physiotherapists and chiropractors used manipulations and physical therapy. Anesthetists were interested in perioperative and postoperative pain relief and their interest in regional blocks evolved into interventional management of more chronic forms of pain.

Bonica stressed the importance of multidisciplinary teams, with several different specialties working together. He knew that no one single therapist or specialist could muster all of the necessary knowledge to assess and treat patients comprehensively, and we all agree with this view.

Pain is complex, multidimensional, and can be very difficult to treat. The biopsychosocial model described by Engel at the University of Rochester, and first discussed in *Science* in 1977, has been widely espoused for the management of chronic pain. However it is regrettable that some practitioners have forgotten the importance of assessing each individual patient for the "bio-" part of the model: that is, identifying the specific pathological causes (both nociceptive and neuropathic) for the chronic pain problem, which can sometimes be addressed and successfully treated.

Anesthetists and neurosurgeons started by trial and error, trying different types of procedure for different types of patient, empirically, and just seeing what worked. In the early days at the Walton Centre, Sam Lipton used percutaneous cordotomy for many patients with unilateral pain. We rapidly discovered that patients who had a normal life expectancy often developed dysesthesia and bothersome neuropathic pain within a few months, which was more troublesome than the original problem, so cordotomy became a treatment for those with only a short-term life expectancy.

As time has passed, the development of evidence-based medicine has meant careful evaluation of medication in large, randomized controlled trials with many patients. Interventions for pain relief have come under attack because of a lack of scientific evidence to prove efficacy. There are still too many procedures being performed – some on empirical grounds without there being much hope of them working, others because that is the way the practitioner was taught, and others done by doctors without the adequate training and knowledge to achieve a successful outcome.

Failed interventions because of faulty technique are simply unacceptable. Performing the wrong technique on the wrong patient is also unacceptable. This type of behavior by uninformed, inadequately trained specialists puts the future of interventional procedures in pain medicine in jeopardy.

To ensure the future of interventional procedures and to secure the place of anesthetists in the management of chronic pain, it is essential that we use evidence-based principles where these exist. We need to have a thorough understanding of the assessment of the patient (both from the physical and psychological point of view), the anatomy, and the physics behind the treatments we use.

This book addresses these important issues. Packed with wonderful illustrations, it describes basic principles of interventional techniques, physical and psychological assessment of the patient, preparation of the patient for treatment, and monitoring during and after therapy. It discusses radiation safety and the importance of imaging, including fluoroscopy and ultrasound. The various different methods of intervention are described, including use of local anesthetics and neurolytic agents, steroids, and the different forms of radio frequency.

It goes on to describe in detail the various different types of procedure that might be performed, in a full and comprehensive manner. In all, there are 18 chapters and over 50 techniques are described.

There are three types of illustration. There are pictures of patients, separate three-dimensional computed tomography scans, and fluoroscopic pictures for each technique, showing each procedure step by step.

The authors know their subject thoroughly, not only from extensive knowledge of the literature and research but most importantly the practical aspect of performing these procedures over many years and on many patients. They have been key figures in many of the inter-national groups mentioned, and have published and taught extensively over decades. The reader will gain a constructive and effective knowledge of the many proce-dures that can be used to aid chronic pain sufferers. In particular, this is an important guide for those who wish to get a higher degree in the subject of pain manage-ment and the Fellowship of Interventional Pain Practice (FIPP).

Dr J. C. D. Wells
President Elect, EFIC

Preface

There is consensus in the pain management community that the practice of pain management has now become a specialty on its own and requires careful nurturing of its growth, training of pain physicians, and the creation of acceptable standards of practice guidelines for the physicians.

This complex task, to define standards of pain practice, is extremely difficult and differs among all the specialists who manage patients with pain in their professional practice. For instance, if one asks the anesthesiologist to describe their plan of pain management, they would invariably describe the performance of regional anesthesia techniques as their primary requirement, with a secondary requirement of pharmacotherapeutics, psychiatric modalities, and functional restoration algorithms. This concept is almost always challenged by psychiatrists, physiatrists, neurologists, and even neurosurgeons.

Whichever direction this debate takes us in the standards of pain practice, it is absolutely necessary that all specialties should agree a multidisciplinary approach is essential. This multidisciplinary approach should consist of knowledge of anatomy and physiology of pain mechanisms, knowledge of pain syndromes, diagnosis and management by conventional methods, and, when necessary, use of interventional techniques including minimal invasive surgery.

Although there are now a multitude of text books on the management of pain, publications of specialized techniques in pain management are still few and far between. This is certainly true of the books pertaining to interventional pain procedures. In the past decade, radiographic imaging techniques in pain management have been published; these include two editions by Raj et al., Rathmel, and Waldman. They have been accepted as valuable books for the study and training of interventional pain physicians.

Interventional pain procedures are now evolving, increasing in their complexities; strict protocols are now required to maintain the standards of practice. Fellowship certification for interventional pain physicians is provided by an examination globally by the World Institute of Pain and by the American Board of Interventional Pain Physicians for US candidates. Physicians who are eligible to take the examination have to show training in interventional procedures in a curriculum acceptable to governing agencies.

Pain-Relieving Procedures: The Illustrated Guide is conceived to fill a void in the existing literature. It is an illustrative guide for all currently performed interventional procedures as approved by the experts in the field.

We conceived to present this book to the reader as a step-by-step guide to perform all interventional techniques in an easily understood, simple style. It took 3 years to complete and contains over 1000 figures.

The chapters are divided in two sections. The first is the general section, where the essential basic knowledge for interventional pain physicians is provided. The second section describes all commonly performed techniques, arranged simply and topographically from head to pelvis. To cover all procedures, a special chapter is provided for specialized techniques, such as continuous analgesia, spinal cord and sacral stimulation, vertebroplasty, and kyphoplasty. Modalities of radiofrequency and ultrasonography are presented wherever indicated, along with their basics of physics and mechanisms.

The chapters are straightforward and simply written, to inform basic and essential knowledge about the general requirements for interventional pain physicians and to provide steps to learn the techniques in a standardized manner. The strength of this book is the preparation of the figures, which are outstanding. The uses of three-dimensional computed tomography anatomical images presented in color are unique and easy to understand. The authors reviewed figures from experts all over the world who could enhance the quality of the book by their original publications. We are indebted to Professor J. Taylor from Western Australia for his exceptionally unique figures depicting the various regions of spinal anatomy in full color. Similarly, we thank James Heavner for his epiduroscopy figures, and Sang Chul Lee for his ultrasonography pictures.

The format of the chapters is uniformly written under the headings of history, anatomy, indication, contraindication, technique, complications, and helpful hints. Chapters do not cite references in the text; however, conveniently, a further reading section is provided at the end of each chapter. We believe that we have achieved the objectives set out by the publisher: to provide an illustrated guide to interventional procedures in a clear, simple step-by-step instruction to the physician who wishes to perform the chosen procedure. The current standard of practice is always kept in mind. We hope that the reader will find this book easy to read and learn from when they train to be specialists in interventional pain practice.

Finally, there is still a disparity between education and training of pain physicians all over the world for interventional pain practice. The publication of this book is a small attempt to minimize this discrepancy. There should be standardized guidelines for interventional pain practitioners.

We hope this book will help physicians set appropriate guidelines. Guidelines need to be established based on best evidence and clinical experience, and should be periodically reviewed. We also hope that pain fellowship programs will make this book part of their curricula for interventional pain procedures.

P. Prithvi Raj
Serdar Erdine

Acknowledgments

This book would not have been completed without special assistance from our colleagues who worked diligently in their specified tasks. We acknowledge special contributions from the following colleagues.

Selcuk Dincer MD from the Department of Algology, Medical Faculty of Istanbul University, Turkey, for his tireless expertise in the design of the three-dimensional computed tomography scans of anatomy, which are the unique features of this book. We thank the team of the Medical Faculty of the Department of Algology, Istanbul University, Turkey, and the team of Istanbul Pain Center, for providing the database of the patients treated in their facilities. We thank all patients, who gave us permission to use their pictures in the book.

We thank Bill Naughton; the graphics designer who collated and formatted over 1000 figures with great expertise and finalized the figures to conform with the publisher's guidelines.

Finally, we thank Susan Raj for being a coordinator for this book; her efforts in triaging the various materials that moved between the authors at two locations and the graphics designer were outstanding.

1 General Principles

1   History of Interventional Pain Medicine

Formative years

The contemporary era in pain management really began with the discovery of nitrous oxide and its analgesic properties in the late 18th century. This was soon followed by scientific investigation of the anesthetic properties of nitrous oxide and ether on animals, and the use of these substances in human patients. Surgical anesthesia was first publicly demonstrated at Massachusetts General Hospital in 1845 and 1846. The discovery and use of anesthetics changed the perception of pain (Fig. 1.1). In the 1850s Charles Gabriel Pravaz, a French surgeon, and Alexander Wood of Edinburgh independently invented the syringe (Fig. 1.2a,b), which allowed injections of morphine. By the 1860s the efficacy of locally applied opiates, especially morphine, directly to the skin or nerves for pain relief was widely accepted. The effects of pre- and intraoperative administration of morphine to the area of incision or amputation were investigated. When cocaine became available as a local anesthetic, owing to the work of Sigmund Freud and, especially, Karl Koller, this soon resulted in its use as a local anesthetic in diverse procedures (Fig. 1.3a,b).

Surgical techniques for pain relief represented another great medical advance during the 19th century. With the advent of antiseptic surgery, procedures became less life threatening, allowing investigation of pain relief techniques involving permanent interruption of afferent pathways. Innovative techniques were developed for treating trigeminal neuralgia, in addition to procedures such as retrogasserian neurectomy and cordotomy, ablation of the sympathetic nervous system, sympathectomy for visceral pain and angina pectoris, and surgical management of neuralgia.

Pain mechanisms

Little was understood about pain mechanisms at the beginning of the 19th century. Many questions such as how sensibility related to movement, whether separate sensory and motor nerves existed, and whether single nerves could perform different functions were still unanswered. Early researchers tried to explain pain by concentrating on the specialization of functions in different parts of the brain. Animal experiments investigating the function of spinal nerve roots were more successful, significantly contributing to medical knowledge during this period. Investigators such as Claude Bernard, Charles Bell, and Francois Magendie developed innovative experimental procedures that allowed differentiation of sensation from movement and between functions of anterior and posterior spinal nerve roots. A significant impetus to the perception of the nervous system as a system involving the transmission of sensations from the periphery to the center through a system of complex relays was provided by the work of German physiologist and comparative anatomist Johannes Muller (Fig. 1.4).

Muller proposed a connection between the anatomic pathway of a fiber and perception of sensation, stimulating further research on specific fibers for pain and nociception. As a result of such work, an entirely new school of physiologic research was founded. Soon nerve structures were identified in the dermis, leading to investigation of dissociation of sensations in that region, such as sensation of touch, pressure, and pain; and the spinal cord was more realistically appraised as a central processor with the ability itself to affect the transmission of sensations. Other noteworthy contributions were made by Waller, who developed a sectioning technique allowing observation of fatty degeneration of a fiber, leading to an awareness of ascending and descending pathways and the origin of nerve fibers.

There were many other pioneers who, through work with patients in pain or self-experimentation, contributed to the general body of medical knowledge: Weir Mitchell's work with neuritis, neuralgia, and causalgia, Henry Head's discovery of two different types of nerve fiber, and Sherrington's notion of an integrated nervous system were major advances establishing a firm foundation for an understanding of pain

Pain-Relieving Procedures: The Illustrated Guide, First Edition. P. Prithvi Raj and Serdar Erdine.
© 2012 John Wiley & Sons, Ltd. Published 2012 by John Wiley & Sons, Ltd.

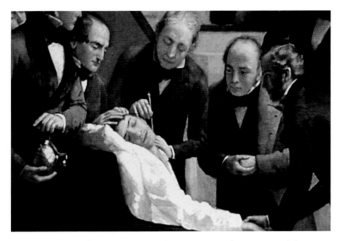

mechanisms and more effective approaches to treatment (Fig. 1.5).

We are indebted to Melzack and Wall for perhaps the most significant leap in understanding, the gate control theory. This explanation located both facilitators and inhibitory influences on the cells of the substantia gelatinosa of the spinal cord; with large-diameter, fast-conducting touch fibers suppressing, and smaller-diameter, slower-conducting pain fibers increasing, central output. Because nerve lesions usually involve smaller fibers, they result in over-activity of the substantia gelatinosa. Scar formation at the site of nerve injury causes complications, increasing nerve excitability at the site of the lesion (Fig. 1.6).

Figure 1.1 The first surgical anesthesia in Massachusetts General Hospital in 1845.

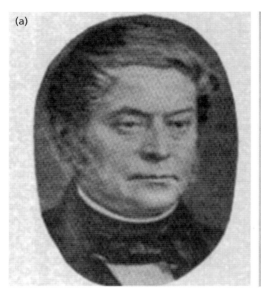

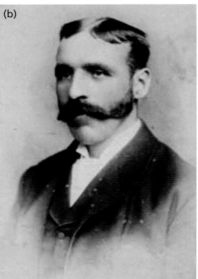

Figure 1.2 (a) Gabriel Pravaz, courtesy of Wellcome Library, London. (b) Alexander Wood, reproduced with permission from Peter Stubbs (www.edinphoto.org.uk).

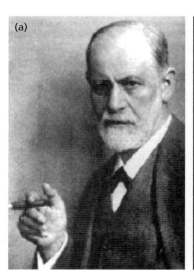

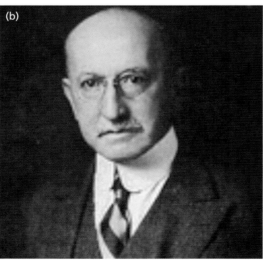

Figure 1.3 (a) Sigmund Freud, (b) Karl Koller (courtesy of the Wood Library Museum of Anesthesiology, Park Ridge, IL, USA).

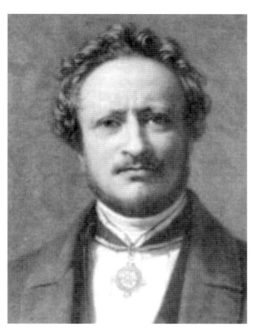

Figure 1.4 Johannes Muller.

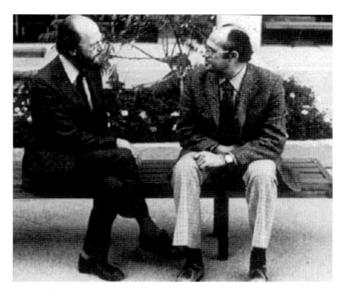

Figure 1.6 R. Melzack and P. Wall. (Courtesy of Dr. Ronald Melzack.)

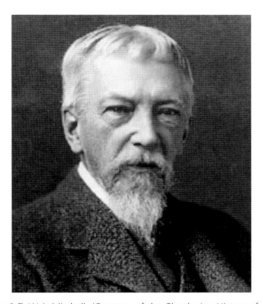

Figure 1.5 Weir Mitchell. (Courtesy of the Clendening History of Medicine Library, University of Kansas Medical Center.)

Establishment of interventional pain medicine

Greater understanding of pain mechanisms has resulted in the development of devices offering innovative therapeutic approaches. For instance, dorsal column stimulators were a direct result of the gate control theory. The efficacy of treatment relies on stimulation of low-threshold primary afferent fibers, which causes central inhibition of pain signals. Dorsal column stimulators are now an effective means of treating patients with chronic neuropathic and vascular pain. In addition, peripheral nerve stimulators have been used to manage chronic pain after peripheral nerve injury. Deep brain stimulation is a newer technique, still somewhat uncertain in terms of efficacy of pain relief.

New treatment techniques represent another beneficial byproduct of pain-related research. For instance, the discovery of opioid receptors in the central nervous system provided a rationale for the development of intrathecal and epidural administration of opioids. These now active techniques have resulted in the formation of a new sub-specialty under the umbrella of primary specialists of pain medicine. This sub-specialty has been called interventional pain medicine.

Biotechnology allows drugs targeted towards specific physiological processes to be developed, sometimes designed for compatibility with the body to reduce side effects. Genomics and knowledge of human genetics is having some influence on medicine, as the causative genes of most monogenic disorders have now been identified. In addition, the development of techniques in molecular biology and genetics is influencing medical technology, practice, and decision-making.

Evidence-based medicine is a contemporary movement to establish the most effective algorithms of practice through the use of systematic reviews and meta-analysis. The movement is facilitated by modern global information science, which allows all evidence to be collected and analyzed according to standard protocols, which are then disseminated to healthcare providers. One problem with this "best practice" approach is that it could be seen to stifle novel approaches to treatment. The Cochrane Collaboration leads this movement.

Defining a pain specialist

John Bonica was the first anesthesiologist who experienced the difficulties of pain management during his years in the army as he was treating the wounded soldiers from the Pacific. He felt strongly that no one particular physician is capable of looking after a patient with pain. He proposed the first concept of multidisciplinary approach to pain management.

What defines a "pain specialist?" Rollin Gallagher stated, "specialties define themselves [in] many ways: by age group (pediatrics), organ system (cardiology), specific constellation of illnesses or diseases (infectious diseases), type of procedure (surgery), or practice setting (emergency medicine)." Held to this definition, pain management becomes a unique specialty indeed. Although pain management is concerned with the diagnosis, treatment, and rehabilitation of a singular sensory symptom, it is essential that practitioners undertake a multidisciplinary approach to achieve these ends. They must also be well versed in the study of pain and its prevention. Although more than 60% of pain specialists originate from the field of anesthesiology, they can also come from a variety of other disciplines such as interventional radiology, physical therapy, psychiatry, primary care medicine, and neurology. In addition, pain specialists must possess a keen understanding of the variety of conditions and causes associated with pain. This broad range of training and knowledge allows the practitioner to achieve their ultimate goal: the management of a patient's pain. Despite these extensive requirements, pain management remains classified as only a subspecialty of anesthesiology under the certification of the American Board of Anesthesiology (ABA) in the United States. The American Academy of Algology in 1983, now the American Academy of Pain Medicine (AAPM), has strived to create a separate specialty of pain medicine, but without success so far.

Education and training of interventional pain physicians

With increasing recognition of pain management as a specialty, there is early development and formalization of curricula and training programs. Noteworthy among accomplishments in this area are development by the American Board of Anesthesiology of a course of training in pain for anesthesiology residents, formulation of guidelines by the Accreditation Council for Graduate Medical Education for

the approval of pain fellowship programs, and the establishment of a core curriculum for the study of pain by the International Association for the Study of Pain (IASP). Postgraduate fellowship training programs are now widely available. The American Board of Anesthesiology certifies anesthesiologists, physiatrists, and neurologists for added qualification in pain management after they have taken their pain management certification examination. The American Board of Pain Medicine certifies physicians of all specialties when they take a written examination. Similar action has also been taken in the United Kingdom and is spreading to other countries such as the Netherlands, Australia, and Turkey. In addition, the study of pain has altered the way many physicians manage their patients, increasing awareness of opportunities for alleviating pain and the necessity of early intervention.

Competency and certification of pain physicians

Effective pain management requires that physicians take a multidisciplinary approach to their evaluation, diagnosis, treatment, and rehabilitation of pain problems. They must not only draw from several medical disciplines, but must also understand the complex nature of pain. This distinction makes pain medicine a unique specialty compared with more specific medical fields such as cardiology and pediatrics. Even so, pain medicine continues to develop gradually as a specialty in North America and Western Europe, with other countries being left behind.

However, because pain practitioners are required to possess such a broad skill set, medical schools have found it difficult to develop effective curricula and credentialing methods for this subspecialty. The inadequacy of education in pain management can, and has, led to the poor treatment of pain disorders, especially those of a chronic nature. Although the link between inadequate education and improper treatment is well understood, studies suggest that disparities in pain education continue to exist.

The current problem in educating a pain specialist is, therefore, a two-fold issue. First, the existing pain medicine education disparity must be addressed. The development of effective and relevant curricula will provide future pain specialists with adequate training. Second, in addition to curriculum development, the program must have a thorough and integral assessment method to determine competency properly. Credentialing is vital for upholding precise standards within pain medicine.

Several organizations, such as the American Board of Anesthesiology, the American Academy of Pain Medicine, and the World Institute of Pain, have begun to address the disparity and credentialing issues.

Present status of interventional pain medicine

Can we, today, looking back over history, state that we have finally conquered pain? The answer has to be the following: in some ways, yes; in some ways, no. We have certainly conquered surgical pain, the pain of childbirth, and perhaps pain due to trauma. Unfortunately, we have not progressed a great deal in the areas of chronic and cancer pain.

Chronic pain remains a taxing and frustrating situation for both the patient and the clinician. Despite our concern and advanced knowledge, we are still unable to help the patient who comes to us with increasing pain, decreased function, and debilitating psychological difficulties, such as feelings of low self-worth, depression, and inability to cope.

One should emphasize the importance of pain management, its advances as a discipline, and the options we now have available to treat a patient with moderate-to-severe pain. The discovery of opioid receptors, a taxonomy of classification of pain, a multidisciplinary and multimodal treatment approach, and the establishment of curricula and training are spectacular advances in pain medicine. It is not surprising, therefore, that these advances have contributed significantly to the practice of medicine.

Pain societies and education

Over the past few decades, several organizations have been created, with the primary purpose of expanding pain management education in the United States and the world. These organizations include the following.
• The American Society of Regional Anesthesiology and Pain Medicine (ASRA). Organized in 1976, the ASRA is an affiliation of anesthesiologists and other physicians who have strived to advance scientific knowledge through education about and research of regional anesthesia. Pain control has become a major area of interest of the society.
• The International Association for the Study of Pain (IASP). Founded in 1973, the IASP has become the largest multidisciplinary international association in the field of pain. Its purpose is to encourage pain research, promote education, facilitate the exchange of information, encourage education of the public regarding pain issues, encourage the development of a data bank, and to advise political agencies on standards of pain treatment.
• The World Institute of Pain (WIP). With the development of pain medicine into a subspecialty, it was recognized that links between the international pain centers also needed to be developed. The WIP was created to accomplish this goal. In addition to this mission, the WIP strives to educate and train personnel of member pain centers, develop common protocols for efficacy and outcome studies, categorize and credential pain centers, and develop examination processes for pain centers in testing trainees.

Credentialing

Even if medical schools adopt and maintain effective pain management curricula, the establishment of clinical reliability for pain specialists is only half-complete. There remains the essential task of credentialing. An effective and objective system for determining competency must also be developed.

The World Institute of Pain

The Fellow of Interventional Pain Practice (FIPP) Examination Board provides an examination in interventional techniques and attempts to establish clinical competency further in interventional pain practice. Eligibility for the certification examination requires the following:
• licensure;
• completion of a 4-year Accreditation Council for Graduate Medical Education (ACGME)-approved residency (or equivalent), that included pain management;
• American Board of Medical Specialties board certification or equivalent;
• a minimum of 24 months of clinical practice experience in pain medicine; and
• upon certification, strict adherence to ethical and professional standards set by the WIP and its Section of Pain Practice.

The Examination in Interventional Techniques consists of three sections: theoretical examination, practical examination, and oral examination.

Although certification programs do recognize accepted levels of knowledge and expertise in pain management, it is generally agreed that they cannot guarantee competence or successful treatment of the patient to the public. Nor can they guarantee that certification examinations will properly reflect state-of-the-art knowledge and procedures, owing to the rapid changes in the field of pain medicine. However, these certification programs strive to establish clinical reliability for a specialty that requires advanced training, experience, and knowledge.

Conclusion

A review of the history of pain demonstrates that until the time of Bonica, pain management was considered to be unimodal, unidisciplinary, and managed without any clear structural organization. Today, new drugs and creative techniques and procedures have expanded the scope of pain medicine into a multidisciplinary field of clinical practice.

Pain management practitioners must possess a broad skill-set, advanced training and knowledge, and, perhaps above all else, clinical experience. Even so, there remain undeniable disparities in pain management education. Now that we recognize that the problems exist, further efforts must be made by our community to establish and assure clinical reliability and competency in the practice of pain medicine. As pain medicine expands as a subspecialty, so too must educational efforts.

Further reading

Brown, D.L. & Fink, R.B. (2009) The history of regional anesthesia. In *Neural Blockade in Clinical Anesthesia and Pain Medicine* (ed. Cousins, M. & Bridenbaugh, P.), 4th edition, pp. 1–23. Philadelphia, PA: Wolters Kluwer.

Paradise, L.A. & Raj, P.P. (2004) Competency and certification of pain physicians. *Pain Practice* **4**(3), 235–244.

Parris, W.C.V. & Johnson, B. (2008) The history of pain medicine. In *Raj's Practical Management of Pain*, 4th edition (ed. Benzon, H.T.), pp. 3–12. Philadelphia, PA: Mosby.

Raj, P.P. (1996) Advances in the practice of pain medicine: contributions of pain management. Distinguished Academician 1995 Lecture. *Annals, Academy of Medicine Singapore* **25**(1), 152–159.

Raj, P.P. (2002) Historical aspects of regional anesthesia. In *Textbook of Regional Anesthesia* (ed. Raj, P.P.), pp. 3–21. New York: Churchill Livingstone.

Raj, P.P. (2010) The 2009 John J. Bonica Award Lecture: the impact of managing pain in the practice of medicine through the ages. *Regional Anesthesia and Pain Medicine* **35**(4), 378–385.

2 Principles for Performing Percutaneous Invasive Procedures

A percutaneous invasive procedure for pain relief in patients suffering from intolerable and intractable pain is commonly performed globally today. The physician needs to be trained and skilled in these procedures. Unfortunately, physicians from different specialties with poor training and skills continue to perform such procedures. To maintain the best standard of practice in interventional pain procedures, it is imperative that basic principles for performing the procedures are followed. They are described below.

Preprocedure due diligence

1. Is the physician eligible to perform the invasive procedure? The patient and/or the family should know that performing a technically complex invasive procedure requires the physician to be trained and eligible to do it. In advanced countries such as the United States or Europe, the protocol requires a credentialing process. This is to protect the patients' safety. Unfortunately, globally this credentialing process is not available. Patients and their families should make every effort in their local communities to ensure that the physician has a satisfactory reputation to perform these procedures, and that their training is accepted by local regulatory bodies. One example of acceptable training is obtaining a Fellow of Interventional Pain Practice (FIPP) Certificate from the World Institute of Pain (WIP).

2. Have a thorough history and the physical examinations been done on the patient and are there any contraindications to perform the procedure? It is the obligation of the physicians to obtain and assess the previous history of a patient's health and illness at the first appointment. In addition, the physician should himself examine the patient thoroughly. This examination includes not only a general examination but also extensive neurological examination, especially directed to the painful areas. After the examination is completed, the physician should, if indicated, obtain laboratory studies relevant to the pain syndrome. At this point, the physician should inform the patient of the procedure they recommend and the contraindications, if any.

3. What is the objective of the physician in performing this procedure? It is the responsibility of the physician to explain to the satisfaction of the patient why a certain procedure needs to be considered, its expected result and its effects on the pain syndrome. This is presented in the form of **"informed consent"** in advanced countries. The patient agrees to have the procedure done by signing an official document.

4. Does the physician have knowledge of the anatomy of the procedure? It is the responsibility of the hospital or institution where the physician practices to determine whether they have experience and knowledge of the anatomy of the region for the invasive procedure about to be performed. This responsibility also lies with the patient or the family or both, who must determine by their own due diligence the physician's capabilities. The hospital or the institution should only allow the physician to perform the procedure if they are satisfied with the physician's eligibility.

5. Does the physician have knowledge of the needles, devices, and drugs to be used for the procedure? It is the responsibility of the hospital and institutions to evaluate and certify that the physicians who will perform the procedure have obtained adequate knowledge of the needles, devices, and drugs to be used in this procedure. This is usually done by the credentialing committee of the institution.

6. Is there an assistant in the room who is familiar with the procedure? Invasive procedures are complex and require other personnel to help the physician perform the procedure. The assistant, who should be familiar with the procedure, is valuable in monitoring the patient's vital functions and assisting in equipment readiness and availability during the procedure.

Pain-Relieving Procedures: The Illustrated Guide, First Edition. P. Prithvi Raj and Serdar Erdine.
© 2012 John Wiley & Sons, Ltd. Published 2012 by John Wiley & Sons, Ltd.

During the procedure

7. Is the patient prepared appropriately? The first step is to position the patient appropriately for the procedure. Then, the patient should be prepared by placing an intravenous catheter and infusion system for drug injection. In addition to the common general set up, there should be an entry point in the tubing to inject the desired drug when it is required. All of this set up should be secured with adhesive tape in a sterile fashion.

8. Is the sedation adequately provided to the patient during the procedure? It is important to assess at this stage of procedure that the patient is comfortable and prepared to accept the procedure. If the patient is highly anxious, appropriate sedation to calm their anxiety is necessary. For instance, if the patient has to be kept awake to respond to the physician's questioning during the procedure, then a very judicious dose of the sedative drug should be used. On the other hand, if being awake is not necessary, a safe, larger dose can be injected for the comfort and amnesia of the procedure.

9. Are the devices and machines tested before the procedure? As the patient is positioned and prepared, the physician should follow the checklist of required devices and machines to be used for the procedure. It is imperative that all devices are tested for correct functioning (e.g. radiofrequency equipment). Needles and devices should be readied for use in a sterile fashion.

10. Is there a trained assistant available for the procedure? A trained nurse or skilled assistant is necessary for moderate to complex invasive procedures such as trigeminal nerve lesioning or lumbar sympathetic ganglion lesioning. The assistant will not only help the physician during the procedure but also monitor the vital functions, assuring and calming the patient, and, when necessary, injecting the drugs.

11. Is the point of entry marked after the imaging machine is set in the correct position? After correct positioning of the patient and after obtaining intravenous access, the radiographic imaging machine should be tested and placed for the expected views needed for the procedure (i.e. posteroanterior–lateral oblique views).

The skin entry (of the needle) should be marked and confirmed by the imaging technique. After a correct confirmation of the needle entry, sterile draping of the region should be done, and the procedure started with injection of a local anesthetic. (Note: the physician must be appropriately protected from radiation and have sterile attire and gloves for the procedure.)

12. Once the needle is placed in the correct position, what are the appropriate steps taken to confirm it? When the physician determines that the needle is in the correct position, the next step should be to aspirate for fluid (blood or cerebrospinal fluid). If the aspiration is negative, confirm in all radiological views that the needle's tip is in the correct position. After that is done, a diagnostic (local anesthetic) or therapeutic (neurolysis or radiofrequency) lesioning can be done. One should always use a contrast solution injection (iohexol) with radiographic image before therapeutic lesioning.

After the procedure

13. Is the postprocedure planned? It is essential that the patient, after the procedure, is taken to a place for monitoring (wherever possible in the recovery room or, alternatively, where vital functions can be monitored). The usual time for any postprocedure to be monitored is 30 minutes, but one should note that most complex procedures require up to 2 hours for patients' vital functions to be stable.

14. Has the postprocedure family counseling been arranged? The patient, if cognitively stable, and the family should be counseled about the procedure just done, its expectations and side effects.

15. Have discharge instructions been given to the patient, family, or both? At discharge, the patient and family should be instructed when and how they should contact the physicians at the pain centre, if significant side effects occur from the procedure. The contact person's telephone number should be available on a 24-hour basis. If everything is considered routine in the postprocedure period, then, at the time of discharge, a follow-up appointment should be given in writing (usually 2 weeks in the future).

16. What is the postprocedure follow-up? At 2 weeks (first follow-up), the progress of the patient should be assessed and documented to assess the efficacy of the procedure, the change in intensity of the pain before the procedure, and any side effects.

It is mandatory that the physician who performed the procedure send a detailed note to the referring physician of the procedure's outcome, at the first follow-up. The note should also state if the physician plans further procedures on the patient in the future. If no other procedures are planned then the patient should be discharged back to the referring physician for further care.

It might be helpful for the patient and the family, hospital or institution, the physicians who perform the procedure, and for the personnel in the pain center to have a checklist of their responsibilities, before, during, and after the procedure.

Further reading

Boswell, M. et al. (2007) Interventional techniques: evidence-based practice guidelines in the management of chronic spinal pain. *Pain Physician* 10, 7–111.

Braxton, K. (2008) Basic risk management for interventional procedures. In *Interventional Pain Management, Image Guided Procedures*
(ed. Raj, P. et al.), 2nd edition, pp. 71–74. Philadelphia, PA: Saunders Elsevier.

Manchikanti, L. (1999) The role of evaluation and management
services in pain management. *Pain Physician* **2**(3), 10–32.

Van Kleef, M., Mekhail, N. & Van Zundert, J. (2009) Evidence-based
guidelines for interventional pain medicine according to clinical
diagnoses. *Pain Practice* **9**(4), 252–259.

3

Physical and Psychological Assessment of the Patient with Pain

A detailed clinical history and assessment of the patient is essential before any intervention. The assessment should not be based on "is the procedure appropriate for the patient?" but "what type of treatment or interventional procedure is appropriate for the patient?"

Successful evaluation depends on the development of a mutually trusting relationship between the physician and the patient. The complaints and the expectations of the patient should be adequately analyzed. The physician should allot a minimum of 30 minutes at the first visit. If the patient is accompanied by a relative or a friend, it may be useful to get more information about the patient and their environment. The steps for the evaluation of the patient are as follows.

Step 1. Pain history
1. Detailed information about pain and associated symptoms since the very beginning.
2. Duration, intensity, frequency, and progress of pain.
3. The nature of pain, such as burning, stabbing, squeezing.
4. Factors that increase or decrease the pain.
5. Associated symptoms with pain.
6. Previous consultations or diagnosis related with pain.
7. Previous medications or treatments and the outcomes.
8. Current medications and other treatment modalities.

Step 2. General history of the patient
1. Other diseases (hypertension, diabetes, cardiovascular disease, renal failure, etc.).
2. Medications other than related with pain treatment.
3. Other treatments including surgery.
4. Addiction; smoking, use of alcohol, or drugs.

Step 3. Physical examination
1. General examination.
   (a) Mental status; level of consciousness, ability to reply to questions, concentration, mood, neurovegetative symptoms.
   (b) General appearance.
   (c) Blood pressure, heart rate, fever, weight, height.
   (d) Gait.
2. Musculoskeletal examination.
   (a) Posture.
   (b) Alignment of spine, shoulders, arm, lower back, and lower extremities.
   (c) Deformities.
   (d) Joints and bursa; tenderness, swelling, pain; especially temporomandibular joint, shoulder, elbow, wrist, coxofemoral, knee.
   (e) Myofascial trigger points; trapezius, splenius capitis, supraspinatus, temporalis, sternocleidomastoid, masseter, others.
3. Neurological examination.
   (a) Cranial nerves, especially trigeminal and glossopharyngeal nerve.
   (b) Motor examination: function of the upper and lower extremities, fingers, and toes should be checked. Muscle strength is assessed by the Medical Research Council Scale. The muscle strength should correspond to the nerve roots and peripheral nerves.
   (c) Sensorial examination, sensorial loss, and paresthesia according to the dermatomal chart should be carefully checked. The lesions may be central, dermatomal (spinal), or peripheric nerve lesions.
   (d) Reflex testing: deep tendon reflexes may be a guide to the anatomical location of the lesion. Grading of the deep tendon reflexes is from 0 to 4+. Common reflex testers are biceps, triceps, patellar, and achilles.

Physical examination of different regions of the body

Face
The first step is the inspection of the face: changes on the face caused by herpes, sudomotor changes, trauma, and

Pain-Relieving Procedures: The Illustrated Guide, First Edition. P. Prithvi Raj and Serdar Erdine.
© 2012 John Wiley & Sons, Ltd. Published 2012 by John Wiley & Sons, Ltd.

mass lesions should be noted. The patient should also be checked intraorally for any lesions within the oral cavity.

Sensory testing is essential to verify any lesions of the cranial nerves.

Trigeminal neuralgia and glossopharyngeal neuralgia may be identified by palpation. Percussion of the sinuses will confirm sinusitis.

Neck, shoulder, and upper extremities

The second step is the examination of the neck, shoulder, and upper extremities.

The first aspect of this step should be the physical examination and inspection of the spine, which provides information on the posture and alignment of the patient. Kyphosis, lordosis, or scoliosis may be seen.

Tenderness during the palpation of the spine may indicate vertebral compression fracture, tumors, or abscess. Palpation may also indicate myofascial trigger points and facet arthropathy.

Normal range of motion of the cervical spine is 60° forward flexion, 75° of extension, 45° of lateral flexion, and 80° of lateral rotation.

Normal range of motion of the thoracolumbar spine is 90° forward flexion, 30° back extension, 25° of lateral flexion, and 60° of lateral rotation.

Pain provoked by back extension and lateral rotation may indicate facet arthropathy. Pain provoked by back flexion may indicate discogenic pain or pain originating from the vertebral body.

During inspection of the upper extremities, sudomotor changes, edema at the fingers, or swelling of the hands may indicate signs of complex regional pain syndromes.

Motor and sensorial testing and testing of the deep tendon reflexes are also important for the upper extremities.

For the shoulder joint, asymmetry, the deltoid muscles, and posture should be inspected. The sternoclavicular joint, clavicle, acromioclavicular joint, glenohumerol joint, and the scapular spine should be palpated. The range of motion is very important for diagnosing several pathologies including "frozen shoulder." The range of motion for the shoulder joint is 180° of flexion and extension with the sagittal plane, 180° of abduction and adduction with the frontal plane, 90° of external rotation, and 40° of internal rotation. Arthritis of the joints, subacromial and subdeltoid bursitis, supraspinatus and bicipital tendinitis, and rotator cuff tears and frozen shoulder are the common etiologies.

For the elbow joint, the range of motion is 30° of extension and 180° of flexion at the humeroulnar joint, and 170° of pronation and supination at the radioulnar joint. Lateral and medial epicondylitis are the common etiologies at the elbow joint.

The range of motion at the wrist is 60° of extension, 70° of flexion, 20° of abduction, and 30° of adduction. The most common etiology is carpal tunnel syndrome, which can be diagnosed by Tinel's sign where percussion of the proximal volar wrist crease produces paresthesia in the thumb, index, and middle fingers, whereas Phalen's sign is when the patient flexes both wrists against each other for one minute, and dysethesia in the thumb, index, and middle fingers begins.

Thorax and abdomen

Inspection of the thorax should include herpetic lesions, traumatic lesions, masses, echymotic lesions, thoracic kyphosis, or scoliosis.

Although very rarely seen, discal hernia may also occur in the thoracic spine and dermatomal sensorial testing is necessary.

Palpation is more important for the abdomen to differentiate visceral and superficial pain.

Lumbosacral region

The lumbosacral region is perhaps the most important region for interventional procedures. Thus a thorough assessment of the patient is crucial. The physician should not try to fit the patient for a specific procedure: instead, try to find the best procedure and implement it only if it is necessary.

Examination of the lumbosacral region will begin by inspection. A global inspection will include the patient's gain, posture, lumbar scoliosis, kyphosis, degree of spinal curvature, and lordosis. Signs of infection, herpes, and masses should also be inspected. The main structures that may be sources of pain are the intervertebral discs, facet joint, sacroiliac joints, and coccyx. The hip joint and bursitis of the trochanter major are also pain sources.

The range of motion for the lumbar spine is flexion to 90°, extension to 30°, bilateral lateral flexion up to 25°, bilateral rotation up to 60°.

The motor and sensory examination and examination of the deep tendon reflexes will reveal important information about the pain sources.

There are specific nerve-root tests. They are the heel test, which shows the L4–L5 function, and the toe walk, which tests the S1–S2 junction. Both are very important for decision-making for a transforaminal procedure.

Examination of the hip joint is also important. The range of motion is 100° of flexion, 30° for extension, 20° for adduction, and 40° for abduction. When the hip is flexed 45°, the range of motion is 45° for internal rotation and 40° for external rotation.

Trochanteric bursitis is also a pain source. There is tenderness during palpation over the trochanter major.

There are several special tests such as the straight leg raise test for nerve root pathology or piriformis syndrome, Patrick's test for the sacroiliac joint, and the back extension test for facet arthropathy.

The physical examination of the patient should overlap with the pain history and radiological findings. One of the serious mistakes in decision-making is only to rely on the radiological image.

Psychological assessment (contributed by Özlem Sertel-Berk)

Currently, since the interacting effects of biological, psychological, and social factors on the pain process have been realized, the psychological preparedness of the patient with chronic pain is of great importance when the extent of that pain requires an invasive intervention either for diagnostic purposes or extenuating pain. This necessity of searching for adequateness for surgical operations stems from the fact that if the patients are not good candidates, the interventions may result in inflations in the severity of pain or multiple somatic complaints in various body sites. Moreover, surgical operations may adversely affect the biopsychosocial functioning of the individual. As a result of these factors, there is a tremendous increase in research concerning biopsychosocial factors predicting the success rates of invasive procedures when chronic pain patients are evaluated.

Within the scope of these parameters, practical issues about the assessment of the most crucial biopsychosocial variables in predicting the adequateness of patients with chronic pain for surgical interventions will be addressed in two major topics: first, which pain patients are better for referral for psychological assessment; second, what the points of emphasis should be during psychological assessment.

Conditions requiring psychological assessment before surgical intervention
Which pain patients should be the candidates for psychological assessment intending to schedule for an invasive procedure? What are the criteria by which the assessment is made?

Scope of psychological assessment
What is meant by convenience for candidacy is by no means based solely on the psychological assessment. First, a comprehensive psychological assessment is required to capture not only the psychological characteristics but also the sociological/cultural environmental issues affecting the patient with pain; moreover, and, significantly, the biological features of the pain experience itself should also be assessed. However, is it necessary to refer every single patient who is planned for an invasive procedure for psychological assessment? Epker and Block (2001) suggest cost-effectiveness as one of the criteria. In line with this suggestion, the referring physician should consider if such an evaluation before an invasive procedure will determine the outcome of the procedure. Several criteria can be formulated to evaluate this factor, based upon Sternbach's (1986) "abnormal pain

behavior" and Engel's (1959) "pain prone patient" conceptualizations, which are as follows.
1. A past history of numerous medical investigations and poor effectiveness of those treatments.
2. Poor compliance in recommended pre-procedure execution of pain algorithms; i.e., irrational utilization of pain medicine, frequent drop-outs and/or analgesic abuse.
3. An excessive verbiage of pain (how frequently does the patient talk about his/her pain, pain discourse).
4. An exaggerated postural behavior or facial expression due to pain (a skewed or hunchbacked position, hobbling, frowning, depressive look).
5. Poor daily functioning, which is not explainable.
6. A history of comorbid interactive pain.
7. An incongruence between the descriptions of pain and scientific and/or clinical recognitions of pathophysiology and pathoanatomy of the pain in question.
8. Patient's poor cognitive grasp of the complexity of pain.

If one or more of the above observations are evident, regardless of an objective organic pathology underlying their pain, these patients need to be referred for a comprehensive psychological assessment.

Explaining the need for a psychological assessment
All of the above criteria bring out the issue of how the physician should communicate the information to the patient that he or she will primarily be referred for a psychological evaluation. First, because it has been reported that for many patients the phrase "psychological evaluation" can be challenging, within the field of health psychology the term "behavioral medicine consultation" is offered instead. Substituting this phrase may decrease the patient's resistance to a referral.

Nevertheless, when asked for a referral, whether for a psychological assessment or for a behavioral medicine consultation, patients should not get the impression that the reason is because nothing was observed about the organic origins of their pain complaint, and that therefore they are not suitable for a surgical intervention.
1. From the beginning, the patient should be told that the purpose behind sending them to a psychologist is the necessity for evaluating the degree of benefits they will get from a surgical implementation.
2. The conversation between the physician and the patient should aim to clarify the psychological issues that may hinder a positive outcome, where the patient can be further informed that in some cases psychological preparation can even lead to improved outcomes.
3. Therefore, it is crucial for the physician to explain and discuss the biopsychosocial nature of pain with the patient, even before any medical assessment is used. If this is not the case, the patient is likely to hold a negative belief that the physician thinks the pain is not real, which further increases

the likelihood of a defensive attitude toward any psychological intervention.

4. It should, therefore, clearly be emphasized to the patient that the "gold standard" for the treatment of chronic pain is a multidisciplinary approach, which involves the physicians, psychologists, and other caregivers, and that offering the patient less than this would be care of a low standard.

The psychological assessment: special issues of emphasis

Within a biopsychosocial perspective, the psychological assessment should primarily use a functional analysis approach where the antecedents, predisposing factors, and consequences of the pain experience are questioned in a comprehensive, causal manner. The assessment should never depend solely on standardized inventories that evaluate personality, level of depression, or anxiety, as they are criticized for not being specifically developed for grasping the problems underlying pain; nor merely on a clinical interview as issues of subjectivity are questioned. Therefore, for cross validation, the information should be gathered from various sources, i.e., from clinical interview with the patient and family members, from psychometric testing, and, if possible, from in vivo observations of daily life activities and encounters.

On the other hand, a hierarchy of major factors is listed in the literature as predictors of poor outcomes of surgical operations; these are high levels of depression, anxiety, somatization, pain intensity, number of pain sites, low level of job satisfaction, poor functioning, high degree of absenteeism, low level of education, poor coping, litigation for workers' compensation, high neuroticism, childhood history of neglect, abuse, or trauma, the reinforcing role of the spouse or the perceived neglect/lack of support from spouse, preoperative poor level of health perception, fear of movement and re-injury, negative treatment outcome expectations, and job stress, according to the degree of variance they explain.

Therefore, during psychological assessment the following considerations are necessary.

1. Consider psychopathology

The psychologist should carefully consider psychopathological conditions, primarily depression, anxiety, and somatoform disorders that may precede or succeed chronic pain.

In situations where there is a real necessity for the success of the invasive procedure, the dominating factoring assessment should be evaluated for the pre-operative evaluation of psychopathology.

2. Consider intensity of pain

The features of pain, especially the intensity, should be taken into account.

There is evidence that the outcomes are poorer for those patients who describe their pain as more intense and who have a higher number of painful body sites. These may be signs for somatization and therefore should be handled before any surgical intervention.

3. Consider secondary gain

Occupational or familial secondary gain should be looked for.

Increased level of absenteeism or severance as a function of pain implicates a necessity for questioning the gains behind the actions. People exhibiting these characteristics often declare that the only condition in which they can start working is the time they are "ever free of pain." Alternatively, pain may serve to receive attention from close family members who are otherwise often neglectful or as an exemption from household roles. A psychotherapeutic intervention is necessary before a surgical intervention in dealing with and replacing the issues of secondary gains with more effective coping mechanisms.

4. Consider coping skills

The active or passive coping mechanisms specific to pain need to be assessed.

The question "what do I do when I feel in pain?" gives clues about how the individuals cope with their pain. If the "initial" answers denote passive mechanisms such as "lying down," "taking pills," or "leaving workplace," the physicians should be cautious in planning an invasive intervention. If there is urgency for such an intervention, then the patients should at least be encouraged to learn relaxation techniques.

5. Consider personality characteristics

Personality characteristics, specifically neuroticism, should be evaluated.

Those who are high in neuroticism often ask "why me?", perceive their pain as a threat, and possess a more negative attitude towards the treatment agents. These points are reported to complicate the outcomes of surgical procedures.

6. Consider history of abuse

Childhood history of neglect, abuse, and trauma need to be taken into account.

This is not easy and requires a sensitive assessment. However, those with such a history view their pain as more severe and are reported to benefit less from interventions.

7. Consider excessive expectations of the patient in their daily life

Health perceptions and behaviors need to be investigated.

There is a group of patients who overwork, with an expectancy that they should keep on working even though they have pain. For this purpose, they may be consuming more painkillers, and they may take the signs of slight relief as a complete recovery, which results in them quitting treatment. These patients benefit less from surgical operations and should be made aware of this at the preoperational period.

8. Consider negative self-efficacy beliefs

Individuals who believe that they do not have the capacity for maintaining well-being after the intervention (i.e., "I cannot do the exercises") gain less from interventions. Such automatic self-efficacy beliefs should be tested and replaced with more positive beliefs before the operation.

Special consideration on psychometric testing: advantages and disadvantages

Apart from the clinical interview, the criteria listed as having adverse effects on the surgical outcome can be investigated through a battery of valid and reliable assessment tools, so that the issues addressed during the interview can be validated. These instruments should include those measuring personality (i.e., the MMPI: Minnesota Multiphasic Personality Inventory), mood states such as depression and anxiety (i.e., the Beck or Zung Depression Inventories; BAI: Beck Anxiety Inventory; STAI: State Trait Anxiety Inventory), coping skills (the Coping Styles Inventory), level of perceived social support (i.e., the Perceived Social Support Inventory), disability (the Oswestry Disability Inventory), quality of life (MOS SF-36), pain characteristics (i.e., the McGill Pain Questionnaire), psychiatric symptoms (Symptom Checklist-90), pain or health beliefs (i.e., the Pain Beliefs and Perceptions Inventory, the Health Locus of Control Questionnaire), and self-efficacy (i.e., the Self-Efficacy Scale).

Psychological testing surely adds an objective database to the psychological evaluation. However, in determining the necessity for and composition of a test battery, the following major considerations should be taken into account:

1. the psychometric adequacy of the measures being considered;
2. the congruence of the theoretical orientations of these measures with the referral questions;
3. the likelihood that these measures will add to the decision-making process; and,
4. the confirmatory and complementary functions that individual measures are likely to serve when used jointly.

Given these conditions, the use of a comprehensive battery of this type can help to determine which way to proceed, together with the other sources of psychological assessment.

Communicating the outcomes of psychological assessment to the multidisciplinary treatment team

The primary consideration is the means of informing the physician and the treatment team about the results of psy-

chological evaluation. To protect confidentiality, a brief report sent to the physician may be preferred. However, for the good of the patient, it seems more appropriate to get the informed consent of the patient for communicating the outcomes to the treatment team. If consent is given, a detailed report followed by a discussion with the physicians concerning the interactional effects of the medical and psychological investigations, is the most valuable source of surgical decision.

The psychological report should be designed to address issues about the pain problem, mood states and signs of psychopathology, current psychological state of the patient concerning coping skills, level of social support, the predisposing, precipitating, and maintaining factors, and the consequences of pain. Special sections should be allocated for summarizing results of psychometric testing, and for a concluding section where a behavioral formulation can be set depending on the strengths and weaknesses based on the topics covered in the report.

Conclusion

It is not infrequent that individuals with pain possess more than one of the above variables, which complicates the picture even more. If such a multifactor predisposition is the case, the patient, family members, and physician must be informed and educated about the potential negative impact of certain psychological states on the patient's responsiveness to and acceptance of surgical interventions. For example, somatizing patients who are oversensitive to internal sensations may have problems in coping with the postoperative complications. Nevertheless, before deciding not to "touch" the patient, regardless of the urgency, as the invasive intervention may result in increased levels of pain, and referring the patient for a psychological intervention beforehand, it is important to recognize that these factors are based on theory and experience, and not all stem from controlled experimental or clinical studies. There have been studies where patients with elevated Minnesota Multiphasic Personality Inventory profiles benefited from invasive procedures whereas those with normal profiles had a poorer outcome. Some patients, even though they may not seem suitable, can be helped by psychological or pharmacological intervention to become better candidates.

Therefore, the assessment of these interdependent variables in a multidisciplinary manner may add to the process of deciding if the patient is suitable; if not, it may help them become suitable for invasive treatment for their pain and for taking necessary action such as short-term goal-specific psychotherapy. As Doleys (2002) says, "Successes are created not just discovered."

Further reading

Abrams, B. (2000) History taking in the patient in pain. In *Practical Management of Pain*, 3rd edition (ed. Raj, P.P.), pp. 333–338. Philadelphia, PA: Mosby.

Bruns, D. & Disorbio, J.M. (2009) Assessment of biopsychosocial risk factors for medical treatment: a collaborative approach. *Journal of Clinical Psychology in Medical Settings* **16**, 127–147.

Carragee, E.J. (2001) Psychological screening in the surgical treatment of lumbar disc herniation. *Clinical Journal of Pain* **17**, 215–219.

Crews, J. & Chan, V. (2009) Perioperative management of patients and equipment selection for neural blockade. In *Neural Blockade in Clinical Anesthesia and Pain Medicine*, 4th edition (ed. Cousins, M., Carr, D., Horlocker, T. & Bridenbaugh, P.), pp. 160–180. Philadelphia: Wolters Kluwer, and Lippincott, Williams and Wilkins.

den Boer, J.J., Oostendorp, R.A., Beems, T., Munneke, M., Oerlemans, M. & Evers, A.W. (2006) A systematic review of biopsychosocial risk factors for an unfavourable outcome after lumbar disc surgery. *European Spine Journal* **15**, 527–536.

Doleys, D.M. (2002) Preparing patients for implantable technologies. In *Psychological Approaches to Pain Management: A Practioner's Handbook*, 2nd edition (ed. Turk, D.J. & Gatchel, R.J.), pp. 334–347. New York: Guilford Press.

Doleys, D.M. & Doherty, D.C. (2000) Psychological and behavioral assessment. In *Practical Management of Pain*, 3rd edition (ed. Raj, P.P.), pp. 408–426. St Louis, MO: Mosby.

Engel, G.L. (1959) Psychogenic pain and the pain-prone patient. *American Journal of Medicine* **26**, 899–918.

Epker, J. & Block, A.R. (2001) Presurgical psychological screening in back pain patients: a review. *Clinical Journal of Pain* **17**, 200–205.

Gatchel, R.J. (2001) A biopsychosocial overview of pretreatment screening of patients with pain. *Clinical Journal of Pain* **17**, 192–199.

Groth-Marnat, G. (2003) *Handbook of Psychological Assessment*, 4th edition. New Jersey: John Wiley.

Lalani, I. & Argoff, C. (2008) History and physical examination of the pain patient. In *Raj's Practical Management of Pain*, 4th edition (ed. Benzon, H., Rathmell, J., Wu, C., Turk, D. & Argoff, C.), pp. 177–188. Philadelphia, PA: Mosby Elsevier.

Mannion, A.F. & Elfering, A. (2006) Predictors of surgical outcome and their assessment. *European Spine Journal* **15**, S93–S108.

Owens, R.G. & Ashcroft, J.B. (1982) Functional analysis in applied psychology. *British Journal of Clinical Psychology* **21**(3), 181–189.

Schade, V., Semmer, N., Main, C.J., Hora, J. & Boos, N. (1999) The impact of clinical, morphological, psychosocial and work-related factors on the outcome of lumbar discectomy. *Pain* **80**, 239–249.

Schofferman, J., Anderson, D., Hines, R., Smith, G. & White, A. (1992) Childhood psychological trauma correlates with unsuccessful lumbar spine surgery. *Spine* **17** (Suppl.), S138–S144.

Simon, S. (2000) Physical examination of the patient in pain. In *Practical Management of Pain*, 3rd edition (ed. Raj, P.P.), pp. 339–359. St Louis, MO: Mosby.

Sternbach, R.A. (1986) *The Psychology of Pain*. New York: Raven Press.

Waldman, S. (2005) *Physical Diagnosis of Pain*. Philadelphia: Elsevier.

4

Preparing the Patient for Interventional Pain Procedures

Preoperative evaluation

Preoperative evaluation of the patient is crucial and can potentially reduce morbidity and enhance outcomes.

The physician should be aware of basic and complex medical diseases and syndromes that may affect the decision-making related to the procedure and the sedation and analgesia used during it.

Current and past medical problems, previous surgeries and types of anesthesia, and any anesthesia-related complications need to be noted.

Diseases or symptoms such as hypertension, diabetes mellitus, coronary artery disease, shortness of breath, or chest pain should also be noted.

Any recent but currently interrupted medications should be included because this may lead to recognition of important issues. It is necessary to inquire about allergies to drugs and substances such as latex or radiographic dye. Frequently, patients claim an allergy to a substance when in reality the reaction was a common, expected, side effect (e.g., nausea or vomiting with narcotics).

Use of tobacco, alcohol, or illicit drugs should be documented. Quantitatively documenting tobacco exposure by pack-years (the number of packs of cigarettes smoked per day multiplied by the number of years of smoking) is best.

A screening review of systems is especially useful to uncover symptoms that may lead to the establishment of previously undiagnosed conditions. During this review, a personal or family history of adverse events related to anesthesia should be investigated; and cardiovascular, pulmonary, hepatic, renal, endocrine, or neurologic symptoms should be noted.

Questioning the patient about snoring and daytime somnolence may suggest undiagnosed sleep apnea.

One should inquire about chest discomfort (pain, pressure, tightness), duration of the discomfort, precipitating factors, associated symptoms, and methods of relief. One should note diagnoses, diagnostic tests, therapies, and names of treating physicians. It is important to note shortness of breath with exertion or when lying flat (orthopnea) or peripheral edema.

A general examination of all organ systems needs to be performed.

The patient should be asked if they have ever had problems with the following:

(1) their heart, lungs, kidneys, liver, or nervous system;

(2) whether they have had cancer, anemia, or bleeding problems;

(3) whether they have ever been hospitalized for any reason – this will often prompt recall of medical problems;

(4) a complete listing of previous surgeries can help complete the medical history.

A review of records from primary care physicians, specialists, or the hospital can reveal issues that the patient may not recall.

Evaluation of the heart, lungs, and skin is necessary, as well as further focus on the organ systems involved with disease as reported by the patient.

A basic neurologic examination to document deficits in mental status, speech, cranial nerves, gait, and motor and sensory function may be indicated, depending on the surgical procedure and patient's history.

Patients require preoperative diagnostic and laboratory studies that are consistent with their medical history and the proposed procedure.

Before getting the informed consent, educating the patient before the procedure can significantly reduce their anxiety and fears of it.

1. Informed consent

Before every procedure, it is necessary to obtain informed consent from the patient. Every patient has the right to have

Pain-Relieving Procedures: The Illustrated Guide, First Edition. P. Prithvi Raj and Serdar Erdine.
© 2012 John Wiley & Sons, Ltd. Published 2012 by John Wiley & Sons, Ltd.

reliable information about the procedures during the decision making.

While obtaining the informed consent, the purpose of the treatment, the expected outcome, the rate of success, risks of the treatment, complications, and other treatment modalities (if there are any) that may be alternative to the procedure should all be considered.

The patient should be informed about the purpose of the treatment in a manner they will be able to understand, including what the treatment will involve, and whether it will cure or minimize the pain, or provide diagnostic information.

The patient should understand and know the expected outcome on a realistic basis, depending on general statistics as well as the pain specialist's personal clinical experience. The patient should be aware that there is no treatment with one hundred percent success.

The patient should be informed about the risks and complications of the treatment in detail. Although the patient authorizes their physician to decide on their behalf, they have the right to know all risks and complications. These should be presented to the patient in a written form for their approval.

The patient should also be informed about other reasonable alternative treatments if there are any, so they can make their own judgments about the social, economic, and personal factors. The patient should be informed about the expected outcome, likelihood of success, and the material risks of the alternative treatments.

The patient should also be given realistic information on the outcome of no treatment. The physician should not exaggerate the results of no treatment.

The patient's consent should be documented, including the information given to the patient, the questions the patient has asked, that the patient understood the procedure, and the risks and complications of the procedure.

It is advisable that a member of the family or a caregiver, witnessing the giving of the consent, should also sign the written consent.

2. Imaging studies

(a) Conventional radiographs
Conventional radiographs are indicated for the diagnosis of osteomyelitis, osteoporosis, fracture, arthritic disorders, arthritic osteophytes, spondylolisthesis, spondylosis, and facet joint abnormalities.

(b) Myelography
Myelography is less commonly used. It may, however, be helpful when primary screening like magnetic resonance imaging (MRI) or a computed tomography (CT) scan cannot be used, for example if a pacemaker is present.

(c) CT scan
A CT scan is used to evaluate bony structures mainly, and soft tissues of the spine, disc hernia, hypertrophy or degeneration of the facet joints. Three-dimensional axial CT scans may provide images of the spinal ligaments and discs.

(d) MRI
MRI provides detailed information about spine pathology, spinal cord, cerebrospinal fluid, discs, disc degeneration, herniated discs, facet joint arthropathy, vertebral or discal infection, spinal stenosis, fracture, neoplasm, and other abnormalities in the soft tissues of the body.

(e) Ultrasound
Ultrasound may be used for the diagnosis of visceral pain of the upper and lower abdomen as well as the pelvic region.

(f) Bone scanning
Bone scanning reveals information about metastasis, osteomyelitis, bone trauma, and arthritis.

(g) PET–CT
Positron emission tomography–computed tomography (PET–CT) may be indicated in patients where a CT scan or MRI does not reveal adequate information.

(h) Discography
Discography is used for the diagnosis of discogenic pain, as a prognostic tool before spinal fusion operations.

(i) Thermography
Thermography may be used in evaluating myofascial pain syndromes and circulatory disorders.

3. Laboratory studies

Laboratory studies are used in diabetes, malnutrition, dysproteinemia, cancer, and immunosuppression. Electrolyte levels should be monitored if indicated based on comorbid illness or medication use, and imbalances corrected before the procedure.

4. Electrodiagnostics

Electrodiagnostics provide information about the functioning of nerve roots, peripheral nerves, and muscles.

5. Preoperative medication

A detailed list of medications, including those available over-the-counter (OTC) and herbal preparations, is important in assessing risks associated with interventional procedures.

Drugs that may affect the procedure include the following:

(1) antihypertensives;
(2) antiplatelet agents, anticoagulants;
(3) corticosteroids;
(4) nicotine;
(5) antineoplastic drugs;
(6) antidiabetics;
(7) antidepressants;
(8) herbal medications.

Propranolol, when used with epinephrine, has been known to cause malignant hypertension and reflex bradycardia. However, rebound hypertension and worsening angina may follow abrupt discontinuation of propranolol or other beta-blockers.

Corticosteroids may decrease fibroblast and epidermal proliferation, formation of granulation tissue, protein and collagen production, decrease the inflammatory response, and increase wound infection rates.

Nicotine may cause vasoconstriction. Patients with heavy smoking habits have a risk during the procedure.

Antineoplastic agents may decrease immune response to infection, interfere with cell division, and increase infection rates.

Abrupt withdrawal of benzodiazepines and antipsychotics may lead to significant hypertension and mental status changes; their use should therefore be continued. Monoamine oxidase inhibitors may interact with epinephrine, phenylephrine, and meperidine, leading to serotonin syndrome (hypertensive crises, mental status changes, fever, muscle cramps, seizures, and coma).

Tricyclic antidepressants or selective serotonin reuptake inhibitors administered for chronic depression need not be discontinued before the procedure because this may worsen anxiety, agitation, and depressed mood.

Potential complications of herbal supplements include coronary ischemia, stroke, bleeding, and interactions with anesthetic agents.

Vitamin E, ginkgo biloba, ginseng, and garlic all inhibit platelet aggregation and increase risk of bleeding and hematoma.

Colchicine, penicillin, and phenytoin may interfere with cellular turnover.

6. Assistive devices

Elderly patients may have eyeglasses, hearing aids, dentures, pacemakers, or prosthetic joints. During the assessment of these patients, the physician should check if these devices are compatible with MRI or other evaluative tools.

For patients with pacemakers, radiofrequency lesioning should be avoided as the currents may interfere with the pacemaker.

Antibiotic prophylaxis

Antibiotics to prevent wound infection are probably indicated even in clean wounds in the oral cavity, axilla, and perineum, or when there are minor breaks in aseptic technique.

7. Preoperative evaluation of patients with coexisting disease

Cardiovascular diseases

Hypertension

Preoperative evaluation identifies causes of hypertension, other cardiovascular risk factors, end-organ damage, and therapy.

It is generally recommended that elective surgery be delayed for severe hypertension (diastolic blood pressure (BP) >115 mm Hg, systolic BP >200 mm Hg) until BP is less than 180/110 mm Hg. A careful history and physical examination to determine cardiac, neurologic, or renal disease is important.

For a BP lower than 180/110 mm Hg, there is no evidence to justify cancellation of surgery, although interventions preoperatively are appropriate.

Frequently, anxiety increases BP, and therefore antianxiolytics can be used as adjunctive therapy. BP should not be lowered too rapidly. Continuation of antihypertensive treatment preoperatively is critical.

Ischemic heart disease

The goals of preoperative evaluation are to identify the risk for heart disease based on risk factors, to identify the presence and severity of heart disease from symptoms, physical findings, or diagnostic tests, to determine the need for preoperative interventions, and to modify the risk for perioperative adverse events.

The risk cardiac index consists of high-risk surgery (intraperitoneal, intrathoracic, or suprainguinal vascular procedures), ischemic heart disease, history of congestive heart failure, history of cerebrovascular disease, diabetes mellitus requiring insulin, and creatinine levels more than 2.0 mg/dl.

Respiratory diseases

1. Patients with moderate to severe chronic obstructive pulmonary disease (COPD) and smokers without demonstrable airflow limitation are at high risk for postoperative pulmonary complications (PPCs). Patients with asthma should also be carefully evaluated.

2. Patients at greater risk for elevated carboxyhemoglobin levels are those who smoke avidly late at night and then undergo an early morning operation. Therefore, it is recommended that smokers stop smoking 12 to 18 hours preop-

eratively (if not permanently) to allow three half-lives of time for carboxyhemoglobin clearance.

3. Smoking may be associated with increased pulmonary complications when the patient is older, has smoked longer, is currently smoking, and perhaps already has significant underlying lung disease.

4. Nicotine has concentration-dependent effects on the cardiovascular system. It can cause systemic vasoconstriction and increase both heart rate and systemic blood pressure. Abstinence from smoking for 20 minutes is followed by a decrease in heart rate, blood pressure, and systemic catecholamine level. These cardiovascular effects of nicotine may contribute to perioperative morbidity in smokers, and short-term abstinence may be beneficial.

5. Patients with obstructive sleep apnea and chronic obstructive pulmonary disease: risk factors for PPCs are related to general health and nutritional status and include advanced age, COPD, congestive heart failure, lower albumin level, dependent functional status, and weight loss.

6. Patients with upper respiratory infections. Afebrile patients with symptoms of an uncomplicated upper respiratory infection, including clear secretions, should be able to undergo interventional procedures.

The preoperative evaluation distinguishes patients with more severe symptoms, including purulent secretions, productive cough, temperature higher than 38°C, or signs of pulmonary involvement, and elective surgery should be postponed for about 4 weeks.

Patients with allergies

The patient's history of allergies and adverse drug reactions should be carefully documented. True anaphylactic reactions should be distinguished from adverse side effects. The patient's definition of allergy may be very different from the true clinical definition, and patients may incorrectly think that previous perioperative difficulties are due to "allergies" to anesthetic or pain medications.

Allergies to preservatives such as para-aminobenzoic acid used with esters are more common. Patients may perceive, especially with dental procedures, adverse side effects from epinephrine in local anesthetic solutions as allergies, and this needs to be carefully distinguished. Similarly, true allergies to opioids are rare, and opioid side effects, such as nausea and emesis, may be misinterpreted as allergies. Skin testing can be used to determine the presence of a true allergy. Allergies to muscle relaxants are more common; there are no reports of anaphylaxis to volatile anesthetics.

Penicillin is the most common cause of anaphylaxis. There is a small risk of cross-reactivity with cephalosporins, but most of these reported reactions involve rashes and not anaphylaxis. Anaphylactic reactions to solutions such as bacitracin or providone-iodine have only rarely been reported;

contact dermatitis in association with these agents is a more common reaction.

Morbidly obese patients

Obesity is associated with an increased incidence of risk factors, including diabetes and cardiovascular disease. These patients have a higher incidence of difficult tracheal intubation, decreased arterial oxygenation, increased gastric volume, decreased gastric pH, postoperative wound infection, pulmonary embolism, and sudden death.

Diabetic patients

Diabetics are at risk for multiorgan dysfunction, with renal insufficiency, stroke, peripheral neuropathy, autonomic dysfunction, and cardiovascular disease being most prevalent. Delayed gastric emptying, retinopathy, and reduced joint mobility occur in these patients.

Patients with psychiatric disorders

Key issues in the preoperative assessment of patients with psychiatric disorders include assessing cognitive capacity, obtaining an accurate psychiatric history, evaluating the patient's capacity to give informed consent, and assessing the impact of psychotropic medications.

Patients with cancer

Patients with a history of cancer may have complications related to the disease or the treatment. Typically, patients will be aware of the side effects of treatment that they have experienced or are at risk of having. Asking them if any "unexpected complications" occurred or if chemotherapy or radiotherapy had to be interrupted because of adverse effects is important. A hypercoagulable state is common in patients with cancer, particularly those with advanced disease and primary brain tumors, ovarian adenocarcinoma, and pancreatic, colon, stomach, lung, prostate, and kidney cancer. Patients with cancer have a sixfold increased risk for thromboembolic events, and active cancer accounts for 20% of new episodes of thromboembolism.

Patients with human immunodeficiency virus (HIV) and acquired immune deficiency syndrome (AIDS)

HIV can affect all organs and cause multiple complications. Myocarditis, dilated cardiomyopathy, valvular disease, pulmonary hypertension, pericardial effusions, and tamponade are possible. Antiretroviral-induced lipodystrophy causes coronary artery disease (CAD).

The preoperative evaluation may elicit a history of thrush, fever of unknown origin, chronic diarrhea, lymphadenopathy, or herpes zoster in more than one dermatome.

Patients with known HIV infection will frequently require further evaluation, including an electrocardiogram (ECG), complete blood count (CBC) with platelets, determination of electrolytes, blood urea nitrogen (BUN), and creatinine, liver function tests (LFTs), and a chest radiograph, depending on the procedure. Determining the CD4[+] lymphocyte cell count and viral load, which reflects the patient's immunologic status during the previous 3 months, can have prognostic value.

Patients with a history of substance abuse

The preoperative evaluation allows an opportunity to obtain a detailed history of addiction and recovery. Addictive disease is considered permanent, even in patients who have had long periods of abstinence. If a patient is in recovery, knowledge of the dosages and effects of medications used for maintenance of recovery is essential.

Clinicians may have prejudicial attitudes and may lack the educational background to formulate appropriate plans for pain management. Pain medication may be inadequate and restricted because of concern about provoking a relapse. Identifying these at-risk patients during the preoperative evaluation and involving the acute pain service to assist in management may be helpful.

Patients who are actively abusing cocaine and amphetamines are at significant risk during anesthesia because of intraoperative hemodynamic instability.

Patients who are currently substance abusers have a variety of clinical manifestations, depending on the drug abused. The preoperative period should be used to plan for appropriate management. Heroin addicts may require substitution with methadone, and those addicted to alcohol, sedatives, or hypnotics may require stabilization with benzodiazepines. Discussion of regional techniques, avoidance of inadequate analgesia, and optimization of analgesia with nonopioids is essential. Inadequate analgesia can potentially activate addiction. All information and potential management plans should be clearly transmitted to members of the operative team.

Alcohol abusers are specifically at risk for potentially life-threatening withdrawal with autonomic instability and hyperpyrexia. Cocaine and amphetamine addicts can have cerebrovascular accidents, cardiomyopathy, and arrhythmias. Additionally, cocaine and amphetamine inhibit the uptake of sympathomimetic neurotransmitters, increase BP, raise heart rate (HR), and can cause paranoia, anxiety, seizures, angina, and myocardial infarction (MI).

Marijuana can affect the cardiovascular and autonomic nervous systems and result in tachycardia, dysrhythmias, and ECG abnormalities.

8. Bleeding risks associated with interventional procedures

All interventional pain procedures carry an inherent risk of major or minor bleeding. Understanding the physiology of bleeding is important, to identify patients at risk for bleeding before performing the invasive procedure. Bleeding is considered as major if it is intracranial, intraspinal, intraocular, mediastinal, retroperitoneal, or if the bleeding results in death, hospitalization, or transfusion. Significant incidences of bleeding occur in the epidural space, owing to prominent epidural venous plexuses. Spinal subarachnoid or subdural bleeding is usually due to trauma of radicular vessels.

The bleeding risk status can be determined in a patient undergoing an invasive procedure by making some assumptions, i.e., the risk of significant bleeding is dependent on the underlying hemostatic problems and which particular technique is used. An overall bleeding risk can be calculated based on an evaluation of **technique-specific** and **patient-specific** factors (Tables 4.1 and 4.2). Such careful determination may help in decisions to avoid, abort, or proceed with the procedure.

Technique-specific bleeding risk. The risk of significant bleeding from an interventional pain procedure can be based on several factors including the presence of blood spontaneously at the needle hub following aspiration. The factors are those that influence the risk of bleeding (sharp needle, multiple passes, large needle gauge), the severity of the consequences of bleeding (proximity to neurological structures,

---

Table 4.1 Technique-specific bleeding risks

- Needle tip's proximity to an important vascular structure
- Needle's proximity to a major neurological structure
- The needle location within a confined space
- The use of a sharp needle
- The need for multiple passages
- The availability of fluoroscopy equipment
- The availability of radiopaque contrast material
- The expected use of a large- rather than small-diameter needle
- The catheter is in continuous use for a prolonged time

Table 4.2 "Patient-specific" bleeding risks

Patients are at risk of bleeding if they
- present with a current or previous history of bleeding (previous surgical bleeds, recurrent or prolonged epistaxis, hematuria, gastrointestinal bleeding, bleeding after circumcision);
- report easy and excessive bruising or bleeding, either without antecedent trauma or with minor trauma, such as injections, small cuts, or tooth extractions;
- have never had previous bleeding problems, but present with a new abnormal bleeding episode;
- have an underlying medical condition, such as renal failure, liver failure, malignancy, or systemic lupus erythematosus, which poses an increased bleeding risk or increased likelihood of abnormal coagulation studies;
- have an unreliable, family history of bleeding and are going to undergo an invasive procedure.

target in a confined space), and whether bleeding is unrecognized. Together, these factors help guide the clinician in predicting, detecting, and differentiating bleeding episodes that are less significant. Technical difficulties have been implicated as a factor in major and minor bleeding events, following invasive procedures. These technical difficulties can be classified as **non-neuroaxial** or **neuroaxial**.

Non-neuroaxial techniques
Retrobulbar blocks may cause hemorrhage, which is typically venous, with an incidence ranging from 0.5 to 3%. Hemorrhages are more common in the elderly and in those with vascular disease.

Trigeminal ganglion balloon decompressions may develop a facial weakness.

Sphenopalatine ganglion radiofrequency thermocoagulation has been associated with cheek hematomas and epistaxis.

Other non-neuroaxial techniques in thoracic, abdominal, and peripheral regions have not produced enough data for description here.

Neuroaxial techniques
These techniques include epidural, subdural, subarachnoid, and selective paraspinal injections. Significant bleeding can occur involving these procedures. They cause hemorrhages, hematomas, and may lead to significant neurological catastrophe or death. These are detailed later in this section.

Patient's previous drug intake history
Bleeding risk during or after an invasive procedure is quite often based on the patient's physical condition and/or the use of drugs that interfere with bleeding and clotting mechanisms.

Aspirin. This drug is considered the "reference standard" for antiplatelet agents. It is a potent cyclo-oxygenase inhibitor that suppresses thromboxane A2 production. Increased doses of aspirin increase major bleeding risk. Aspirin is commonly used by patients who are scheduled for an invasive procedure. Aspirin therapy has been implicated as a risk factor in interventional procedures. Preoperative antiinflammatory consumption of other anticoagulant drugs may increase bleeding during these procedures

Warfarin. Another drug that is commonly prescribed for patients is warfarin. It is typically prescribed for patients at risk for arterial or venous thromboembolism, venous thromboembolism prevention and treatment in patients with deficiencies of protein S and C, atrial fibrillation, prosthetic heart valves, and acute myocardial infarctions complicated by ventricular mural thrombi. Oral anticoagulants like warfarin exert their anticoagulant effect by interfering with the gamma carboxylation of vitamin-K-dependent coagulation factors. The liver enzyme epoxide reductase is blocked and thus the regeneration of reduced vitamin K is prevented.

The vitamin-K-dependent coagulation factors II, VII, IX, X, S, and C are functionally depleted.

The intensity of the anticoagulant (warfarin) regimen depends on the proportion of inactive factors and the duration of effect depends on factor half-life. If less than 40% of any particular factor is present, bleeding may occur. After administration of an effective dose of warfarin, the coagulant activity of the blood decreases to about 50% of normal by the end of 12 hours and to about 20% of normal by the end of 24 hours. The coagulation process is not blocked immediately but must await the natural consumption of prothrombin and other affected coagulation factors already present in the plasma. The use of multiple anticoagulants increases the risk of significant bleeding, especially if their actions are synergistic. Intraoperative bleeding, from a continuous spinal infusion, can cause severe hypotension.

Herbal medications. A spontaneous epidural hematoma can occur after garlic consumption. The American Society of Anesthesiology recommends discontinuing herbal medicines for 2–3 weeks before elective procedure. Herbal medications, such as garlic, ginseng, ginger, and ginkgo, may be a risk factor for spinal bleeding, especially if patients are consuming other anticoagulants.

Tests of clotting function. Clotting tests commonly performed for patients scheduled for an invasive procedure are **platelet count (PC)**, **bleeding time (BT)**, **activated partial throboplastin time (aPTT)**, and **prothrombin time (PT)**; the **international normalized ratio (INR)** is calculated from PT.

PC. The normal concentration of platelets in the blood is between 140,000 and 445,000 per microliter. The PC is an extremely important routine investigation, as platelet deficiency (thrombocytopenia) will increase bleeding tendency. Thrombocytopenia is defined as a PC of fewer than 150,000 per microliter.

Bleeding time. The bleeding time is an indicator of primary hemostasis in vivo. Bleeding time prolongation occurs in patients with quantitative and qualitative platelet disorders.

aPTT and **PT.** aPTT and PT are measures of the intrinsic and extrinsic pathways. Both pathways result in the generation of factor Xa. PT reveals disorders in the extrinsic pathway. It is a simple test based on incubation of patient plasma, calcium, and tissue thromboplastin (tissue factor). The addition of tissue factor accelerates the normal clotting time for plasma from 5 minutes to about 10 seconds.

INR. Normal PT is about 12 seconds. In each laboratory, a curve relating prothrombin concentration to PT is drawn for the method used, so that the prothrombin in the blood can be quantified. However, variations between laboratories in PT values have led to the development of the INR. The INR simplistically converts the ratio of PT of the patient to a PT-mean normal, to the value expected if the World Health Organization reference for thromboplastin were used.

PT and INR are most sensitive to the activity of the factors with the shortest half-lives, VII and X, but least to the factor with the longest-half life, II. When factor VII activity is reduced to 55% of baseline, the INR will exceed 1.2. When factor VII activity is reduced to 40% of baseline, the INR will exceed 1.5. Hemostasis is presumed to be normal when the INR is less than 1.5, because factor levels exceed 40%. This applies to INR values upon initiation of warfarin therapy. Factor II and X levels will take longer to normalize and may not be adequate even if the INR is less than 1.4 typically. An INR value that is within the normal range implies that there are sufficient levels of vitamin-K-dependent clotting factors, and coagulation returns to normal within 1–3 days after discontinuing warfarin therapy.

Diagnosis of bleeding and management. Significant bleeding after an invasive pain procedure is an extremely rare event. Tools to help predict these events would be helpful to pain physicians performing interventional procedures.

Signs and symptoms of occult bleeding. Symptoms depend on the location and the temporal qualities of the hematoma. For example, back pain and neurological dysfunction are the typical pre-monitory symptoms in lumbar and thoracic spinal hematomas. Progressive sensorimotor loss occurs in 68% of patients and bowel/bladder dysfunction in 8% of patients, but back and radicular pain are less common. In the cervical spine, patients have presented with Brown–Sequard syndrome. Cervical myelopathy or flaccid tetraparesis increases radicular/neck pain. The bleeding and its sequelae can be immediate or delayed. This delay can be as long as several days.

Diagnosis of anticoagulant (warfarin) overdose. A **warfarin** overdose manifests as **ecchymosis** formation, **mucosal hemorrhage**, and **subserosal** bleeding into the wall of the gastrointestinal tract. The PT is markedly prolonged in the presence of an anticoagulant (warfarin) overdose. If an anticoagulant expansile hematoma occurs after an invasive procedure, in the presence of anticoagulation with warfarin, urgent care is warranted. Close monitoring of vital signs, PT, and hematocrit (Hct) are imperative, and surgical intervention may be necessary to prevent further sequelae.

Management of overdose of anticoagulants. Recommendations for perioperative management of oral anticoagulation have been made based on the type of thromboembolic event (venous versus arterial) and specific risk factors for thromboembolism. If an invasive procedure is planned within the first month after an acute venous thromboembolic episode, then the major invasive procedure should be postponed. If this is not possible, anticoagulant (warfarin) should be held, and intravenous heparin should be administered whenever the INR falls below 2. Intravenous heparin should be held 6 hours before and restarted 12 hours after the procedure, without a bolus. Heparin may have to be held even longer if there is bleeding at the procedure site. If oral anticoagulation has been administered for more than 1 month, but less than 3 months, after venous thromboembolism, preoperative intravenous heparinization is not needed. Postoperative heparinization is needed. However, if oral anticoagulation has been administered for more than 3 months, only postoperative venous thromboembolism prophylaxis is necessary.

Administration of fresh frozen plasma and vitamin K is necessary to reverse the effects of warfarin. There is no consensus on the optimal management of patients receiving oral anticoagulants in the perioperative period. Once the INR reaches 1.5, certain types of procedure may proceed uneventfully. If warfarin is held for 4 days before procedure and re-started the night of the procedure, then the actual time frame within which patients are exposed to thromboembolism risk would only be 1 day before and 1 day after the procedure. Joint injections, subcutaneous nerve, or fascial injections do not increase the risk of joint or soft tissue hemorrhage.

Hemostatic drugs. Hemostatic drugs deserve brief mention owing to their potential role as therapeutic agents for acquired and congenital coagulation disorders and for major bleeding episodes. Synthetic amino acids, such as **aminocaproic acid** and **tranexamic acid**, may interfere with fibrinolysis by reversibly binding to plasminogen and preventing its transformation to plasmin. Tranexamic acid is more potent than aminocaproic acid and has a longer half-life. These agents can reduce blood loss in primary menorrhagia, gastrointestinal bleeding, urinary tract bleeding, oral bleeding in hemophiliacs, oral bleeding after dental extractions in patients receiving oral anticoagulant therapy, cardiac surgery, thrombocytopenia, patients receiving thrombolytics, joint replacement, and liver transplants. The dose of tranexamic acid is typically 10–15 mg/kg. Side effects are typically dose dependent.

Further reading

We acknowledge that portions of this section have been taken from the following review article:

Raj, P.P. et al. (2004) Bleeding risk in interventional pain practice: assessment, management, and review of the literature. *Pain Physician* **7**, 3–51.

Fischer, S., Bader, A. & Sweitzer, B. (2009) Preoperative evaluation. In *Miller's Anesthesia*, 7th edition, pp. 1001–1065. Philadelphia, PA: Churchill Livingstone.

White, P.F., Kehlet, H., Neal, J.M., et al. (2007) The role of the anesthesiologist in fast-track surgery: from multimodal analgesia to perioperative medical care. *Anesthesia & Analgesia* **104**, 1380–1396.

5 Monitoring the Patient Before, During, and After the Procedure

Interventional pain procedures should be considered as minimal invasive surgery. Thus monitoring of the patient before, during, and after the procedure has to be planned thoroughly.

The goals of monitoring pain relief procedures are as follows:

- monitoring the hemodynamic and metabolic response to the procedure of the patient;
- neurophysiologic monitoring and documenting the efficacy of pain relief;
- functional restoration: monitoring the patient as well as work-status restoration;
- global outcome monitoring.

Monitoring before the procedure

The physician

The physician should first check if complete resuscitation facilities are available. The facilities must include the following equipment:

- positive-pressure oxygen devices;
- suction apparatus;
- intubation equipment with appropriate laryngoscope blades and handles already tested to be in working order, appropriate sizes of endotracheal tubes and oral airways;
- emergency drugs (appropriately labeled and stored in a cart);
- electrocardiograph (ECG) monitoring, heart rate, blood pressure;
- respiratory rate, oxygen saturation monitors;
- monitor for baseline level of consciousness, pulse oximetry, and vital signs.

The nurse

Before the procedure, the nurse should obtain and document the following:

- an allergy;
- record baseline vital signs including pulse, oxygen, temperature parameters;
- pain intensity;
- the nurse should have a working knowledge of the anatomy and physiology of the region to be blocked and the pharmacology of the drugs to be used;
- the nurse should know the drug complications and side effects of the procedure about to be performed; this is imperative to anticipate problems and deal with emergencies.

The patient

Preparation of the patient should include the following:

- a complete explanation of the procedure to be performed and the informed consent obtained before the patient is brought to the procedure room;
- the patient should know what to expect at each step of the procedure;
- an informed patient is less likely to make sudden, unexpected movements;
- the patient must be NPO (nothing by mouth) for at least 6 hours before the procedure.

Monitoring during the procedure

The physician

- The physician should be well trained to perform the procedure.
- A well-trained faculty member should always be present to monitor the procedure done by the physician and assist if necessary.

The nurse

At the beginning and during the procedure, the nurse should do the following:

- monitor and set up equipment on a sterile table for the procedure;

Pain-Relieving Procedures: The Illustrated Guide, First Edition. P. Prithvi Raj and Serdar Erdine.
© 2012 John Wiley & Sons, Ltd. Published 2012 by John Wiley & Sons, Ltd.

- help to position the patient;
- monitor vital signs;
- help the patient relax and anticipate the needs of the patient;
- start a functioning intravenous catheter;
- provide premedication if necessary;
- monitor the level of consciousness.

Monitoring of the patient during the procedure may vary depending on the technique used during the procedure.

Sympathetic blocks

- Sympathetic denervation produces arterial and arteriolar vasodilation.
- Venodilatation and reduced preload result in a reduction in cardiac output and can cause significant hypotension.
- For the stellate ganglion block, because of the proximity of the ganglion to critical vascular structures, a test dose is mandatory. Local anesthetic, 0.25 mL, should be administered and the patient should be continuously monitored for any type of toxic reaction.
- The local anesthetic should be injected in divided doses. The patient must be continuously monitored for any change in the level of consciousness or for toxic reaction. Adequate placement of the local anesthetic after the block is performed can be confirmed by presence of an elevated temperature on the blocked side and evidence of a Bernard–Horner syndrome (myosis, ptosis, and enophthalmos).
- Lumbar sympathetic block. Inadvertent intravascular injection can cause seizure and subarachnoid placement of local anesthetic causes total spinal anesthesia; thus, the anesthesiologist must be prepared for this rare outcome.
- The patient should be monitored for changes in lower extremity motor strength and sensation. Monitoring should be continued after the block is complete.
- Celiac plexus block. Before the procedure, an adequate intravenous line should be established and baseline blood pressure, heart rate, respiratory rate, and level of consciousness should be determined.
- Because the sympathetic nervous system supply to the abdominal viscera is interrupted with this block, hypotension is common and must be anticipated.
- Respiratory rate must be determined before the block, and adequacy of ventilation must be monitored continually throughout the procedure.

Intraspinal analgesia

- When spinal narcotics are administered, one should monitor for delayed respiratory depression and sedation or excessive somnolence.
- The respiratory rate and depth of respiration must be followed closely. Pulse oximetry can help detect inadequate arterial oxygenation. Patients should be monitored for at least 12 hours after the last dose of intrathecal opioids is administered.

Head and neck procedures

- The physician should be very careful for inadvertent puncture of blood vessels around the target nerve.
- All procedures need to be performed under fluoroscopy.
- The physician should be aware of all possible complications related with the head and neck procedures.

Radiofrequency procedures

- The physician should monitor the response of the patient during the sensory and motor stimulation.
- The patient should be awake enough to respond to stimulation and sudden changes during the procedures.

Postprocedural monitoring

- Observe the patient for at least 2 hours after the procedure. Monitor vital signs (mandatory). In addition, objectively document the pain relief.
- Observe sensory level by means of neurovascular checks.
- Check if there is abdominal or urinary distention.
- Check that there is no bleeding at the site of entry of the needle.
- Check the blood pressure before discharging.
- Check the level of agitation: whether the patient is asleep or calm, has mild agitation or is hysterical after the procedure.
- Check if the patient responds to questions.

Monitoring during discharging the patient

- After a satisfactory observation, discharge the patient with appropriate and adequate instructions given to the escort. Written instructions are preferable for emergencies, as they are helpful to the patient and the family.
- During the observation, the patient must meet specific criteria before discharge:
  - The patient must be awake.
  - The patient must be oriented to time, place, and person.
  - The patient must have recovered full muscle control as is normal for that person.
  - The patient must have stable vital signs within the normal range.
  - The patient should be ambulated without syncope or significant change in vital signs.
  - The patient should be able to retain small amounts of clear liquid before discharge.
  - The patient will be discharged with a responsible adult companion. A responsible adult is someone of legal age who can act on behalf of the patient.
  - The patient may be taken to the car by wheelchair or ambulation. Either a nurse or a transportation aide may take the patient out to the car, if necessary.

○ The patient should not be allowed to drive home after sedation or the procedure.

○ The nurse should telephone each outpatient the day after their surgery or procedure.

○ The nurse will chart a postprocedure telephone call note based on the information received and any instructions given to the patient, including any referrals made on the patient's chart.

Further reading

American Society of Anesthesiologists (1986) *Standards for Basic Intraoperative Monitoring*. Newsletter, Park Ridge, IL.

Brodsky, J.B. (1999) What intraoperative monitoring makes sense? *Chest* **5**, 101–105.

Helman, J.D. (2001) Monitoring pain management procedures. In: *Clinical Monitoring: Practical Applications for Anesthesia and Critical Care* (ed. Lake, C.L., Hines, R.L. & Blitt, C.D.), pp. 539–552. Philadelphia, PA: W.B. Saunders.

Plancarte, R. & Rivera, F. (2002) Monitoring in regional anesthesia. In *Textbook of Regional Anesthesia* (ed. Raj, P.P.), pp. 157–175. Philadelphia, PA: Churchill Livingstone.

Prause, G. & List, W.F. (1997) The anesthesiologic risk patient. Preoperative evaluation, intraoperative management and postoperative monitoring. *Chirurg* **68**, 775–779.

Raj, P.P. & Johnston, M. (2002) Organization and function of the nerve block facility. In *Textbook of Regional Anesthesia* (ed. Raj, P.P.), pp. 147–156. Philadelphia, PA: Churchill Livingstone.

6 Radiation Safety and Use of Fluoroscopy During Interventional Pain Procedures

History

Fluoroscopy is rooted in the invention of X-rays by W. Conrad Roentgen in 1895. The first fluoroscopy device was developed by Thomas Edison and other scientists and introduced in 1900. However, it was not widely used until World War II as the "image intensifier" had not been developed. During this period, Zworykin's pioneering studies, as well as development of the television monitor and "intensifier," provided the basis for fluoroscopy as it is currently used.

General concepts used in radiation safety

With the common use of fluoroscopy, radiation safety has become a significant issue. During the first half of the 20th century, cancer incidence among physicians using fluoroscopy was higher compared with others. Therefore, training was made mandatory by the US Food and Drug Administration for physicians using fluoroscopy in 1994. Radiation safety should be discussed in terms of physics, biology, engineering, and legal aspects.

Today almost all interventional procedures are accompanied by fluoroscopy. Unfortunately, many physicians performing interventional procedures using fluoroscopy neglect the guidelines of radiation safety.

Radiation is a serious risk factor. Physicians practicing interventional pain procedures by fluoroscopy should, therefore, be aware of basic guidelines of radiology to ensure their own safety, as well as that of other staff and patients. Ideally, the fluoroscope should be used personally by the physician, who can operate the device properly to apply the basic settings, rather than by a technician. This will help to reduce the amount of radiation exposed.

Basic concepts of radiation physics

The smallest building block of material is an atom. The atomic number is the characteristic used for classification of each element, determined by the proton number. Protons are positively charged particles.

Another particle of the atomic nucleus is the neutron, which has no electrical charge. Existing on specific orbits surrounding the nucleus, electrons are the negatively charged particles. Such negative charge holds the electrons in specific orbits surrounding the positively charged atomic nucleus. A substantial amount of energy is needed to break the electrons nearest to the nucleus off their orbits, whereas less energy is required to break those on outer orbits with weaker attaching energy off their locations. Based on this rule, if an electron switches from an orbit with higher energy to one with lower energy, then energy will be released. Another conclusion from such a rule is that the lower the number of electrons in an atom, the lower the attaching energy to the nucleus, whereas the higher the number of electrons (consequently the higher the number of orbits), the higher the energy of attaching of the innermost orbit (orbit K). For example, sodium and tungsten have very different attaching energies for electrons on the innermost orbit.

Typically, an atom is neutral, which means the number of protons in the nucleus and that of electrons surrounding it are equal. When an atom gains or loses an electron, it is ionized.

If an X-ray has sufficient energy to break the electron off the orbit when running through the material, the energy is transferred into the electron, which in turn breaks the electron off the atomic orbit. This results in the occurrence of an ion pair consisting of one negatively charged electron and one positively charged atom, which leads to the ionization process.

Pain-Relieving Procedures: The Illustrated Guide, First Edition. P. Prithvi Raj and Serdar Erdine.
© 2012 John Wiley & Sons, Ltd. Published 2012 by John Wiley & Sons, Ltd.

Radiation is the dispersion of energy through electromagnetic waves or particles. The radiation ionizing the atom by breaking off the electrons from their orbits is called ionizing radiation. An X-ray is ionizing radiation, which causes an atom to be ionized by transferring the energy after colliding with it.

Electromagnetic energy. Electromagnetic energy is a type of energy radiating at light speed in the form of a sine wave, which is classified by its wavelength. The **amplitude** is the height of the wave, while the **wavelength** is the distance between two different waves, and the **frequency** is the number of waves passing through a specific point in a given time period (measured in hertz, symbol Hz). The smaller the wavelength and the higher the frequency is, the larger the electromagnetic energy (measured in kiloelectronvolts, keV). An X-ray is a typical electromagnetic (EM) radiation. However, not all EM radiations are ionizing. Visible light, infrared light, and radio waves are other examples for EM radiation (Fig. 6.1). These differ from each other only in terms of frequency and wavelengths. Waves with longer wavelengths and lower frequencies (e.g. radio waves, visible light) have lower energy levels, whereas waves with shorter wavelengths and higher frequencies (e.g. X-rays) have higher energy levels, which means they are ionizing. In other words, higher frequency corresponds to higher energy. The only ionizing part of the EM spectrum is that with a higher frequency, which consists of X-rays, gamma rays, and cosmic rays.

Fluoroscopy device specifications and settings

Fluoroscopy is a live imaging technique using X-rays (Fig. 6.2).

Fluoroscopy components are as follows.
1. Radiography tube.
2. Attached filter.
3. Collimator.
4. Antiscatter grid.
5. Image receptor.
6. Image intensifier.
7. Flat panel receptor.

1. Radiography tube
In fluoroscopy the radiography tube provides the source of energy to produce X-rays. The amount, energy, and time of radiation from the X-ray tube can be controlled. Voltage is measured in kilovolts (peak kilovoltage, kVp). In the clinic the voltage varies between 50 and 150 kVp.

The flow of electrons from the cathode to the anode is measured in milliamps (mA). In the fluoroscopy device this varies between 1 and 1000 mA. It is possible to get an image during the flow of electrons from the cathode to the anode. The display time is calculated in terms of seconds or minutes.

2. Attached filter
This is a metal disk attached to the edge of the X-ray tube. The purpose of the attached filter is to modify the X-ray energy spectrum. Without this piece, more rays would be used. Ideally a filter would hold low-energy photons while allowing the passage of high-energy photons.

Filtration undergoes a process called photoelectric absorption. Photoelectric absorption of photons varies according to the filter and occurs with low energies. Based on this, photons under 20 keV photons are filtered. Aluminum and copper are generally used as filters.

3. Collimator
A collimator is useful for restricting the area X-rays focus on. In general, X-rays are restricted to a rectangular area.

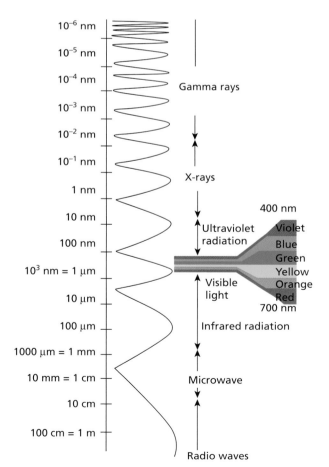

Figure 6.1 Electromagnetic spectrum.

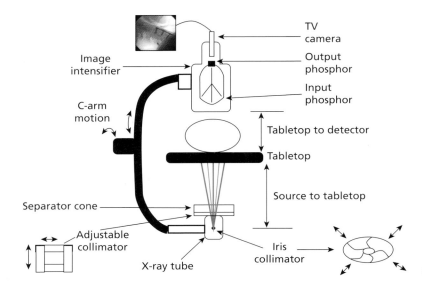

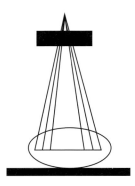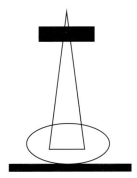

Figure 6.2 Fluoroscopy components.

Figure 6.3 Collimation.

X-rays take up a space immediately below the tube (Fig. 6.3).

A collimator has two purposes: (a) to display the desired target organ exposure to radiation and block the outside body parts from the radiation and (b) to improve image quality.

4. Antiscatter grid

A Bucky is a grid of radiopaque strips located between the radiolucent materials. It is placed between the patient and the image sensor. The purpose of this is to reduce the number of photons scattering on the image receptor. Thus, photons coming directly pass through the grille, and the number of photons that are emitted toward the patient is reduced (Fig. 6.4).

When describing a Bucky grid, specific terminology is used. The grill rate is equal to the thickness of the radiopaque laths divided by the number of spaces between the laths. As the grill rate increases, the ratio of photon scattering being stopped increases. However, as this ratio increases, the ratio of photons supplying imaging decreases. This creates a situation where there is an increase in the number of photons, so providing better imaging results. The second term in defining a Bucky grid is "lines per inch." This displays the number of radiopaque slats in the grid. With more slats, there is a reduction in image quality.

5. Image receptor

Digital technology is now used because of advances in imaging sensor technology.

6. Image intensifier

Image-enhancing technology is a feature that distinguishes a fluoroscopic device from a simple X-ray machine. Because of this, a live image can be taken.

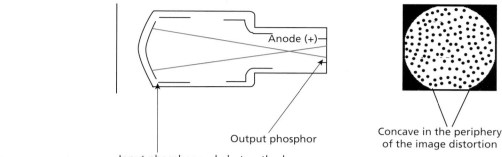

Figure 6.4 Bucky grid.

Input phosphor and photocathode

Output phosphor

Concave in the periphery
of the image distortion

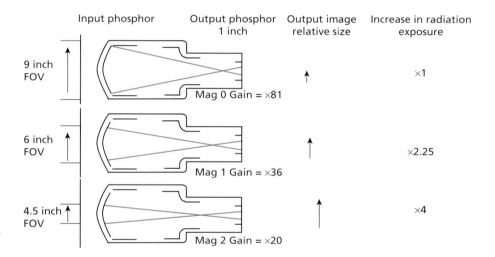

Figure 6.5 Area minimizing radiation. FOV,
field of view.

The image enhancer consists of four parts: the photon and photocathode entrance, the electrostatic focusing lenses, the acceleration mode, and the photon exit. The photon entrance is a fluorescent layer coated with cesium iodide (CsI) crystals. The purpose of the cesium iodide is to stop the photons from entering and exiting the patient and to convert high-energy X-ray photons to visible-light photons. The purpose of the photocathode layer is to convert opaque images in the CsI to images created by free electrons.

The free electrons of the image allow it to become brighter. Electrons have different loads compared with photons. Because of this, they can achieve high speed and high kinetic energy.

The purpose of electrostatic lenses is to magnify the image at different sizes. The acceleration mode allows the image to be magnified up to 50 times. Images can be strengthened in two ways: (a) using kinetic energy to increase the brightness, and (b) electron photon out image area with a smaller recovery (minimization).

This minimization leads to an increase in electrons per unit area providing for 200 times magnification. Using both methods together, the image quality is improved by $200 \times 50 = 10,000$ times (Fig. 6.5).

7. Flat panel receptor

This is a piece that replaces the image booster. It was recently added to the fluoroscopy device. X-rays convert it into an image.

Fluoroscopy operating principles

One of the primary parts of a fluoroscopy device is the X-ray tube. X-rays are the result of an evacuated tube and electrons that come out of heated cathodes colliding with anodes.

X-ray acquisition

An X-ray tube is composed of a cathode and anode. The electron source is the cathode tube. Direct current applied at the cathode heats up the filament and makes it incandescent. In this way, the electrons that make up an atom are freed in a process called thermionic emission. Filaments are generally produced from heavy metals like tungsten, which are resistant to high heat. The melting point of tungsten is about 3400 °C. Another reason tungsten is preferred is that it is able to create more thermionic emission.

The focusing heads around the filaments allow the electron beam to be redirected in the desired direction. With the high voltage generated between the cathode and anode, electrons accelerate from the cathode to the anode and gain kinetic energy.

When discharged electrons from the cathode hit the anode, they abruptly stop and their kinetic energy is transformed into another type of energy. This energy is 99.8% heat and 0.2% defined as the **breaking** and the **characteristic X-ray radiation**. Seventy-five to eight-five percent of the X-ray radiation is breaking radiation and 15–30% is characteristic radiation.

When the voltage to the cathode or the atomic number of the anode material increases, the breaking radiation also increases. The X-ray that is created in the tube is directed to the target area and the image booster provides radiographic images.

Factors affecting X-ray quality

X-rays travel at the speed of light and are ionizing. They are invisible, do not show deviation in a magnetic field, and decrease in density in proportion to the square of the distance they travel. The quality of the X-ray is dependent on the penetration capability, i.e. the beam passing through the material. The factors affecting this are X-ray energy, filtration, and the structure of the X-ray tube's anode. X-ray energy depends on the energy of the electrons emitted from the cathode. The energy of the electrons is directly proportional to their speed. To increase the speed of the X-rays, their energy, penetration, and thus improve their quality, the power supply (in other words, the voltage (kV)) must be increased.

Factors affecting X-ray quantity

Quantity relates to the amount of X-rays beamed from the tube and can be used in place of beam density or exposed radiation. Factors affecting X-ray quantities are the current intensity (mA) of the tube, its voltage (kV), the distance, and the filtration.

There is a direct proportion between the amounts of X-rays that are obtained and current intensity (mA). The milliampere setting that regulates the voltage in the tube and the heat in the cathode determines the number of free electrons joining the event, in other words X-ray density. When the current is doubled, the quantity of X-rays also doubles.

An increase in tube voltage (kV) will increase the quantity of X-ray images. When the X-ray leaves the tube, it is filtered

before it is redirected toward the patient. The purpose of this is to obtain the X-ray beams from the bundle of other beams that do not contribute to the diagnosis, and to eliminate low-energy X-rays and thus increase the quality and quantity of the X-rays.

Collimation settings (which narrow the beam) are used to keep the radiation beam at the lowest possible levels. Another setting on the fluoroscopy control panel is the time counter. Usually the alarm is set to 5 minutes, because time is the definitive factor that is used for the X-ray exposure.

Scattered radiation

There are three types of X-rays: **primary X-rays** are released from the X-ray tube; **scattered X-rays** are scattered from the primary substance and occur as a result of collision of electrons; and **residual radiation** is X-rays that pass through the patient and strengthen the image.

The primary beam interacts with the patient after exiting the tube. Part of the radiation is absorbed, some of it is transmitted, and some of it is scattered from the patient to the surroundings by primary scattering. **Secondary radiation** occurs when scattered X-ray radiation passes through an object. **Primary scattering** occurs in all directions from the patient.

The greatest danger to staff from the fluoroscopy process is the radiation risk from exposure to patients during treatments. The amount of scattered radiation is determined by the voltage used, collimation area, and the thickness of the tissue. Intervention of the secondary radiation before an operation requires the narrowing of the diameter of the X-ray beam. Collimators are used for this purpose. Reduction of power reduces the scattered radiation. However, this situation lowers X-ray penetration and reduces quality so is not a preferred method.

The patient becomes the primary source of the scattered radiation during exposure time. Primary scattered radiation also interacts with other objects and so secondary scattered radiation increases. **Secondary scattering** is at very low levels of intensity during primary radiation. Obese patients, compared with thinner patients, will need to have more primary radiation for a satisfactory image.

Another factor that affects the scattering quantity to someone working with a fluoroscopy device is the point at which the beam goes through the patient. The patient's body is held to the side near where the beam would be to the patient's midsection; consequently, the beam scatters less.

Back scattering radiation. Back scattering radiation is a type of beam that is scattered backwards from the surface that it penetrates. The use of some of the fluoroscopy C-arm positions can create a serious risk of back scattering radiation to the user.

If the X-ray tube is on the patient and at eye level to the physician performing the scanning, and the image intensifier is under the patient, the physician's face is relatively close to the X-ray tube and is unprotected against **radiation leaks scattered from the tube**. The image booster, if it is positioned above the patient, also serves as a barrier to protect the physician's face. In addition, because in this position the tube is placed below the patient, back scattering also occurs toward the ground.

Collimation

If there is insufficient collimation (beam diameter restriction), then the estimated area of radiation will be larger. This is a factor that increases dosage for the patient as well as for staff. If possible, collimation should be done on the smallest possible area; this will reduce the volume of scattered radiation and increase image quality. Fluoroscopy devices that automatically determine the beam settings also automatically adjust the tube potential (kV) with increasing thickness of the patient's body.

With an increase in tube potential, the force of the primary beam increases and scattering radiation will be more penetrating.

Despite the X-ray tube casing being lined with lead, some radiation still leaks out. This radiation is more penetrating then the equivalent radiation kilowattage that is emitted from the patient.

When the X-ray tube is used as described above and at an angle, the physician applying the device should be careful of scattered radiation as well as radiation from the source (leakage radiation).

Fluoroscopy usage types

1. Continuous fluoroscopy. This is found in all the old machines, and is still a format that is used. Fluoroscopy continues as long as the pedal is held down. This format is used incorrectly by many physicians. From the aspect of radiation safety, this is very dangerous.
2. High-speed fluoroscopy. This is used in situations where normal fluoroscopy is inadequate. However, it is not recommended.
3. Pulsed fluoroscopy. The image speed and frames per second rate (fps) is selected. This is the most advantageous format.

Fluoroscopy table

A fluoroscopy table has different characteristics than other tables. There should be as few metal parts as possible and the section the patient lies on should consist of carbon fibers.

The effects of radiation on biological systems

Radiation effects on biological systems are divided into two groups, determining and cytocastic.

Determining (direct, definitive) effect. For this to be evident the threshold of a certain dose of radiation should be reached. The effects of the force of the radiation can be determined beforehand. The determining effects of radiation are evident with the result of dying cells. As radiation doses increase, so does the ratio of dying cells. Findings have revealed that cataracts, infertility, hair loss, and skin issues are the determining effects of radiation.

Cytocastic (indirect, nondefinitive) effect. There is no threshold dose of radiation for cytocastic effects. The severity of the effect is unrelated to the dose of radiation exposure. The development effect of the "all or nothing law" applies. The effects of radiation developing in someone at a certain dosage cannot be predicted. This effect is similar to buying a lottery ticket: the more tickets that are bought, the better are the chances of winning and the larger the amount to be won. The cytocastic effects of radiation are the ones that cause mutagenic effects like cancer and leukemia.

Radiation causes neuroplasticity, which initiates DNA damage. During a radiological examination, the photons that pass through the body cause damage to the body's DNA by ionization. The carcinogenic effects of ionizing radiation, caused either directly or as a result of ionization, depend on the effect occurring on free radicals or other chemical products. Damage to a cell's DNA is either immediately repaired or eliminated through programmed cell death (apoptosis). In the rare event that a mistake occurs in the repairing mechanism or the repair is not made, part of the chromosomes are changed (mutation) and tumor induction will start.

There may be a long latent period between X-ray exposure and tumor formation. There is no concept of a threshold for ionizing radiation. Despite all the protective measures that can be taken, there is always the risk of cancer. No matter how small, any exposure to radiation causes a risk. This risk is believed to be proportional to the total exposure dose. The effects of radiation are shown in Tables 6.1, 6.2, and 6.3.

Radiation safety

In situations where a radiological image is to be used, first the necessity for imaging or the procedure should be assessed, including the effectiveness of the procedure,

Table 6.1 Radiation exposure and dose units

Term	Traditional unit	SI unit	Conversion
Exposure	Röntgen (R)	Coulomb/kg (C/kg)	$1R = 2.5 \times 10^{-4}$ C/kg
Absorbed radiation dose	Rad	Gray (Gy)	100 rad = 1 Gy
Radiation equivalent	Rem	Sievert (Sv)	100 rem = 1 Sv

Table 6.2 Yearly maximum radiation dosages

Area/organ	Permissible yearly maximum doses
Thyroid	50 rem (500 mSv)
Extremities	50 rem (500 mSv)
Ocular lens	15 rem (150 mSv)
Sex glands	50 rem (500 mSv)
Full body	5 rem (50 mSv)
Pregnancy	0.5 rem to fetus (5 mSv)

Table 6.3 Minimal pathological dose to target organ and effects

Target organ	Dose*(rad)	(Gy)	Results
Ocular lens	200	(2)	Cataract
Skin	500	(5)	Erythema
Skin	700	(7)	Permanent alopecia
Full body	200–700	(2–7)	Death due to hematopoietic failure in 4–6 weeks
Full body	700–5000	(7–50)	Death due to gastrointestinal failure in 3–4 days
Full body	5000–10000	(50–100)	Death due to cerebral edema in 1–2 days

Source: Scott et al. (2002).

personal dose limits, and a risk assessment. If the decision is made to perform the procedure, then radiation protection should take into account three basic rules. These are time, distance, and the use of protective materials (shielding) against ionizing radiation.

Other fundamental principles that can be added to this are not to interfere with the primary beam path and to use the lowest possible dose.

The dose received is proportional to the radiation exposure period.

On many devices during fluoroscopy, the voltage and current are adjusted automatically. The physician only controls the X-ray exposure time. The numbers of photons in the X-ray beam are controlled by voltage (kV), tube current (mA), and irradiation time in the tube. Low-energy X-rays, if aimed at the patient, can cause higher doses on the skin. Higher voltages, on the other hand, reduce the skin dose and lead to higher depth doses and more scattered X-rays. As voltage applied to the tube is increased, the X-ray beam energy penetrating the body will increase. However, this will also reduce image contrast. For dose analysis that can be done manually, to acquire the image desired, the highest voltage and the smallest current should be preferred.

Fundamental principles of radiation protection

1. Hold the tube low. When the radiation is scattered within the patient, it loses its energy rapidly. The scattered radiation level of the primary beam at the point where it comes in contact with the patient, in other words the side the X-ray tube is located, is 985 times higher than where the X-ray beam exits. For this reason, the X-ray tube should be kept under the table or patient. In this position most of the scattered beam is pointed downwards and will provide relative protection to the physician's body, head, and neck. Physicians using the fluoroscopic device routinely insert their hands in the primary beam when holding the X-ray tube on the patient. This causes epidermal degeneration and

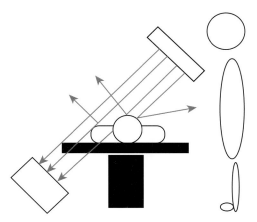

Figure 6.6 If the X-ray tube is above the practitioner, they will be exposed to more radiation.

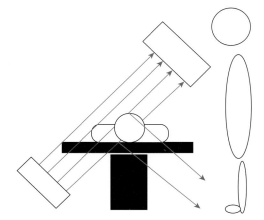

Figure 6.7 If the image booster is above the physician who is applying the procedure, it doubles as a protective function to the neck and head.

(a)   (b)

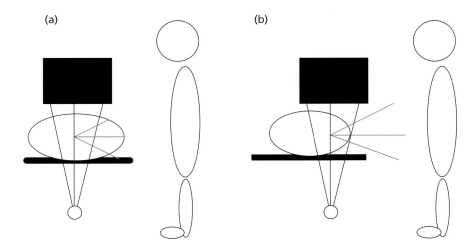

Figure 6.8 (a,b) If the primary beam passes close to the center, the exposure to scattered radiation will be less.

browning of the fingernails in the hands. To obtain the image safely, the most appropriate position is to move the X-ray tube away from the patient and the image amplifier close to them. The severity of the scattered radiation that enters the patient is thus minimized (Figs 6.6 and 6.7).

2. Keep away from sources of radiation. The intensity of electromagnetic radiation that is emitted from the source (power) is reduced in inverse proportion to the square of the distance. In space, X-rays beams move away from each other and cover a wider area. The reverse frame rate, which is determined by the X-ray area covered by the expanded X-ray photons, highlights the fact that the concentration is decreased in inverse proportion to distance. In other words, when radiation distance from its source is doubled, the radiation density is reduced by one-quarter (Fig. 6.8). This rule is not applicable if the source of the radiation is not from a point source. Electromagnetic radiation has an infinite range in space. For this reason, only when it interacts with another

substance will the force be reduced. This means that as the distance to the light source increases, in reality the force does not decrease because of beam dispersion; however, that lowers the amounts of radiation that reach the target. The common method of protecting from ionizing radiation is to use distance. So, what is a safe distance? The answer lies in understanding the relationship between the distance from the irradiation and the intensity of the radiation source. Even if not necessary, one should stand 3 meters away from the table to reduce the beam level that can be absorbed to an acceptable level. The best place to stand for staff is where the X-ray scatters twice before it reaches them. In this situation, the radiation intensity decreases approximately 1000 times with each scattering event. With the first scattering the irradiation value is reduced to 0.0001 milliröntgen (mR), in other words one-millionth of the original value.

3. Consider the scattering profile. When the C-arm of the fluoroscopy unit is angled, the scattered radiation is also angled and the amount of radiation that can reach the physician at the oblique angle can be up to four times. The situation becomes more prominent for the person operating the image intensifier portion of the fluoroscopy device from a distance, and an unprotected head and neck will get more radiation. If the profile is applied in the manner described and if the physician is unable to move away from the scattered radiation that is used, they should use thyroid-protective lead and special lead-sided protective glasses. When an X-ray passes through an object, it is reduced owing to energy absorption and scattering. The amount of reduction depends on the material's atomic coefficient, its density, and photonic energy of the material that it is passing through. As noted previously, the source of radiation for medical personnel is the patient themselves. During fluoroscopic investigations, the amount of radiation scattered from the patient will be very high near the table, in other words the place the person is standing during monitoring will have high radiation levels. Low voltages have more back scattering, whereas higher voltages have more forward scattering. During scattering the wavelength and energy of photons will change. For example, when a primary photon beam of 110 keV is scattered at an angle of 90°, approximately 17% of the energy of the scattered photon beam is lost and 91 keV of the photon beam will strike a physician standing beside the table. For this reason, if the physician has not adhered to the basic rules of protection from radiation, despite wearing a lead apron they will be exposed to the primary beam (Fig. 6.9).

4. Keep the beam time brief. The longer a person is exposed to a radiation field, the more beams they will absorb

and the more the consequences of this can be seen. The way to reduce ionizing radiation received during fluoroscopy is to use the scope intermittently to take a snapshot, to take the final shot into memory, and to refrain from taking long, continuous images.

Every fluoroscopy operator should do the following.

1. Track the beam time. The C-arms of fluoroscopy devices have an irradiation alarm that sounds for every 5 minutes of irradiation. For the individual who is operating the fluoroscopy device, this must be kept in mind when determining the total fluoroscopic time.

2. Save the last image. When a fluoroscopy operator is working on a still image, or if procedures require intermittent imaging, it is more appropriate to return recorded images and use them. Pressing the pedal for a long time is not a factor in increasing quality, the image brightness, or contrast. For this reason, short-term snapshots can be used for the same purpose. Storing the last image in memory in this manner will significantly reduce the radiation dose.

3. Use the pulse mode. Fluoroscopy devices use two different modes, continuous and pulse. In pulse-mode imaging, intermittent versus continuous radiation is provided. This mode reduces the irradiation time by up to two to five times.

4. Limit the beam size (collimation). In general, fluoroscopy users tend to set the largest dimension of an X-ray area. As a result, a larger area can be displayed. This type of usage leads the patient and physician to receive unnecessarily more X-rays than needed, because the beam size is proportional to the amount of radiation emitted. If possible, the person operating the fluoroscopy device should restrict the irradiated area by reducing the diaphragm or with the collimator. This process reduces the amount of scattered radiation and improves the image quality. The use of the collimator improves the resolution of other tissues by blocking the bright areas.

5. Set the appropriate geometry. Just as much as the thickness of a patient's skin, distance plays an important role in determining X-ray dose limitations. Owing to X-ray beam divergence, the increase in tube–patient distance and the divergence in patients will reduce the irradiated volume. The C-arm fluoroscope is used most effectively within the manufacturer's stated focus distance. If the X-ray tube is brought too close to the patient, it can cause skin burns during long-term applications. On the other hand, if the X-ray tube is too far from the patient, this can increase the size of the image. In this case, the fluoroscopy device will try to increase the amount of radiation emitted to maintain the image quality and brightness. As a rule, doubling the focus distance increases the rate of exposure to radiation fourfold. For this reason, the growth mode should only be used when it is really needed. The distance between the image intensifier and the patient should be the lowest possible because this will reduce the patient's skin dosage. This

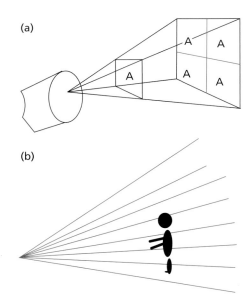

(a)

(b)

Figure 6.9 (a,b) Exposure to X-rays is inversely proportional to the square of the distance.

will occur with the reduction of radiation exiting from the automatic brightness control system.

6. Eliminate X-rays from the outside. Outside light barriers interacting with the fluoroscopy device can block the image details from being seen. In such a case, the fluoroscopic image needs to be enlarged or the amount of scattered light increased.

7. The device should undergo technical checks. Technical control is very important for devices that are used in fluoroscopy. As the image intensifier ages and loses effectiveness, the automatic brightness control mode will increase the irradiation of the primary beam and its duration automatically to maintain an adequate beam level in the camera. To determine the potential damage to performance, a periodic examination is required. The brightness stabilization system automatically adjusts the degree of image brightness and, according to the tissue thickness, the attenuation of photons passing through tissue. The two basic control mechanisms that adjust the brightness are the variable voltage and the variable tube current (mA).

8. Wear protective clothing. Shielding in the most general sense means putting obstacles between the ionizing-radiation sources and the object to reduce the effect of radiation. Elastic protective clothing such as aprons, vests, shirts, skirts, thyroid protectors, and gloves, as well as side-protective glasses, are used in stationary or moving environments without shielding. Radiation barriers such as lead aprons will reduce the amount of radiation reaching the person wearing it; however, they will never completely stop X-rays, only reduce them to an acceptable level. At 100 kV, 3.2% of the beam will pass through a 0.5 mm lead shirt, and at 70 kV 0.36% will pass. Even if the physician wears a lead apron and gloves but stands in the way of the primary radiation path, full security is not guaranteed. For this reason the three main principles of time, distance, and shielding should be considered together for radiation protection. The biggest mistake in shielding is placement. These types of lead material were designed to be used under primary beams. For example, a person wearing lead gloves should leave their hand in this area for as short a time as possible. This is not to say that there is no point to using protective materials. On the contrary, for someone whose hands are exposed to a primary beam, they should also wear a ring or bracelet dosimeter and have this monitored. A lead apron used correctly can offer 80% protection to active blood-producing organs. A well-chosen apron should start just below the manubrium sternum to include the pubis symphysis index down to just above the knee. However, for the protection to be effective, the face of the person must be turned toward the scattering source. The physician who is implementing the fluoroscopy procedure should not turn their back on the beam. Aprons are in general made of a thin material with the insides being of reinforced or equivalent materials that are filled with lead, copper, barium, and tungsten. These aprons should not be folded or wrinkled, and should not be thrown around randomly. In addition, they should be checked every year, including vital areas to ensure there are no cracks or breaks. The organ that is exposed to radiation the most, apart from organs protected by an apron, is the thyroid. Therefore, everyone who uses a fluoroscopy device should use a thyroid protector and increase the distance as much as possible to minimize radiation exposure. To protect against scattered radiation from the patient, two hanging lead curtains next to the sides of the fluoroscopy tables can be used (Fig. 6.10).

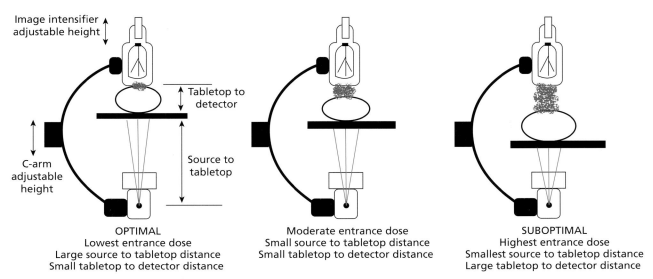

OPTIMAL
Lowest entrance dose
Large source to tabletop distance
Small tabletop to detector distance

Moderate entrance dose
Small source to tabletop distance
Small tabletop to detector distance

SUBOPTIMAL
Highest entrance dose
Smallest source to tabletop distance
Large tabletop to detector distance

Figure 6.10 Fluoroscopy operation.

Personal radiation measurement devices

Medical personnel who use a fluoroscopy device are exposed to long-term chronic low-dose radiation. The International Committee for Radiation Protection (ICRP) has determined that the maximum tolerable radiation dose (the permissible maximum dose) does not cause somatic and genetic effects, and is the yearly permissible radiation dose.

The maximum permissible annual dose of total body radiation should be 50 millisieverts (mSv), and for a 5-year average it should be a maximum of 20 mSv per year. The annual dose for the lens is 150 mSv and for the skin is 500 mSv. In addition to the mutagenic effects from chronic radiation exposure, immunosuppressant and atherosclerosis risks increase.

Dosimeters are devices carried by personnel who work with radiation to determine radiation exposure. To protect the dosimeter from the scattered beam, it must be worn on the chest pocket under the iron apron. If, during an application, the hand is exposed to radiation, a ring dosimeter should be worn under the glove. It is recommended that the complete blood count and biochemical values of individuals working with radiation should be regularly monitored, and an antioxidant diet followed including refraining from tobacco and drugs that increase the oxidative burden.

Film dosimeters measure 3 cm × 4 cm. They consist of a hard plastic protective cover where the film is placed. Radiation density absorption is measured with the help of the film densitometer. The disadvantage of these dosimeters is that X-rays of different energies can be affected to varying degrees, and the dosimeter is sensitive to changes in atmospheric temperature and humidity.

Pen dosimeters are portable, pen-shaped, pocket dosage-measuring tools. They allow radiation levels to be monitored by people who are exposed to radiation doses daily or weekly. Their disadvantages are they are expensive and prone to vibration and shock. In addition, higher radiation doses resulting from acute exposure doses may not show up on the indicator.

Dose optimization rules for fluoroscopy use

The basic rules in clinical applications for patients and staff to optimize image quality and dose optimization are explained below.

1. An increase in body mass in turn increases the amount of scattered radiation, which also increases the doses that staff receive.
2. The tube current (mA) values should be set as low as possible.
3. The highest tube voltage (kV) should be selected to give the best combination of the lowest possible dose to the patient with the optimal image quality.
4. The space between the X-ray tube and the patient should be the maximum distance possible. Also, this maximum distance should not obstruct the procedure that is being performed.
5. The space between the image magnifier and the patient must be the minimum distance possible.
6. The zoom mode should not be used unless essential.
7. Always use the narrowest collimation.
8. If possible, on anteroposterior imaging, place the X-ray tube toward the lower part of the patient.
9. Lateral or oblique imaging should be avoided if possible; if this is not possible, it should stand on the image booster side.
10. All employees should have protective goggles, thyroid protectors, wear uniforms, use a dosimeter, and position themselves in ways so that they receive minimum doses from the system.
11. Irradiation should be kept within the minimum time possible. Because the last image is stored and snapshots are taken, the procedure of choice is pulsed fluoroscopy because it reduces the time exposed to radiation. Radiation dose is directly related to time. When the irradiation time is cut in half, the radiation dose is also halved.
12. The person using the fluoroscopy device should be trained on it for their own safety and that of the patient.
13. Finally, the radiation risk should be assessed from the standpoint of the benefit of the procedure that will be provided; the planned intervention should be decided accordingly.

Results

One of the cornerstones of interventional procedures is fluoroscopy. As important as it is, it also brings many risks and dangers with it. For this reason, one must be very careful when using fluoroscopy. The initiative on implementing the fluoroscopy should be with the physician. This shortens the duration of application and reduces the dose of radiation the physician is exposed to. Fluoroscopy is neither a television nor a video camera. For this reason, it should only be used for the shortest possible period. Under no circumstances should the hand be under the beam when fluoroscopy is being used. This is the most common error when a doctor applies this initiative.

Further reading

Brateman, L. (1999) Radiation safety considerations for diagnostic radiology personnel, imaging and therapeutic technology. *Radiographics* **19**, 1037–1055.

Bushong, J.T., Seibert, J., Leidholdt, Jr, E.M., et al. (1994) *The Essential Physics of Medical Imaging*, pp. 169–192. Baltimore, MD: Williams & Wilkins.

Bushong, S.C. (2004) *Radiologic Science for Technologists*, 8th edition, pp. 357–370. St. Louis, MI: Elsevier Mosby.

Carlton, R.R. & Adler, A.M. (2001) The cathode assembly. In: *Principles of Radiographic Imaging*, pp. 111–114. Stamford, CT: Delmar.

Davros, V. (2007) Fluoroscopy: basic science, optimal use, and patient/operator protection. *Techniques in Regional Anesthesia and Pain Management* **11**, 44–54.

National Council of Radiation Protection and Measurements (1987) Recommendations on Limits for Exposure to Ionizing Radiation. NCRP Report No. 91. Washington, DC.

Nicholas, J.R.T. (2004) Protection and safety from energies used in X-ray, CT, nuclear medicine and PET, and MRI Part III cardinal principles of radiation protection. Available at http://www.radiographicceu.com/article9.html.

Raj, P.P., Lou, L., Erdine, S., Staats, H. & Waldman, S. (2003) *Radiological Imaging for Regional Anesthesia and Pain Management*. Philadelphia, PA: Churchill Livingstone.

Scott, F.M., Howard, S., Alec, M. & Anthony, S.J. (2002) Radiation safety in pain medicine. *Regional Anesthesia and Pain Medicine* **27**(3), 296–305.

Stojanovic, M.P. (2007) Basic pain management interventions using fluoroscopy: targets and optimal imaging of lumbar spine. *Techniques in Regional Anesthesia and Pain Management* **11**, 55–62.

Wagner, L.K., Eifel, P.J. & Geise, R.A. (1994) Potential biological effects following high x-ray dose interventional procedures. *Journal of Vascular and Interventional Radiology* **5**, 71–84.

Zhou, Y.L. (2005) Fluoroscopy radiation safety for spine interventional pain procedures in university teaching hospitals. *Pain Physician* **8**, 49–53.

7 Sedation and Analgesia for Interventional Pain Procedures

Most interventional procedures are performed under sedation and analgesia. Sedation and analgesia decrease pain and anxiety during the intervention; they also sedate the patient afterwards. An intervention in the prone position creates a separate problem for the patient. Therefore, it is necessary to know the principles of sedation and analgesia.

Most drugs used for sedation and analgesia can lead to depression of the respiratory, cardiovascular, and central nervous systems. For this reason, patients who undergo sedation and analgesia interference will require monitoring of cardiovascular and pulmonary systems.

It is important to keep in mind the characteristics of the population of patients on whom the intervention has been performed. For example, elderly or cancer patients should be given more consideration because of their condition.

At this point, the reader should know terms associated with sedation and analgesia.

Anxiolysis. Reducing the status of anxiety without affecting consciousness.

Analgesia. Reducing the pain while leaving the mental state unchanged.

Sedation. A controlled reduction of consciousness.

Sedation and analgesia are the terms given to the agents that remove the anxiety and pain from a patient during a procedure without disturbing cardiorespiratory functions. In 2001, the American Society of Anesthesiologists (ASA) classified sedation by categorizing it into four levels: minimal sedation, moderate sedation, deep sedation, and general anesthesia (Fig. 7.1).

When ketamine and similar agents are used, they are referred to as dissociative sedation.

Minimal sedation

During minimal sedation, the patient can yield responses to verbal commands. Even if cognitive functions and coordina-

tion have slightly deteriorated, cardiovascular and respiratory functions are not affected.

Moderate sedation

The conscious is under slight pressure during moderate sedation. Patients respond to verbal commands or touch. Airway or respiratory support is not required. Cardiovascular functions follow a normal course.

Deep sedation

Deep sedation describes a drug-induced depression of consciousness during which patients cannot be easily aroused but respond purposefully after repeated or painful stimulation. The ability to maintain ventilatory function independently may be impaired. Cardiovascular functions are not usually impaired.

General anesthesia

Under general anesthesia, the patient's consciousness is completely lost. The patient cannot be aroused, even by painful stimulation. The ability to maintain ventilatory function independently is often impaired. Patients often require assistance in maintaining a clear and open airway, and positive-pressure ventilation. There is also drug-induced neuromuscular function. Cardiovascular functions are not usually impaired.

Dissociative sedation is the resulting cataleptic state when ketamine is used. Respiratory reflexes, spontaneous respiration, and cardiovascular stability are not impaired.

Pain-Relieving Procedures: The Illustrated Guide, First Edition. P. Prithvi Raj and Serdar Erdine.
© 2012 John Wiley & Sons, Ltd. Published 2012 by John Wiley & Sons, Ltd.

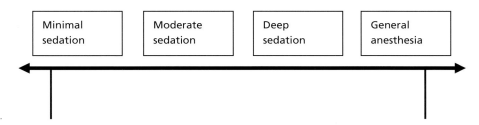

Figure 7.1 Classification of sedation.

Table 7.1 The patient's physical status related to the American Society of Anesthesiologists classification

Classification	Description	Example	Sedation risk
I	Normal and healthy person	No past history of illness	Minimal
II	Mild systemic disease without functional limitations	Slight asthma, controlled diabetes	Low
III	Severe systemic disease with functional limitation	Pneumonia, difficult to control seizures	Middle
IV	Continuous life-threatening illness	Advanced cardiac problems, renal failure, sepsis	High
V	Requiring intervention in patients with serious risk of death	Septic shock, serious trauma	Very high

The advancing process from minimal sedation to general anesthesia shows variation from patient to patient. It is a dynamic process of sedation and analgesia that is bound to the knowledge and skills of the applying physician. There are no obvious transition points between the levels, and depending on the patient's characteristics the transitions can be abrupt.

Evaluation of the patient from the standpoint of sedation and analgesia

Sedation and analgesia may carry increased risks of adverse events in those of extreme age, patients with anatomical abnormalities, those unable to lie in the prone position, or those on whom the face mask does not fit. The patient's general status is determined by ASA criteria (Table 7.1). The patient's age, general condition, diseases, drug allergies, present and previously used drugs, alcohol and smoking habits, and previous applications of sedation and analgesia should be recorded. The patient should also be examined physically.

The possible risks and side effects of sedation and analgesia should be explained to patients and their relatives. The patient's, and possibly a relative's, written consent must also be obtained. The ASA recommends that 6 hours of fasting from solid food should occur before the intervention, and 2 hours fasting from water and other beverages, although there is no consensus on this issue. For this reason, patients should fast for a period of at least 4 hours.

The fasting period carries more importance if the patient is lying in the prone position. An anesthesiologist must perform sedation and analgesia allowing for the possibility of cardiopulmonary resuscitation in the operation theater. This includes ensuring that all devices and equipment for allergic reactions, excessive sedation, respiratory depression, and (however rare) cardiopulmonary arrest (oxygen tube, respirator, cardiopulmonary monitor, defibrillator, laryngoscope, intubation tube, Ambu equipment, aspirator, etc.) are available.

Monitoring

Monitoring is one of the most important issues in analgesia and sedation. And one of the most important areas of monitoring is the patient's face. If the intervention does not concern the head area, then the face should be open. The degree of sedation can be controlled according to whether the individual does or does not respond to commands, the color of their face, and cyanosis.

The patient's oxygenation should not be the only item observed through a monitor: respiration should be tracked as well. The blood pressure, heart rate, and respiratory rate should be continuously tracked through the monitor.

The most significant side effects after sedation and analgesia occur within 5–20 minutes. The patient should be monitored for a period of at least 1 hour after the last injection.

The patient should be tracked after the awakening period until they are in a state to respond consciously to all verbal commands.

Before being discharged from the hospital, the patient's motor functions, mental status, and other parameters should be reevaluated.

Sensory and motor assessments of the patient should be made, especially after spinal injections. The patient must be discharged with a companion. The patient should not drive for at least 12–24 hours, and if any unexpected side effects occur during this time the patient should be advised to consult immediately with a physician.

Drugs used in sedation and analgesia

When choosing medications to be used in sedation and analgesia, the patient's general condition and the risks and benefits of the drugs to be used should be taken into account. The ideal agent is a drug that can provide for adequate analgesia, anxiolysis, amnesia, and somnolence. Usually a single agent is not enough and a combination of drugs is used. The effects, side effects, administration format, advantages, and exposure times for drugs used in sedation and analgesia are indicated in Tables 7.2 and 7.3.

The path selected for sedation and analgesia should be the fastest, most reliable, and the most appropriate for titration of drugs. Generally, for sedation and analgesia the intravenous route is taken. Other ways should only be considered if the intravenous method is not used.

When using the intravenous route, the drug should be administered with a very slow infusion, or a bolus should be given in small doses. This method can avoid respiratory depression. Particular attention should be paid to high-risk patients. Coming to the desired impact level should not be rushed, and time should be given to allow the drug to show its effects.

Opioids
The most commonly used opioids are fentanyl and morphine, used in combination with midazolam for sedation. Propofol can also be added to this combination. Meperidine is no longer available owing to a long-lasting toxic metabolite, normeperidine.

Fentanyl is the most commonly used opioid for sedation and analgesia. It is preferred because of its rapid onset of effect, short duration of action, and it not leading to the release of histamines. It passes through the blood–brain barrier quickly, and its effects start almost immediately. Duration of action is 30–40 minutes. It can be repeated if there is a prolongation of the intervention.

Usually 1–2 μg/kg are given. In obese patients, the effect can last longer owing to accumulation in fatty tissue. It can be used in combination with midazolam. Fast and high injection doses can cause respiratory depression afterwards. However, for the elderly and for patients in poor condition, even with low doses, respiratory depression could develop and should be kept in mind. At high doses hypotension and bradycardia may develop. The side effects of fentanyl can be reversed with naloxone.

Morphine is rarely used. Owing to its low solubility in fat, it passes through the blood–brain barrier more slowly. It takes at least 30 minutes to take effect. The starting dose is determined as 0.1 mg/kg. Because histamine secretion is increased, the risk of hypotension is greater.

Benzodiazepines
Benzodiazepines have strong amnesic, hypnotic, and anxiolytic properties. There are no analgesic effects. For this reason, they are given in conjunction with opioids to help

Table 7.2 Drugs used in sedation and analgesia

Drug	Classification	Primary effect	Administration method	Beginning dose
Fentanyl	Opioid	Analgesia	i.v.	1 μg/kg
Morphine	Opioid	Analgesia	i.v.	0.1 mg/kg
Midazolam	Benzodiazepine	Sedation; amnesia	i.v.	0.05 mg/kg
Ketamine	Phencyclidine derivatives	Disassociation; analgesia; sedation; amnesia	i.v. i.m.	1–2 mg/kg; 4–5 mg/kg
Etomidate	Imidazole derivatives	Sedation; amnesia	i.v.	0.1 mg/kg
Propofol	Alkyl phenol derivatives	Sedation; amnesia; antiemetic	i.v.	0.5 mg/kg
Nitrous oxide	Anesthetic gas	Analgesia	Inhalation	30–70%

i.m., intramuscular; i.v., intravenous.

Table 7.3 Benefits and side effects of sedation and analgesia agents used

Drug	Administration method	Time to begin effects (minutes)	Exposure time (minutes)	Advantages	Side effects
Fentanyl	i.v.	1–2	30–40	Rapid effect; short-term; ↓ secretion of histamine; minimal cardiovascular effects;	Respiratory depression
	i.m.	10–30	60–120		
Morphine	i.v.	10	240–360	Long acting	Hypotension; respiratory depression
Midazolam	i.v.	1–2	30–60	Fast acting; short-term effect; easy titration; can be administered in different ways	Respiratory depression
	i.m.	10–15	60–120		
	p.o.	15–30	60–90		
	p.r.	10–30	60–90		
	i.n.	10–15	45–60		
Ketamine	i.v.	1	15	Airway reflexes are preserved; no respiratory depression	Emesis; laryngospasm; ICP↑ and IYOP↑
	i.m.	5	15–30		
	p.o.	30–45	120–240		
	p.r.	5–10	15–30		
	i.n.	5–10	30–120		
Etomidate	i.v.	<1	5–10	Fast; short-term effect; minimal cardiovascular effect	Respiratory depression; myoclonus; adrenal suppression
Propofol	i.v.	<1	8–10	Fast; short-term effect; antiemetic	Respiratory depression; hypotension; burning during injection
Nitrous oxide	Inhalation	1–2	3–5	Fast; short-term effect; minimal KV effect	Expansion in closed body cavities; emesis

i.m., intramuscular; i.n., intranasal; i.v., intravenous; p.o., per oral; p.r., per rectal.

with sedation. Intravenous, intramuscular routes are preferred. The most frequently used agent is midazolam. It is preferred over other benzodiazepines because of its fast onset and short duration. The initial dose is 0.05 mg/kg. The effects begin within 1–2 minutes and continue for 30–60 minutes. The side effects are dose-dependent hypoventilation and hypoxemia if used in conjunction with analgesics in low doses. Older patients should be given special consideration. For chronic users of alcohol, higher doses may need to given to achieve the same effect.

Propofol

Propofol in recent years has been the most frequently used short-acting sedative and is a hypnotic agent. With very rapid effects, it has a short duration of action and provides for deep sedation. Sedation is resolved quickly. It has antiemetic properties. It also reduces intracranial pressure.

If used with opioids, it increases the risk of respiratory depression. The starting intravenous bolus dose is 0.5 mg/kg. It can be repeated every 3–5 minutes, and given as an infusion. Sedation begins in 1 minute and lasts for 10 minutes.

For interventions that will take more than 10 minutes, infusions of 3–6 mg/kg/hour can be administered. The side effects are dose-related respiratory depression, apnea, and hypotension. If used with opioids these complications can be seen more frequently; it can also lead to short-term hypotension. Bolus doses should be given quickly. The most complained about side effect from patients is severe pain along the vein during injection. To reduce this pain during the propofol injection, an injection of 1–2 cm³ of 1% lidocaine may be injected beforehand.

Ketamine

Ketamine is a phencyclidine derivative drug that induces dissociative anesthesia. Thalamocortical connections between the limbic system are temporarily cut off at the upper portion of the visual, sensory cortex and prevent responses to painful stimuli. This can lead to analgesia, amnesia, and catalepsy. Respiratory depression is not seen. Airway reflexes are preserved. Blood pressure is not reduced. The most serious side effect is the development of hallucinations in patients when they wake up. This may continue for a few days. Psychiatric problems may occur. These problems can be prevented by benzodiazepines.

Etomidate

Etomidate is a short-acting sedative hypnotic agent. There is no analgesic effect. The effects on the respiratory and cardiovascular systems are low. The effects begin within 1 minute and continue for 5–10 minutes. The starting dose is 0.1 mg/kg. Every 2–3 minutes an additional dose of 0.05–0.01 mg/kg may be given. Side effects such as apnea, respiratory depression, myoclonus, nausea, vomiting, and adrenal suppression may occur.

Nitrous oxide

Nitrous oxide (N_2O) is an inhalation agent that has been known for a long time. It is a very good analgesic in conjunction with oxygen. The effects begin within 1–2 minutes and continue for 3–5 minutes. It is given with oxygen in 30–70% concentrations. The ratio of oxygen to prevent hypoxemia must be at least 30%. It must be administered by an anesthesiologist.

Antidotes for drugs used in sedation and analgesia

Drugs used in sedation and analgesia should be titrated very carefully. This way, side effects are significantly prevented. Because the drugs that are being used have short effect times, the side effects such as oxygenation, ventilation, and fluid replacement can be eliminated rather quickly. However, if the effects in some patients last longer, opioids and benzodiazepines antidotes should be used.

Naloxone

Naloxone is used to antagonize respiratory depression due to opioids during intervention. Effects start fast, the half-time is 45 minutes, and the effect lasts for 15–30 minutes. Patients given naloxone should be observed for a period of at least 1 hour. In general it is usually administered intravenously. Naloxone is also titrated. Initially 0.1–0.2 mg is given. Observation of the patient is continued while the dosage is being administered. The administered total should not exceed 1–2 mg.

Flumazenil

Flumazenil is an antagonist to benzodiazepine. It antagonizes sedation and is used against respiratory depression. Flumazenil is administered if excessive sedation accidentally occurs. Effects begin in 1–2 minutes and reach their highest level within 5–10 minutes. The half-time is 45–90 minutes. The patient should be observed after flumazenil is administered. When the effects have worn off, re-sedation and side effects may occur. The initial dose is 0.1–0.2 mg. The maximum dose is 1 mg. It should be used with caution in patients addicted to benzodiazepines: it may lead to a seizure or epilepsy crises in these patients.

Considerations during sedation and analgesia

1. Sedation and analgesia while performing interventional procedures require specific knowledge and skills.
2. The most commonly used agents are propofol, fentanyl, and midazolam.
3. Propofol provides deep sedation.
4. Fentanyl provides analgesia.
5. The patient should be continuously monitored during sedation and analgesia.
6. Sedation and analgesia should occur in environments where cardiopulmonary resuscitation opportunities exist.
7. Sedation and analgesia should be applied by or under the supervision of an anesthesiologist.
8. Antidotes for drugs used in sedation and analgesia must be available.
9. After sedation and analgesia, the patient should be in a position to be able to respond to any verbal command, to stand on their own, walk, and meet their own personal needs.
10. When a patient who has had sedation and analgesia is discharged, they should be warned against the possible effects of hypotension and other side effects.

Further reading

American College of Emergency Physicians (2005) Procedural sedation in the emergency department. *Annals of Emergency Medicine* **46**, 103–104.

American Society of Anesthesiologists (1996) Practice Guidelines for Sedation and Analgesia by Non-anesthesiologists. A report by the American Society of Anesthesiologists Task Force on Sedation and Analgesia by Non-Anesthesiologists. *Anesthesiology* **84**, 459–471.

American Society of Anesthesiologists Task Force on Sedation and Analgesia by Non-Anesthesiologists (2002) Practice Guidelines for Sedation and Analgesia by Non-anesthesiologists. *Anesthesiology* **96**, 1004–1007.

Bahn, E.L. & Holt, K.R. (2005) Procedural sedation and analgesia: a review and new concepts. *Emergency Medicine Clinics of North America* **23**, 503–517.

Benzon, H. (2008) Pain treatment and procedural sedation. In *Raj's Practical Management of Pain* (ed. Benzon, H., Rathmell, J., Wu, C., Turk, D. & Argoff, C.), 4th edition, pp. 1146–1150. Philadelphia, PA: Mosby.

Berde, C.B. & Strichartz, G.R. (2000) Local anesthetics. In *Miller's Anesthesia*, 5th edition (ed. Miller, R.D.), pp. 491–522. Philadelphia, PA: Churchill Livingstone.

Colson, J.D. (2005) The pharmacology of sedation. *Pain Physician* **8**, 297–308.

Fanning, R.M. (2008) Monitoring during sedation given by non-anaesthetic doctors. *Anaesthesia* **63**(4), 370–374.

Frazee, B.W., Park, R.S., Lowery, D., et al. (2005) Propofol for deep procedural sedation in the ED. *American Journal of Emergency Medicine* **23**, 190–195.

Godwin, S.A., et al. (2005) Clinical policy: procedural sedation and analgesia in the emergency department. *Annals of Emergency Medicine* **45**, 177.

Green, S.M. (2007) Research advances in procedural sedation and analgesia. *Annals of Emergency Medicine* **49**(1), 31–36.

Green, S.M., et al. (2007) Fasting and emergency department procedural sedation and analgesia: a consensus-based clinical practice advisory. *Annals of Emergency Medicine* **49**, 454–461.

Joshua, P., Prager, J.P. & Aprill, C. (2008) Complications related to sedation and anesthesia for interventional pain therapies. *Pain Medicine* **9**(1), 121–127.

Levine, D.A. & Platt, S.L. (2005) Novel monitoring techniques for use with procedural sedation. *Current Opinion in Pediatrics* **17**, 351–354.

Miller, R.D. (2005) *Miller's Anesthesia*, 6th edition, chapter 10. Philadelphia, PA: Churchill Livingstone.

Smally, A.J. & Nowicki, T.A. (2007) Sedation in the emergency department. *Current Opinion in Anaesthesiology* **20**, 379–383.

Symington, L. & Thakore, S. (2006) A review of the use of propofol for procedural sedation in the emergency department. *Emergency Medicine Journal* **23**, 89–93.

8 Drugs Used During Interventional Pain Procedures

Local anesthetics

Local anesthetic agents are classified as either ester or amide agents. Clinically useful agents in the ester group are cocaine, procaine, 2-chloroprocaine, and tetracaine. In the amide group, they are lidocaine, mepivicaine, bupivacaine, ropivacaine, and recently synthesized agents (Table 8.1).

Ester group

Cocaine

Chemistry
Cocaine occurs in abundance in the leaves of the coca shrub and is an ester of benzoic acid and methylecgonine. Ecgonine is an amino alcohol base closely related to tropine, the amino alcohol in atropine. It has the same fundamental structure as synthetic local anesthetics.

Pharmacological actions
The clinically desired actions of cocaine are the blockade of nerve impulses and local vasoconstriction secondary to inhi-

bition of local norepinephrine reuptake. Toxicity and the potential for abuse have steadily decreased the clinical uses of cocaine. Its high toxicity is due to block of catecholamine uptake in both the central nervous system (CNS) and peripheral nervous system. Its euphoric properties are due primarily to inhibition of catecholamine uptake, particularly dopamine, at CNS synapses. Other local anesthetics do not block the uptake of norepinephrine and do not produce the sensitization to catecholamines, vasoconstriction, or mydriasis characteristic of cocaine. Currently, cocaine is used primarily to provide topical anesthesia of the upper respiratory tract, where its combined vasoconstrictor and local anesthetic properties provide anesthesia and shrinking of the mucosa with a single agent. Cocaine hydrochloride is used as a 1, 4, or 10% solution for topical application. For most applications, the 1 or 4% preparations are preferred to reduce toxicity. Because of its abuse potential, cocaine is listed as a schedule II drug by the US Drug Enforcement Agency.

Procaine
Procaine (Novocain), introduced in 1905, was the first synthetic local anesthetic and is an amino ester. Although it formerly was used widely, its use now is confined to infiltration anesthesia and, occasionally, diagnostic peripheral nerve blocks. This is because of its low potency, slow onset, and short duration of action. Although its toxicity is fairly low, it is hydrolyzed in vivo to produce *para*-aminobenzoic acid (PABA), which inhibits the action of sulfonamides. Thus, large doses should not be administered to patients taking sulfonamide drugs.

Chloroprocaine
2-Chloroprocaine (Nesacaine), an ester local anesthetic introduced in 1952, is a chlorinated derivative of procaine. Its major assets are its rapid onset and short duration of action and its reduced acute toxicity due to its rapid metabo-

Table 8.1 Comparison of local anesthetics by potencies

Local anesthetic	Potency	Duration of local anesthetic effect
Procaine	1	Short
Chloroprocaine	2–4	Medium
Lidocaine	4	Medium
Mepivacaine	3–4	Medium
Prilocaine	3–4	Medium
Bupivacaine	16	Long
Ropivacaine	14–16	Long
Levobupivacaine	16	Long
Tetracaine	16	Long

Pain-Relieving Procedures: The Illustrated Guide, First Edition. P. Prithvi Raj and Serdar Erdine.
© 2012 John Wiley & Sons, Ltd. Published 2012 by John Wiley & Sons, Ltd.

lism (plasma half-life approximately 25 seconds). Enthusiasm for its use has been tempered by reports of prolonged sensory and motor block, after epidural or subarachnoid administration of a large dose.

This toxicity appears to have been a consequence of low pH of the local anesthetic solution and the use of sodium metabisulfite as a preservative in earlier formulations. There are no reports of neurotoxicity with newer preparations of chloroprocaine, which contain calcium ethylenediaminetetraacetic acid (EDTA) as the preservative, although these preparations also are not recommended for intrathecal administration. A higher-than-expected incidence of muscular back pain after epidural anesthesia with 2-chloroprocaine has also been reported. This back pain is thought to be due to tetany in the paraspinal muscles, which may be a consequence of calcium ion (Ca^{2+}) binding by the EDTA included as a preservative; the incidence of back pain appears to be related to the volume of drug injected and its use during skin infiltration.

Pharmacological actions
2-Chloroprocaine is procaine with the addition of a chlorine group to the benzene ring. This drug has a very rapid onset of action and a short duration of activity (30–60 minutes). Once absorbed into the circulation, the drug is rapidly metabolized. The approximate half-life in plasma in adults is 45 seconds to 1 minute; hence, it is the most rapidly metabolized local anesthetic currently used. Because of this extremely rapid breakdown in plasma, it has very low potential for systemic toxicity and has been particularly attractive to obstetric anesthesiologists for use when elevated maternal blood levels of local anesthetic can cause major problems for the fetus and mother. This drug is also frequently used for epidural and peripheral blocks in an ambulatory care setting when short duration of anesthesia is needed and rapid recovery is highly desirable.

The epidural use of this drug, however, has been limited because of several reported problems. Prolonged and profound motor and sensory deficits occurred with the unintentional subarachnoid injection of the original commercially prepared 2-chloroprocaine local anesthetic solution with the preservative bisulfite. The classic work by Gissen and co-workers and Wang and colleagues demonstrated that bisulfite in the presence of a highly acidic solution releases sulfur dioxide (SO_2), which equilibrates in solution into sulfurous acid, which is neurotoxic. Gissen postulated that the injection of the highly acidic commercial 2-chloroprocaine (PH_3) solution into the spinal intrathecal space resulted in the slow formation of, and prolonged exposure to, sulfurous acid, causing spinal cord damage. More recently, a 2-chloroprocaine preparation was released in clinical use, from which the bisulfite was removed and EDTA was substituted as the preservative. This change, however, has not been satisfactory because there appears to be a significant occurrence of

back muscle spasm after epidural application of this formulation. It has been postulated that the EDTA in this commercial preparation binds to calcium and causes spasm in the paraspinal muscles.

A new 2-chloroprocaine commercial preparation has been released from which all preservatives have been removed. Initial studies with this formulation appear to be promising. No preparations of 2-chloroprocaine are recommended for either spinal or intravenous regional anesthesia.

Tetracaine
Tetracaine is the butylamino derivative of procaine (Pontocaine). It was introduced in 1932, as a long-acting amino ester. It is significantly more potent and has a longer duration of action than procaine.

Tetracaine has an increased toxicity because it is metabolized more slowly than the other commonly used ester local anesthetics. Currently, it is widely used in spinal anesthesia when a drug of long duration is needed. Tetracaine is incorporated into several topical anesthetic preparations. With the introduction of bupivacaine, tetracaine is rarely used now in peripheral nerve blocks, because of its slow onset and toxicity.

Tetracaine is a potent long-acting local anesthetic and has been widely used, mainly for spinal anesthesia in a dose of 6–15 mg in adults. Clinically, such drug administration produces a high degree of motor blockade. Tetracaine has also been used as a 0.2–0.5% solution for epidural anesthesia; however, it is not considered adequate for this purpose because of its slow onset of action and its tendency to produce spotty sensory anesthesia. Many otolaryngologists use this drug to produce topical anesthesia for the upper airway.

Amide group

Lidocaine
Lidocaine (Xylocaine), introduced in 1948, is now the most widely used local anesthetic.

Pharmacological actions
The pharmacologic actions that lidocaine shares with other local anesthetic drugs have been described widely. Lidocaine produces faster, more intense, longer lasting, and more extensive anesthesia than does an equal concentration of procaine. Unlike procaine, it is an aminoethylamide and is the prototypical member of this class of local anesthetics. It is a good choice for individuals who are sensitive to ester-type local anesthetics.

Absorption, fate, and excretion
Lidocaine is absorbed rapidly after parenteral administration and from the gastrointestinal and respiratory tracts. Although it is effective when used without any vasoconstrictor, in the presence of epinephrine, the rate of absorption and the

toxicity are decreased, and the duration of action usually is prolonged. Lidocaine is dealkylated in the liver by mixed-function oxidases to monoethylglycine xylidide and glycine xylidide, which can be metabolized further to monoethylglycine and glycine xylidide. Both monoethylglycine xylidide and glycine xylidide retain local anesthetic activity. In human beings, about 75% of xylidide is excreted in the urine as a secondary metabolite, 4-hydroxy-2,6-dimethylaniline.

Toxicity

The side effects of lidocaine seen with increasing dose include drowsiness, tinnitus, dizziness, and twitching. As the dose increases, seizures, coma, and respiratory depression and arrest will occur. Clinically significant cardiovascular depression usually occurs at serum lidocaine levels that produce marked CNS effects. The metabolites monoethylglycine xylidide and glycine xylidide may contribute to some of these side effects.

Clinical uses

Lidocaine has a wide range of clinical uses as a local anesthetic; it can be used in almost any application in which a local anesthetic of intermediate duration is needed. Lidocaine also is used as an antiarrhythmic agent.

Mepivacaine

Mepivacaine (Carbocaine), introduced in 1957, is an intermediate-acting amino amide. Its pharmacologic properties are similar to those of lidocaine. Mepivacaine, however, is more toxic to the neonate and thus is not used in obstetric anesthesia. The increased toxicity of mepivacaine in the neonate is related to its slower metabolism in the neonate, owing to ion trapping of this agent at the lower pH of neonatal blood and the dissociation constant (pK_a) of mepivacaine. Despite its slow metabolism in the neonate, it appears to have a slightly higher therapeutic index in adults than lidocaine. Its onset of action is similar to that of lidocaine and its duration slightly longer (about 20%) than that of lidocaine in the absence of a coadministered vasoconstrictor. Mepivacaine is not effective as a topical anesthetic.

Prilocaine

Prilocaine (Citanest) is an intermediate-acting amino amide It has a pharmacologic profile similar to that of lidocaine. The primary differences are that it causes no vasodilatation and thus can be used without a vasoconstrictor. Its increased volume of distribution reduces its CNS toxicity, making it suitable for intravenous regional anesthesia. It is unique among the local anesthetics for its propensity to cause methemoglobinemia. This effect is a consequence of the metabolism of the aromatic ring to a-toluidine. Development of methemoglobinemia is dependent on the total dose administered, usually appearing after a dose of 8 mg/kg. In healthy persons, methemoglobinemia is usually not a problem. If

necessary, it can be treated by the intravenous administration of methylene blue (1–2 mg/kg). Methemoglobinemia after prilocaine administration has limited its use in obstetric anesthesia because it complicates evaluation of the newborn. Also, methemoglobinemia is more common in neonates because of decreased resistance of fetal hemoglobin to oxidant stresses and the immaturity of enzymes in the neonate that convert methemoglobin back to the ferrous state. The amino amide agents are metabolized primarily in the liver. Patient age may influence the physiologic disposition of local anesthetics.

Bupivacaine

Bupivacaine (Marcaine, Sensorcaine), introduced in 1963, is a widely used amide local anesthetic; its structure is similar to that of lidocaine, except the amine-containing group is a butyl piperidine. It is a potent agent capable of producing prolonged anesthesia. Its long duration of action plus its tendency to provide more sensory than motor block, has made it a popular drug for providing prolonged analgesia during labor or the postoperative period. With use of indwelling catheters and continuous infusions, bupivacaine can be used to provide several days of effective analgesia.

Bupivacaine was developed as a modification of mepivacaine. Its structural similarities to mepivacaine are readily apparent. Bupivacaine has a butyl (four-carbon substitution) group on the hydrophilic nitrogen.

Bupivacaine has made a contribution to regional anesthesia second in importance only to lidocaine. It is one of the first of the clinically used local anesthetic drugs to provide good separation of motor and sensory blockade after administration. The onset of anesthesia and the duration of action are long and can be further prolonged by the addition of epinephrine in areas with a low fat content. Only small increases in duration are seen when bupivacaine is injected into areas with a high fat content. For example, a 50% increase in duration of brachial plexus blockade (an area of low fat content) occurs after the addition of epinephrine to bupivacaine solutions; in contrast, only a 10–15% increase in duration of epidural anesthesia results from the addition of epinephrine to bupivacaine solutions, because the epidural space has a high fat content.

Toxicity

Bupivacaine is more cardiotoxic than equieffective doses of lidocaine. Clinically, this is manifested by severe ventricular arrhythmias and myocardial depression after inadvertent intravascular administration of large doses of bupivacaine. The enhanced cardiotoxicity of bupivacaine probably is due to multiple factors. Lidocaine and bupivacaine both block cardiac sodium channels rapidly during systole. However, bupivacaine dissociates much more slowly than lidocaine during diastole, so a significant fraction of Na^+ channels remain blocked at the end of diastole (at physiologic heart rates) with bupivacaine. Thus, the block by bupivacaine is cumulative and substantially greater than would be predicted by its local anesthetic potency. At least a portion of the cardiotoxicity of bupivacaine may be mediated centrally, because direct injection of small quantities of bupivacaine into the medulla can produce malignant ventricular arrhythmias. Bupivacaine-induced cardiotoxicity can be very difficult to treat, and its severity is enhanced in the presence of acidosis, hypercarbia, and hypoxemia.

Clinical uses

In the United States, bupivacaine is used mainly for obstetric anesthesia and postoperative pain control when analgesia without significant motor blockade is highly desirable and achievable with low bupivacaine concentrations. In contrast to lidocaine, however, when high blood levels occur with bupivacaine, a higher incidence of cardiotoxic effects is seen. Bupivacaine has a poorer therapeutic index than lidocaine in producing electrophysiologic toxicity of the heart. Although bupivacaine metabolism is slower in the fetus and newborn than in the adult, active biotransformation is accomplished by the fetus and newborn.

A second major role of bupivacaine is in subarachnoid anesthesia. It produces very reliable onset of anesthesia within 5 minutes, and the duration of anesthesia is approximately 3 hours. In many ways, it is similar to tetracaine; however, the dose of bupivacaine required is somewhat larger, specifically, 10 mg of tetracaine is approximately equal to 12–15 mg of bupivacaine. The onset of sympathetic blockade after spinal anesthesia appears to be more gradual with bupivacaine than with tetracaine. Also, the sensory blockade produced by bupivacaine lasts longer than the motor blockade, which is in contrast to what occurs with etidocaine and tetracaine. Bupivacaine can be used for subarachnoid anesthesia in either the glucose-containing hyperbaric solution (0.75%) or with the isobaric solution by using the drug packaged for epidural use as a 0.25 or a 0.5% concentration.

Etidocaine

Etidocaine (Duranest), introduced in 1972, is a long-acting amino amide. Its onset of action is faster than that of bupivacaine and comparable with that of lidocaine, yet its duration of action is similar to that of bupivacaine. Compared with bupivacaine, etidocaine produces preferential motor blockade. Thus, although it is useful for surgery requiring intense skeletal muscle relaxation, its utility in labor or postoperative analgesia is limited. Its cardiac toxicity is similar to that of bupivacaine.

Etidocaine is structurally similar to lidocaine, with alkyl substitution on the aliphatic connecting group between the hydrophilic amine and the amide linkage. This increases the drug's lipid solubility and results in a drug more potent than lidocaine that has a very rapid onset of action and a pro-

longed duration of anesthesia. Because etidocaine produces rapid profound motor and sensory blockade at all of its clinical concentrations, it is unacceptable for obstetric anesthesia when motor blockade is undesirable. In addition, motor blockade has been observed in many instances to far outlast sensory blockade, thus causing significant postoperative patient anxiety during recovery.

Some physicians have found it helpful to take advantage of the rapid onset of anesthesia and the significant motor blocking effect associated with etidocaine administration by using it for lengthy procedures to induce epidural anesthesia and then substituting bupivacaine or lidocaine for subsequent doses to maintain an adequate sensory level without undue prolongation of motor block on recovery. The addition of epinephrine to etidocaine solutions produces a 50% increase in duration of brachial plexus blockade but only a 10–15% increase in duration of epidural blockade. This effect, as with bupivacaine, stems from significant solubility into the high fat content of the epidural space by a highly lipid-soluble drug.

Newer local anesthetics: chiral forms

An area of newfound importance for anesthesiologists is the use of stereoisomers of drugs to take advantage of differences in activity or toxicity of the isomers. For stereoisomerism to be present, an asymmetrical carbon (a carbon atom in the molecule that has four distinctly different substitution groups) must be present in the molecule. Stereoisomers are possible for the local anesthetics etidocaine, mepivacaine, bupivacaine, prilocaine, and ropivacaine, and some of these drugs have differences in potency or toxicity for the isomers.

In the older literature, isomers were described as levo and dextro on the basis of chemical configuration and as (+) or (−) on the basis of topical rotation (i.e., L [+] or D [−]). More recent literature describes isomers as R or S, and the optical rotation is still included in parentheses as (+) and (−). R and S basically correspond to the D and L in the older nomenclature.

As a rule, when differences between the activity of isomers are present for local anesthetics, the S form is less toxic and has a longer duration of anesthesia. For instance, anesthesia produced by bupivacaine infiltration was of longer duration compared with the R isomer when the S isomer was used. Also, the S isomer had lower systemic toxicity. The mean convulsant dose of R-bupivacaine was 57% of the S-bupivacaine convulsant dose. When the isomers of ropivacaine were evaluated, the S isomer of the drug had a longer duration of blockade and a lower toxicity than its R isomer. Additionally, when cardiac electrophysiologic toxicity was evaluated in animal studies, ropivacaine (the commercial preparation is the S form of drug) at equipotent nerve-blocking doses appeared to have a safety margin that was almost twice that of commercial bupivacaine, which is a mixture of the R and S isomers. Studies with the R and S bupivacaine isomers indicate that the R form is apparently more arrhythmogenic and more cardiotoxic. Further evaluation of the isomers of bupivacaine is necessary before commercial use can be achieved.

Ropivacaine

The cardiotoxicity of bupivacaine stimulated interest in developing a less toxic, long-lasting local anesthetic. The result of that search was the development of a new amino ethylamine, ropivacaine, the S-enantiomer of 1-propyl-2′,6′-pipecolocylidide. The S-enantiomer, like most local anesthetics with a chiral center, was chosen because it has a lower toxicity than the R isomer. This is presumably because of slower uptake, resulting in lower blood levels for a given dose. Ropivacaine is slightly less potent than bupivacaine in producing anesthesia. In several animal models, it appears to be less cardiotoxic than equieffective doses of bupivacaine. In clinical studies, ropivacaine appears to be suitable for both epidural and regional anesthesia, with duration of action similar to that of bupivacaine. Interestingly, it seems to be even more motor-sparing than bupivacaine.

Ropivacaine is a long-acting, enantiomerically pure (S-enantiomer) amide local anesthetic with a high pK_a, and low lipid solubility, which blocks nerve fibers involved in pain transmission (A-delta and C fibers) to a greater degree than those controlling motor function (AB fibers). The drug was less cardiotoxic than equal concentrations of racemic bupivacaine but moreso than lidocaine (lignocaine) in vitro and had a significantly higher threshold for CNS toxicity than racemic bupivacaine in healthy volunteers (mean maximal tolerated unbound arterial plasma concentrations were 0.56 and 0.3 mg/L, respectively).

Extensive clinical data have shown that epidural ropivacaine (0.2%) is effective for the initiation and maintenance of labor analgesia, and provides pain relief after abdominal or orthopedic surgery, especially when given in conjunction with opioids (coadministration with opioids may also allow lower concentrations of ropivacaine to be used). The drug had efficacy generally similar to that of the same dose of bupivacaine for pain relief but caused less motor blockade at low concentrations.

Lumbar epidural administration of 20–30 ml ropivacaine (0.5%) provided anesthesia of a similar quality to that achieved with bupivacaine (0.5%) in women undergoing cesarean section, but the duration of motor blockade was shorter with ropivacaine. For lumbar epidural anesthesia for lower limb or genitourinary surgery, comparative data suggest that higher concentrations of ropivacaine (0.75 or 1.0%) may be needed to provide the same sensory and motor blockade as bupivacaine (0.5 and 0.75%). In patients about to undergo upper limb surgery, 30–40 mL of ropivacaine (0.5%) produced brachial plexus anesthesia broadly similar to that achieved with equivalent volumes of bupivacaine (0.5%), although the time to onset of sensory block tended to be faster and the duration of motor block shorter with ropivacaine.

Ropivacaine had an adverse event profile similar to that of bupivacaine in clinical trials. Several cases of CNS toxicity were reported after inadvertent intravascular administration of ropivacaine, but only one case of cardiovascular toxicity has been reported to date. The outcome of these inadvertent intravascular administrations was favorable.

The conclusion is that ropivacaine is a well-tolerated regional anesthetic with an efficacy broadly similar to that of bupivacaine. However, it may be a preferred option because of its reduced CNS and cardiotoxic potential and its lower propensity for motor block.

Ropivacaine appears to be less cardiotoxic than equal concentrations of racemic bupivacaine (because of its faster dissociation from cardiac Na^+ channels) but more cardiotoxic than lidocaine (lignocaine). The drug had a smaller effect on QRS prolongation than bupivacaine in healthy volunteers (+2.4% versus +6%: $P < 0.05$). CNS toxicity occurs at lower plasma concentrations than cardiotoxicity with all local anesthetics; ropivacaine and bupivacaine caused seizures at lower concentrations than lidocaine in dogs.

In healthy volunteers, ropivacaine had a significantly higher threshold for CNS toxicity (lightheadedness, tinnitus, and numbness of the tongue) than bupivacaine, with mean maximum tolerated unbound arterial plasma concentrations of 0.56 and 0.3 mg/L, respectively ($P < 0.001$).

Ropivacaine has a biphasic vascular effect, causing vasoconstriction at low concentrations but not at higher concentrations. Importantly, epidural ropivacaine 0.5% did not compromise uteroplacental circulation in healthy pregnant women.

After epidural administration in women undergoing cesarean section, mean maximum plasma concentrations C_{max} of 1.1–1.6 mg/L were reached after administration of 20–28 ml ropivacaine (0.5 or 0.75%). The drug also underwent a degree of systemic absorption after intercostal, subclavian perivascular, peribulbar, intraarticular, or local administration. However, because ropivacaine is extensively (90–94%) bound to plasma proteins after systemic absorption, C_{max} for unbound drug remains well below the threshold for CNS toxicity.

Levobupivacaine

Levobupivacaine is the S enantiomer of bupivacaine. It is included in the amide group of local anesthetics. Almost all of it is metabolized, and excreted in urine and feces.

Levobupivacaine is a long-acting local anesthetic. Exposure time depends on the dose.

The effects begin in 15 minutes; it takes longer than bupivacaine. During an epidural application it was shown in practice to provide less motor blockage in ratio to bupivacaine. It has similar effects if it is in the peripheral nerve block. In clinical practice, levobupivacaine and bupivacaine showed similar effects.

In normal doses, no significant CNS and electrocardiography (ECG) side effects were observed. The most common side effect of levobupivacaine is hypotension.

Metabolism of local anesthetics

The metabolic fate of local anesthetics is of great practical importance, because their toxicity depends largely on the balance between their rates of absorption and elimination. As noted earlier, the rate of absorption of many anesthetics can be reduced considerably by the incorporation of a vasoconstrictor agent in the anesthetic solution. However, the rate of destruction of local anesthetics varies greatly, and this is a major factor in determining the safety of a particular agent. Because toxicity is related to the free concentration of drug, binding of the anesthetic to proteins in the serum and to tissues reduces the concentration of free drug in the systemic circulation and, consequently, reduces toxicity. For example, in intravenous regional anesthesia of an extremity, about half of the original anesthetic dose is still tissue-bound 30 minutes after release of the tourniquet; the lungs also bind large quantities of local anesthetic.

Ester local anesthetics

Ester-linked local anesthetics are hydrolyzed at the ester linkage in plasma by the plasma pseudocholinesterase. This plasma enzyme also hydrolyzes natural choline esters and the anesthetically administered drug succinylcholine. The rate of hydrolysis of ester-linked local anesthetics depends on the type and location of the substitution in the aromatic ring. For example, 2-chloroprocaine is hydrolyzed about four times faster than procaine, which in turn is hydrolyzed about four times faster than tetracaine. In the case of 2-chloroprocaine, the half-life in the normal adult is 45 seconds to 1 minute. In individuals with atypical plasma pseudocholinesterase, the rate of hydrolysis of all the ester-linked local anesthetics is markedly decreased, and a prolonged half-life of these drugs results. Therefore, whereas the potential for toxicity from plasma accumulation of the ester-linked local anesthetics (e.g., 2-chloroprocaine) is extremely remote with repeated dosing of the drug in normal individuals, this likelihood should be considered with the administration of large doses or repeated doses to individuals with the atypical pseudocholinesterase enzyme.

The hydrolysis of all ester-linked local anesthetics leads to the formation of para-aminobenzoic acid (PABA) or a substituted PABA. PABA and its derivatives are associated with a low but real potential for allergic reactions. A history of an allergic reaction to a local anesthetic agent should be considered primarily as resulting from the presence of PABA or derived from ester-linked local anesthetics. Allergic reactions may also develop from the use of multiple-dose vials of amide-linked local anesthetics that contain PABA as a preservative. Allergic reactions to amide-linked local anesthetics without preservatives are rare.

Amide local anesthetics

In contrast to the ester-linked drugs, the amide-linked local anesthetics must be transported by the circulation to the liver before biotransformation can take place. The two major factors controlling the clearance of amide-linked local anesthetics by the liver are (l) hepatic blood flow (delivery of the drug to the liver) and (2) hepatic function (drug extraction by the liver). Factors that decrease hepatic blood flow or hepatic drug extraction result in an increased elimination half-life.

For example, drugs such as general anesthetics, norepinephrine, cimetidine, propranolol, and calcium channel blockers (e.g., diltiazem) can all decrease hepatic blood flow and increase the elimination half-life of the amide-linked local anesthetics. Similarly, decreases in hepatic function caused by a lowering of body temperature, immaturity of the hepatic enzyme system in the fetus, or liver damage (e.g., cirrhosis) lead to a decreased rate of hepatic metabolism of the amide local anesthetics.

Renal clearance of unchanged local anesthetics is a minor route of elimination. For example, the amount of unchanged lidocaine excretion in the urine in the adult is small, roughly 3–5% of the total drug administered. For bupivacaine, the renal excretion of unchanged drug is also small but somewhat higher, in the 10–16% range of the administered dose.

Lidocaine metabolism occurs after uptake of the drug by the liver. The primary biotransformation step for lidocaine is a dealkylization reaction in which an ethyl group is cleaved from the tertiary amine. Interestingly, this primary step in lidocaine's biotransformation appears to be only slightly slower in the newborn than in the adult, indicating functional maturity of this particular enzyme system in the newborn. However, an approximately twofold increase in the elimination half-life of lidocaine is seen in the newborn, which is believed to result not from enzymatic immaturity but, instead, to reflect the larger volume of distribution for lidocaine in the newborn. A larger volume of distribution means that a given dose of drug achieves a lower plasma concentration; thus, fewer drugs would be delivered to the liver for metabolism per unit time and to the kidney for excretion. Thus, it takes longer to clear a drug from the body when the drug has a larger volume of distribution.

As with the biotransformation of lidocaine, that of bupivacaine progresses with a dealkylization reaction as the primary step. Again, in the newborn, an increased volume of distribution is present for bupivacaine and a longer half-life is thus anticipated compared with those expected in the adult. Other reactions in the biotransformation of amide-linked local anesthetics include hydrolysis of the amide-link portion and oxidation of the benzene-ring portion of the drug. The metabolites thus formed can be cleared by the kidney as unchanged or conjugated compounds. For example, when hydroxy derivatives are formed from the oxidation of the benzene ring, they are conjugated and excreted as the glucuronide or sulfate conjugate.

With mepivacaine, the primary metabolic pathway is the oxidation of the benzene ring portion of the molecule, producing 3- and 4-hydroxymepivacaine. Because this oxidation metabolic pathway is less well developed in the newborn, mepivacaine metabolism occurs more slowly in the newborn than in the adult.

Ropivacaine metabolism in humans has been studied extensively. At low plasma concentrations, the drug is primarily metabolized and excreted in the urine. Significantly less drug is metabolized by dealkylation at low concentrations to pipecolylxylidine (PPX). At high concentrations in vitro, dealkylation to PPX becomes an important pathway. The metabolites formed are much less active than ropivacaine, the parent compound. Renal clearance of ropivacaine also is relatively small, with only about 1% of the administered dose excreted unchanged in the urine.

Undesired effects of local anesthetics

In addition to blocking conduction in nerve axons in the peripheral nervous system, local anesthetics interfere with the function of all organs in which conduction or transmission of impulses occurs. Thus, they have important effects on the CNS, the autonomic ganglia, the neuromuscular junction, and all forms of muscle. The danger of such adverse reactions is proportional to the concentration of local anesthetic achieved in the circulation.

Side effects of local anesthetics

Side effects during regional anesthesia administration or after related to local anesthesia are as follows:

(1) by direct effect of the drug;
(2) physiological changes caused by the drug or secondary to the block;
(3) develops independently from the drug or the block;
(4) direct effects of the drug.
Side effects seen directly from the effect of drugs can be divided into local and systemic.

Local effects

It is believed that local anesthetics on the market are not considered cytotoxic. The stabilizer that is added to local reactions is widely known to be originated from bacteriostatic agents and heavy metals. In addition, tissue damage may occur because of traumatic injection, a high drug concentration in the tissue, poor blood supply, and for mechanical reasons. The most commonly seen reaction is local tissue allergy.

Systemic effects

Local anesthetics are absorbed in the area that they are applied, affecting various organs and causing side effects. The local anesthesia concentrated in the blood, if excitable cells have increased enough to cause membrane stabilization, will affect the CNS, heart and respiratory centers, and vital organs, depending on the concentration. This will be influenced by the rate of increase in plasma concentration of local anesthetic, the protein attached to the local anesthetic drug (free drug concentration), and, in the CNS, the combined use of depressants.

This situation is usually a result of absorption with too much circulation of an overdose of a local application drug or accidental injection into a vein.

To avoid these side effects, pay attention to local anesthetic and vasoconstrictor dose, use the most diluted dose possible, and, to prevent injection into a vein, perform an aspiration test.

Local anesthetics, especially the plasma proteins alpha-1 acid glycoprotein (AAG), are connected to albumin to a lesser extent. For patients who have a low AAG level, the lidocaine-free fractions will be higher. For CNS and CVS toxicity to be bound less to acidosis and proteins depends on the elevation of the local anesthetic free fraction. Surgical stress may affect AAG levels. These drugs should be used very carefully in children and adolescents.

Toxicity

Mixing in high rates of local anesthetics into the systemic circulation or overdose can cause toxicity to the CNS and CVS. In its general meaning, toxicity is a drug that damages living cells. Toxicity may be secondary or indirect. Drugs may not always be toxic, and sometimes the expected pharmacological effects of the drug may cause some pathological events to occur. The entire body may be affected, causing the development of systemic toxicity. As noted above, toxicity may be dose-related and symptoms might be found if there are high levels of the drug in the plasma. Immune response disorders in some patients may be due to toxicity. Here, as a result of the exposure to the antigen and development of sensitivity, the toxic effect occurs.

Toxicity may be absolute or relative. The absolute toxicity of the drug refers to its potential harm. Relative toxicity is expressed when taking into consideration the therapeutic values of similar drugs. For example, the milligram base toxicity of lidocaine is approximately twice that of procaine. If the absolute toxicity of procaine is said to be 1, the absolute toxicity of lidocaine will be 2. If lidocaine is twice as toxic as procaine, a similar block should be half the necessary dose of procaine. Thus, the relative toxicity of lidocaine to procaine will be equal.

CVS toxicity

There are three potential mechanisms to explain CVS toxicity mechanisms.

1. Sodium channel block, deceleration, bradycardia, and "re-entry" predisposition to dysrhythmias.

2. CNS autonomic discharge, arrhythmias, or medication directly to "re-entry" to warn dysrhythmias.

3. Sarcolemma or endoplasmic reticulum Ca^{2+} is shown to suppress translocation.

The currently accepted view is that the start of toxicity is the inhibition of intracellular energy production.

Local anesthetics on the heart and vascular smooth muscle directly develop depression on the cardiac conduction system. The effect of this mechanism explains the deterioration in the smooth muscle and conduction system with disruption to the ionic system. Here again, the main cause is the degradation of Na^+ transport in the foreground.

With the toxic doses, the first PR on ECG as prolongation of the QRS are seen as an expansion and as sinus bradycardia. When there is an increase in the level of the local anesthetic, decreased myocardial contractility inhibition of intracellular Ca^{2+} liberalization occurs which leads to a decrease in cardiac heartbeat.

Cardiovascular toxicity is proportional to the potency of drugs. In addition, the CVS is more resistant than other systems against the potential effects of local anesthetics, and the toxic symptoms can rise to higher blood levels. The cardiovascular toxicity of long-lasting drugs such as bupivacaine and etidocaine is much more than short acting drugs such as lidocaine.

Bupivacaine has been reported in cases of malignant ventricular fibrillation. In experimental studies, bupivacaine concentrations rose rapidly in plasma, and its myocardial distribution was found to be very rapid.

Depression induced by long-effecting drugs caused by their excessive tissue binding brings no response from resuscitation owing to the long length of time required.

Local anesthetic drugs, by acting directly on vascular smooth muscles, usually cause vasodilatation and the development of hypotension.

Treatment. Systemic local anesthetic toxicity is more difficult to treat. The first step is to apply basic life support and to start treating acidosis if it is present. During hypotension, the legs must be lifted and intravenous fluid must be given. For bradycardia, 0.01 mg/kg atropine is administered intravenously. Use adrenaline (0.1–1 µg/kg, intravenously) for cardiac depression and hypotension to obtain (+) inotropic and vasoconstrictor effects. If necessary, cardioversion can be performed on ventricular arrhythmias. As an antiarrhythmic, bretilium is more effective. For cardiac arrest, cardiopulmonary resuscitation is applied.

CNS toxicity

In the CNS, toxicity is first seen in inhibition of cortical inhibitory synapses. Later, it affects the excitatory neurons and creates a general depression. Thus, an excitation phase with the inhibition of inhibitory neurons, then a generalized depression including the respiratory and circulatory centers, develop.

If the intravenous injections are too rapid, depression could set in before the excitation phase is seen. This depression is long acting and with potent local anesthetics can last longer. Cerebral perfusion maintenance ensures that the brain is not injured. The early symptoms of CNS toxicity are somnolence, feeling of weight on the head, and deterioration of postural stability. Later, perioral paresthesia, tinnitus, dizziness, fatigue, hallucinations, visual disturbances, dysarthria, nystagmus, and tremors occur. Tonic–clonic convulsions occur with the rise in blood pressure. CNS depression develops later. Without lidocaine and procaine, excitation phase depression has been reported to develop.

After applying local anesthesia, the patient should be continuously monitored. If sedation is administered before intervention, the first symptoms of toxicity are eliminated. The first indications of the excitation period may be disorientation, nausea, and vomiting. The patient should be carefully monitored for any changes of behavior. This period should not be confused with hysterical reactions from the patient. Afterwards, the excitation period continues with small muscle twitching, which causes tonic–clonic convulsions. An early diagnosis of toxic symptoms can assist development of adequate oxygenation and anticonvulsant therapies applied to the patient, which can prevent more serious problems from occurring.

Treatment. Treatment with an anticonvulsant, a short-lasting barbiturate (thiopental 4 mg/kg, intravenously), or benzodiazepines (diazepam 0.1 mg/kg intravenously, midazolam 0.05–0.1 mg/kg intravenously) is used. If necessary, it can be repeated within intervals of a few minutes until the convulsions stop. It should be noted that benzodiazepines will bind to the plasma proteins, leading to an increase in free fractions of local anesthetics. In the meantime, respiration should be continued and adequate oxygenation provided. If it is necessary to do so, apply artificial respiration.

Local toxicity

Local toxicity is toxicity of the drug injection or the drug's cytotoxic effect in the contact area. In this kind of local damage, the actual toxicity of the drug, to be tolerated at the top level of concentration, hypo- or hyperosmolarity, of drugs may be responsible in local ischemia with prolonged contact time. Local toxicity can also occur on the surfaces of the body, skin, and mucous membranes, and may be due to an allergic response. This phenomenon is referred to as delayed hypersensitivity.

Allergic reactions

Allergic reactions to local anesthetics occur more in ester groups. In the amide group, the allergic response is usually against a preservative substance (methylparaben, etc.). The composition of the allergic reaction can vary from anaphylaxis to a simple skin reaction. Treatment for mild reactions is provided through antihistamines; for more advanced cases, adrenaline, steroids, and volume resuscitation are used.

Methemoglobinemia

Methemoglobinemia occurs when prilocaine is used at 8 mg/kg or more in healthy individuals. This event depends on the procaine metabolites o-toluidine, nitrozotoluidin, p-hidroksitoluidin in the body.

The clinical signs are cyanosis. Methemoglobinemia develops at low doses before cyanosis becomes significant. For heart and lung patients and for those with severe anemia, it impairs oxygen transportation. Prilocaine should not be used in these patients.

Methemoglobinemia may not just appear through injection with prilocaine, but also with compounds containing a eutectic mixture of local anesthetics (EMLA) transdermal in a high dose or with reuse. For treatment, either methylene blue (1% solution of 1–2 mg/kg, intravenously) or ascorbic acid (vitamin C, 2 mg/kg, intravenously) is used.

Special attention should be paid to techniques to avoid local anesthetic toxicity; the smallest amount of drug for a minimum dose should be used. Despite the drugs that have appeared on the market in recent years having little toxic effect, any drug used in high-enough dosage or injected intravenously risks being toxic. For this reason, physicians need to know the techniques that they will use very well and, if needed, the specifications of the local anesthesia that they will be using. In addition, evaluation of the patient before and during the procedure and in follow-up is greatly important in preventing toxicity.

Intolerance

Intolerance is effective below the analgesic concentration in the plasma of the local anesthetic. This is rare. Much depends on the patient's general condition more than any inherited sensitivity. Acidosis, alkalosis, dehydration, febrile conditions, and intolerance can lead to liver failure.

Tolerance and tachyphylaxis

It is not correct to address both tolerance and toxicity together. The term tolerance is applied when the local anesthetic dosage in a normal physiological concentration does not produce the usual effect of analgesia. It is not structural but functional. The development of tolerance can change, based on the drug's chemical composition and physiological activity.

When tolerance to local anesthetics decreases, the situation is called intolerance. An intolerance symptom or response may be treated by reducing the dose of the local anesthetic.

Tachyphylaxis is the progressive decrease in the effectiveness of a specific drug when it is reused. It is also referred to as acute tolerance. The effect that each dose becomes less than the previous one, may be due to the chemical structure of the drug, its concentration, and changes in local tissue. The underlying mechanism is not known. Some drugs, often at short intervals after exposure, develop a refractory situation and their effectiveness is reduced. Another meaning for tachyphylaxis is when it is used to increase the dosage after chronic drug use. The response is normal, but the dose still needs to be increased. However, tachyphylaxis occurs acutely, its effect is reduced, and it is not affected even in very high doses.

Idiosyncrasy

Idiosyncrasy is a qualitative reaction. The allergic reaction is thought to be hereditary. The side effects can be produced from eye drops containing lidocaine which may lead to a loss of consciousness. This can be explained as an idiosyncratic event.

Secondary effects

This group of effects includes hypotension as a result of a local anesthetic block developing into a sympathetic block, respiratory depression due to paresis, and a burning sensation due to vasodilatation.

Effects unconnected to local anesthetics or blocks

Conditions that may arise which do not depend on regional anesthesia during surgery include syncope, mania, hysteria, heart failure, brain hemorrhage, and coronary spasm.

Neurolytic drugs

Neurolytic drugs provide long-term or permanent effects on nerve conduction. This effect is called neurolysis. Neurolytic blocks should be used more for cancer pain.

Neurolytic drugs have different physical and chemical properties. The mechanism of action and the resulting neural damage as well as their side effects also differ. Currently, ethyl alcohol, phenol, glycerol are used. Other drugs (such as silver nitrate, osmic acid, intrathecal hypertonic sodium chloride, and cold serum physiologic applications) were abandoned owing to the numerous side effects. Table 8.2 gives information on neurolytic drugs.

Ethyl alcohol

As one of the oldest neurolytic drugs, alcohol is applied in 50–95% concentrations. The hypobaric structure of alcohol (density 0.80) provides quick distribution for the area it is injected into. Alcohol is prepared in 2–5 ml or 10 ml colorless ampoules sterilized in an autoclave. Alcohol absorbs mois-

Table 8.2 Frequently used neurolytic drugs

Drug name	Concentration	Application	Specifications
Alcohol	50–100%	Gasser ganglion; celiac plexus; sympathetic chain	Hypobaric; painful injection; spreads easily
Phenol	6% aqueous, 10% glycerin	Sympathetic chain; celiac plexus; peripheral nerve	Hyperbaric; difficult deployment; painless injections; vascular graft injury
Glycerol	50%	Gasser ganglion; peripheral nerve	Viscous

ture from the atmosphere, so an opened ampoule should be used immediately. High concentrations (75–95%) are used for intrathecal or peripheral blocks and low concentrations (50–75%) for a sympathetic block. Its injection is painful and a local anesthetic should be injected before the block. Percutaneous alcohol injection leads to degeneration of nerves. After nerve damage a painful complication called neuritis may develop. The incidence for neuritis following the injection of alcohol in the peripheral nerves is between 10 and 66%. The direct injection of alcohol into the nerve tissue creates a conduction block. The nature of the effect changes depending upon the structure of the nerve tissue. In sensorial nerves, hypoesthesia or anesthesia is seen; in motor nerves, paralysis or paresis is evident; and in mixed nerves, both are observed. Alcohol is the agent used for Gasser ganglion block, a variety of peripheral nerve blocks, celiac plexus, and lumbar sympathetic blocks.

Side effects
For disulfiram users after an injection of alcohol, related side effects such as aldehyde dehydrogenase enzyme inhibition may develop. Users of beta-lactamase antibiotics, metronidazole, chloramphenicol, tolbutamide, or chlorpropamide may see the occurrence of sweating, flushing, dizziness, nausea, and vomiting after the injection of alcohol. A high-dose injection of alcohol, depending on the blood concentration, can cause a CNS depressive effect.

Phenol
Phenol is a neurolytic drug that is widely used. It easily spreads to all the tissues, affecting them all, including the skin. It also disrupts protein structures. Concentrations of phenol of 5% or higher lead to necrosis on skin contact. It has a biphasic effect on nerve tissue, having both the effect of a local anesthetic and neurolytic. Therefore its injection is painless.

Solubility in water is performed at most to a 1:15 ratio and concentrations of 6–7%. For higher concentrations,

small amounts of glycerin and/or a radiopaque substance are added. It must not come in contact with plastic or rubber material during preparation and is sterilized in an autoclave. Vials of it are dark-colored, stored in a refrigerator. After preparation, it remains stable for a period of 1 year.

Phenol causes protein coagulation in the nerves, which is similar to the effects of alcohol. High concentrations can cause excessive fibrosis and thickening of the arachnoid. The damage phenol does can be characterized by Waller degeneration and segmental demyelination.

Side effects
Phenol initially causes stimulation and later depression in the CNS. In humans, the stimulation phase is short. Systemic absorption into circulation suppresses the myocardium and the toxic effect in small vessels leads to hypotension.

Chronic phenol poisoning can cause the development of skin rashes, gastrointestinal disturbances, and renal damage. When applied as a neurolytic and injected at 2–20 cm^3 of blood levels at 6–10% concentrations, a toxic blood level cannot be reached. In addition, there is a strong antipyretic effect. A significant portion (80%) is expelled through the kidneys and the remainder (20%) is oxidized from the liver. The effect of phenol on vascular structures is greater than that of neurophospholipids on nerve tissue. For this reason, high volumes of phenol cannot be applied to vascular structures; for example, for a celiac ganglion block, alcohol is preferred.

Glycerol
Glycerol's neurolytic properties were discovered during use for another purpose by Hakanson in 1981. Within a short time, glycerol became the drug of choice over other neurolytic drugs, especially in treating trigeminal neuralgia. Glycerol, owing to its viscosity during a Gasser ganglion application, does not spread to the surrounding tissue and

does not create permanent damage. Thus with most patients sensorial faculty loss is prevented.

It is quite difficult to inject extremely viscous glycerol with specifically thin needles. To make the injection easier to administer into the peripheral nerves, the drug is divided into $0.1\,cm^3$ volumes.

Complications of neurolytic drugs

1. Neuritis
Neuritis, a major complication that develops after nerve blockage, has an observed rate of 2–28% of peripheral nerve damage.

2. Paresthesia, hypesthesia
In fact, paresthesia and hypesthesia result from the application of neurolytic blocks. For patients for whom a neurolytic block is being considered, they should be warned about paresthesia and hypesthesia, and their approval for the use of the block should be sought. It is better yet to apply the block with local anesthetics in the patient to make them aware of how it will feel.

3. Paralysis
Paralysis is the most serious complication of neurolytic block applications. It is related to giving incorrect intrathecal ranges of neurolytic drugs inadvertently. Intrathecal neurolysis, which was used in the past, will not be discussed here.

4. Anesthesia dolorosa
This is another important complication seen after the neurolytic block. It is more common after Gasserian ganglion block. It may also occur after intercostals block and other peripheral nerve blocks.

5. Nerve damage due to injection
The needle can also lead to nerve damage during injection. The needle tip can lead to a decrease in local blood flow, and defects to the perineurium and endoneurium. In addition, needle trauma can damage the surrounding tissue and the injected drug concentration in the targeted tissue can cause a decrease in efficiency. The development of blunt needles that cause far less trauma, the development of impedance-measuring electrodes and stimulation techniques, and the use of imaging reduce the likelihood of nerve damage.

Rules when applying neurolytic blocks
Neurolytic blocks are widely applied in the treatment of cancer and noncancer pain. Complications can occur during neurolytic blocks. Consider the basic rules when choosing the most appropriate method to prevent complications that may occur, such as the following.

1. Neurolytic blocks should only be applied by experienced, skilled clinicians with relevant training in these practices.
2. Neurolytic blocks should be applied as part of multimodality treatment planning for patients with severe cancer pain or noncancer chronic pain.
3. Patient selection must be made very carefully and the most appropriate neurolytic block with the least risk of side effects should be considered. Detailed questioning about the type of pain, extent, severity, progression, and disease-related information should be performed. The patient's expected life expectancy is important in choosing the method.
4. All the possible side effects and complications of the method described should be explained to the patient and relatives.
5. For all patients who will have a neurolytic block applied, a prognostic or diagnostic block should also be applied.
6. The evaluation of neurolytic block covers the full period of time from the interruption of nociceptive conduction and the pain-free period. Evaluation should not only be done by physicians, but also by nurses and patients' relatives. Review the patient's verbal response, as well as duration of sleep, appetite, general activity, and the reduction in the requirement of analgesic medication. However, the evaluation of neurolytic blocks of patients with physical dependencies on opioid analgesics is difficult. A neurolytic drug should be applied at the lowest concentration and the lowest volume known to be effective.

Contrast agents

Implementation of interventional procedures with fluoroscopy has made it mandatory to use contrast agents. Contrast agents are widely used, especially in interventions aimed at the spine.

Classification of contrast agents
Contrast agents can be classified in two ways.
1. Positive and negative contrast agents.
   (a) Positive-contrast agents: by absorbing X-rays, a more pronounced image of the desired tissue is revealed. Non-ionic and ionic substances used for treatment of pain are in this group.
   (b) Negative contrast agents: these are more transparent than the other agents. This group includes air, nitrogen, carbon dioxide, helium, oxygen, nitrous oxide, and xenon.
2. Contrast agents by chemical structure.
   (a) Ionic contrast agents.
   (b) Non-ionic contrast agents.

(a) Ionic contrast agents
Contrast agents are materials such as barium and iodine containing radiopaque agents. Iodine-based contrast agents

provide for X-ray absorption through the tri-iodinate benzoate anion. The osmolarity of free ion amounts in ionic solutions is increased, leading to eight times the hyperosmolarity amounts for normal plasma osmolarity. Ioxaglate can be given as an example of an ionic drug. Ionic drugs with high and low osmolarity properties can be handled in two separate groups. However, this hyperosmolar structure increases the contrast material's risk of toxicity.

(b) Non-ionic contrast agents

All drugs contain organic iodine, which accounts for the contrast appearance. Non-ionic contrast agents are more hydrophilic than ionic drugs. Owing to this hydrophilic feature, the toxic effects are reduced when given to the subarachnoid space or intravenously. The osmolarity of non-ionic drugs is low. This also reduces any side effects. Drugs used during interventional methods are non-ionic. Examples of non-ionic drugs are iohexol, iopamidol, iodixanol, and ioversol.

Rules when using contrast agents

1. Informed consent must be taken pre-intervention from the patient and the side effects of the contrast agents must be explained.
2. Patients' allergies, especially iodine allergy, should be investigated.
3. A contrast agent taken with an injector should not be confused with others. For this, a label can be pasted onto it. A more practical method is to control the injector under the fluoroscopy before it is used.
4. Low concentrations of contrast agents containing iodine are safer and have a better imaging capability.
5. For concentrations of contrast agents, a range of $200 \, mg/ml$ to $300 \, mg/cm^3$ should be used. The total dose of daily iodine is 3 grams. Using a 25% contrast material mixed with saline may provide a better image.
6. Metformin should be discontinued temporarily.
7. Contrast agents are discharged from the kidneys and this can lead to sudden changes in renal functions. In patients using high doses of metformin, lactic acidosis may develop.

Side effects of contrast agents

Side effects are difficult to predict beforehand. Nevertheless, it is important to determine if a patient has an allergic make-up or not. Side effects can be classified as follows.
1. Allergic reactions.
2. Reactions based on chemical make-up.
  (a) Hyperosmolarity related reactions
  (b) Toxicity:
    (i) chemotoxicity;
    (ii) osmotoxicity;
    (iii) ion toxicity.
Chemotoxicity occurs when the enzymes bind to the proteins and the molecules bind to the cell structures through cell membranes. Chemotoxic reactions may be associated with osmotic side effects. Among some of the side effects are arrhythmia and ECG changes such as cardiac depression. Water-soluble angiographic contrast agents can cause spinal cord damage.

Inadvertent injection of the contrast material in the subarachnoid space is possible during transforaminal injection or epidurography. The contrast agent's osmotoxicity depends on hyperosmolarity. There is a significant osmolarity difference between ionic and non-ionic contrast agents. Osmolarity for ionic substances is 600–2400 mOsm/kg, whereas the level for non-ionic substances is 300 mOsm/kg.

Side effects can be seen in a broad context from mild to severe. Most side effects subside without treatment. After injection of ionic substances, mild side effects such as pain, flushing, heat sensation, and vasodilatation, as well as more serious side effects such as erythrocyte aggregation and vascular endothelial injury, may occur. The most frequently seen side effects are nausea, vomiting, and musculoskeletal pain. Side effects start 1–1.5 hours after the injection and decrease within 24 hours. Low back pain, tinnitus, sweating, and seizures are seen infrequently. In rare cases, this may develop into peripheral neuropathy. Side effects such as sensory and motor disorders, myelitis, motor weakness in leg muscles, muscle cramps, fasciculations, and spasticity, progressing to paralysis, occur very rarely.

In particular, the use of ionized drugs with high osmolarity may result in acute renal failure (Table 8.3).

Table 8.3 Contrast agents' side effects

Mild side effects
Nausea, vomiting
Feeling of warmth, blushing
Chills
Chest pain
Facial swelling, edema
Abdominal pain
Pain during injection
Urticaria
Hoarseness, cough

Severe side effects
Dyspnea
Hypotension
Loss of consciousness
Paresthesia
Convulsions
Tissue necrosis
Cardiac arrest
Paralysis

Source: Chopra & Smith (2004). Reproduced with permission from American Society of Interventional Pain Physicians.

Precautions

1. Medical history. The patient's allergy history should be researched. Care must be taken with patients who have seafood allergies. Other risk factors include renal failure, heart failure, multiple myeloma, diabetics using methylmorphine, liver failure, and excessive alcohol use.

2. Hydration. In particular, prehydration should be provided to patients before the application of intravenous contrast agents.

3. All types of resuscitation equipment should be available.

4. Corticosteroids, antihistamines, and adrenaline should be available.

Corticosteroids

Hollander in 1951 described the use of hydrocortisone and cortisone injections into the joints with painful arthritis. Then spinal injections using steroids were introduced. With the application of neuroaxial steroid injections, complications began to emerge. The most commonly used steroids are methylprednisolone acetate, triamcinolone, betamethasone acetate, and dexamethasone.

Pharmacology of steroids

There are many pharmacologic effects of corticosteroids. They can be classified as corticosteroids, glucocorticoids, and mineralocorticoids. In addition, they can be classified according to their effect on sodium retention, carbohydrate metabolism and anti-inflammatory effects. Glucocorticoids are produced in the zona fasciculata of the adrenal cortex. They are under the "negative feedback" control of the hypothalamus and pituitary gland. The hypothalamus secretes a "corticotrophin releasing hormone." This stimulates the pituitary "adrenal corticotrophin hormone" (ACTH), which provides synthesis. The ACTH endogenous glucocorticoid provides for cortisol production. Glucocorticoid encourages immunological activity and accelerates wound healing. They are also necessary for normal carbohydrate, lipid, and protein metabolism Daily glucocorticoid secretion of 20–30 mg of oral hydrocortisone is estimated to be equal to 5–7 mg of oral prednisolone. During excessive stress, cortisol synthesis may be up 10-fold.

Mineralocorticoids are produced by stimulation of the renin–angiotensin system in the zona glomerulosa of the adrenal gland. The basic mineralocorticoid is aldosterone and plays a role in maintaining sodium–potassium balance. Glucocorticoids suppress the secretion of pituitary ACTH. Externally given steroids have the same effect and they inhibit the secretion of endogenous corticosteroids in the adrenal cortex. This also leads to secondary adrenal cortical insufficiency. The degree of this insufficiency depends on the route by which the steroids are administered as well as on the duration of the treatment. Corticosteroids are used to take advantage of their anti-inflammatory effects for the treatment of pain. All the steroids used in spinal injections are prednisolone derivatives.

Methylprednisolone is a methyl derivative of prednisolone. Betamethasone, dexamethasone, and triamcinolone are fluoride derivatives of prednisolone. Betamethasone is an isomer of dexamethasone. Particulate compounds, triamcinolone acetonide, betamethasone sodium phosphate, and acetate betamethasone can show an effect for a longer time. However, using particulate steroids in the cervical region would not be correct, owing to the risk of embolism.

Evaluation of steroids based on their size

Dexamethasone

Dexamethasone particles are $0.5\,\mu m$ and have a diameter 5–10 times smaller than red blood cells. Dexamethasone is soluble in water. There is no aggregation property. Dexamethasone when mixed with other anesthetics has an increase in viscosity and does not demonstrate aggregation features. The effects start faster and sooner than for other agents, which are less soluble in water. However, recent studies on this subject have shown that there are no big differences between the duration of effect. Because these drugs do not have particles, the use of dexamethasone, especially in the cervical region, would be more appropriate.

Triamcinolone

Triamcinolone particles vary in size between 0.5 and $100\,\mu m$. Large-scale particles are 12 times larger than a mid-sized red blood cell. They cause over-aggregation.

Betamethasone

Betamethasone particles vary. There are very small particles, as well as particles over $100\,\mu m$. They cause over-aggregation.

Methylprednisolone

Methylprednisolone particles have a uniform composition and most have smaller diameters than red blood cells. Despite the possibility of aggregation being very low, there is still the risk of embolism. The injectable forms of steroids are composed of various buffer solutions such as polyethylene glycol, benzyl alcohol, and benzalkonium chloride. Related to this, neurotoxity may develop. These toxic effects may occur much later.

Various theories have been proposed about the place of corticosteroids in invasive pain procedures. Corticosteroids reduce the inflammation caused by mechanic compression, ischemia and chemical irritation.

Corticosteroids disrupt the PLA2 cascade, arachidonic acid metabolites, and reduce prostaglandins and leukotrienes, which facilitate the emergence of pain. These inflammatory

Table 8.4 Relative doses of steroids and efficiency

Drug	Anti-inflammatory potency	Effect time (hours)	Equivalent dose (mg)
Cortisol	1	8–12	20
Triamcinolone	5	12–36	4
6-Methylprednisolone	5	12–36	4
Betamethasone	25	36–72	0.75
Dexamethasone	25	36–72	0.75

Source: Kushnerik et al. (2009).

mediators lead to intraneural edema and venous congestion. Corticosteroids suppress the autoimmune response triggered by glycoproteins.

Local injection of corticosteroids to mesodermal elements, arachnoid tissue, and fibrous tissue are more effective than a systemic injection. Adhesion and fibrosis can be prevented. Corticosteroids have a stabilizing effect on the nerve membrane. Thus, the ectopic discharge in the nerve root can be blocked. Corticosteroids slow down the conduction in C fibers. This may play a role in their analgesic effect. They also have local anesthetic properties. They may have an effect on the central mechanisms of pain. They may reduce the sensitization in the dorsal horn neurons. In addition, they may have a direct effect on the CNS by effecting the production of neurotransmitters in the brain stem and spinal cord. Corticosteroids that are given into the epidural space temporarily reduce the levels of plasma cortisol and ACTH (Table 8.4).

In general, the most widely used drug is methylprednisolone. The dose is between 40 and 80 mg. A local anesthetic can be added to extend the duration of effect.

Complications

1. Ophthalmologic reactions
Steroid-induced chorioretinopathy has been reported However, this is rare.

2. Local complications

3. Epidural lipomatosis
This may develop due to epidural steroid injections. The cause is unknown. Increase in fat tissue within the epidural space can lead to spinal cord compression.

4. Systemic complications
(a) Increase in blood pressure. Systolic pressure increases temporarily owing to corticosteroids' mineralocorticoid effects.

Table 8.5 Toxic effects of exogenous corticosteroids

1. Hyperglycemia, impaired glucose tolerance impairment
2. Lipogenesis, the increase in circulating fatty acids
3. Lipomatosis
4. Obesity
5. Muscle catabolism, myopathy
6. Skin atrophy, wrinkling, telangiectasia
7. Glucocorticoid induced osteoporosis
8. Aseptic osteonecrosis
9. Proliferation of lymphoid tissue
10. Growth delay
11. Peptic ulcer
12. Hypertension
13. Decrease in resistance to infections
14. Electrolyte imbalance
15. Mental disorder
16. Cataract formation
17. Cushing's syndrome

(b) Hyperglycemia. This should especially be considered in diabetic patients. The patient should be warned in advance.

(c) Fluid retention. Peripheral edema or further complications may arise.

(d) Suppression in the hypothalamo–adrenal axis. This can be seen in patients undergoing consecutive epidural steroid injections. Serum cortisol levels decrease temporarily and for several weeks.

(e) Cushing's syndrome. Facial edema, facial skin wrinkling, and skin lesions may occur (Table 8.5).

Authors' notes

Physicians should follow all current developments with regard to drugs used in interventional methods. The number of drugs used with the development of interventional techniques has also constantly increased.

Further reading

Abdi, S., Datta, S., Trescot, A.M., et al. (2007) Epidural steroids in the management of chronic spinal pain: a systematic review. *Pain Physician* **10**, 185–212.

Berde, C.B. & Strichartz, G.R. (2000) Local anesthetics. In *Miller's Anesthesia*, 5th edition (ed. Miller, R.D.), pp. 491–522. Philadelphia, PA: Churchill Livingstone.

Bettmann, M.A., Heeren, T., Greenfield, A., et al. (1997) Adverse events with radiographic contrast agents: results of SCVIR contrast agent registry. *Radiology* **203**, 611–620.

Boswell, M., Trescot, A. & Datta, S. (2007) Interventional techniques: evidence-based practice guidelines in the management of chronic spinal pain. *Pain Physician* **10**, 7–111.

Butterworth, J.F. & Strichartz, C.R. (1990) The molecular mechanisms by which local anesthetics produce impulse blockade: a review. *Anesthesiology* **72**, 711–734.

Carpenter, R.I. & Mackey, D.C. (1992) Local anesthetics. In *Clinical Anesthesia*, 2nd edition (ed. Barash, P.C., Cullen, B.F. & Stoelting, R.K.), pp 509–541. Philadelphia, PA: JB Lippincott.

Chopra, P. & Smith, H. (2004) Use of radiopaque contrast agents for the interventional pain physician. *Pain Physician* **7**, 459–463.

De Jong, R.H. (1994) *Local Anesthetics*, 2nd edition. St. Louis, MO: CV Mosby.

Derby, R., Lee, S.H., Date, E.S., Lee, J.H. & Lee, C.H. (2008) Size and aggregation of corticosteroids used for epidural injections. *Pain Medicine* **9**(2), 227–234.

Hadzic, A. (editor) (2007) *Textbook of Regional Anesthesia and Acute Pain Management*. New York: McGraw-Hill.

Heavner, J.E. (1996) Neurolytic agents. In *Pain Medicine: A Comprehensive Review* (ed. Raj, P.P.), pp. 285–286. St. Louis, MO: Mosby.

Huntoon, M.A. (2007) Complications associated with chronic steroid use. In *Complications in Regional Anesthesia and Pain Medicine* (ed. Neal, J.M. & Rathmell, J.P.), pp. 331–339. Philadelphia, PA: WB Saunders.

Jain, S. & Gupta, R. (2001) Neurolytic agents in clinical practice. In *Interventional Pain Management*, 2nd edition (ed. Waldman, S.D.), pp. 220–225. Philadelphia, PA: WB Saunders.

Kushnerik, V., Altman, G. & Gozenput, P. (2009) Pharmacology of steroids used during epidural steroid injections. *Techniques in Regional Anesthesia and Pain Management* **13**, 212–216.

Lasser, E.C. (1992) Mechanisms of contrast media reactions III. In *The Contrast Media Manual* (ed. Katzberg, R.), pp. 171–179. Baltimore, MD: Williams & Wilkins.

Manchikanti, L. (2002) Role of neuraxial steroids in interventional pain management. *Pain Physician* **5**, 182–199.

Raj, P.P. & Patt, R.B. (1996) Peripheral neurolysis. In *Pain Medicine: A Comprehensive Review* (ed. Raj, P.P.), pp. 288–296. St. Louis, MO: Mosby.

Salinas, F.V. (2007) Pharmacology of drugs used for spinal and epidural anesthesia and analgesia. In: *Spinal and Epidural Anesthesia* (ed. Wong, C.A.), pp. 75–109. New York: McGraw-Hill.

Schimmer, B.P. & Parker, K.L. (2001) Adrenocorticotropic hormone; adrenocortical steroids and their synthetic analogs; inhibitors of the synthesis and actions of adrenocortical hormones. In: *Goodman & Gilman's The Pharmacological Basis Of Therapeutics* (ed. Hardman, J.G. & Limbird, L.E.), 10th edition, pp. 1649–1677. New York: McGraw-Hill.

Wood, K.A. (1978) The use of phenol as a neurolytic agent: a review. *Pain* **5**, 205–229.

9 Tools and Equipment Used in Interventional Pain Procedures

Pain centers performing interventional procedures should have all the necessary facilities, equipment, and devices available to perform these procedures safely and precisely. Interventional pain procedures vary widely from simple nerve blocks to radiofrequency techniques and neuromodulation. Most pain centers have limited facilities and perform a limited number of procedures such as those targeting the spine. There are very few pain centers performing all procedures.

In this chapter, it will be appropriate to show and describe the equipment, devices, and the set up available in interventional pain centers. The following should be available in an interventional pain center.

1. Procedure room.
2. Procedure table.
3. Operating light.
4. Fluoroscopy device.
5. Radiation gown, radiation gloves, thyroid shield, radiation eyeglasses.
6. Cardiopulmonary monitor.
7. Pulse oximeter.
8. Anesthesia device.
9. Suction device-aspirator.
10. Sphygmomanometer.
11. Emergency set up, drugs.
12. Defibrillator.
13. Laryngoscope and blades.
14. Ambu bag.
15. Needles.
    (a) Epidural.
    (b) Spinal.
    (c) Radiofrequency electrodes.
16. Radiofrequency generator.
17. Catheters.
    (a) Epidural.
    (b) Spinal.
18. Stimulating devices.
19. Epiduroscope.
20. Ultrasound device.
21. Intradiscal procedure kits.
22. Intrathecal–epidural port and pumps.
23. Spinal cord stimulator kit and electrodes.
24. Vertebroplasty kit.
25. Set of equipment for surgery.
26. Stretcher.

Procedure room (Fig. 9.1)

The interventional procedures can be performed safely in a procedure room having all facilities for emergency set up. Interventional pain medicine should be considered as minimal invasive surgery and the physician and staff should be prepared accordingly.

All personnel attending the procedure should be attired in a sterile manner. The sterilization of the procedure room should be checked regularly.

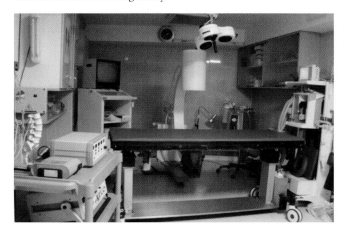

Figure 9.1 Procedure room.

Pain-Relieving Procedures: The Illustrated Guide, First Edition. P. Prithvi Raj and Serdar Erdine.
© 2012 John Wiley & Sons, Ltd. Published 2012 by John Wiley & Sons, Ltd.

Procedure table (Fig. 9.2)

The procedure table is different than other surgical tables. Because of the use of fluoroscopy, the procedure table should be radiolucent.

The height and the width of the table should be appropriate for free movement of the C-arm of the fluoroscope.

Movement of the table is important. The table should be designed to have up and down movements, rotation to left and right, and Trendelenburg and reverse Trendelenburg positions.

The table should have add-on devices for cervical, head, and neck procedures.

The fluoroscope (Fig. 9.3)

The fluoroscope is one of the indispensable tools for interventional pain procedures. All procedures should be performed under visualization by fluoroscopy, computed tomography (CT), or ultrasound. The most frequently used tool for visualization is still the fluoroscope. The fluoroscope comes in two parts: the monitor and the C-arm (which produces the radiation). The monitor may have one or double screens so that the images can be saved before each step during the procedure.

The physician should be trained in radiation safety and hazard prevention.

Radiation gown, thyroid shield, radiation eyeglasses, radiation gloves (Fig. 9.4)

The physician performing the interventional procedure should always wear a gown, a thyroid shield, radiation eyeglasses, and radiation gloves in order to protect from radiation hazard. For protection, gowns should contain 0.3–0.5 mm

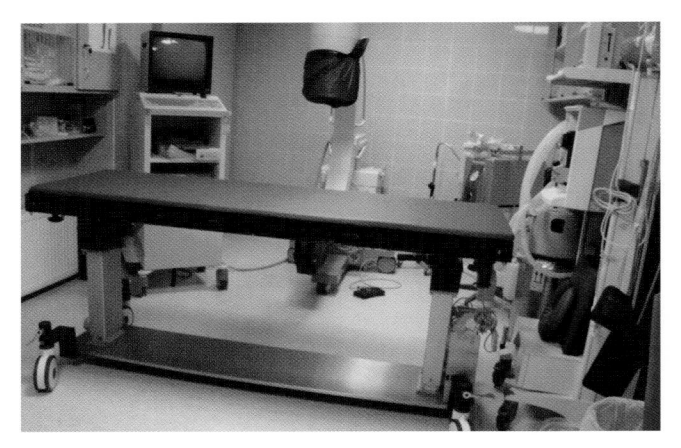

Figure 9.2 Procedure table.

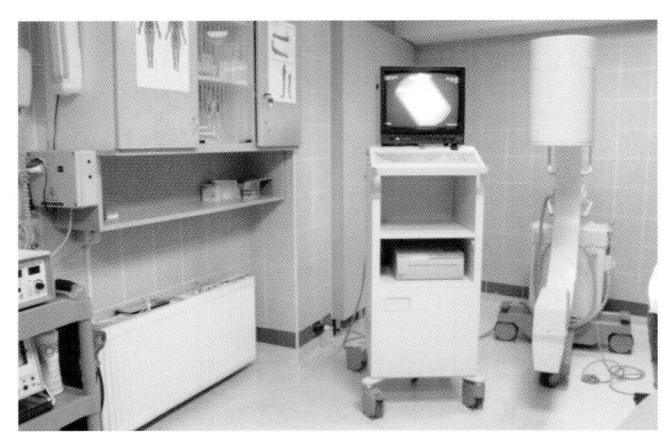

Figure 9.3 Fluoroscope.

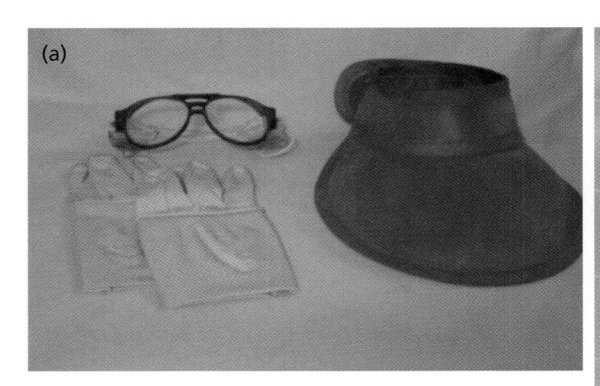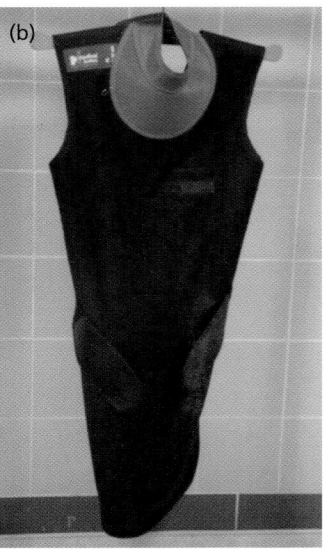

Figure 9.4 (a,b) Radiation gown, thyroid shield, radiation eyeglasses, radiation gloves.

thick lead. The gowns should be worn tightly and appropriately. The gown should not be folded, as it will break the lead. Breaking the lead will not provide protection from radiation.

The thyroid gland is sensitive to radiation. Poor coverage or lack of coverage of the thyroid gland may result in hypothyroidism. Thus the physician should wear the thyroid shield during the procedure.

There is also a risk for the lens of the eyes from radiation. Some physicians wear radiation eyeglasses to protect from cataract changes.

One should not forget that the lead gloves are radiation resistant, although not entirely protective. Further, the physician should be aware of the radiation safety rules of the institution.

Resuscitation facilities (Fig. 9.5)

During interventional pain procedures, the patient needs to be sedated. During sedation and analgesia, all facilities for resuscitation should be available in the procedure room. Sedation should be conducted by an anesthesiologist.

The facilities should include the following equipment:
• positive-pressure oxygen device;
• suction assembly;
• intubation kit with appropriate laryngoscope blades and handles already tested for working order, variously sized endotracheal tubes, and oral airways;
• emergency drugs;
• electrocardiograph (ECG) monitoring, heart rate, blood pressure monitor;
• devices to monitor respiratory rate and oxygen saturation if sedative drugs or opioid analgesics are to be given before or during the procedure.

Radiofrequency generators (Fig. 9.6)

Radiofrequency lesioning and pulsed radiofrequency are commonly performed in interventional pain procedures. Many generators are available for this purpose. The generators should allow sensory and motor testing, impedance monitoring, and temperature monitoring.

Generators are now available that perform both conventional radiofrequency lesioning and pulsed radiofrequency.

Physicians who intend to perform these procedures should be appropriately trained for decision making on when to use them, as well as their side effects and complications.

Needles (Fig. 9.7)

Most interventional pain procedures are performed by needles and/or needle-like electrodes. Blunt needles have been developed to decrease the risks of serious injury. There are also specialized needles for procedures that require special equipment. The most commonly used needles for spinal procedures are the Quincke needles. Spinal needles are also used for peripheral nerve blocks. The most common epidural needle used is the Tuohy needle in various lengths and bevels. The Racz needle is designed to introduce the Racz catheter during epidural neuroplasty. Radiofrequency electrodes are needles designed for radiofrequency lesioning. They are insulated, except for the "active tip" of different lengths (1 mm, 2 mm, 5 mm). Radiofrequency electrodes are designed to be of different lengths, for different procedures.

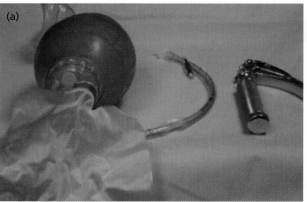
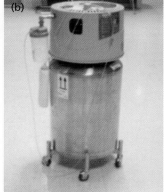
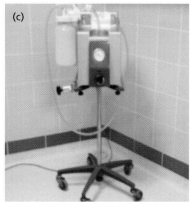

Figure 9.5 (a–c) Resuscitation facilities.

Catheters (Fig. 9.8)

Catheters are used for epidural or intrathecal procedures. Racz catheters are used for epidural neuroplasty. Epidural or intrathecal catheters are also used for epidural access ports or intrathecal pump systems, and drug delivery systems.

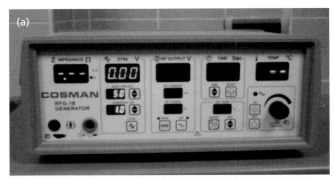
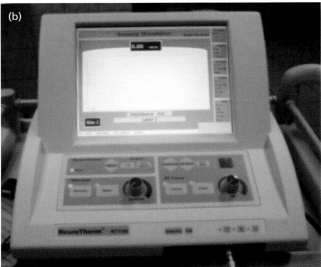

Figure 9.6 (a,b) A variety of radiofrequency generators.

Catheters can also be used for continuous peripheral nerve blocks.

Nerve stimulator (Fig. 9.9)

Nerve stimulators are used to confirm the final position of the tip of the needle during selective transforaminal cervical and epidural blocks as well as for periphera nerve blocks. The device requires motor stimulation at 2 Hz and sensory stimulation at 50–100 Hz.

Epiduroscope (Fig. 9.10)

An epiduroscope can be used only at comprehensive pain centers that perform epiduroscopy. An epiduroscopy set consists of a special monitor, dilator, introducer cannula, and epiduroscope.

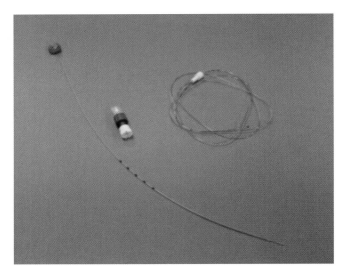

Figure 9.8 Catheters.

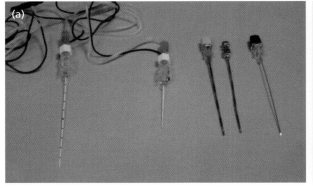
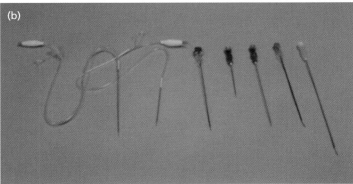

Figure 9.7 (a,b) Needles and electrodes at different sizes.

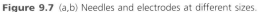

Equipment for intradiscal procedures (Fig. 9.11)

Equipment necessary for intradiscal procedures such as intradiscal electrothermal annuloplasty (IDET), discTRODE, or nucleoplasty consists of introducers, intradiscal electrothermal catheters, or electrodes. This equipment should be available in centers performing these procedures.

Epidural or intrathecal drug delivery systems (Fig. 9.12)

Epidural or intrathecal drug delivery systems have been developed for prolonged intraspinal analgesia both for chronic and terminal pain relief. These systems vary widely, from simple access ports to programmable intrathecal pumps. Each system has advantages and disadvantages, which are discussed in their respective manuals and in Chapter 18.

Equipment for spinal cord stimulation (Fig. 9.13)

Equipment for spinal cord stimulation consists of trial electrodes, permanent electrodes, and the neurostimulator. There are different types of equipment in the market place.

Vertebroplasty set (Fig. 9.14)

Vertebroplasty equipment is required only in pain centers where these procedures are performed.

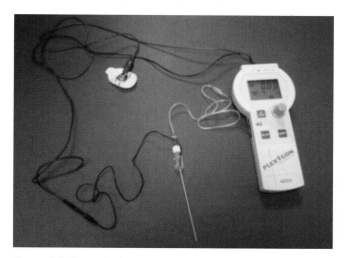

Figure 9.9 Nerve stimulator.

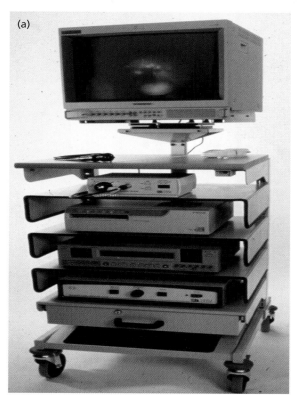

(a)

(b)

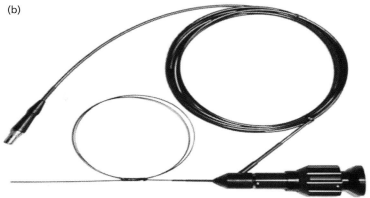

Figure 9.10 (a,b) Epiduroscope.

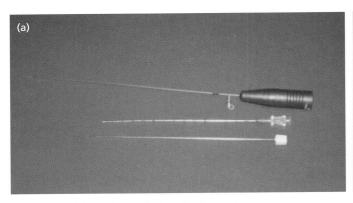
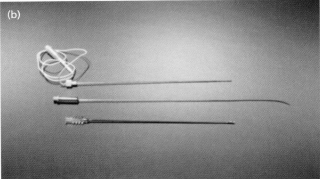

Figure 9.11 (a,b) Equipment for intradiscal procedures.

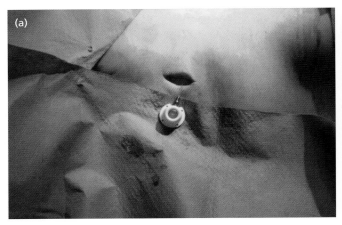
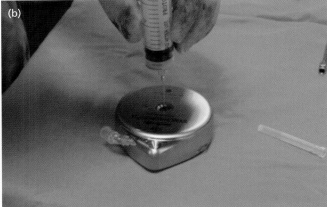

Figure 9.12 (a,b) Port and pump systems.

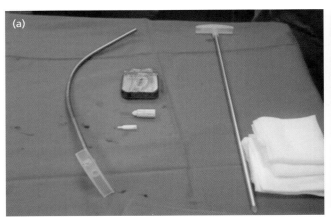
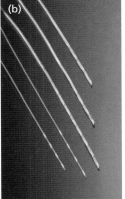

Figure 9.13 (a,b) Equipment for spinal cord stimulation.

CHAPTER 9 Tools and Equipment Used in Interventional Pain Procedures

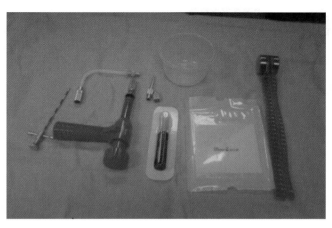

Figure 9.14 Vertebroplasty set.

Further reading

Mathis, J. (2010) Materials used in image-guided spine interventions. In *Image-Guided Spine Interventions*, 2nd edition (ed. Mathis, J.M. & Golovac, S.), pp. 29–38. New York, Dordrecht, Heidelberg, & London: Springer.

Rodriguez, J., Lou, L. & Loretz, S. (2002) Interventional pain practice equipment and devices. In *Interventional Pain Management, Image-Guided Procedures* (ed. Raj, PP. et al.), pp. 597–610. Philadelphia, PA: Saunders Elsevier.

Principles and Descriptions of Special Techniques

Radiofrequency lesions (contributed by Eric R. Cosman Sr and Eric R. Cosman Jr)

The radiofrequency (RF) technique was first put into clinical practice for making controlled therapeutic lesions in the nervous system in the early 1950s. It has remained an important methodology to this day. The first part of this chapter summarizes the physical principles of the RF lesion method and describes the accepted rules for RF lesion generation that have been verified over the years by clinical experience.

A brief history of RF lesion making

Although there have been many contributors to the progress made in the use of the RF technique, there are two names that stand out as particularly significant for their early work in the field and for the historic magnitude of their contributions: William H. Sweet and Bernard J. Cosman (Fig. 10.1). Sweet wrote a landmark paper in 1953, coauthored by Vernon Mark, which showed that the use of very high frequency current (in the RF range) for lesion production has decisive advantages over the then established direct current lesion methods. Sweet made a second major advance to the field a few years later when he performed the first temperature-controlled RF lesions in the trigeminal ganglion for the treatment of trigeminal neuralgia.

Bernard J. Cosman made parallel pioneering contributions to the design and engineering of RF lesion generators and electrodes. Prototype RF generators were made by Cosman in collaboration with the neurosurgical group at the Massachusetts General Hospital in Boston in the early 1950s. Shortly thereafter, Cosman introduced the first commercial RF lesion generator, the Radionics Model RFG-2, for sale in the USA. For the next 40 years Bernard Cosman, with one of the present authors, his son, Eric Cosman Sr, continued to make major advances in RF generator and electrode tech-

nology. Their designs dominated the field for decades, being offered by their company Radionics.

Modern RF lesion generators and electrode designs are elaborate and sophisticated. Figure 10.2 shows two of the latest RF generators, the Model RFG-1A and the Model G4 Graphics-Four (Cosman Medical, Burlington, Massachusetts, USA). They both incorporate multiple functions and circuitry, including an impedance monitor, wide-range stimulator, recording outputs and input connections, temperature monitors, continuous RF and pulsed RF generator circuits, automatic temperature control, and lesion timers. They have built-in microprocessors and computers that can provide automatic functions for the lesion process as well as safety checks to guard against untoward effects during the procedure. The Model G4 unit enables use of up to four RF electrodes to be applied to the patient at the same time, which has use, for example, in treating multiple-level medial branches for spinal pain. It has full color graphic display of the electrode functions with touch-screen features such as built-in standard procedure menus, recording memory, and printout records of procedure parameters, which are helpful, for example, in a busy pain clinic where the throughput of patients being treated for spinal pain is high.

Modern RF electrodes are also far more elaborate and sophisticated than in the early days of RF technology. Because the RF electrode can be made in a wide variety of shapes and configurations, a large range of styles has been developed for use at specific target sites.

Physical principles of RF heat lesion generation

The proper use of the RF lesion method requires a basic understanding of the physical processes involved. Figure 10.3 shows the basic RF lesioning circuit. The RF generator is the source of an RF voltage that is impressed across its output terminals. The terminals are in turn connected by cables to the so-called active electrode and the dispersive

---

Pain-Relieving Procedures: The Illustrated Guide, First Edition. P. Prithvi Raj and Serdar Erdine.
© 2012 John Wiley & Sons, Ltd. Published 2012 by John Wiley & Sons, Ltd.

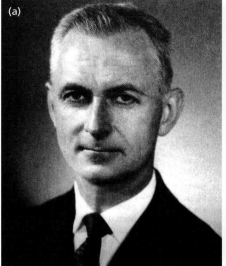
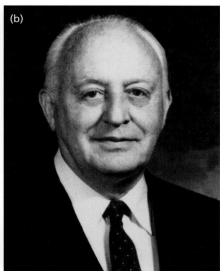

Figure 10.1 Two pioneers of radiofrequency surgery. William H. Sweet (a) of the Massachusetts General Hospital wrote the landmark paper in 1953 that described the decisive advantages of the radiofrequency lesion. Bernard J. Cosman (b) was the electrical engineer who built and perfected the earliest commercial radiofrequency lesion generators in the early 1950s, working with Dr Sweet and Dr Thomas Ballantine.

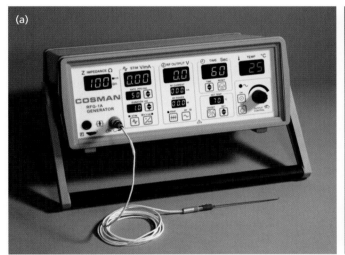
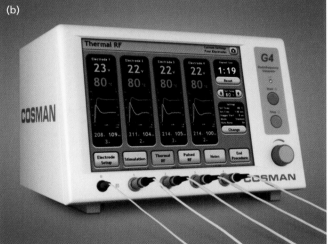

Figure 10.2 Two modern RF lesion generators. The Cosman Model RFG-1A (a) incorporates multiple functions and controls, digital readouts, and computer controls for effective and safe lesion making. The Cosman Model G4 "Graphics Four" (b) has a touch screen interface, the ability to store settings and procedure records, and both digital and graphic screen representations for the function processes. It also has four electrode output jacks so that as many as four electrodes can be used at the same time during a procedure. Multiple electrode usage provides time efficiency in some pain treatments; for example, performing multiple segmental medial branch RF heat lesions during the same patient treatment session.

electrode (often called a reference electrode). The active electrode produces the heat lesion, and the dispersive electrode is typically a large-area electrode that is not intended to produce heating, but serves as a return pathway for the RF current. Electrical metering can monitor the RF power, current, and voltage. Appropriate metering can also monitor the impedance and temperature at the active electrode tip.

Figure 10.4 illustrates how the RF current flows through the body between the active and dispersive electrodes. The total RF current I_{RF} in the cables reaches the electrodes and

spreads out in space in the electrolytic medium of the body. This is illustrated by lines of RF current density **j**, whose patterns are governed by the laws of electricity. The greatest heating takes place in the region of highest current density, which is near the tip of the active electrode. If the dispersive electrode has a significantly large area, the current density near it is low and heating nearby is minimal. For this reason, large-area dispersive electrodes with an area of at least $110\,cm^2$ and an ample amount of conductive gel between the electrode and the patient's skin are recommended to avoid

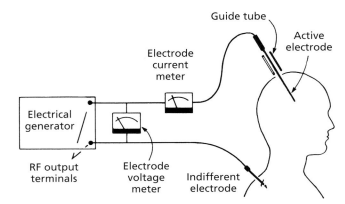

Figure 10.3 The basic RF circuit.

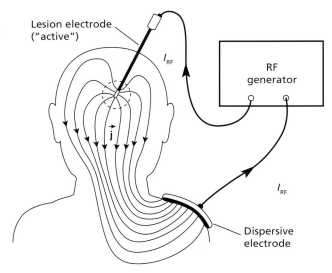

Figure 10.4 The RF current patterns in the tissue between the active lesion electrode and the dispersive electrodes.

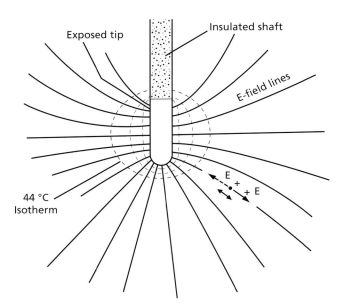

Figure 10.5 The electric field line patterns in tissue around the RF electrode, and the associated isotherm surfaces (dashed lines). The RF current lines follow the same pattern and the electric field lines.

any chance of skin burns. The dispersive, or reference, electrode is typically placed on the skin surface over an area of musculature, not far from the site of the active electrode. For example, an active electrode used in the brain may be accompanied by a reference electrode attached and taped to the patient's shoulder. Galvanic potentials can arise if active and reference electrodes are made from different metals. Thus, when the active lesion tip is made of stainless steel, which is a common type of electrode material, the base material of the reference electrode should also be made of stainless steel to prevent any transient potentials arising between the active and reference electrodes when the electrodes are first connected to the patient and the RF generator.

Figure 10.5 shows the pattern of the electric field and current density near the uninsulated active electrode tip. The mechanism for heating near the tip arises from the RF voltage that is created on the active electrode by the RF

generator output. This voltage creates a distribution of the electric field E in the space around the electrode, shown by the E-field lines in Fig. 10.5. The electric field at any given point in space oscillates with the RF frequency and causes the nearby charged ions in the electrolyte to move back and forth in space at the same high frequency, which is typically about 500,000 Hz for most modern generators. This ionic oscillation is called the ionic current density $\mathbf{j}$, and the pattern of the $\mathbf{j}$-field lines in space around the electrode tip follows the same pattern as the E-field lines shown in Fig. 10.5. It is the frictional heating within the tissue resulting from the RF ionic oscillation, i.e. the current density $\mathbf{j}$, that is the basic mechanism by which the tissue heats up, and, accordingly, by which the RF heat lesion is made. The ionic oscillations and current density are strongest near the electrode tip because the electric field is strongest there. Thus, the power deposition and tissue temperatures are highest adjacent to the electrode tip. The tissue that is heated by this mechanism in turn heats up the RF electrode tip, and so, by monitoring the tip temperature, an accurate measure of the nearby tissue temperature, and thus the progress of the RF lesioning, is obtained. Temperature monitoring during the RF lesion making is an essential for control, consistency, and safety of the procedure.

The dashed lines in Fig. 10.5 illustrate the surfaces of constant temperature, which are referred to as isotherms. The 45–50 °C isothermal surface is critical, because within that surface the tissue will be hotter than 45–50 °C and will be permanently killed. That then defines the heat lesion volume. It can be shown that at equilibrium, in a homogeneous

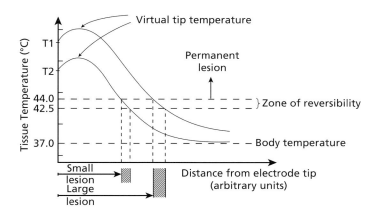

Figure 10.6 Temperature falloff as a function of nominal distance from the RF electrode tip.

medium, and for a specific tip size and tip temperature, the isotherm dimensions are roughly independent of the electrical and thermal conductivities. For a fixed tip size, a higher tip temperature produces a larger 45 °C isotherm surface; that is, the lesion volume is larger. However, for a given tip temperature, the lesion size is also dependent on the size of the electrode tip, with larger tips producing larger lesions.

Figure 10.6 is a schematic diagram of the temperature falloff in the tissue as a function of nominal distance from the electrode tip. This curve can now be calculated by modern computer methods. Predicted lesion sizes agree with experimentally and clinically observed data. Certain qualitative features are notable. The highest temperatures occur in the tissue near the tip. The specific shape of the curve, and thus the lesion volume, depend on specific parameters such as the following: the electrode tip dimensions; the temperature that is maintained in the tissue near the electrode tip (by control of the RF voltage on the electrode); and the electrical conductivity, thermal conductivity, and fluid convection of the surrounding tissue. As shown in Fig. 10.6, the higher the measured tip temperature, the larger the distance associated with the 45 °C isotherm. It is believed that in the range between 42 and 44 °C, neural tissue can sustain "reversible" damage by heating. Thus, there may be a zone of reversibility for a given tip temperature corresponding to the shell of tissue near the 45 °C isotherm that can be stunned, but not killed, by thermal lesioning. Measurement of the electrode tip temperature not only quantifies the lesion size but also avoids the tissue near the electrode tip reaching the 100 °C point, and thus avoids the catastrophic effects of boiling, explosive gas formation, and searing and charring of the tissue. This dangerous condition can be avoided through careful elevation and monitoring of the tissue temperature to prevent temperature runaway to boiling.

Figure 10.7 illustrates another important aspect of the lesion making: the time progression toward an equilibrium lesion size. This figure shows the increase of the transverse dimension of the lesion as a function of the time during which the electrode tip temperature is held at a fixed value. The size of

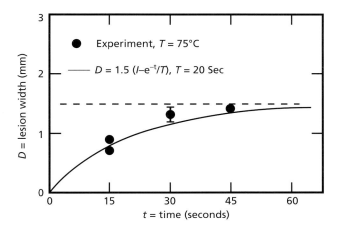

Figure 10.7 Dorsal root entry zone lesion width versus time. The equilibrium lesion size is achieved after 35–45 seconds for an approximately constant temperature at the electrode tip.

the lesion increases until it reaches its asymptotic value. Once this value has been approached, no substantial increase of the lesion size occurs. For consistent lesion making, it is desirable to achieve this equilibrium situation, because it avoids some of the uncertainties associated with variability in tissue impedance, vascularity, and proximity to cerebrospinal fluid (CSF), bone, and other heat sinks. The typical time to reach the asymptotic temperature is 30–60 seconds for electrode tip sizes that are typically used in neurosurgery and pain therapy and for relatively uniform soft-tissue environments.

The above discussion can be summarized by some simple rules associated with RF lesion making.

Rule 1. The RF current heats the tissue, and the tissue in turn heats the RF electrode tip.

Rule 2. Temperature is the basic lesioning parameter, and it should be measured and controlled for consistent and safe RF lesioning. The measurement of electrode tip temperature is directly related to tissue temperature and lesion size.

Rule 3. Achievement of an equilibrium lesion as a function of time for a fixed tip temperature produces a more consistent lesion size than lesions that are stopped while still expanding. It is desirable to hold the proper tip temperature for 30–60 seconds to achieve the equilibrium lesion size.

Rule 4. The proper electrode size and tip temperature should be selected for a given target site to achieve a consistent and desired lesion size.

Specific factors that are difficult to predict or quantify can give rise to variations in the simplified picture of the RF lesion process from one patient to the next. Among these factors are the inhomogeneities in the tissue medium itself. Figure 10.8 schematically illustrates examples. The proximity of the electrode to CSF bodies such as the ventricles can provide a low-impedance shunt pathway for the RF current density **j**, and thus sink the heat away and cause irregular lesion shapes and sizes. An example of this situation is RF lesioning in the trigeminal ganglion. The proximity of large blood vessels also has an inhomogeneous cooling effect on the tissue near them. The placement of the RF electrode near a bony structure may have the opposite effect, since a bony mass is an insulator with lower blood circulation. Examples of this are the RF heating of an intervertebral disc or of the space between other joints in the body.

Despite the uncertainties caused by tissue in homogeneities, however, the above rules for homogeneous tissue and for nominal conditions have worked well over the past decades, as attested by a mass of successful clinical data using the RF heating method.

Typical lesion sizes as a function of electrode geometries and tip temperatures

It is important to have a sense of the size of the lesion that is being made for a given electrode tip geometry and tip temperature. An extensive discussion of this issue is given in papers by Cosman et al. (see Further reading section), and only summary information will be given here. Table 10.1 shows lesion sizes in the human brain reported by several stereotactic neurosurgeons using conventional electrodes of straight, cylindrical tip geometry. These data for the most part were accumulated in postmortem studies at varying times after the lesion was made, and some variation in the lesion size might be expected as a function of time. As an example from Table 10.1, it is seen that for thalamotomies performed using electrode tips with a diameter of 1.1 mm and a tip length of 3–5 mm and tip temperatures of 65–75 °C, lesion sizes of approximately 3 mm minor in diameter and 4–7 mm in length can be achieved. Lesions for cylindrical electrode tip shapes are typically prolate ellipsoids of revolution. It is also seen that larger lesions can be made in the brain with larger electrode tips and higher temperatures. For example, lesions made in the cingulum with electrodes having 1.6 mm diameter and 10 mm tip length at 80–90 °C have dimensions of typically 10 mm in minor diameter and 12 mm in length. Electrodes of greater diameter and length for equivalently high temperatures are accordingly larger. Table 10.1 shows the range of parameters used by several stereotactic neurosurgeons to produce thalamic lesions. This suggests that some variation in lesion size has been used successfully in RF thalamotomies, but also that there is a reasonable norm for acceptable lesion parameters.

A summary of these data is shown in Fig. 10.9. The transverse lesion diameter, which is equivalent to the width of

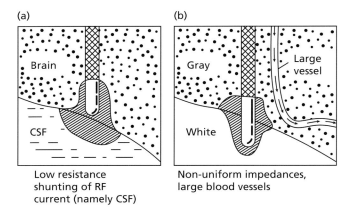

(a)   (b)

Brain

CSF

Gray   White   Large vessel

Low resistance shunting of RF current (namely CSF)   Non-uniform impedances, large blood vessels

Figure 10.8 (a,b) Irregularities of RF heating can be caused by inhomogeneities in nearby tissue structures and fluid bodies.

Table 10.1 Postmortem lesion sizes versus heating parameters

	Electrode tip*		Temperature and times			Lesion size (mm)	
Lesion size	Diameter (mm)	Length (mm)	Temperature (°C)	Time (seconds)	Time (postmortem)	A	B
Thalamus	1.1	5	72	360	2 years	3	7
Thalamus	1.2	3	65	120	?	2	4
Cingulum	1.6	5	70	60	5 months	8	8
Cingulum	1.6	10	80–90	60	6 months	10	10–12
Cingulum	1.6	10	80	60	6 months	10	12

*Straight stereotactic electrodes as shown in Fig. 10.17.

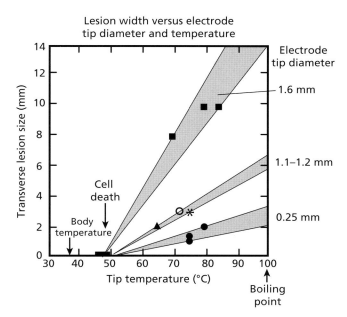

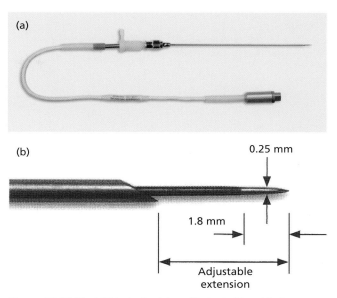

Figure 10.9 The canonical curves of lesion diameter versus tip temperature as a function of the electrode tip diameter (top). The dimensions of the heat lesion and the electrode tip (bottom).

Figure 10.10 The LCE Levin Cordotomy Electrode (a) and its tip geometry (b).

the prolate ellipsoidal lesion, is plotted as a function of the tip temperature for various electrode diameters. The length of the lesion can be assumed to be approximately 1–3 mm longer than the exposed length of the RF electrode, assuming substantially cylindrical electrode tip geometry with either a hemispherical or a sharpened tip end shape. Although this graph may supply canonical curves for lesion size, it must be recognized that the unpredictable factors of tissue inhomogeneity, inhomogeneous conductivities and convectivities, and proximity to bony structures can all produce significant variations in the shape and size of lesions in a given situation.

Electrodes with more complex geometries, such as those having side-outlet electrode tip extensions, have also been used for more precise or more asymmetric targeting in the region of the thalamus, in cases where physiological testing indicates that the initial electrode placement is not ideal.

Information on lesion size for very small RF electrodes, such as those used in the spinal cord, is rare but does exist. Cosman et al. (1984) reported that electrodes with tip diameters of 0.25 mm and tip lengths of 2 mm, raised to a temperature of about 80 °C and for a lesion time of approximately 15 seconds, will produce lesion sizes of about 2 mm in width and 2 mm in length.

RF electrode configurations for specific clinical procedures

In addition to the choice of the proper RF electrode size and tip temperature, safe and effective lesion making is dependent on the following conditions:

1. the proper placement of the electrode in the target region;

2. adequate physiological testing using stimulation and recording to assess that the target is correct and assure that untoward effects will not occur from encroachment in non-target volumes;

3. proper configuration of the electrode as adapted for a particular target region.

The reader is referred to many articles and procedure technique monographs for specific recommendations on these points for the various RF lesion sites. A brief description is given below of successful RF electrode geometries for specific procedures to illustrate the great range of such designs.

Spinal cord electrodes

Targets in the spinal cord are discrete and critical. Associated RF electrodes must be appropriately small, with temperature monitoring, despite the fact that their historical forerunners, such as the cordotomy electrodes of Rosomoff, Lin and associates, Mullan, and others, were of relatively larger size and of a nontemperature-measuring variety.

Figure 10.10 shows the pointed tip configuration for the Levin-Cosman Cordotomy Electrode (LCE) Kit (Cosman Medical), which has an approximately 0.25 mm tip diameter and 2.0 mm tip exposure with an indwelling surface-mounted thermocouple. The electrode can penetrate the pia and make very precise and discrete lesions in the spinothalamic tract for the treatment of intractable pain. The unique design of a surface thermocouple sensor within the

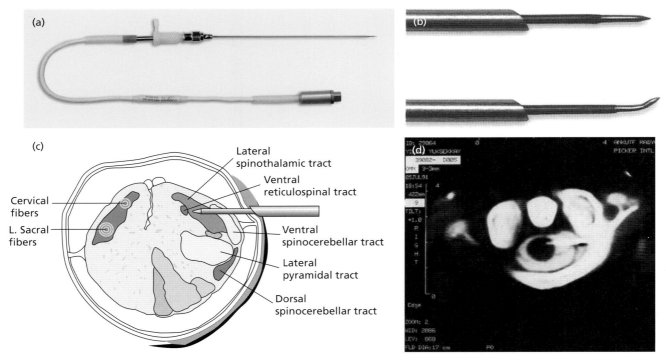

Figure 10.11 The KCTE Kanpolat Cordotomy Electrode (a). The KCTE tip includes a straight tip and an angled tip (b) to enable adjustment of the tip position in the spinal cord variations. The diagram (c) illustrates the approach to the lateral spinothalamic tract under CT control. A CT scan (d) shows the KCTE electrode in the spinal cord.

sharpened tip allows rapid and faithful lesion temperature readings, which are essential in such tight geometries.

Figure 10.11 illustrates the tip geometries for the KCTE Kanpolat CT Radionics electrodes, which have both straight and bent-tip geometry. These electrodes are used for percutaneous cordotomy and spinal tractotomies and embody the important innovation of being computed tomography (CT)-compatible. Kanpolat and associates demonstrated that, with the use of proper materials, a CT image of the electrode in place in the spinal cord can be made for direct visualization of the positioning of the electrode tip in the lateral spinothalamic tract.

RF electrodes for lesioning in the trigeminal ganglion

In the 1950s, W.H. Sweet and coworkers at the Massachusetts General Hospital in Boston revolutionized the treatment of facial pain from tic douloureux through the use of temperature-monitoring RF electrodes inserted percutaneously into the trigeminal ganglion and posterior rootlets through the foramen ovale.

Figure 10.12 shows the earliest electrode system for this procedure: the Cosman TIC Kit. It evolved from Sweet's original concepts and was designed by B.J. Cosman; it is still offered by Cosman Medical and used by many neurosur-geons. The set has four insulated cannulas with a removable obdurating stylet. The cannulas have exposed tip lengths of 2, 5, 7, and 10 mm. In practice, a cannula, with a stylet in place, is inserted into the trigeminal ganglion; the stylet can be removed, and a thermocouple (TC) temperature electrode can be inserted. The TC electrode is connected to the RF generator, and physiologic testing is done using the stimulation signal output from the generator's stimulator circuitry. Once the proper target position is thereby confirmed, the RF signal output from the RF generator is applied to the electrode, and the heat lesion is made while monitoring electrode tip temperature on the generator's readout display. In this way, Sweet and other clinicians have reported excellent results for the relief of trigeminal pain since the early 1970s.

The straight electrodes of the TIC Kit, which have been adequate for most trigeminal neuralgia procedures, are sometimes inadequate to reach selectively the first division of the trigeminal nerve. Therefore, a modification of the TIC Kit was built to overcome this limitation. Figure 10.13 shows the Tew Kit that was developed by John M. Tew and Eric Cosman Sr. The Tew Kit includes an insulated cannula through which either an obdurating stylet, a straight emergent RF electrode, or a flexible side-outlet emergent RF electrode can be passed. The tip configurations for the

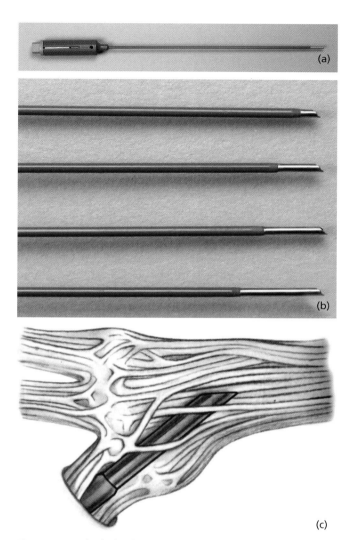

Figure 10.12 (a–c) The classic TIC Kit electrodes for trigeminal nerve RF lesioning. The upper figure shows the temperature sensor probe inserted into a cannula. The middle figure shows the different available cannula tip lengths. The lower figure shows the electrode cannula's tip within the trigeminal rootlets.

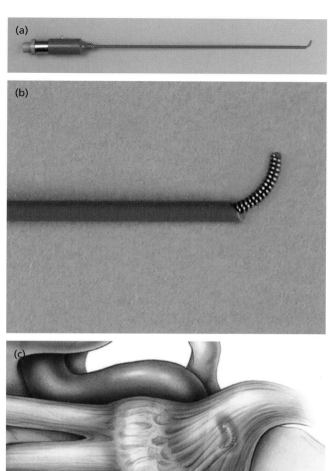

Figure 10.13 The Tew electrode accommodates straight and curved RF lesioning tips for use in the trigeminal ganglion. (a) Tew cannula with a curved temperature sensor inserted within it. (b) Curved spring electrode tip emerging from the cannula's distal end. (c) Curved electrode tip within the posterior rootlets of the trigeminal nerve. The curved tip can be angled upward or downward to reach the painful trigeminal division better.

straight and curved Tew electrodes are also shown in Fig. 10.13. Both electrodes have TC temperature sensors built into their tip ends. The curved spring electrode is inserted, for making off-axis tip extensions. This gives the clinician the capability of searching in the space of the trigeminal rootlets with the electrode to find the desired trigeminal division corresponding to the trigeminal pain as determined by sensory stimulation.

RF lesion electrodes for the spine to relieve neck and back pain

In the early 1970s, C.N. Shealy proposed a technique of percutaneous RF rhizotomy of the medial branch to relieve

mechanical lower back pain associated with the lumbar facet joints. The original SRK Shealy Rhizotomy Kit was developed by E.R. Cosman Sr and B.J. Cosman. It had a set of 14-gauge spinal needles that could be inserted percutaneously to approach the area proximate the suspected pain facets. A 16-gauge RF electrode, insulated except for an exposed 7 mm distal tip, could then be passed through the 14-gauge spinal needle, and could be advanced so that the electrode tip contacts the medial branch innervating the selected facet joint. This electrode was designed to produce a heat lesion with temperature control near the medial branch. There were encouraging successes in the early days of the technique, but the results were not always consistent. A variant of the SRK electrode, referred to as the RRE Ray Rhizotomy Electrode Kit, was designed by E.R. Cosman and produced by Radionics in association with C. Ray. Because this electrode had a tissue-penetrating tip, an insulated shaft, and integrated temperature sensor, it eliminated the need for the spinal needles. The RRE electrode is still offered by Cosman Medical, and it is still preferred by some pain clinicians because of the large lesions it produces and because of its especially rigid shaft.

In the late 1970s, M. Sluijter and E.R. Cosman developed a more discrete set of electrodes, referred to as the SMK Kit, having finer gauge cannulas for the purpose of treating spinal facet pain in a similar manner to that proposed by Shealy. Sluijter's approach used somewhat different target positions and electrode trajectories (Fig. 10.14). Because of its finer gauge electrodes, Sluijter used the system to treat pain in the lumbar as well as the cervical areas. A modern-day version of this electrode system is the CSK Kit (Cosman Medical), shown in Fig. 10.15.

The CSK Kit (Cosman Spinal Kit) contains, in one of its versions, 22-gauge (approximately 0.7 mm diameter) disposable cannulas, which are offered with uninsulated tip lengths of 2, 4, 5, and 10 mm tip exposures. Other versions of the CSK Kit are offered with 21-, 20-, or 18-gauge cannulas, with shaft lengths of 5, 10, 15, or 20 cm, and with a variety of tip lengths to accommodate different target sites and patient sizes. The finer cannulas have the great advantage, over the Shealy and Ray designs, of minimizing the discomfort and problems of percutaneous insertion. The larger gauge CSK cannulas (20- and 18-gauge) are preferred by some clinicians over the 22- and 21-gauge types because they can make larger heat lesions in the lumbar and the sacral regions, or because they can be used to produce multiple heat lesions for sacroiliac joint denervations.

Pulsed RF technique

In modern RF generators, such as shown in Fig. 10.2, there are two modes of RF output that are commonly used for

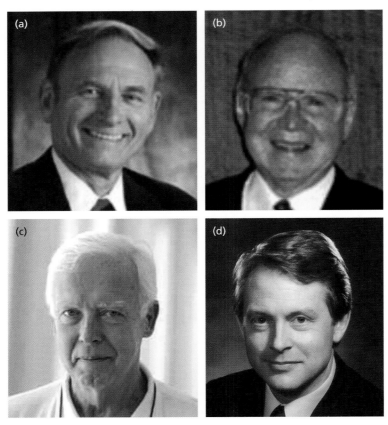

Figure 10.14 (a) Dr C. Norman Shealy performed the first RF facet denervation or rhizotomy in 1971; (b) Dr Charles Ray developed a simpler one-piece electrode system for RF facet denervations in 1974; (c) Dr Menno Sluijter developed a 22-gauge RF electrode system for performing RF procedures in the spine, including the facets, in the late 1970s; (d) Professor Eric R Cosman Sr collaborated with these clinicians to develop the SRK, RRE, and SMK electrode systems.

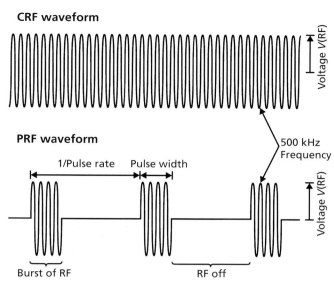

Figure 10.16 The RF waveforms for continuous (CRF) and pulsed RF mode (PRF). Axes are not to scale.

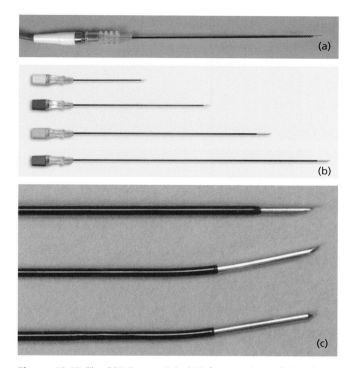

Figure 10.15 The CSK Cosman Spinal Kit for procedures of the spine such as the RF medial branch or DRG procedures. (a) CSK cannula with the temperature sensing TC probe inserted in it. (b) The range of shaft lengths to accommodate cervical to sacral approaches in the spine for all size patients. (c) The straight and curved tips and the sharp and blunt points available to suit clinicians' approaches, insertion techniques, and injection criteria.

pain therapy. The output waveforms for these two modes are shown schematically in Fig. 10.16. The first mode is the conventional, thermal (or heat) RF mode, which has been described so far in this chapter. It uses a continuous sinusoidal RF waveform output, commonly referred to as continuous RF, or CRF. The second mode, which was first reported on by M. Sluijter, E.R. Cosman, and coworkers in 1998, uses a series of pulsed bursts of RF signal, referred to as pulsed RF, or PRF. To date, PRF has been used primarily to treat peripheral nerves and the dorsal root ganglions (DRGs), and most commonly it has been applied to treat back and neck pain and neuropathies. The results have been very good and have now been the subject of a large published literature and several clinical trials. One popular advantage of PRF over CRF is that it can be done with little or no pain to the patient as the PRF output is being delivered. This is in contrast to some CRF applications in which there is considerable pain and discomfort to the patient during the RF heating of the neural tissue. To date, there have been limited attempts to use PRF in the central nervous system, although if it were to have success there, it could have significantly expanded potential.

In both the continuous and the pulsed RF modes, the amplitude of the RF voltage, $V(RF)$, of the RF waveforms as shown in Fig. 10.16, is measured in units of volts (V). As described above, for the continuous RF waveform, a heat lesion is produced by the action of ionic friction of the RF currents in the tissue caused by the voltage $V(RF)$ on the electrode. This means that the neural tissue near the uninsulated, metal electrode tip is heated continuously to destructive temperatures (greater than 45–50 °C). Thus, the CRF lesion volume includes all tissue within the 45–50 °C isotherm boundary, which tends to have an ellipsoidal shape that encompasses the electrode tip. Within this lesion volume, all cell structures are macroscopically destroyed by heat.

The action of pulsed RF on neural tissue is different from continuous RF. Because the RF output is delivered in bursts of short duration relative to the intervening quiescent periods, the average temperature of the tissue near the electrode is not raised continuously or as high as for continuous RF for the same RF voltage $V(RF)$. Because the PRF voltage is typically regulated to keep the average tip temperature in a nondestructive range, other mechanisms must produce the clinically observed pain-relieving effects.

The electric field, E, is the fundamental physical quantity that governs all the actions of RF output on neural tissue, both for pulsed RF and for continuous RF modes. The electric field is created in space around an RF electrode that is connected to the output voltage $V(RF)$ from an RF generator. This is illustrated in Fig. 10.5, and is shown in Fig. 10.17 for a pointed electrode that is commonly used for percutaneous pain procedures. E is represented by an arrow (vector) at every point in space around the electrode tip, indicative of the magnitude and the direction of the force it will

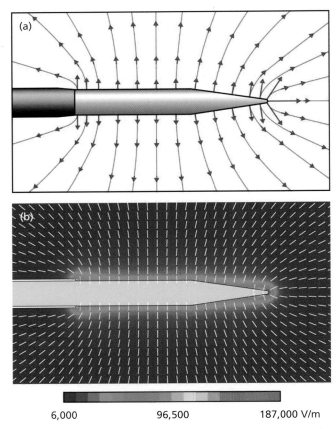

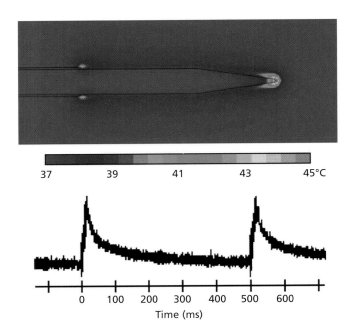

Figure 10.18 Hot flashes during a PRF pulse.

Figure 10.17 Schematic *E*-field patterns around a pointed RF electrode (a); and the calculated *E*-field strength distribution (b) in tissue for a 22-gauge, 5 mm tip electrode at *V*(RF) = 45 V.

produce on charged structures and ions in the tissue. The *E*-field produces various effects on tissue including the following: oscillations of charges, ionic currents, charge polarizations, membrane voltages, and structure-modifying forces. For continuous RF mode, the dominant consequence of these effects is the production of heat in the tissue caused by frictional energy loss due to the ionic currents that are driven by the *E*-field. However, for pulsed RF, the effects of the *E*-field are more complex and varied, and range from heat flashes, to modification of neuron ultrastructure, to neural excitation phenomena. All of these effects can play a role in neuronal modification, though exactly how they produce antinociception in PRF treatments is a subject of active scientific investigation.

Two consequences of theoretical predictions of the electric field in tissue during PRF are supported by experimental and clinical observations. The first is that, as a consequence of the very high *E*-fields at the electrode tip, there are hot flashes at the electrode tip that can be thermally destructive to neurons. The second is that there are significant nonthermal effects of the *E*-field on neurons at positions away from

the point of the tip that are certainly related to the pain-relieving effects of PRF.

During the brief RF pulse, a hot spot occurs at the tip which can be 15–20 °C above the average temperature of the tissue that remains near body temperature of 37–42 °C, as shown in Fig. 10.18, top. This has been confirmed by ex vivo measurements (Fig. 10.18, bottom) and by finite-element calculations. The intense *E*-field and hot flashes could be expected to have destructive effects on neural tissue very near the tip point. Evidence for such destruction has been observed *in vitro* (Cahana et al. 2003). This may play a role in PRF's clinical effect when the electrode point is in the nerve or pressing against it. However, it is unlikely that such focal effects can account for all PRF pain relief, because the regions of extremely high *E*-fields and *T* hot flashes are likely confined to less than about 0.2 mm radius from the electrode point.

There is evidence that direct, nonthermal effects are important in PRF. It is known that pain relief can be achieved when the side of the electrode tip, not the tip point, is next to an axon or dorsal root ganglion (DRG). Although the hot flash fluctuations are less than 1 °C at 0.5 mm from the tip in any direction for typical PRF voltages, at lateral distances of greater than 1 mm, the magnitude of the electric field is still large in biological terms. For example, finite-element computation of the *E*-field for *V*(RF) = 45 V predicts that *E* is 20,000 V/m at 0.5 mm, and 12,000 V/m at 1.0 mm laterally (Fig. 10.19). Thus, neuronal modifications in this *E*-field range should be significant.

Comparisons of *E* and *T* strengths between typical CRF and PRF waveforms show striking differences between these RF

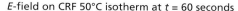

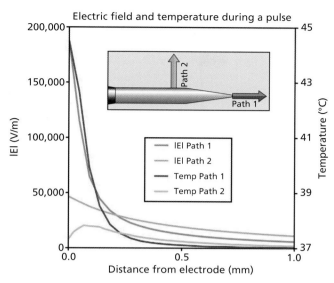

Figure 10.19 Electric field strength and temperature field strength distributions for the first PRF pulse around a 22-gauge, 5 mm tip pointed electrode at $V(RF) = 45$ V and a pulse width of 20 ms.

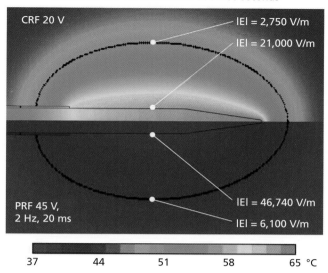

Figure 10.20 E-fields dominate over T-fields in PRF. The opposite is true for CRF.

modes (Fig. 10.20). Calculations predict that after 60 seconds of CRF at $V(RF) = 20$ V, $E = 21,000$ V/m and $T = 60–65$ °C at the lateral tip surface, and $E = 2,750$ V/m and $T = 50$ °C at 1.8 mm away. In contrast, after 60 seconds of PRF with $V(RF) = 45$ V, $E = 46,740$ V/m and $T = 42$ °C at the lateral tip surface, and $E = 6,100$ V/m and $T = 38$ °C at 1.8 mm away. In other words, in PRF, the direct electric field effects are more prominent, whereas in CRF, the thermal fields are more prominent and largely mask the E-field effects.

Combined with the understanding that PRF has a clinical effect even when the electrode is not placed on the nerve directly, these physical observations suggest that the E-field is directly involved in the analgesic effect of PRF. It is known that PRF E-fields produce significant transmembrane potentials on the neuron membrane and organelles. The E-field can also penetrate the membranes of axon and the DRG soma to disrupt essential cellular substructures and functions. For example, PRF done on the DRG of rabbits causes pronounced neuron ultrastructural modifications that are seen only under electron microscopy (Erdine et al., 2005) and that are likely to modify or disable the cell's function. This would suggest that PRF can produce subcellular, microscopic lesions on neurons in a volume around the electrode, possibly resulting in reduction of afferent pain signals. PRF membrane potentials are also capable of neural excitations (action potentials) by a process called membrane rectification. Because the PRF pulse rate is similar to that of classical conditioning stimulation (1–2 Hz), it has been proposed that PRF may have a similar action. Conditioning stimulation is capable of suppressing synaptic efficiency of A-delta and C-fiber afferent nociception signals, a phenomenon known

as long-term depression. Therefore, the PRF might be reducing transmission of pain information by long-term depression of synaptic connections in the dorsal horn. The appropriate exposure of PRF for a given pain syndrome and anatomical target, either for microscopic or long-term depression mechanisms, should be governed by the PRF "E-dose." E-dose provides a parametric measure of E-field strength and integral pulse/time exposure.

Principles of ultrasonography

This section of the chapter is adapted from a presentation entitled "Ultrasound Guided Pain Management" given by Sang Chul Lee at the 15th Annual Advanced Interventional Pain Conference in Budapest, Hungary, in 2010.

History

Ultrasound brings a new dimension to intervention in pain management. Kapral et al. (1995) described ultrasound-guided supraclavicular brachial plexus block. Since then, the number of publications in the field of ultrasonography has exceeded 1000. There had been only three publications related to ultrasound-guided techniques in chronic pain management before 2000. Again Kapral et al. (1995) described ultrasound imaging for stellate ganglion block. However, the acceptance has been much slower, perhaps because of technical limitations of ultrasound, lack of experience, and lack of formal training. There have been 42 publications since 2003, and numbers are growing rapidly. Ultrasound systems are more available and affordable

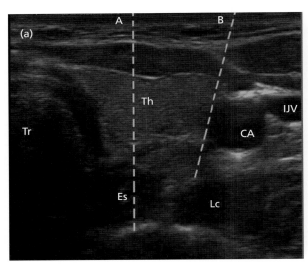 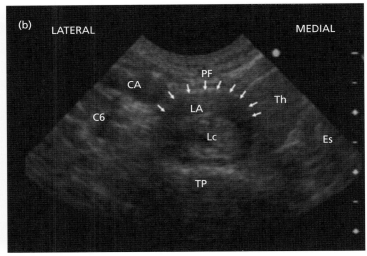

Figure 10.21 (a,b) Two lines of approach with ultrasound technique of stellate ganglion block. CA, carotid artery; C6, cervical 6 vertebra; Es, esophagus; IJV, internal jugular vein; LA, local anesthetic; Lc, longus colli muscle; PF = prevertebral fascia; Th, thyroid; TP, transverse process; Tr, trachea.

nowadays. Portable devices provide high-resolution and high-quality pictures. Ultrasound imaging allows real-time visualization of the needle and surrounding structures during the procedure on the target site, for example the stellate ganglion (Fig. 10.21).

The use of ultrasonography or ultrasound has produced a conceptual change in the way the imaging technique is performed for interventional procedures. This change is because the technique is performed under direct puncture visualization and, therefore, constitutes a much more anatomical approach. During ultrasound guidance, the structures through which the needle is inserted are identified, and the target site is directly localized; the consequence of this is a reduction in complications.

Physics of ultrasonography

Ultrasonography (or echography) is the result of technological developments in the application of ultrasound to imaging diagnosis. Sound is a vibratory phenomenon where frequency defines the number of vibrations, oscillations, or cycles per second (measured in hertz, where 1 Hz = one oscillation per second). Ultrasound is defined as sound at a frequency above the human auditory threshold (over 20,000 Hz). The piezoelectric principle allows the generation of ultrasound with applications to imaging techniques. This effect is based on the capacity of certain crystals (piezoelectric crystals) to generate mechanical energy in the form of ultrasound waves in response to the application of electric energy, and vice versa.

The physical characteristics of ultrasound are defined by the **wavelength, period, amplitude, frequency**, and **velocity** of the waves. The **wavelength** is the distance traveled by sound in the course of a single cycle, and is measured in millimeters (mm). The **period** is the time required to complete a full cycle, and is measured in seconds (s), whereas the **amplitude** corresponds to the square root of the energy of the wave, and **frequency** is the number of periods per second. Ultrasound frequency in turn depends on the generating piezoelectric material used. The frequencies employed in clinical practice range from 1 to 20 MHz, whereas in application to brachial plexus block the range is typically 3.5–10 MHz (Figs 10.22 and 10.23). **Wave velocity** is the displacement of sound per unit time (measured in m/s); it depends on the medium through which the sound travels, approximately 1540 m/s in the case of biological tissues.

Echogenicity is the capacity of structures standing in the way of the ultrasound beam to reflect the waves back to their source. This **capacity** depends not only on the characteristics of the ultrasound waves but also on the properties of the medium through which the sound travels. The **interface** is the limit or contact zone between two distinct media that transmit sound at different velocities. The acoustic impedance is in turn defined as the resistance of the medium to the passage of sound. When an ultrasound beam penetrates a given structure, the beam intensity decreases as a result of attenuation on one hand, and wave reflections on the other. Attenuation represents the loss of wave amplitude (energy) on traveling through a medium, and depends on the wavelength, the density of the medium or tissue, and the heterogeneity (number and type) of the interface present (attenuation being 1 dB/MHz on average). Wave reflection in turn conditions the formation of ultrasound images; it is proportional to the differences in acoustic impedance between two media that form an interface standing in the

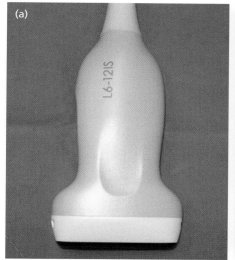 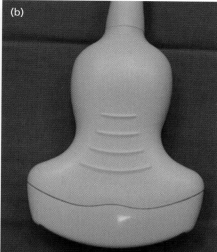

Figure 10.22 (a,b) Two types of ultrasound probe.

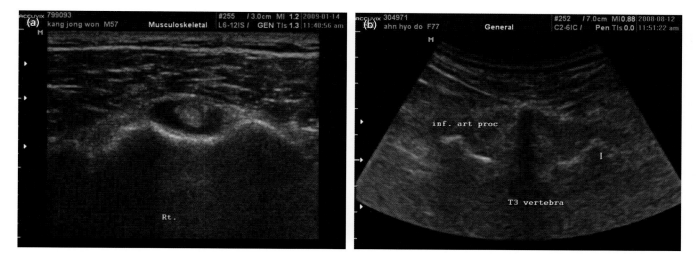

Figure 10.23 (a) Linear penetration with a 5–15 Hz probe. (b) Linear penetration with a curved probe.

way of the ultrasound beam. In terms of reflectivity, the resulting images can be regarded as hyperechogenic, normo-echogenic or hypoechogenic (Figs 10.24 and 10.25). In turn, hypoechogenic structures may appear anechogenic (anechoic) when ultrasound is completely attenuated or transsonorous when the waves are neither attenuated nor reflected back toward the emitting source.

A characteristic of ultrasound echoes applied in the clinical setting is the so-called **Doppler effect**, which occurs when the ultrasound beam encounters a moving structure in its path. As a result of such contact, the frequency of the reflected echo is modified, and an analysis of the corresponding frequency difference can inform us of the velocity of the moving structure (e.g. blood within the vascular lumen).

The images seen on the echograph screen can depend upon the tissue through which the sound travels (tissue images), or on the separation zones between tissues (contour images). In turn, contour images can be (a) anatomical (or wall) images, when two tissues are separated by an anatomically identifiable structure with a distinct acoustic impedance; or (b) interface (or separation) images, in the presence of different acoustic impedances without any actual anatomical separation between them. On the other hand, tissue images can exhibit (a) fluid patterns, characterized by the absence of echoes with posterior enhancement and lateral shadowing (e.g., blood vessels), (b) solid patterns, characterized by disperse internal echoes that can be either homo- or heterogeneous, (c) mixed patterns, and (d) acoustic shadows,

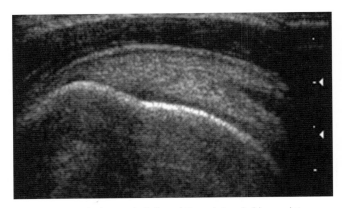

Figure 10.24 The hyperechoic line of the subchondral bone plate.

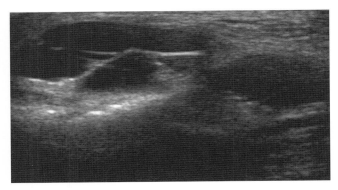

Figure 10.26 Ultrasound image showing the posterior acoustic enhancement artifact in a multiloculated cyst.

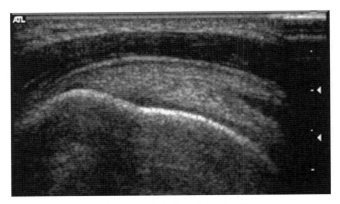

Figure 10.25 (a,b) The hypoechoic line of the shoulder bursa.

beyond which echoes are no longer generated. **Acoustic shadowing** occurs when ultrasound crosses interfaces with great differences in acoustic impedance (e.g. air/bone interfaces) (Fig. 10.26). Water is the body element that best transmits ultrasound waves, generating a black (anechoic) image. Thus highly cellular tissues containing abundant water can be expected to be hypoechoic, whereas more fibrous tissues containing less water and many interfaces are characteristically **hyperechoic**). Beam penetration and an image's resolution have an inverse ratio: the higher the resolution, the lower the working depth (tissue penetration). For deep locations, one needs to use a low-frequency probe (<7 MHz) that will produce poor resolution. On the contrary, for superficial structures (1–2 cm from skin), one needs to use a high-frequency probe (>7 MHz) producing at the same time high-resolution images. The common indications, advantages, and disadvantages of transverse and/or longitudinal techniques are described in Table 10.6.

Equipment for ultrasonography

There are seven ultrasonographic models in clinical use for medical imaging. They are enumerated in Table 10.7. Wynd et al. (2009) reported the models providing excellent care

as the Philips HD11 XE, which had the highest score, followed by GE LOGIQe and Esaote MYLab25, as tested by experienced and inexperienced participants in the study (Fig. 10.27 and Tables 10.2–10.5).

Methods of ultrasonography

Linear array transducer ultrasonography. This method uses a probe containing multiple acoustic transducers to send pulses of sound into body tissue. Whenever a sound wave encounters a material with a different density (acoustic impedance), part of the sound wave is reflected back to the probe and is detected as an echo. The time it takes for the echo to travel back to the probe is measured and used to calculate the depth of the tissue interface causing the echo. The greater the difference between acoustic impedances, the larger the echo is. If the pulse hits gases or solids, the density difference is so great that most of the acoustic energy is reflected and it becomes impossible to see deeper. The frequencies used for medical imaging are generally in the range of 1–18 MHz. Higher frequencies have a correspondingly smaller wavelength, and can be used to make sonograms with smaller details. However, the attenuation of the sound wave is increased at higher frequencies, so to have better penetration of deeper tissues, a lower frequency (3–5 MHz) is used. The speed of sound varies as it travels through different materials, and is dependent on the acoustic impedance of the material. However, the sonographic instrument assumes that the acoustic velocity is constant at 1540 m/s. An effect of this assumption is that in a real body with nonuniform tissues, the beam becomes somewhat defocused and image resolution is reduced.

To generate a **two-dimensional image**, the ultrasonic beam is swept. A transducer may be swept mechanically by rotating or swinging; or a one-dimensional phased array transducer may be used to sweep the beam electronically. The received data are processed and used to construct the image. The image is then a two-dimensional representation of the slice into the body.

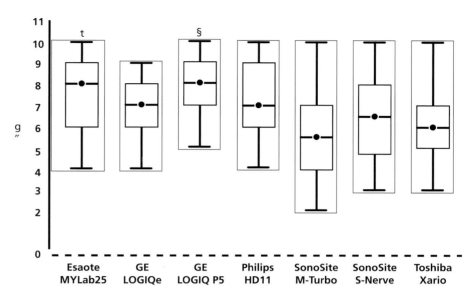

Figure 10.27 Phantom image quality ratings of experienced and inexperienced providers. Box plots summarize the distribution of points at each factor level. The ends of the box are the 25th and 75th quartiles, and the difference between the quartiles is the interquartile range. The line identified with a bullet point indicates the *n* value. Whiskers extend from the ends of the box to the outermost data point that falls within the distances computed as [lower quartile − 1.5 × (interquartile range) to upper quartile + 1.5 × (interquartile range)]. t, $P < 0.001$ versus SonoSite M-Turbo and 0.002 versus Toshiba Xario. §, $P < 0.001$ versus SonoSite M-Turbo, SonoSite S-Nerve, and Toshiba Xario.

Table 10.2 Basic knowledge of ultrasound principles and familiarity with equipment is mandatory

1. Ultrasound imaging is based on sound waves that are transmitted from, and received by, an ultrasound utilizing frequencies of 2–15 MHz.
2. The sound waves travel into the body and hit a boundary between tissues (e.g., between fluid and soft tissue, soft tissue and bone).

Table 10.3 Potential advantages of ultrasound

1. Visualization of nerves and surrounding structures: vessels, muscles, bone and viscera pleura, lung, peritoneum, bowel.
2. Diagnostic: recognizing anatomical variability and pathology.
3. Real-time visualization of needle trajectory, needle–nerve contact, and injectate spread.

Table 10.4 Definitions commonly used in ultrasonography

Hypoechoic. Dark structures.
Hyperechoic. Bright structures.
Anisotropy. The image is highly dependent on the angle to ultrasound beam. Some nerves are more anisotropic than others. Ninety degrees gives the best picture.
Air. Ultrasound beams will not pass through air. Be generous with gel to provide air-free contact with skin.
Acoustic shadowing. Highly reflective surfaces (bone) reflect almost all of the entire sound beam, throwing a shadow over all deeper structures.
Post-cystic enhancement. Increased brightness behind a fluid-filled structure.
Arteries. Anechoic, pulsatile.
Veins. Anechoic, compressible.

Table 10.5 Performing the block: advantages and disadvantages of transverse or longitudinal techniques

Advantages of transverse technique
- Short-axis technique (transverse) typical entry point.
- Shortest distance.

Disadvantages of transverse technique
- Needle only seen as a bright dot while within the beam.
- Poor vision of needle–nerve contact.
- Long-axis technique (longitudinal).

Advantages of longitudinal techniques
- Tunnel for catheter placement.
- Good vision of needle–nerve contact.
- Needle visualized in entire length*.

Disadvantages of longitudinal techniques
- Uncommon needle entry.
- Longer distance skin–nerve.
- More painful.

*Note the deeper the structure, the less perpendicular your needle will become and the more parallel to the beam. At an angle less than 60° you are likely to lose the needle image and then the benefits of the "in plane" technique.

Table 10.6 Ultrasound machine models

Esaote MYLab25
GE LOGIQe
GE LOGIQ P5
Philips HDII XE
SonoSite M-Turbo
SonoSite S-Nerve
Toshiba Xario

Table 10.7 Common pain procedures where ultrasound is possible

Table: head and neck
Occipital nerve
Extraforaminal cervical nerve roots
Superficial cervical plexus
Cervical medial branch/facet
Stellate ganglion
Suprascapular nerve
Lumbar spine
Facet joints
Medial branch of posterior ramus
Paraspinal muscle injection
Erector spinae
Quadratus lumborum
Psoas
Sacroiliac joint
Piriformis muscle
Pudendal nerve
Lower limb
Femoral nerve
Lateral cutaneous of the thigh saphenous nerve
Sciatic/popliteal
Hip joint
Knee

Three-dimensional images can be generated by acquiring a series of adjacent two-dimensional images. Commonly a specialized probe that mechanically scans a conventional two-dimensional image transducer is used. However, because the mechanical scanning is slow, it is difficult to make three-dimensional images of moving tissues.

Recently, two-dimensional phased-array transducers that can sweep the beam in three-dimensions have been developed. These can image faster and can even be used to make live three-dimensional images of a beating heart.

Doppler ultrasonography is used to study blood flow and muscle motion. The different detected speeds are represented in color for ease of interpretation, for example leaky heart valves: the leak shows up as a flash of unique color. Colors may alternatively be used to represent the amplitudes of the received echoes.

Modes of sonography. Several different modes of ultrasound are used in medical imaging. They are as follows.

A-mode. A-mode is the simplest type of ultrasound. A single transducer scans a line through the body with the echoes plotted on screen as a function of depth. Therapeutic ultrasound aimed at a specific tumor or calculus is also A-mode, to allow for pinpoint accurate focus of the destructive wave energy.

B-mode. In B-mode ultrasound, a linear array of transducers simultaneously scans a plane through the body that can be viewed as a two-dimensional image on screen.

C-mode. A C-mode image is formed in a plane normal to a B-mode image. A gate that selects data from a specific depth from an A-mode line is used; then the transducer is moved in the two-dimensional plane to sample the entire region at this fixed depth. When the transducer traverses the area in a spiral, an area of $100\,cm^2$ can be scanned in around 10 seconds (Lee 2010).

M-mode. M stands for motion. Ultrasound pulses are emitted in quick succession each time, and either an A-mode or B-mode image is taken. Over time, this is analogous to recording a video in ultrasound. As the organ boundaries that produce reflections move relative to the probe, this can be used to determine the velocity of specific organ structures.

Doppler mode. This mode makes use of the Doppler effect in measuring and visualizing blood flow.

Color Doppler. Velocity information is presented as a color-coded overlay on top of a B-mode image.

Pain procedures under ultrasound guidance

Ultrasound might have a potential usefulness in interventional pain management (Table 10.7). Possible applications are nerve blocks of the cervical and lumbar zygoapophysial joints, stellate ganglion block, intercostal nerve blocks, peripheral nerve blocks of the extremities, blocks of painful stump neuromas, caudal epidural injections, and injections of tender points. Ultrasound can be used for local anesthetic injection procedures, and for destructive procedures, such as cryoanalgesia, RF lesions, or chemical neurolysis (Figs 10.28–10.32).

Recently, an ultrasound-guided lumbar zygoapophysial joint has been described. Lee (2010) used a curved array ultrasound transducer with a frequency between 2 and 6 MHz to guide the needle to the L2–L4 medial branches (Fig. 10.31b,c). Accuracy of ultrasound-guided T12–L4 medial branch blocks was recently confirmed in a cadaver study by CT control, with a rate of over 90% of successful needle placements. This procedure has limitations, because it is difficult to identify the bony landmarks to block the medial branch at L5 at the junction between the ala and the superior articular process of the sacrum. In the obese patient, poor ultrasound image quality is obtained, considering a significant increase in skin-to-target distances from the third to the fifth lumbar vertebrae.

In the treatment of patients suffering from vascular diseases, sympathetically maintained pain of the head or the upper extremity, ultrasound allows the visualization of all relevant anatomical structures of the stellate ganglion region (Fig. 10.21). Kapral et al. compared stellate ganglion block either by ultrasound guidance or by a blind standard technique and found a reduction in the amount of local anesthetic to 5 ml was achieved, and no hematoma in the ultrasound group was recorded. There are no published data on ultrasound-guided intercostal nerve blocks, basically

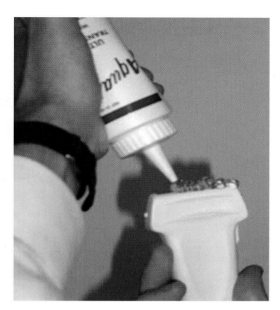

Figure 10.28 The use of gel during ultrasonography.

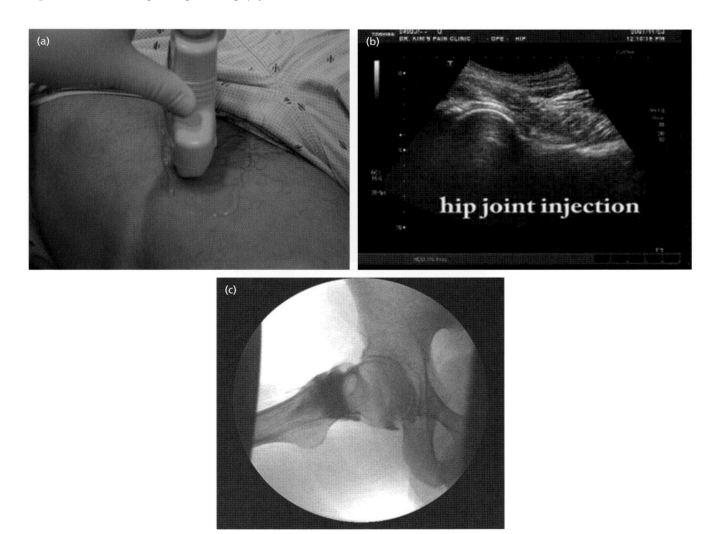

Figure 10.29 (a) The ultrasound transducer placed on the surface of the skin for hip joint injection. (b) The ultrasound image during the hip joint injection. (c) The fluoroscopic image of the same hip joint after injection.

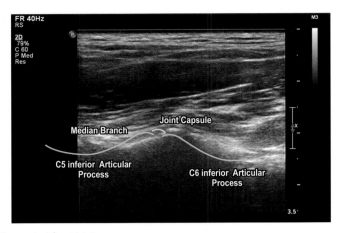

Figure 10.30 Ultrasound image of the cervical facet joint.

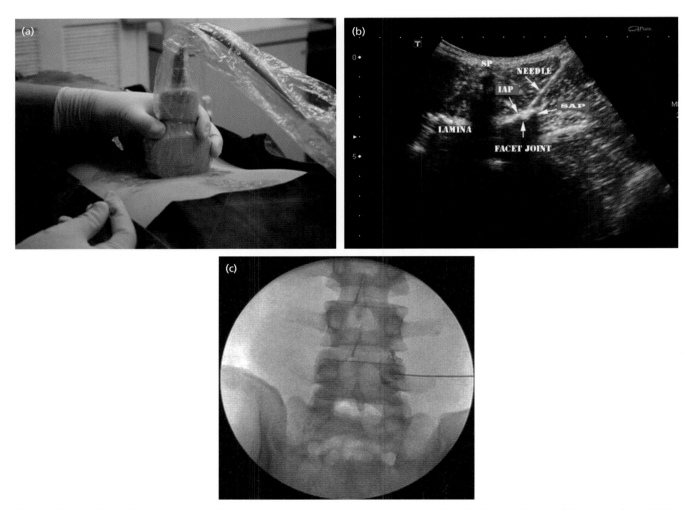

Figure 10.31 (a) The surface application of ultrasound transducer during lumbar facet joint injection. (b) Ultrasound image of the lumbar facet. (c) The fluoroscopic view of the lumbar facet.

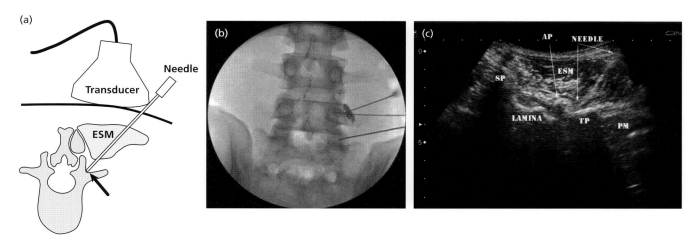

Figure 10.32 (a–c) The technique of lumbar medial branch block with ultrasound compared with the fluoroscopic view.

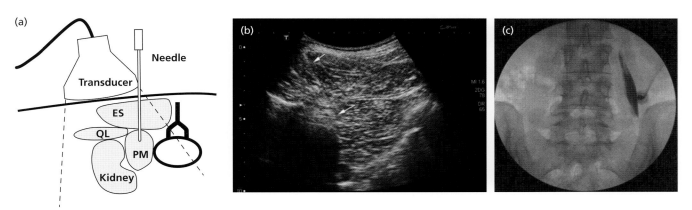

Figure 10.33 (a–c) The ultrasound image during psoas muscle injection compared with the fluoroscopic view. ES, esophagus; QL, quadratus lumborum, PM, psoas major.

because the nerves are rarely seen as they are lying close to or recovered by the caudal edge of the rib. Eichenberger et al. (2004) have stated that 2 ml of local anesthetic is sufficient to fill the intercostal space, and the spread of the injected solution can mostly be seen clearly by ultrasound during the injection. These authors add the concept of dosing based on observed clinical anatomy considering the width of the intercostal space may vary and sometimes more volume has to be applied to fill the intercostal space. The ilioinguinal and the iliohypogastric nerves are often blocked without the use of an imaging technique for postoperative pain relief, but most importantly for chronic pain relief after inguinal hernia repair. Ultrasound offers a perspective of precise percutaneous approach to these nerves using high-resolution probes. With some anatomical variations on the location, they lie between the external and internal oblique or the internal oblique and transverse abdominal muscles,

just medial and cranial to the superior iliac crest. The genitofemoral nerve, probably because of its deep course, is unlikely to be displayed by ultrasound. In peripheral nerves, the treatment of stump neuroma after amputation is made using initially diagnostic blocks. Using ultrasound can help to identify the anatomical source of pain in these patients. For caudal injection of steroids, the point of entrance of sacral hiatus may be difficult to identify and ultrasound may be a useful tool for appropriate caudal needle placement (Figs 10.33–10.36). In patients with a diagnosis of chronic pain of myofascial origin, a trigger point may be defined as a focal, hyperirritable spot located in a taut band of skeletal muscle. According to Eichenberger et al. (2004), in the performance of trigger/tender point infiltrations under ultrasound visualization, it is possible to see a muscle twitch when the needle is entering the trigger point in the target muscle. Montero Matamala et al. (1989) described the

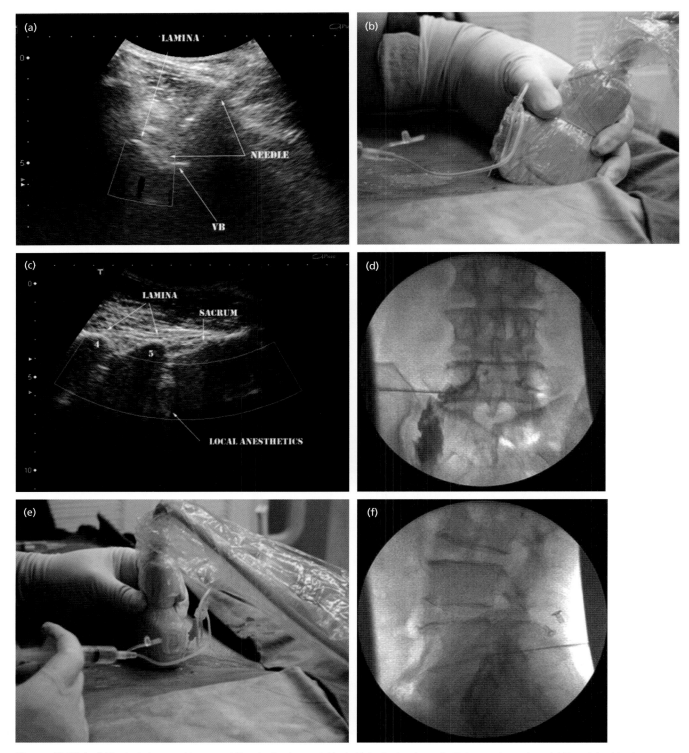

Figure 10.34 (a–f) The technique and images of Doppler lumbar root block. Note the local anesthetic image shown in red. VB, vertebral body.

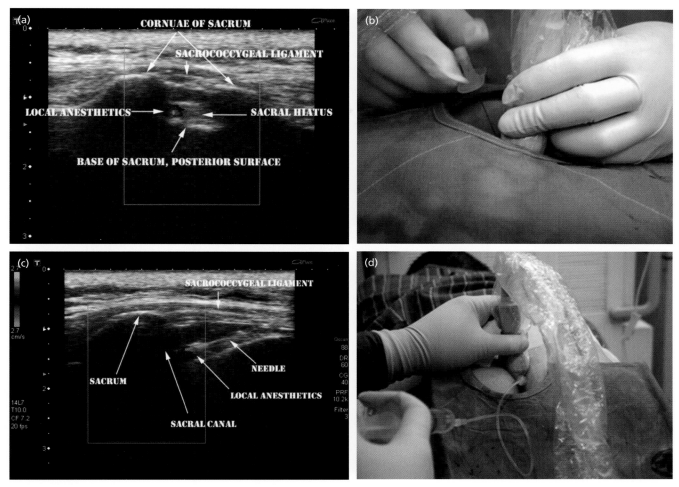

Figure 10.35 (a–d) The technique of color Doppler caudal epidural injection.

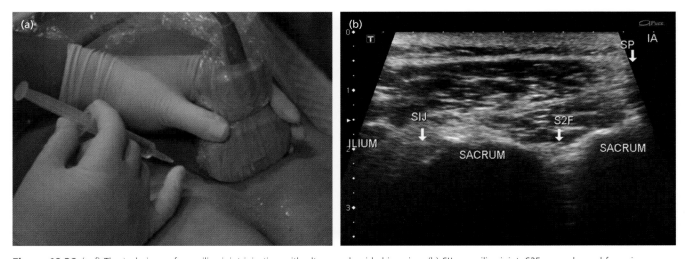

Figure 10.36 (a–f) The technique of sacroiliac joint injection with ultrasound-guided imaging. (b) SIJ, sacroiliac joint; S2F, second sacral foramina. (c) SA, sacrum; SIJ, sacroiliac joint; IL, ilium. (d) TR, transducer; SIJ, sacroiliac joint; SP, spinous process.

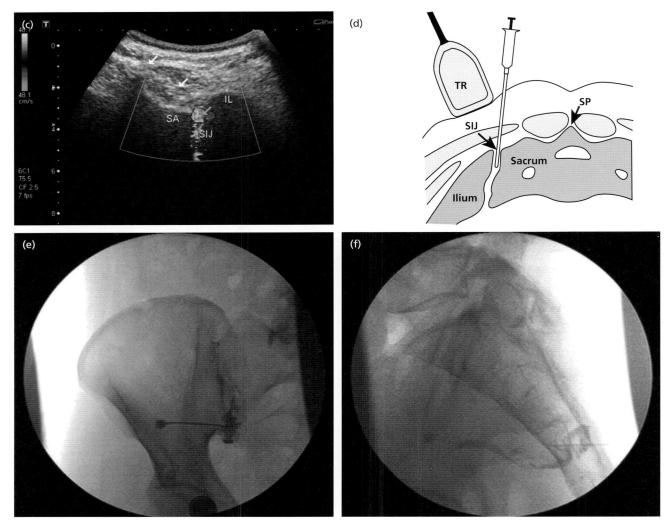

Figure 10.36 *(Continued)*

neurolytic block of the celiac plexus through the anterior abdominal wall using ultrasonic guidance. Since this publication, the usefulness of sonographically guided percutaneous neurolysis of the celiac plexus in patients with abdominal tumors or chronic pancreatitis has been evaluated in several papers. The ultrasonic-guided anterior approach was used for needle placement and examination of the spread of injection. The aorta and discharge of the truncus celiacus or the arteria lienalis, respectively, are ultrasonographically presented, and the celiac plexus as echogenic foci were observed around the origin of the celiac trunk and superior mesenteric artery in all cases.

Acknowledgment: Figures 10.21 to 10.36 are reproduced with permission from 2010 Advanced Interventional Pain Conference Inaugural Lecture Series (www.worldinstituteofpain. org).

Further reading

Cahana, A., Vutskits, L. & Muller, D. (2003) Acute differential modification of synaptic transmission and cell survival during exposure target position pulsed and continuous radiofrequency energy. *Journal of Pain* **4**(4), 197–202.

Chen, C.P., Tang, S.F., Hsu, T.C., et al. (2004) Ultrasound guidance in caudal epidural needle placement. *Anesthesiology* **101**, 181–184.

Cosman, B.J. & Cosman, E.C. (1974) Guide to radiofrequency lesion generation in neurosurgery. Radionics Procedure Technique Series Monographs. Burlington, MA: Radionics.

Cosman, E.R. & Cosman, B.J. (1984) Methods of making nervous system lesions. In *Neurosurgery*, vol. 1 (ed. Wilkins, R.H. & Rengachary, S.S.), pp. 2490–2498. New York: McGraw-Hill.

Cosman, E.R., Nashold, B.S. & Ovelman-Levitt, J. (1984) Theoretical aspects of radiofrequency lesions in the dorsal root entry zone. *Neurosurgery* **15**, 945–950.

Cosman, E.R. Jr & Cosman, E.R. Sr (2005) Electric and thermal field effects in tissue around radiofrequency electrodes. *Pain Medicine* **6**(6), 405–424.

Eichenberger, U., Greher, M. & Curatolo, M. (2004) Ultrasound in interventional pain management. *Techniques in Regional Anesthesia and Pain Management* **8**, 171–178.

Erdine, S., Yucel, A., Cunan, A., et al. (2005) Effects of pulsed versus conventional radiofrequency current in rabbit dorsal root ganglion morphology. *European Journal of Pain* **9**(3), 251–256.

Gimenez, A., Martinez-Noguera, A., et al. (1993) Percutaneous neurolysis of the celiac plexus via the anterior approach with sonographic guidance. *American Jounal of Roentgenology* **161**(5), 1061–1063.

Grau, T., Leipold, R.W., Conradi, R., et al. (2001) Ultrasound imaging facilitates localization of the epidural space during combined spinal and epidural anesthesia. *Regional Anesthesia and Pain Medicine* **26**, 64–67.

Kanpolat, Y. & Cosman, E.R. (1996) Special radio frequency electrode system for computed tomography-guided pain-relieving procedures. *Neurosurgery* **38**, 600–603.

Kapral, S., Krafft, P., Gosch, M., et al. (1995) Ultrasound imaging for stellate ganglion block: direct visualization of puncture site and local anesthetic spread. A pilot study. *Regional Anesthesia* **20**, 323–328.

Lee, S.C. (2010) Ultrasound guided pain management. Paper presented at the 15th Annual Advanced Interventional Pain Conference, Budapest, Hungary, 2010.

Levin, A.B. & Cosman, E.R. (1980) Thermocouple-monitored cordotomy electrode. *Journal of Neurosurgery* **53**, 266–268.

Marhofer, P., Greher, M. & Kapral, S. (2005) Ultrasound guidance in regional anaesthesia. *British Journal of Anaesthesia* **94**, 7–17.

Montero Matamala, A., Vidal Lopez, F., Aguilar Sanchez, J.L., et al. (1989) Percutaneous anterior approach to the coeliac plexus using ultrasound. *British Journal of Anaesthesia* **62**(6), 637–640.

Peng, W.H. & Narouze, S. (2009) Ultrasound-guided interventional procedures in pain medicine: a review of anatomy, sonoanatomy, and procedures. *Regional Anesthesia and Pain Medicine* **34**(5), 458–474.

Narouze, S. & Peng, W.H. (2010) Ultrasound-guided interventional procedures in pain medicine: a review of anatomy, sonoanatomy, and procedures, part II: axial structures. *Regional Anesthesia and Pain Medicine* **35**(4), 386–396.

Ray, C.D. (1982) *Percutaneous Radio-Frequency Facet Nerve Blocks: Treatment of the Mechanical Low-Back Syndrome*. Radionics Procedure Technique Series. Burlington, MA: Radionics.

Rosomoff, H.L., Carroll, F., Brown, J. & Sheptak, T. (1965) Percutaneous radiofrequency cervical cordotomy: technique. *Journal of Neurosurgery* **23**, 639–644.

Sandkuhler, J., Chen, J.G., Cheng, G. & Randic, M. (1997) Low frequency stimulation of the afferent A-delta fibers induces long-term depression at the primary afferent synapses with substantia gelatinosa neurons in the rat. *Journal of Neuroscience* **17**, 6483–6491.

Schafhalter-Zoppoth, I., McCulloch, C.E. & Gray, A.T. (2004) Ultrasound visibility of needles used for regional nerve block: an in vitro study. *Regional Anesthesia and Pain Medicine* **29**, 480–488.

Shealy, C.N. (1975) Percutaneous radiofrequency denervation of spinal facets and treatment for chronic back pain and sciatica. *Journal of Neurosurgery* **43**, 448–451.

Sites, B.D., Chan, V.W., Neal, J.M., et al. (2009) The American Society of Regional Anesthesia and Pain Medicine and the European Society of Regional Anaesthesia and Pain Therapy Joint Committee Recommendations for Education and Training in Ultrasound Guided Regional Anesthesia. *Regional Anesthesia and Pain Medicine* **34**(1), 40–46.

Sites, B.D., Gallagher, J.D., Cravero, J., et al. (2004) The learning curve associated with a simulated ultrasound-guided interventional task by inexperienced anesthesia residents. *Regional Anesthesia and Pain Medicine* **29**, 544–548.

Sluijter, M.E. (1990) *Radiofrequency Lesions in the Treatment of Cervical Pain Syndromes*. Radionics Procedure Technique Series. Burlington, MA: Radionics.

Sluijter, M.E. & Mehta, M. (1981) Treatment of chronic back and neck pain by percutaneous thermal lesions. In *Persistent Pain, Modern Methods of Treatment*, vol. 3 (ed. Lipton, S. & Miles, J.), pp. 141–179. London: Academic Press.

Sluijter, M.E., Cosman, E.R., Rittman, W.J. & Kleef, M. (1998) The effects of pulsed radiofrequency fields applied to the dorsal root ganglion – a preliminary report. *Pain Clinic* **11**(2), 109–118.

Sweet, W.H. & Wepsic, J.G. (1974) Controlled thermocoagulation of trigeminal ganglion and rootlets for differential destruction of pain fibers: I. Trigeminal neuralgia. *Journal of Neurosurgery* **39**, 143–156.

Tew, J.M. Jr & van Loveren, H. (1988) Percutaneous rhizotomy in the treatment of intractable facial pain (trigeminal, glossopharyngeal and facial nerves). In *Operative Neurosurgical Technique* (ed. Schmidek, H.H. & Sweet, W.H.), pp. 1111–1123. Orlando, FL: Grune & Stratton.

White, J.C. & Sweet, W.H. (1969) *Pain and the Neurosurgeon: A Forty-Year Experience*, pp. 169–197, 607–609. Springfield, IL: Charles C. Thomas.

Wynd, K.P., Smith, H.M., Jacob, A.K., Torsher, L.C., Kopp, S.L. & Hebl, J.R. (2009) Ultrasound machine comparison: an evaluation of ergonomic design, data management, ease of use, and image quality. *Regional Anesthesia and Pain Medicine* **34**(4), 349–356.

2 Description of Specific Techniques

11 Simple, Frequent Procedures in the Musculoskeletal Region

INJECTIONS INTO UPPER EXTREMITY JOINTS

Shoulder joint

Anatomy
The shoulder joint is formed by three bones: the clavicle, the scapula, and the humerus, and their associated muscles, ligaments, and tendons. The major joint of the shoulder is the glenohumeral joint. In human anatomy, the shoulder joint comprises the part of the body where the humerus attaches to the scapula.

Joints of the shoulder
There are three joints of the shoulder: the glenohumeral, acromioclavicular (AC), and the sternoclavicular joints. The sternoclavicular joint is not relevant for shoulder joint block, hence it will not be described here.

Glenohumeral joint
The glenohumeral joint is the main joint of the shoulder. It is a ball and socket joint that allows the arm to rotate in a circular fashion or to hinge out and up away from the body. It is formed by the articulation between the head of the humerus and the glenoid fossa of the scapula. The "ball" of the joint is the rounded, medial anterior surface of the humerus; the "socket" is formed by the glenoid fossa, the dish-shaped portion of the lateral scapula. The shallowness of the fossa and relatively loose connections between the shoulder and the rest of the body allow the arm to have tremendous mobility.

The capsule at the glenohumeral joint is a soft tissue that envelops the joint and attaches to the scapula, humerus, and head of the biceps. It is lined by a thin, smooth synovial membrane. This capsule is strengthened by the coraco-humeral ligament, which attaches the coracoid process of the scapula to the greater tubercle of the humerus. There are also three other ligaments that attach the lesser tubercle of the humerus to the lateral scapula; they are collectively called the glenohumeral ligaments.

There is also a ligament called the semicirculare humeri, which is a transversal band between the posterior sides of the greater and lesser tubercules. This band is one of the most important strengthening ligaments of the joint capsule.

The acromioclavicular (AC) joint
The AC joint is a joint at the top of the shoulder. It is the junction between the acromion (part of the scapula that forms the highest point of the shoulder) and the clavicle. It is stabilized by three ligaments: the AC ligament attaches the clavicle to the acromion of the scapula; the coracoacromial ligament runs from the coracoid process to the acromion; and the coracoclavicular ligament, which itself consists of two ligaments, the conoid and the trapezoid ligaments.

Rotator cuff
The rotator cuff is an anatomical term given to the group of muscles and their tendons that act to stabilize the shoulder. It is composed of the tendons and muscles (supraspinatus, infraspinatus, teres minor, and subscapularis) that hold the head of the humerus (ball) in the glenoid fossa (socket) (Figs 11.1 and 11.2).

Indications
- Frozen shoulder.
- Bursitis.
- Impingement syndrome.
- Adhesive capsulitis.

Contraindications
- Local or systemic infection.
- Coagulopathy.

Pain-Relieving Procedures: The Illustrated Guide, First Edition. P. Prithvi Raj and Serdar Erdine.
© 2012 John Wiley & Sons, Ltd. Published 2012 by John Wiley & Sons, Ltd.

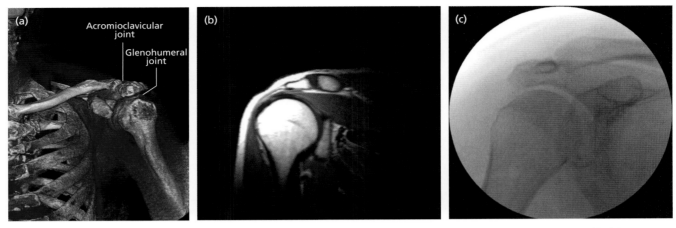

Figure 11.1 (a) Three-dimensional computed tomography scan showing the shoulder joint. (b) MRI scan showing the shoulder joint. (c) Plain radiograph showing the shoulder joint.

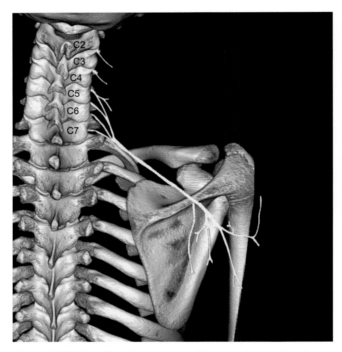

Figure 11.2 Three-dimensional computed tomography scan showing the innervation of the shoulder joint.

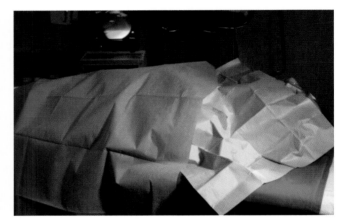

Figure 11.3 Place and prepare the patient in supine position.

Technique of three in one block of the shoulder

Glenohumeral joint block

Step 1. Prepare the patient before the procedure
The type of analgesia or sedation needs to be ascertained before performance of the invasive procedure. If a local anesthetic block is planned, mild sedation is all that is necessary.

Step 2. Positioning and monitoring the patient (Fig. 11.3)
1. The patient is placed in a supine position on the table.
2. Obtain an intravenous access if drugs need to be administered.
3. Monitoring of vital signs is mandatory in unstable patients.
4. The area for needle entry is prepared in a sterile fashion.

Step 3. Drugs and equipment for the block
Prepare and confirm that the following equipment, needles, and drugs are ready to be used for the procedure:
• 1½ inch, 25 gauge needle for skin infiltration;
• 5 ml syringe containing local anesthetic solution;
• 22 G 3½ inch needle for the nerve block;
• 5 ml of 1% lidocaine;
• preferred steroid solution (decadron or equivalent);
• 2 ml of 6% phenol (usually prepared in iohexol).

Step 4. Visualization

1. Prepare and drape the area in a sterile fashion.

2. Place the C-arm in the posteroanterior (PA) position centered on the shoulder joint, inclined slightly caudally (10°) (to visualize the AC joint); the elbow is rotated in 90° flexion with the hand on the stomach until the greater tuberosity is clearly visualized (Fig. 11.4).

Step 5. Direction of the needle

1. The entry point is just above the AC joint.

2. Infiltrate the skin with local anesthetic.

3. Insert a 10 cm, 22 gauge needle under fluoroscopic guidance through the AC joint and subacromial space to the superior part of the glenohumeral joint.

Note: there is a loss of resistance when entering the glenohumeral joint (Fig. 11.5).

Step 6. Confirm the position of the needle and the block

1. Inject 2–3 ml contrast material into the glenohumeral joint. A semicircular image should appear under fluoroscopy. Inject 5 ml of the combination of 5 ml of 0.5% bupivacaine, 40 mg methylprednisolone, and 4 ml saline into the joint (Fig. 11.6).

2. Gradually withdraw the needle to the middle third of the subacromial space. Two milliliters of contrast material is injected to confirm that the needle is in the subacromial space. Inject 4 ml of the combination into the subacromial space (Fig. 11.7).

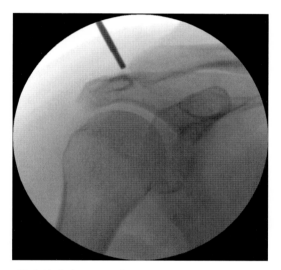

Figure 11.4 Mark the entry point.

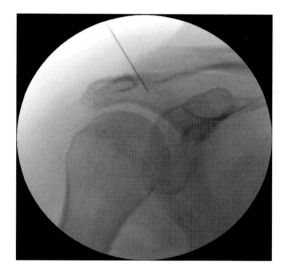

Figure 11.5 Direct the needle through the AC joint.

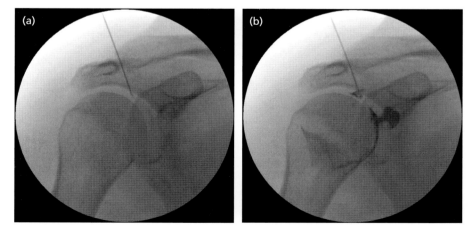

Figure 11.6 (a,b) Direct the needle toward the glenohumeral joint, and inject contrast material to confirm the position of the needle.

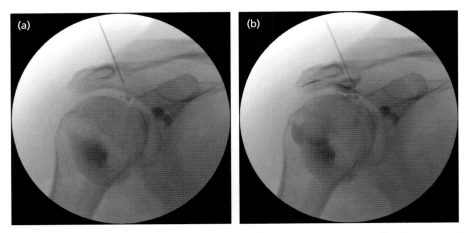

Figure 11.7 (a,b) Withdraw the needle upward to the subacromial space, and inject contrast material to confirm the correct placement of the needle.

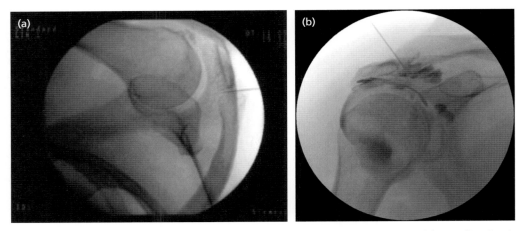

Figure 11.8 (a,b) Withdraw the needle further upward to the midway of the AC joint, and inject contrast material to confirm the placement of the needle.

3. Withdraw the needle further upwards again under continuous imaging to the midway of the AC joint. Inject 1 ml contrast material to confirm the correct placement of the needle. Inject 1 ml of the solution into the AC joint (Fig. 11.8).

4. In some cases, the needle may pass with difficulty through the AC joint. Then, under PA view, mark the glenohumeral joint under fluoroscopy. Insert the needle perpendicular to the skin. There will be a loss of resistance when entering the glenohumeral joint under live imaging. There will be a semi-crescent image under fluoroscopy (Fig. 11.9).

Note: some physicians perform pulsed radiofrequency of the glenohumeral and AC joints. However, there is no consensus on this approach.

Step 7. Postprocedure care
After the procedure is completed, the patient needs to be observed for up to 2 hours. Monitoring of vital signs is man-

datory. In addition, the pain relief should be objectively documented. After a satisfactory observation, the patient should be discharged with appropriate and adequate instructions given to the escort. Written instructions are preferable for emergencies; this is helpful to the patient and the family.

Complications
Pain during injection: the block should be performed under sedation, otherwise it is painful.
Infection: the infection risk is the same as with other procedures.

Helpful hints
The three in one block facilitates functional improvement during physiotherapy of the frozen shoulder. The patient should avoid repetitive overhead loading for 3 months and use compensating techniques during abduction movements.

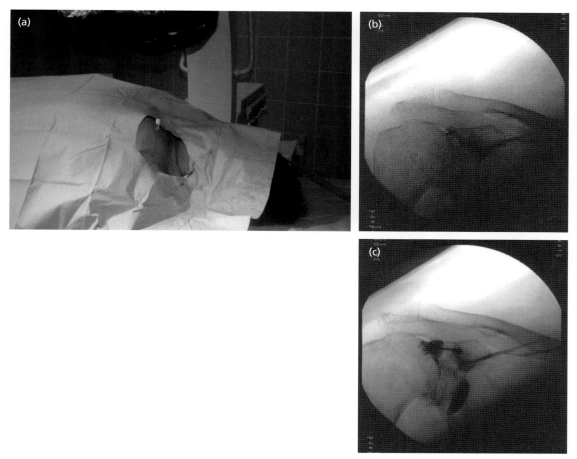

Figure 11.9 (a–c) Perpendicular approach and the needle in place.

Elbow joint

Anatomy

The human elbow is a hinge joint in the middle of the upper extremity. Three bones form the elbow joint: the humerus and the paired radius and ulna of the forearm. The bony prominence at the very tip of the elbow is the olecranon process of the ulna, and the inner aspect of the elbow is called the antecubital fossa.

Ligaments

The trochlea of the humerus fits into the semilunar notch of the ulna. The capsule and ligaments of the humerus articulate with the fovea on the head of the radius. The articular surfaces are connected together by a capsule, which is thickened medially and laterally, and, to a less extent, in front and behind. These thickened portions are usually described as distinct ligaments.

The major ligaments are the ulnar collateral ligament, radial collateral ligament, and annular ligament.

Synovial membrane

The synovial membrane is very extensive. It extends from the margin of the articular surface of the humerus, and lines the coronoid, radial and olecranon fossae of the ulna; the capsule is reflected over the deep surface of the capsule and forms a pouch between the radial notch, the deep surface of the annular ligament, and the circumference of the head of the radius. Projecting between the radius and ulna into the cavity is a crescentic fold of synovial membrane, dividing the joint into two: one the humeroradial, the other the humeroulnar.

Between the capsule and the synovial membrane are three masses of fat: the largest, over the olecranon fossa, is kept in the fossa by the triceps brachii during flexion; the second fat mass is over the coronoid fossa, and the third fat mass is over the radial fossa; they are kept in place by the brachialis in their respective fossae during extension.

The muscles closely related with the elbow joint are as follows: the brachialis anteriorly; the brachioradialis posteriorly; the triceps brachii and anconaeus laterally; the supinator and the common tendon of origin of the extensor

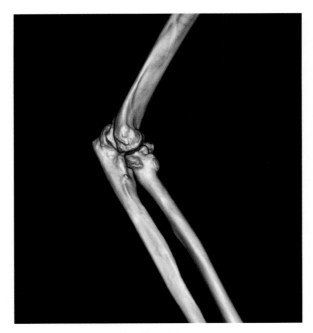

Figure 11.10 Anatomy of the elbow joint.

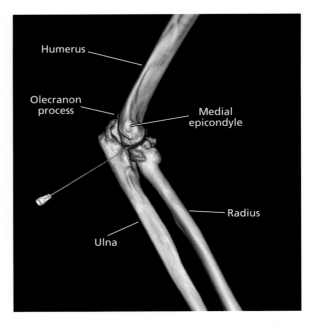

Figure 11.11 Three-dimensional computed tomography scan showing the direction of the needle during the elbow joint injection.

muscles medially; the common tendon of origin of the flexor muscles, and the flexor carpi ulnaris (Fig. 11.10).

Indications
- Acute capsulitis.
- Chronic capsulitis.

Contraindications
- Local or systemic infection.
- Coagulopathy.

Elbow joint block

Step 1. Prepare the patient before the procedure
Mild sedation may be necessary in some patients. Obtain an intravenous access if drugs need to be administered.

Step 2. Positioning and monitoring the patient
1. Patient sits with the elbow supported at 45° flexion.
2. Monitoring of vital signs is mandatory in unstable patients.
3. The area for needle entry is prepared in a sterile fashion.

Step 3. Drugs and equipment for the elbow joint block
Prepare and confirm that the following equipment, needles, and drugs are ready to be used for the procedure:
- 1½ inch, 25 gauge needle for skin infiltration;
- 5 ml syringe containing local anesthetic solution;
- 22 G 3½ inch needle for the nerve block;
- 5 ml of 1% lidocaine;
- preferred steroid solution (decadron or equivalent).

Step 4. Surface landmark for needle entry
Identify the head of the radius posteriorly and the space between the radius and humerus.

Step 5. Direction of the needle
Insert the needle perpendicular to the head of the radius, advance until it penetrates the capsule of the joint (Fig. 11.11).

Step 6. Elbow joint block
Inject 20 mg of deposteroid together with 5 ml of 1% lidocaine (Fig. 11.12).

Step 7. Postprocedural care
Apply icepack for 10 minutes after the injection. After several days the patient should be advised to start exercise to increase the range of motion if pain is relieved.

Complications
Serious complications are not expected to occur. Pain at the injection site may last for a few days. The risk of infection is very low.

Injection technique for tennis elbow (lateral epicondylitis)

Anatomy
The supinator muscle spirals around the outer side of the radius to attach to the dorsal surface of the ulna, the lateral epicondyle of the humerus, the lateral and ventral ligaments

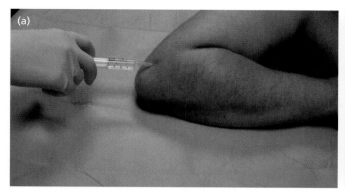
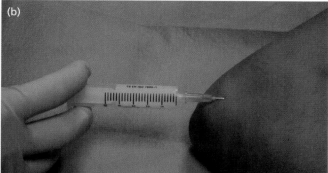

Figure 11.12 (a,b) Elbow joint injection.

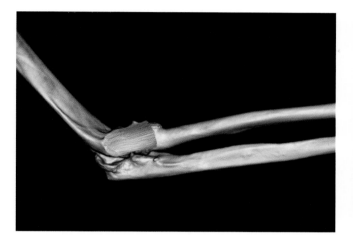

Figure 11.13 Tennis elbow, structures in close vicinity.

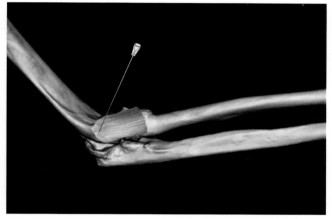

Figure 11.14 Direction of the needle for tennis elbow injection.

of the radioulnar joint, and the anterior capsule of the humeroulnar joint.

Lateral epicondylitis is a painful condition at the epicondyle of the long bone of the forearm.

It occurs at the teno-osseous origin of the common extensor tendon at the elbow.

Lateral epicondylitis (also known as tennis elbow, shooter's elbow, and archer's elbow) is a condition where the outer part of the elbow becomes sore and tender. It is commonly associated with playing tennis and other racquet sports, though the injury can happen by itself or through other mechanical injuries (Fig. 11.13).

Indications
• Lateral epicondylitis.

Contraindications
• Local or systemic infection.
• Coagulopathy.

Steps 1–3 are as described above in the elbow joint injections.

Step 4. Positioning of the patient
The patient sits, supporting the elbow bent at a right angle and the forearm supinated to relax the tendon.

Step 5. Surface landmark
Identify the facet lying anteriorly on lateral epicondyle.

Step 6. Direction of the needle
Insert the needle in line with cubital crease perpendicular to the facet until it touches the bone (Fig. 11.14).

Step 7. Tennis elbow injection
Inject 1–2 ml of 1% lidocaine with 10–20 mg of deposteroid solution (Fig. 11.15).

Injection technique for golfer's elbow

Anatomy
The common flexor tendon arises from the anterior facet on the medial epicondyle. Golfer's elbow is the chronic tendonitis of the common flexor tendon (Fig. 11.16).

Steps 1–3 are as described above.

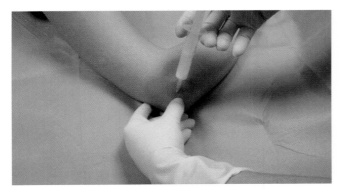

Figure 11.15 Tennis elbow injection.

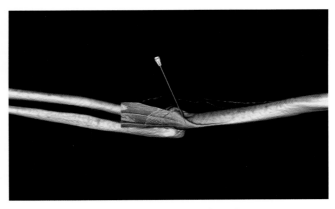

Figure 11.17 Direction of the needle for golfer's elbow injection.

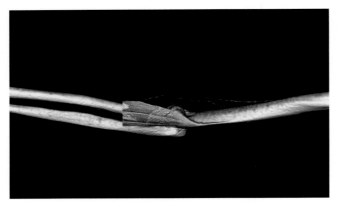

Figure 11.16 Golfer's elbow, structures in close vicinity.

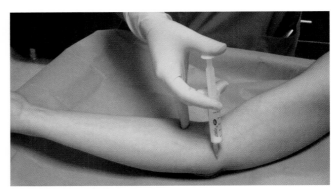

Figure 11.18 Golfer's elbow injection.

Step 4. Positioning of the patient
The patient sits and the arm is supported and extended.

Step 5. Surface landmark
Identify the anterior facet of the medial epicondyle.

Step 6. Direction of the needle
Insert the needle perpendicular to the facet until the bony contact is made (Fig. 11.17).

Step 7. Injection
Inject 1–2 ml of 1% lidocaine with 10–20 mg deposteroid solution (Fig. 11.18).

Wrist joint

Anatomy
The wrist is formed by the carpal bones, which consist of eight bones forming the proximal skeletal segment of the hand, the wrist joint or radiocarpal joint, the joint between the radius and the carpus, the anatomical region surrounding the carpus including the distal parts of the bones of the forearm and the proximal parts of the metacarpus or five metacarpal bones and the series of joints between these bones, thus referred to as wrist joints. This region also includes the carpal tunnel, the anatomical snuff box, the flexor retinaculum, and the extensor retinaculum.

The radiocarpal, intercarpal, midcarpal, carpometacarpal, and intermetacarpal joints often intercommunicate through a common synovial cavity (Fig. 11.19).

Indications
- Acute capsulitis.
- Rheumatoid arthritis.

Contraindications
- Local or systemic infection.
- Coagulopathy.

Step 1. Prepare the patient before the procedure
Mild sedation may be necessary in some patients. Obtain an intravenous access if drugs need to be administered.

Step 2. Positioning and monitoring the patient
1. Patient places hand palm down.
2. Monitoring of vital signs is mandatory in unstable patients.
3. The area for needle entry is prepared in a sterile fashion.

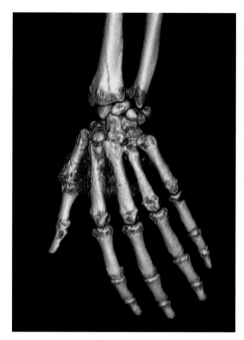

Figure 11.19 Anatomy of the wrist.

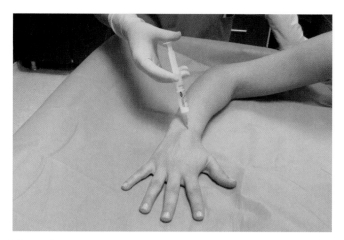

Figure 11.20 Wrist joint injection.

Step 3. Drugs and equipment for the wrist joint block
Prepare and confirm that the following equipment, needles, and drugs are ready to be used for the procedure:
- 1½ inch, 25 gauge needle for skin infiltration;
- 5 ml syringe containing local anesthetic solution;
- 22 G 3½ inch needle for the nerve block;
- 5 ml of 1% lidocaine;
- preferred steroid solution (decadron or equivalent).

Step 4. Anatomical landmark
Identify mid-carpus proximal to hollow dip of capitate.

Step 5. Direction of the needle
Direct the needle at the midpoint of carpus.

Step 6. Wrist joint injection
Inject 2–3 ml of 1% lidocaine with 20 mg of deposteroid solution at different points across the dorsum of the wrist both into the ligaments and into the capsule of the joint (Fig. 11.20).

Step 7. Postprocedural care
A splint is advised until the pain is relieved and the patient begins gentle exercises.

Complications

Serious complications do not occur. Pain at the injection site may last for a few days. The risk of infection is very low.

Injection technique for carpal tunnel syndrome

History

In 1854, Sir James Paget was the first to report median nerve compression at the wrist in a distal radius fracture. Carpal tunnel syndrome was most commonly noted in medical literature in the early 20th century but the first use of the term was noted in 1939. Dr George S. Phalen identified the pathology after working with a group of patients with carpal tunnel syndrome in the 1950s and 1960s.

Anatomy

The carpal tunnel is an anatomical compartment located at the base of the wrist. Nine flexor tendons and the median nerve pass through the carpal tunnel, which is surrounded on three sides by the carpal bones that form an arch. The nerve and the tendons provide function, feeling, and movement to some of the fingers. The finger and wrist flexor muscles, including their tendons, originate in the forearm at the medial epicondyle of the elbow joint and attach to the metaphalangeal, proximal interphalangeal, and distal interphalangeal bones of the fingers and thumb. The carpal tunnel is approximately as wide as the thumb and its boundary lies at the distal wrist skin crease and extends distally into the palm for approximately 2 cm.

The median nerve can be compressed by a decrease in the size of the canal, an increase in the size of the contents (such as the swelling of tissue around the flexor tendons), or both. Simply flexing the wrist to 90° will decrease the size of the canal.

Compression of the median nerve as it runs deep to the transverse carpal ligament causes atrophy of the thenar eminence, weakness of the flexor pollicis brevis, opponens pollicis, and abductor pollicis brevis, as well as sensory loss in the distribution of the median nerve distal to the transverse carpal ligament. There is a superficial sensory branch of the

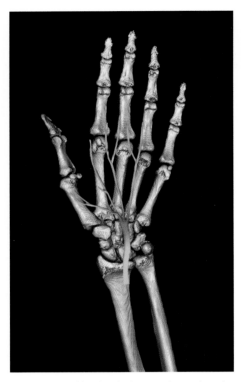

Figure 11.21 Anatomical landmarks for carpal tunnel syndrome.

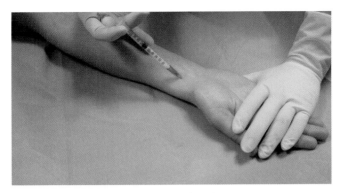

Figure 11.22 Injection for carpal tunnel syndrome.

Step 5. Direction of the needle
Advance the needle at 45° at the proximal wrist crease medial to the flexor carpi radialis tendon.

Step 6. Carpal tunnel injection
Slide distally until the needle point lies under the midpoint of the retinaculum. Parathesia in the median nerve is common. Inject 1 ml of 1% lidocaine together with 20 mg of deposteroid solution (Fig. 11.22).

Step 7. Postprocedural care
A night splint may be helpful after the injection for several days.

Complications
Pain at the injection site may last for a few days. The risk of infection is very low.

INJECTIONS INTO LOWER EXTREMITY JOINTS

Hip joint

Anatomy
The hip joint, anatomically called the acetabulofemoral joint, is the joint between the femur and acetabulum of the pelvic bone.

Articulation
The hip joint is a synovial joint formed by the articulation of the rounded head of the femur and the cup-like acetabulum of the pelvic bone. It forms the primary connection between the bones of the lower limb and the axial skeleton of the trunk and pelvis. Both joint surfaces are covered with a strong but lubricated layer called articular hyaline cartilage. The cup-like acetabulum forms at the union of three pelvic bones – the ilium, pubis, and ischium. The Y-shaped growth

median nerve, which branches proximal to the transverse carpal ligament and travels superficial to it. This branch is therefore spared, and it innervates the palm towards the thumb.

Patients with carpal tunnel syndrome experience numbness, tingling, or burning sensations in the thumb and fingers, particularly the index, middle, and radial half of the ring fingers, which are innervated by the median nerve. Less specific symptoms may include pain in the hands or wrists and loss of grip strength (both of which are more characteristic of painful conditions such as arthritis) (Fig. 11.21).

Indications
• Carpal tunnel syndrome.

Contraindications
• Local or systemic infection.
• Coagulopathy.

Injection for carpal tunnel syndromes
Steps 1, 2, and 3 are as explained in the section on the wrist joint, except that the hand palm is placed supine (vide supra).

Step 4. Surface landmark
Identify the flexor carpi radialis tendon lying on the radial side of the wrist by flexing the wrist against resistance.

plate that separates them, the triradiate cartilage, is fused definitively at ages 14–16. It is a special type of spheroidal or ball and socket joint where the roughly spherical femoral head is largely contained within the acetabulum and has an average radius of curvature of 2.5 cm. The acetabulum grasps almost half the femoral ball, a grip augmented by a ring-shaped fibrocartilaginous lip, the acetabular labrum, which extends the joint beyond the equator. The head of the femur is attached to the shaft by a thin neck region that is often prone to fracture in the elderly, which is mainly caused by the degenerative effects of osteoporosis (Fig. 11.23).

Indications
- Acute capsulitis.
- Osteoarthritis.
- Trauma.

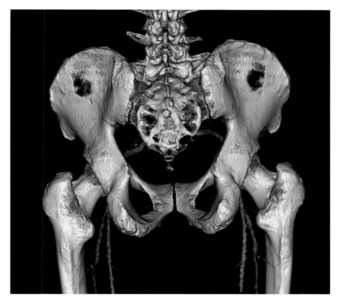

Figure 11.23 Anatomy of the hip joint.

Contraindications
- Local or systemic infection.
- Coagulopathy.
- Unstable joint.
- Intraarticular hip fracture.

Injection technique for hip joint

Step 1. Prepare the patient before the procedure
Type of analgesia or sedation needs to be ascertained before performance of the invasive procedure. Intravenous fentanyl or midazolam may be judiciously used for patient comfort.

Step 2. Positioning and monitoring the patient
1. The patient is placed in a supine position on the table.
2. Obtain an intravenous access if drugs need to be administered.
3. Monitoring of vital signs is mandatory in unstable patients.
4. The area for needle entry is prepared in a sterile fashion.

Step 3. Drugs and equipment for the block
Prepare and confirm that the following equipment, needles, and drugs are ready to be used for the procedure:
- 1½ inch, 25 gauge needle for skin infiltration;
- 5 ml syringe containing local anesthetic solution;
- 22 G 3½ inch needle for the nerve block;
- 5 ml of 1% lidocaine;
- preferred steroid solution (decadron or equivalent).

Step 4. Visualization
Place the C-arm in the lateral position, identify the greater trochanter and head of the femur (Fig. 11.24).

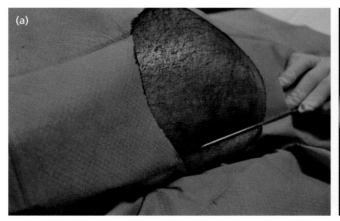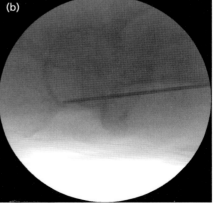

Figure 11.24 (a,b) Identify the greater trochanter and head of femur.

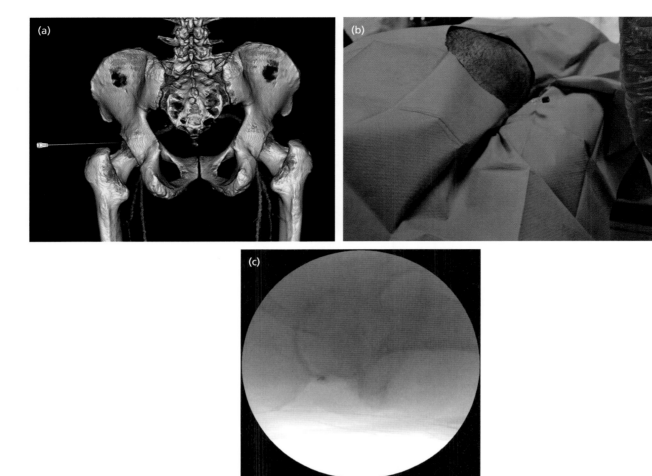

Figure 11.25 (a) Three-dimensional computed tomography scan showing the direction of the needle. (b) Direction of the needle. (c) Direction of the needle in tunneled vision.

Step 5. Direction of the needle

The entry site is immediately cephalad to the greater trochanter, at the mid-level of the anteroposterior dimension of the thigh. Advance the needle in "tunneled vision" until its tip enters the hip joint laterally at the junction of the femoral head and neck. Normally there will be no feeling of penetrating the capsule (Fig. 11.25).

Step 6. Confirm the position of the needle

Inject 1 ml of contrast material to verify the position of the needle. The contrast material should spread within the joint in a circumferential shape (Fig. 11.26).

Step 7. Hip joint injection

Inject 5–10 ml of 1% lidocaine together with 40 mg of depo-steroid solution.

Step 8. Postprocedural care

The patient should be advised not to do weight-bearing exercise.

Complications

1. Local complications.
   (a) Swelling.
   (b) Tenderness.
   (c) Infection.
   (d) Postinjection pain flare-up.
   (e) Soft-tissue atrophy.
   (f) Depigmentation.
   (g) Periarticular calcifications.
   (h) Tendon rupture.
2. Systemic complications.
   (a) Increase in blood glucose.
   (b) Abnormal uterine bleeding.
   (c) Alteration of taste.

Helpful hints

Hip joint injections should be performed under strict aseptic conditions to prevent the risk of infection. There is also potential for systemic effects of the steroids. It is recommended that only one joint be injected each time. The

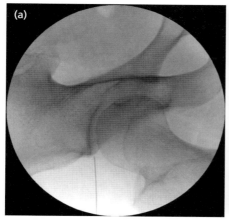
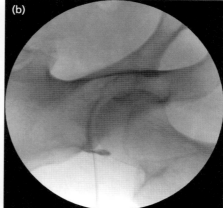

Figure 11.26 (a,b) Confirm the position of the needle.

patient should rest for a while to reduce the possibility of postinjection pain.

Injection technique for trochanteric bursa

Anatomy
The trochanteric bursa lies over the greater trochanter of the femur.

Indications
• Trochanteric bursitis.

Contraindications
• Local or systemic infection.
• Coagulopathy.
• Trochanteric bursa injection.
• Steps 1, 2, and 3 are as explained above (vide supra).

Step 4. Visualization
Place the C-arm in the PA position. Identify the great trochanter.

Step 5. Direction of the needle
1. After infiltrating the skin advance the needle in tunneled vision until a bony contact is made with the tip of the needle.
2. Gently slide the bone approximately 5 mm, without losing the contact with the bone.

Step 6. Confirm the position of the needle
Inject 1 ml of contrast material. It should be confined at the edge of the great trochanter.

Step 7. Trochanter bursa injection
Inject 2 ml of 1% lidocaine together with 20 mg of depo-steroid solution (Fig. 11.27).

Knee joint

Anatomy
The knee is a complex, compound, condyloid variety of a synovial joint. It actually comprises three functional compartments: the femoropatellar articulation consists of the patella, or "kneecap," and the patellar groove on the front of the femur through which it slides; and the medial and lateral femorotibial articulations linking the femur with the tibia. The joint is surrounded by synovial fluid, which is contained inside the synovial membrane called the joint capsule.

The articular bodies of the femur are its lateral and medial condyles. These diverge slightly distally and posteriorly, with the lateral condyle being wider in front than at the back whereas the medial condyle is of more constant width. The radius of the condyle's curvature in the sagittal plane becomes smaller toward the back. This diminishing radius produces a series of involute midpoints (i.e., located on a spiral). The resulting series of transverse axes allow the sliding and rolling motion in the flexing knee while ensuring the collateral ligaments are sufficiently lax to allow the rotation associated with the curvature of the medial condyle about a vertical axis.

The pair of tibial condyles are separated by the intercondylar eminence composed of a lateral and a medial tubercle.

The patella is inserted into the thin anterior wall of the joint capsule. On its posterior surface is a lateral and a medial articular surface, both of which communicate with the patellar surface which unites the two femoral condyles on the anterior side of the bone's distal end. The articular capsule has a synovial and a fibrous membrane separated by fatty deposits. Anteriorly, the synovial membrane is attached on the margin of the cartilage both on the femur and the

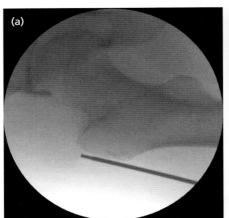
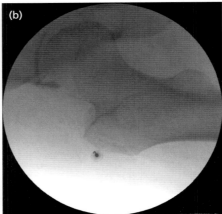
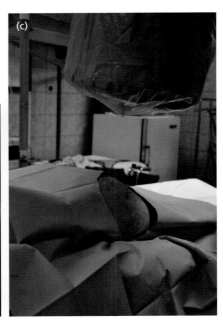

Figure 11.27 (a–c) Trochanteric bursa injection.

tibia; but on the femur, the suprapatellar bursa or recess extends the joint space proximally. The suprapatellar bursa is prevented from being pinched during extension by the articularis genu muscle. Behind, the synovial membrane is attached to the margins of the two femoral condyles, which produces two extensions similar to the anterior recess. Between these two extensions, the synovial membrane passes in front of the two cruciate ligaments at the center of the joint, thus forming a pocket. Numerous bursae surround the knee joint. The largest communicative bursa is the suprapatellar bursa (described above). Four considerably smaller bursae are located on the back of the knee. Two noncommunicative bursae are located in front of the patella and below the patellar tendon, and others are sometimes present.

Cartilage is a thin, elastic tissue that protects the bone and makes certain that the joint surfaces can slide easily over each other. Cartilage ensures supple knee movement. There are two types of joint cartilage in the knees: fibrous cartilage (the meniscus) and hyaline cartilage. Fibrous cartilage has tensile strength and can resist pressure. Hyaline cartilage covers the surface along which the joints move. Cartilage will wear over the years. Cartilage has a very limited capacity for self-restoration. The newly formed tissue will generally consist in large part of fibrous cartilage of lesser quality than the original hyaline cartilage. As a result, new cracks and tears will form in the cartilage over time.

Menisci

The articular discs of the knee joint are called menisci because they only partly divide the joint space. These two discs, the medial meniscus and the lateral meniscus, consist of connective tissue with extensive collagen fibers containing cartilage-like cells. Strong fibers run along the menisci from one attachment to the other, whereas weaker radial fibers are interlaced with the former. The menisci are flattened at the center of the knee joint, fused with the synovial membrane laterally, and can move over the tibial surface.

The menisci serve to protect the ends of the bones from rubbing on each other and effectively to deepen the tibial sockets into which the femur attaches. They also play a role in shock absorption, and may be cracked, or torn, when the knee is forcefully rotated and/or bent.

Ligaments

The knee is stabilized by a pair of cruciate ligaments. The anterior cruciate ligament (ACL) stretches from the lateral condyle of the femur to the anterior intercondylar area. The ACL is critically important because it prevents the tibia from being pushed too far anterior relative to the femur. It is often torn during twisting or bending of the knee. The posterior cruciate ligament (PCL) stretches from the medial condyle of the femur to the posterior intercondylar area. Injury to this ligament is uncommon but can occur as a direct result of forced trauma to the ligament. This ligament prevents posterior displacement of the tibia relative to the femur.

The transverse ligament stretches from the lateral meniscus to the medial meniscus. It passes in front of the menisci. It is divided into several strips in 10% of cases. The two menisci are attached to each other anteriorly by the ligament. The posterior and anterior meniscofemoral ligaments stretch from the posterior horn of the lateral meniscus to

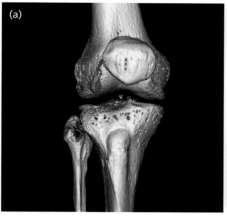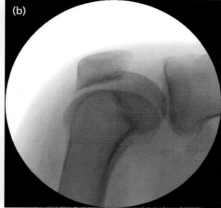

Figure 11.28 (a,b) The anatomy of knee joint. Three-dimensional computed tomography scan and lateral view of the knee in plain radiography.

the medial femoral condyle. They pass posteriorly behind the posterior cruciate ligament. The posterior meniscofemoral ligament is more commonly present (30%); both ligaments are present less often. The meniscotibial ligaments (or "coronary") stretches from the inferior edges of the mensici to the periphery of the tibial plateaus.

Extracapsular ligaments

The patellar ligament connects the patella to the tuberosity of the tibia. It is also occasionally called the patellar tendon because there is no definite separation between the quadriceps tendon (which surrounds the patella) and the area connecting the patella to the tibia. This very strong ligament helps give the patella its mechanical leverage and functions as a cap for the condyles of the femur. Laterally and medially to the patellar ligament, the lateral and medial patellar retinacula connect fibers from the vasti lateralis and medialis muscles to the tibia. Some fibers from the iliotibial tract radiate into the lateral retinaculum, and the medial retinaculum receives some transverse fibers arising on the medial femoral epicondyle.

The medial collateral ligament (also known as the "tibial") stretches from the medial epicondyle of the femur to the medial tibial condyle. It is composed of three groups of fibers, one stretching between the two bones, and two fused with the medial meniscus. The medial collateral ligament is partly covered by the pes anserinus, and the tendon of the semimembranosus passes under it. It protects the medial side of the knee from being bent open by a stress applied to the lateral side of the knee (a valgus force). The lateral collateral ligament (also known as the "fibular") stretches from the lateral epicondyle of the femur to the head of fibula. It is separate from both the joint capsule and the lateral meniscus. It protects the lateral side from an inside bending force (a varus force).

Lastly, there are two ligaments on the dorsal side of the knee. The oblique popliteal ligament is a radiation of the tendon of the semimembranosus on the medial side, from where it is directed laterally and proximally. The arcuate popliteal ligament originates on the apex of the head of the fibula to stretch proximally, crosses the tendon of the popliteus muscle, and passes into the capsule (Fig. 11.28).

Indications
- Osteoarthritis.
- Rheumatoid arthritis.
- Trauma.
- Miscellaneous degenerative and inflammatory conditions of the knee.

Contraindications
- Local or systemic infection.
- Coagulopathy.

Step 1. Prepare the patient before the procedure
Mild sedation may be necessary in some patients. Obtain an intravenous access if drugs need to be administered.

Step 2. Positioning and monitoring the patient
1. Patient sits with the knee in flexion.
2. Monitoring of vital signs is mandatory in unstable patients.
3. The area for needle entry is prepared in a sterile fashion.

Step 3. Drugs and equipment for the knee joint block
Prepare and confirm that the following equipment, needles, and drugs are ready to be used for the procedure:
- 1½ inch, 25 gauge needle for skin infiltration;
- 5 ml syringe containing local anesthetic solution;
- 22 G 3½ inch needle for the nerve block;
- 5 ml of 1% lidocaine;
- preferred steroid solution (decadron or equivalent);
- hyaluronic acid (synvyst or orthovyst).

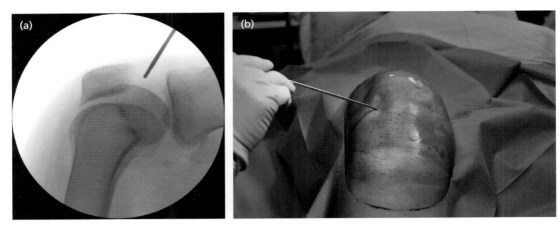

Figure 11.29 (a,b) Identify the medial edge of the patella.

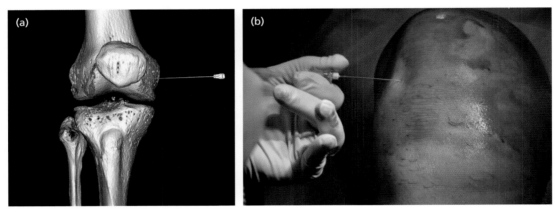

Figure 11.30 (a,b) Direction of the needle for knee joint injection.

Step 4. Visualization
Place the C-arm in the lateral position, identify the patella fluoroscopically in this view (Fig. 11.29).

Step 5. Surface landmark
Place the thumb on the lateral side of the relaxed patella and push medially.

Identify the medial edge of the patella while maintaining the position with the thumb.

Step 6. Direction of the needle
Insert the needle horizontally at the midpoint of the medial edge of the patella between it and the femoral condyle and slide under patella (Fig. 11.30).

Step 7. Confirm the position of the needle
First aspirate to see if there is effusion within the joint. Then inject 2 ml of contrast solution, and view the spread of the contrast material within the joint (Fig. 11.31).

Step 8. Knee joint injection
Inject 2 ml of hyalorunic acid with or without 5 ml of 1% lidocaine together with 20 mg of deposteroid solution.

Step 9. Postprocedural care
Apply icepack for 10 minutes after the injection. The patient should avoid undue weight-bearing activity for one week, then strengthening and mobilizing exercises should be advised.

Ankle joint

Anatomy
The ankle, or talocrural joint, is a synovial hinge joint that connects the distal ends of the tibia and fibula in the lower limb with the proximal end of the talus bone in the foot. The articulation between the tibia and the talus bears greater

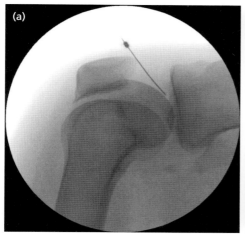 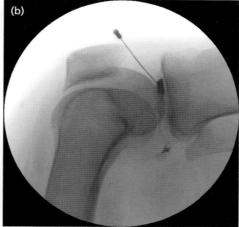

Figure 11.31 (a,b) Direction of the needle within the knee joint, and confirming the position by contrast material.

weight than the articulation between the fibula and the talus.

Tarsal bones consist of the talus, calcaneus, navicular, cuboid, medial or internal cuneiform, middle cuneiform, and lateral or external cuneiform.

The lateral malleolus of the fibula and the medial malleolus of the tibia along with the inferior surface of the distal tibia articulate with three facets of the talus. These surfaces are covered by cartilage. The anterior talus is wider than the posterior talus. When the foot is dorsiflexed, the wider part of the superior talus moves into the articulating surfaces of the tibia and fibula, creating a more stable joint than when the foot is plantar flexed.

The ankle joint is bound by the strong deltoid ligament and three lateral ligaments: the anterior talofibular ligament, the posterior talofibular ligament, and the calcaneofibular ligament. The deltoid ligament supports the medial side of the joint, is attached at the medial malleolus of the tibia, and connects in four places to the sustentaculum tali of the calcaneus, calcaneonavicular ligament, the navicular tuberosity, and to the medial surface of the talus. The anterior and posterior talofibular ligaments support the lateral side of the joint from the lateral malleolus of the fibula to the dorsal and ventral ends of the talus. The calcaneofibular ligament is attached at the lateral malleolus and to the lateral surface of the calcaneus.

The joint is most stable in dorsiflexion and a sprained ankle is more likely to occur when the foot is plantar flexed. This type of injury occurs more frequently at the anterior talofibular ligament, which is also the most commonly injured ligament during inversion sprains (Fig. 11.32).

Indications
- Acute capsulitis due to trauma.
- Chronic capsulitis.
- Traumatic injuries to the ankle.

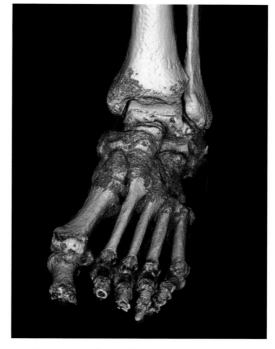

Figure 11.32 Anatomy of the ankle joint.

Contraindications
- Local or systemic infection.
- Coagulopathy.

Injection technique for ankle joint

Step 1. Prepare the patient before the procedure
Mild sedation may be necessary in some patients. Obtain an intravenous access if drugs need to be administered.

Step 2. Positioning and monitoring the patient
1. Patient lies with foot supported in neutral position.
2. Monitoring of vital signs is mandatory in unstable patients.
3. The area for needle entry is prepared in a sterile fashion.

Step 3. Drugs and equipment for the ankle joint injection
Prepare and confirm that the following equipment, needles, and drugs are ready to be used for the procedure:
- 1½ inch, 25 gauge needle for skin infiltration;
- 5 ml syringe containing local anesthetic solution;
- 22 G 3½ inch needle for the nerve block;
- 5 ml of 1% lidocaine;
- preferred steroid solution (decadron or equivalent).

Step 4. Surface landmark for needle entry
Palpate the small triangular space at the junction of the tibia and fibula just above the talus.

Step 5. Direction of the needle
Inject directly into the capsule (Fig. 11.33).

Step 6. Ankle joint injection
Inject 2 ml of 1% lidocaine together with 20 mg deposteroid solution.

Step 7. Postprocedural care
Apply icepack after the injection for 10 minutes. The patient should avoid excessive weight-bearing activities for a week.

Complications
The patient may feel transient pain at the site of injection for a week.

INJECTIONS INTO MYOFASCIAL TRIGGER POINTS

History
Myofascial trigger point injection is a form of soft tissue therapy for somatic dysfunction and resulting pain and restriction of motion. In pain management literature, the term myofascial pain was historically used by Janet Travell, in the 1940s. She was referring to musculoskeletal pain syndromes and trigger points. Travell further used the term "myofascial trigger point" and later published the reference book *Myofascial Pain & Dysfunction: The Trigger Point Manual*. Some clinicians use the term "myofascial therapy" or "myofascial trigger point therapy" to refer to the treatment of trigger points. The phrase has also been loosely used for different manual therapy techniques, including soft tissue manipulation.

Common pain syndromes that cause trigger or tender points in the muscles are myofascial pain syndromes and fibromyalgia.

Myofascial pain syndromes
Myofascial pain syndrome (MPS) is defined as a musculoskeletal pain disorder caused by one or more myofascial trigger points (TPs) and their associated reflexes. MPS typically involves myofascial TPs found within the belly muscle of one or more muscles or muscle groups, but they can also be found in ligaments, periosteum, scar tissue, skin, and tendons. MPS may be the most common cause of persistent musculoskeletal pain, including chronic low back, head, neck, and shoulder pain. This syndrome is also associated with other chronic pain conditions, such as osteoarthritis, rheumatoid arthritis, migraine, and tension-type headaches, complex regional pain syndrome, and whiplash-associated disorders. MPS can be primary (unrelated to medical condi-

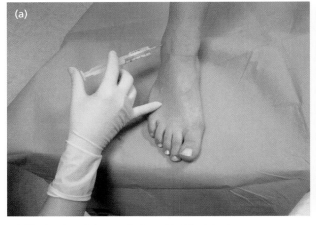
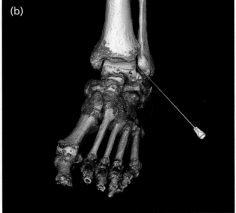

Figure 11.33 (a,b) Direction of the needle for ankle joint injection.

Table 11.1 Comparison of MPS and fibromyalgia

Myofascial pain syndrome	Fibromyalgia
Pain symptoms: acute or chronic; localized or regional distribution directly associated with TP; referred in nature.	Pain symptoms: chronic (present 3+ months); generalized and widespread distribution involving several anatomic sites; migratory in nature.
Systemic symptoms: seldom reported.	Systemic symptoms: frequently reported (including depression, irritable bowel, sleep disruption, and fatigue).
Origin: acute onset from trauma or repetitive injuries.	Origin: insidious onset rarely involving an inciting event.
Trigger points: present with one or more zones of reference. Exhibit palpable local twitch response, referred pain, and taut bands of skeletal muscle.	Trigger points: absent.
Tender points: absent.	Tender points: present in 11 or more of 18 paired tender point sites. Do not exhibit palpable local twitch response, referred pain, and taut bands of skeletal muscle.
Range of motion: restricted.	Range of motion: increased.
Response to TP injection: immediate and amenable.	Response to therapy: poor.

tion) or secondary (related to other medical conditions) in origin, and determining which is vital to proper treatment. Trauma (direct and indirect) and repetitive muscle strain are common causes of MPS.

Fibromyalgia will not be described here but the differences between it and MPS are described below

Differences between MPS and fibromyalgia

Although MPS and fibromyalgia have similar symptoms, they should be considered separately. In MPS taut bands are palpated whereas in fibromyalgia the pain is more diffuse. MPS has an acute characteristic whereas fibromyalgia is more chronic. The number of TPs is much less in MPS and, according to the previous criteria, there should be at least 11 TPs in fibromyalgia. Fatigue and sleeping disorders and irritable colon are more common in fibromyalgia. The differences are described in Table 11.1.

Epidemiology

An estimated 44 million Americans suffer from myofascial pain and MPS may account for 30–93% of the patients presenting with musculoskeletal pain at general medical clinics and specialty pain management centers. Pain specialties continue to recognize MPS as being clinically useful. Women are significantly more likely to suffer from myofascial TPs than men. Epidemiological studies have shown that women aged 30–49 are more likely to exhibit myofascial TPs. Sedentary workers appear more likely to develop myofascial TPs than laborers. Studies suggest that MPS is the most common cause of chronic low-back pain, with 60–97% of patients examined exhibiting myofascial abnormalities. This high prevalence of MPS indicates the need for a proper diagnostic approach when examining a patient suffering from low-back pain with no identifiable organic cause to avoid misdiagnosis.

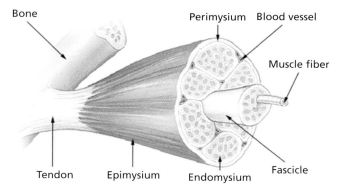

Figure 11.34 Structure of the skeletal muscle.

Anatomy

Because TPs are the hallmark of MPS and they are found in skeletal muscle, it is essential that the structure and function of the muscle should be understood. The structure of skeletal muscle is shown in Figs 11.34–11.37.

The skeletal muscle is formed by muscle sheaths, annulospiral endings, a nuclear bag, motor end plates, and intrafusal fibers.

The muscle sheath is a connective tissue capsule that surrounds the intrafusal muscle fibers of the spindle.

The annulospiral endings are also known as nuclear bag endings. They are large axons with many branches and terminal enlargements. Arborization of this type of ending occurs around the nucleus of intrafusal muscle fibers. These endings have a low threshold to stretch reflex exit action. They discharge when the intrafusal muscle fibers are stretched. The receptors are silent when the extrafusal muscle fibers contract and the intrafusal fibers are relaxed.

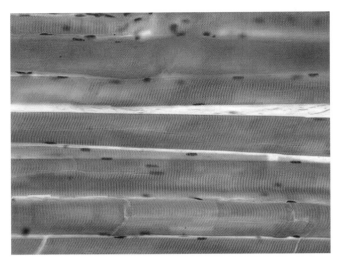

Figure 11.35 Motor end plate, subneural apparatus.

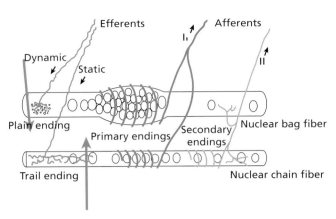

Figure 11.37 Muscle spindle structure and innervation.

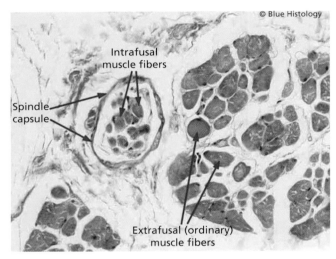

Figure 11.36 Neuromuscular spindle.

Central processes of the annulospiral endings originate in the spinal cord and participate in the monosynaptic (myotatic) reflex.

Nuclear bag muscle fibers are a larger variety of intrafusal muscle fibers. They are enlarged equatorial regions to accommodate numerous small nuclei. It is here that annulospiral endings arborize.

The smaller nerve fibers within the spindle are axons of gamma neurons in the spinal cord. The axons terminate as typical motor end plates on intrafusal muscle fibers.

Intrafusal muscle fibers are small striated muscle fibers rich in sarcoplasm and arranged parallel to the extrafusal skeletal muscle fibers.

Pathophysiology of TPs

TPs are small (2–5 mm in diameter) nodules of hypersensitivity located in taut, "rope-like" bands of skeletal muscle that are detectable through palpatory examination. Palpation of myofascial TPs will produce or increase a referred, radiating pain pattern recognizable by the patient. Pain will be referred to distal or proximal locations. In the "zone of reference," which is the specific region of referred pain, the patient will experience deep pain that ranges in intensity from a dull ache to being severe and incapacitating. Myofascial TPs are clinically defined by their motor and sensory characteristics. "Snapping" palpation or needling of a myofascial TP may provoke an involuntary twitch in the muscle and/or skin. More commonly, the patient will flinch away from the palpation in a reaction known as the "jump sign." Verbalization may accompany the jump sign. Myofascial TP activation may evoke autonomic phenomena, including coryza, dermal flushing, lacrimation, sweating, vasoconstriction (blanching), and temperature changes. Several histopathological mechanisms to TP development have been suggested. Muscle overload, acute trauma, and microtrauma are generally agreed to be the most likely causes of myofascial TP development. Other causes may include muscle deficiency, joint dysfunction, sleep disorders, postural dysfunction, systemic influences, and neurological influences. The most common cause of TP formation is occupational and recreational activity that produces repetitive stress on one or muscles or muscle groups. In the low back, myofascial TP formation may occur owing to "structural inadequacies," such as small hemi-pelvis, short leg or arm, and short first and long second metatarsal bones (Fig. 11.38).

Classification of TPs

Depending on the clinical characteristics, the TP can be classified as either **active** or **latent. Active myofascial TPs**

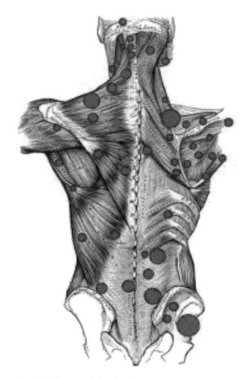

Figure 11.38 TPs all around the body.

Table 11.2 Clinical characteristics of myofascial TPs
Focal exquisite spot tenderness of a nodule in a taut band.
Painful restriction to range of motion.
Patient's recognition of current pain complaint by pressure on the tender nodule (identifies as a TP).
Referred pain to a regional site upon TP activation.
Reproducibility of pain complaints.
Presence of taut band.
Visual or tactile identification of local twitch response on TP activation.
Pain or altered sensation on compression of tender nodule.
Muscle weakness without muscle atrophy.
Jump sign symptoms of autonomic dysfunction (e.g., sweating, localized vasoconstriction, pilomotor activity, etc.).

are associated with a clinical pain complaint and remain symptomatic and painful, even at rest. Taut fibers within a palpable, "rope-like" band will be present in the muscle or muscle group. TPs can be found at the "spot of maximum tenderness" along the taut band. Palpation of active TPs produces local or referred pain (or both) in a predictable pattern specific to the involved muscle or muscle group. Pain will be described as "spreading" or "radiating" and reproduces the patient's pain complaint. The jump sign and local twitch response will also be present. There can be a reduction in range of motion and strength, as well as autonomic phenomena (Table 11.2).

Latent myofascial TPs are not associated with spontaneous pain, but are tender to palpation. They can be inactive for years, precipitated by previous muscular injury. Muscle shortening and weakness, stiffness, and restricted range of motion are present with latent TPs. Unlike active TPs, latent TPs usually do not require treatment unless activated by mechanical overload, stress, and prolonged muscle shortening.

Evaluation of patients for injections into TPs

Before one performs TP injections, it is essential that the patient should be properly evaluated with a correct diagnosis. This process starts with history followed by physical examination and laboratory tests specific for MPS.

History

An evaluation should begin with the patient's complete personal and family history, including medical and surgical history. The practitioner should focus the inquiries around three key points: characteristics of pain, history of onset, and possible contributing causes. Patients should describe the pain's nature (constancy, type, sources of relief, reaction to activity and rest). Illustrating the patient's pain pattern(s) is vital to proper diagnosis of MPS and, therefore, it is strongly indicated that the patient draw their pain pattern on a body form. This illustration should also show the location of different sensations, such as ache, needles, and numbness.

Physical examination

In clinical practice, myofascial pain is diagnosed by a thorough physical examination with an adequate medical history. Depending on the clinical presentation, it may be reasonable to check for indicators of inflammation, assess thyroid function, and perform a basic metabolic panel to rule out a concomitant medical illness.

The physical examination should begin with a general observation of the patient to determine any abnormalities in algometry, gait, muscle strength, muscle tension, posture, or range of motion, specifically in the trunk, thighs, and legs. Denervation, muscle weakness, and restricted range of motion may indicate the presence of myofascial TPs in affected muscles or muscle groups. This visual evaluation is then followed by a physical and systematic search for myofascial TPs through palpation. Previously acquired information about the patient's pain patterns will help in this search by determining which muscles and muscle groups should be examined. Myofascial TPs commonly appear in muscular structures used for posture maintenance. In the instance of low-back pain, specific muscles have been identified as containing myofascial TPs, each exhibiting common pain patterns. Of these, the quadratus lumborum, used for trunk stabilization and posture, is the most common source of myofascial pain, but is also the most overlooked. Myofascial TPs involving the piriformis, the posterior superior iliac spine, the iliac crest, and the posterior sacroiliac line are other common sources of low-back pain.

The patient should be positioned so that the back, buttocks, and thigh muscles are relaxed. If the muscle is tense or in spasm, the physician must wait before proceeding as myofascial TPs cannot be detected during this time. Palpation should begin in the region of suspected TPs, using the flat, pincer, or deep (probing) techniques. Probing palpation is indicated for the evaluation of myofascial low-back pain due to the deep nature of the muscles typically involved (e.g., piriformis and quadratus lumborum). Flat palpation may be used for more superficial muscles. The physician forcefully and deeply palpates the muscle and surrounding area with their fingertip, thumb tip, or a blunt object (3–5 mm in diameter) and compares it with the contralateral muscle. They should also take notice of any autonomic and/or proprioceptive symptoms, such as sweating and temperature variance, in these areas. Affected muscles will contain taut fibers formed in a band among normally pliable fibers. Further palpation is then conducted along the length of the taut band(s) to locate the active myofascial TPs, which are tiny, hyperirritable knots or nodules. The patient will report pain when the myofascial TP is touched, and possibly react physically and/or verbally (jump sign). The local twitch response in the muscle or skin may be elicited by briskly rolling the taut band beneath the finger to cause a sudden pressure change. The recognizable pain will be local and/or be referred to another location, and reproduce the original pain complaint. The physician should then repeat this process until they have examined the patient thoroughly to determine if the low-back MPS is simple (single muscle involvement) or complex (multi-muscle involvement) in origin. It is important to remember that different muscles overlap and, therefore, must be examined to obtain a proper diagnosis of MPS.

Additionally, it is not uncommon that the physician may unintentionally locate latent myofascial TPs during a palpatory examination. Latent myofascial TPs can exhibit tenderness, as well as demonstrate local twitch response. The patient may be unaware of their existence, despite muscle shortening and weakness. The location of all latent myofascial TPs should be noted for later treatment.

The suspected myofascial TPs, active and latent, are marked with a skin pencil for subsequent quantification. Quantification of the myofascial TPs is conducted with a pressure threshold measurement gauge and/or thermography. This will allow the physician to locate the exact location of the point of greatest sensitivity (i.e., the myofascial TP). This will provide the physician with an objective measure for diagnostic, treatment, and medicolegal purposes. It should be noted that latent myofascial TPs will exhibit a lower pressure pain threshold than active TPs (Table 11.3).

Table 11.3 Trigger points versus tender points. Reproduced from Alvarez and Rockwell (2002) with permission from American Academy of Family Physicians

Trigger points	Tender points
Local tenderness, taut band, local twitch response, jump sign	Local tenderness
Singular or multiple	Multiple
May occur in any skeletal muscle	Occur in specific locations that are symmetrically located
May cause a specific referred pain pattern	Do not cause referred pain, but often cause a total body increase in pain sensitivity

Laboratory studies

Myofascial pain traditionally does not produce abnormalities in the results of the patient's laboratory work. Travell and Simons (1983) describe a study looking at lactate dehydrogenase (LDH) isoenzymes. A shift may be noted in distribution of the isoenzymes, with higher levels of LDH1 and LDH2, whereas the total LDH may remain within normal limits.

Imaging studies

Imaging studies often reveal nonspecific change only, and typically are not helpful in making the diagnosis of cervical myofascial pain; however, radiographs and a magnetic resonance imaging (MRI) scan of the cervical spine may be helpful in ruling out other pathology that may be present at the same time.

Other tests

Several research articles have attempted to identify changes on electromyograms/nerve conduction velocity studies that may be unique to patients with myofascial pain. The research has been somewhat contradictory, with some studies finding no real electromyographic activity and others finding nonspecific electrical activity. Studies by Simons et al. (1999) and by Hubbard and Berkoff (1993) described low-amplitude action potentials recorded at the region of the myofascial TP. Spontaneous electrical activity apparently can be detected using high-sensitivity recordings at the site of the TP. The spontaneous electrical activity may be a type of endplate potential.

Causes of MPS TPs

Cervical myofascial pain is thought to occur after either overuse or trauma to the muscles that support the shoulders and neck. Common situations are that the patient was recently involved in a motor vehicle accident or that they performed repetitive upper extremity activities. Trapezial myofascial pain commonly occurs when a person with a desk job does not have appropriate armrests or must type on a keyboard that is too high. Other issues that may play

(a)

(b)

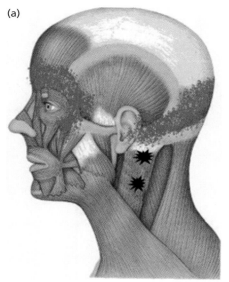
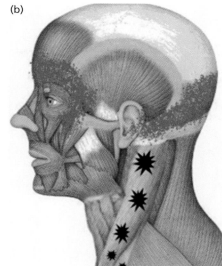

Figure 11.39 (a,b) TPs on the sternocleidomastoid muscle.

a role in the clinical picture include endocrine dysfunction, chronic infections, nutritional deficiencies, poor posture, and psychological problems.

The most frequently seen TPs are in the head and neck. They will be described here as superficial or deep trigger points.

Sternocleidomastoid muscle (Fig. 11.39)

The sternocleidomastoid muscle has sternal and clavicular divisions and contains multiple TPs on both. The sternal division may refer pain to the vertex, occiput, across the cheek, over the eye, to the throat and sternum. The clavicular portion may refer pain to the frontal part of the head and ear.

Referred autonomic symptoms from the sternal division involve the eye and sinuses, while from the clavicular division, proprioceptive dizziness related to the posture and disturbed equilibrium may develop.

Examination of TPs may be performed by turning the head to the opposite side, so that the sternocleidomastoid muscle becomes more prominent

Trapezius muscle (Fig. 11.40)

The trapezius muscle extends in the midline from the occiput to T12 and reaches laterally to the clavicle, to the acromion, and to the spine of the scapula behind.

The trapezius is tripartite, comprising the upper, middle, and lower trapezius. The referred pain arises in the upper trapezius fibers along the posterolateral aspect of the neck, behind the ear and to the temple. Trigger points in the lower trapezius muscle refer to the neck, suprascapular and interscapular regions. The middle trapezius TPs refer pain toward the vertebra and to the interscapular region.

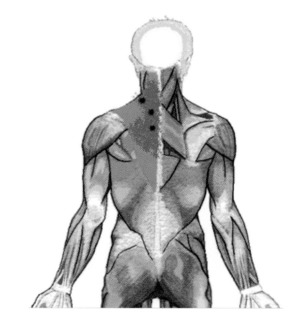

Figure 11.40 TPs on the trapezius muscle.

To approach the upper trapezius TPs, the patient should lie supine, whereas the other trapezius TPs are approached from behind with the patient lying on the opposite side.

Levator scapulae (Fig. 11.41)

The levator scapulae muscle is one of the main causes of "stiff neck." The muscle attaches to the transverse processes of the first four cervical vertebrae above and to the superior angle of the scapula below.

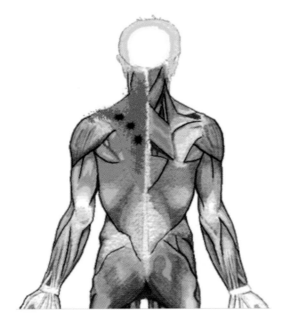

Figure 11.41 TPs on the levator scapulae muscle.

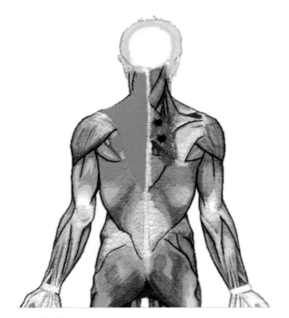

Figure 11.42 TPs on the rhomboid major and minor muscles.

Referred pain from the levator scapulae radiates to the angle of the neck and along the vertebral border of the scapula. It may also project to an area posterior to the shoulder joint.

The patient restricts the neck rotation. The first TP is beneath the trapezius at the angle of the neck. It may be difficult to locate the second TP, which is just above the angle of the scapula.

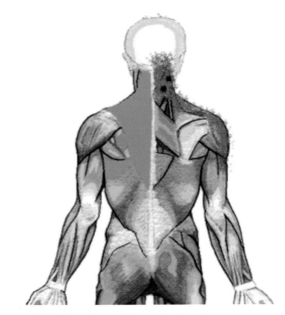

Figure 11.43 TPs on the posterior cervical muscles.

Rhomboideus major and minor muscles (Fig. 11.42)

TPs on the rhomboideus major and minor muscles cause superficial backache and shoulder pain. Referred pain from the rhomboid muscles radiates to the vertebral border of the scapula and extends over the supraspinous area of the scapula. The TPs are medial to the vertebral border of the scapula.

Posterior cervical muscles (Fig. 11.43)

The muscles of the back of the neck are the semispinalis capitis, semispinalis cervices, longissimus capitis, and the multifidus, rotatores, and small sub-occipital muscles which connect the occiput with the first two cervical vertebrae.

Referred pain from these TPs radiates at the C4, C5 level, travels strongly upward to the sub-occipital region and downward over the neck and the posterior occiput. There is a marked restriction of the head and neck flexion, and less severe restriction of the extension and rotation of the head and neck.

During injection of the TP, one should be careful to avoid inadvertent injection into the vertebral artery.

Thoracolumbar paraspinal muscles (Fig. 11.44)

The paraspinal musculature consists of a superficial group of long fibered longitudinal muscles and a deep group of short diagonal muscles. In the superficial group, the longissimus thoracis, iliocostalis thoracic, and iliocostalis lumborum are the most significant muscles having TPs. The deep paraspinal group includes the semispinalis, multifidus, and rotatores.

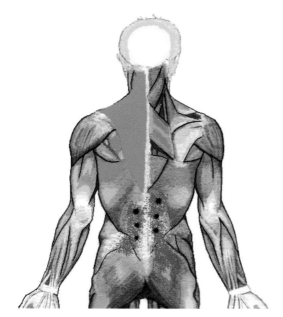

Figure 11.44 TPs on thoracolumbar paraspinal muscles.

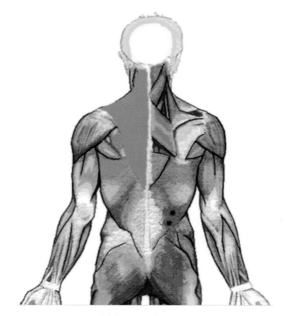

Figure 11.45 TPs on multifidus muscle.

The pain due to TPs in the iliocostalis thoracic is projected laterally across the back of the chest, as well as anteriorly in the abdomen and up toward the back of the shoulder. The lumbar iliocostalis TPs refer pain to the mid-buttock. TPs in the longissimus thoracic muscle at the low thoracic and high lumbar levels also refer pain downward to the sacroiliac region and the buttock. The TPs are at the level of first lumbar vertebra.

Multifidus muscle (Fig. 11.45)

Pain from the multifidus and rotatores muscles centers on the spinous processes at the segmental level of the TP or in the lumbar region, and may be referred to a few caudal segments.

Trigger points on the multifidus muscle are located on the L2, S1, and S2 levels (Fig. 11.45).

One should be careful not to go to deep to cause inadvertent dural puncture at these levels.

Indications

Myofascial TPs in different regions of the body.
- Myofascial pain caused by the following:
  ◦ arthritis;
  ◦ trauma;
  ◦ muscle cramps;
  ◦ acute or chronic muscle strain;
  ◦ soft tissue pain of nonneurogenic origin.

Contraindications
- Local or systemic infection.
- Coagulopathy.

Injection technique for TPs

Step 1. Prepare the patient before the procedure
Increased bleeding tendencies should be explored before injection. Capillary hemorrhage augments postinjection soreness and leads to unsightly ecchymosis. Patients should refrain from daily aspirin dosing for at least 3 days before injection to avoid increased bleeding.

Step 2. Position and monitor the patient
1. Positioning depends on the site of the TP.
2. The patient may either sit, lie supine, or lie prone.
3. Prepare and drape the area in a sterile fashion.

Step 3. Drugs and equipment for TP injections
- 1½ inch, 25 gauge needle for skin infiltration;
- 5 ml syringe for local anesthesia;
- 10 ml syringe for muscle injection;
- 1½–3 inch needles;
- 5 ml lidocaine;
- 40 mg methylprednisolone.
Drugs commonly used include the following.
- Local anesthetics are the most frequent agents used for TP injection. One should not inject more than 1 ml of local anesthetic for each TP.
- Corticosteroids should be used if there is a local inflammation around the area. Corticosteroids may cause myotoxicity.
- Botulinum toxin A or B may be preferred to prolong the effect. A nerve stimulator has to be used and the physician should seek where the motor contraction of the muscle is

the highest. The dose should not exceed 200 units for TP injections.

Step 4. Injection technique for TPs
1. Palpate the TP in the taut band, and place the muscle in a slightly stretched position to prevent it from moving (Fig. 11.46).

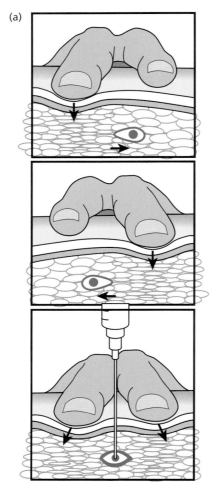

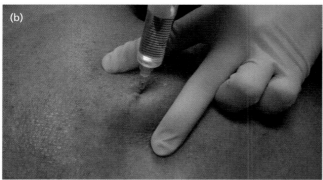

Figure 11.46 (a,b) Palpating the TP and injection.

2. Once a TP has been located and the overlying skin has been cleansed with alcohol, the clinician isolates that point with a pinch between the thumb and index finger or between the index and middle finger, whichever is most comfortable.

Step 5. Needle insertion
1. Using sterile technique, the needle is then inserted 1–2 cm away from the TP so that the needle may be advanced into the TP at an acute angle of 30° to the skin. The stabilizing fingers apply pressure on either side of the injection site, ensuring adequate tension of the muscle fibers to allow penetration of the TP but preventing it from rolling away from the advancing needle. The application of pressure also helps to prevent bleeding within the subcutaneous tissues and the subsequent irritation to the muscle that the bleeding may produce.
2. Before advancing the needle into the TP, the physician should warn the patient of the possibility of sharp pain, muscle twitching, or an unpleasant sensation as the needle contacts the taut muscular band. To ensure that the needle is not within a blood vessel, the plunger should be withdrawn before injection (Fig. 11.47).

Step 6. Inject local anesthetic and/or steroids or other drugs
1. A small amount (0.2 ml) of anesthetic should be injected once the needle is inside the TP. The needle is then withdrawn to the level of the subcutaneous tissue, and redirected superiorly, inferiorly, laterally, and medially, repeating the needling and injection process in each direction until the local twitch response is no longer elicited or resisting muscle tautness is no longer perceived.

Step 7. Postinjection management
After injection, the area should be palpated to ensure that no other tender points exist. If additional tender points are palpable, they should be isolated, needled, and injected. Pressure is then applied to the injected area for 2 minutes

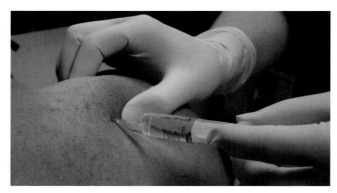

Figure 11.47 TP injection.

to promote hemostasis. A simple adhesive bandage is usually adequate for skin coverage.

One study emphasizes that stretching the affected muscle group immediately after injection further increases the efficacy of TP therapy. Travell and Simons (1983) recommend that this be best performed by immediately having the patient actively move each injected muscle through its full range of motion three times, reaching its fully shortened and its fully lengthened position during each cycle.

Complications
Increased pain in area of injection.
Infection.
Hematoma in the muscles.
Fever, weakness in the muscles, chilling sensation: these appear when botulinum toxin is injected.
Postinjection soreness is to be expected in most cases, and the patient's stated relief of the referred pain pattern notes the success of the injection. Reevaluation of the injected areas may be necessary, but reinjection of the TPs is not recommended until the postinjection soreness resolves, usually after 3–4 days. Repeated injections in a particular muscle are not recommended if two or three previous attempts have been unsuccessful. Patients are encouraged to remain active, putting muscles through their full range of motion in the week following TP injections, but are advised to avoid strenuous activity, especially in the first 3 or 4 days after injection.

Helpful hints

Needle selection
The choice of needle size depends on the location of the muscle being injected. The needle must be long enough to reach the contraction knots in the TP to disrupt them. A 22 gauge, 1.5 inch needle is usually adequate to reach most superficial muscles. For thick subcutaneous muscles such as the gluteus maximus or paraspinal muscles in persons who are not obese, a 21 gauge, 2.0 inch needle is usually necessary. A 21 gauge, 2.5 inch needle is required to reach the deepest muscles, such as the gluteus minimus and quadratus lumborum, and is available as a hypodermic needle.

Using a needle with a smaller diameter may cause less discomfort; however, it may provide neither the required mechanical disruption of the TP nor adequate sensitivity to the physician when penetrating the overlying skin and subcutaneous tissue. A needle with a smaller gauge may also be deflected away from a very taut muscular band, thus preventing penetration of the TP. The needle should be long enough so that it never has to be inserted all the way to its hub, because the hub is the weakest part of the needle and breakage beneath the skin could occur.

Deep muscle TPs

Piriformis muscle

Anatomy
The piriformis is a flat muscle, pyramidal in shape, lying almost parallel with the posterior margin of the gluteus medius.

It is situated partly within the pelvis against its posterior wall, and partly at the back of the hip joint.

It arises from the front of the sacrum by three fleshy digitations, attached to the portions of bone between the first, second, third, and fourth anterior sacral foramina, and to the grooves leading from the foramina: a few fibers also arise from the margin of the greater sciatic foramen, and from the anterior surface of the sacrotuberous ligament.

The muscle passes out of the pelvis through the greater sciatic foramen, the upper part of which it fills, and is inserted by a rounded tendon into the upper border of the greater trochanter behind, but often partly blended with, the common tendon of the obturator internus and superior and inferior gemellus muscles.

The piriformis muscle is part of the lateral rotators of the hip, along with the quadratus femoris, gemellus inferior, gemellus superior, obturator externus, and obturator internus. The piriformis laterally rotates the extended thigh and abducts the flexed thigh. Abduction of the flexed thigh is important in the action of walking because it shifts the body weight to the opposite side of the foot being lifted, which keeps us from falling. The action of the lateral rotators can be understood by crossing your legs to rest an ankle on the knee of the other leg. This causes the femur to rotate and point the knee laterally. The lateral rotators also oppose medial rotation by the gluteus medius and gluteus minimus. At a range of more than 90° the actions of the piriformis are reversed to adduct and internally rotate (medial).

It is occasionally (15–30%) pierced by the common peroneal nerve (fibular) when the sciatic nerve bifurcates before exiting the greater sciatic foramen. Thus, the piriformis is divided more or less into two parts.

It may be united with the gluteus medius, send fibers to the gluteus minimus, or receive fibers from the superior gemellus. It may have one or two sacral attachments; or it may be inserted into the capsule of the hip joint.

Innervation of the piriformis muscle is directly from the first and second sacral nerves. The obturator externus is supplied by the obturator nerve from third and fourth spinal nerves. The remaining short lateral rotators receive innervation through motor nerves that may arise from spinal nerves lumbar 4 to sacral vertebra 5.

Piriformis syndrome
This syndrome occurs when the piriformis irritates the sciatic nerve, which comes into the gluteal region beneath the

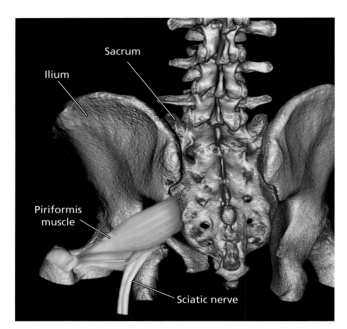

Figure 11.48 The piriformis muscle and structures in close vicinity.

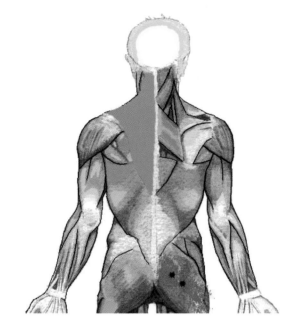

Figure 11.49 TPs on the piriformis muscle.

muscle, causing pain in the buttocks and referred pain along the sciatic nerve. This referred pain is known as sciatica. Fifteen percent of the population have their sciatic nerve coursing through the piriformis muscle. This subgroup of the population is predisposed to developing sciatica. Sciatica can be described by pain, tingling, or numbness deep in the buttocks and along the sciatic nerve. Sitting down, stretching, climbing stairs, and performing squats usually increases pain. Diagnosing the syndrome is usually based on symptoms and on the physical examination. More testing, including MRI, X-rays, and nerve conduction tests can be administered to exclude other possible disorders (Figs 11.48 and 11.49).

Indications
• Piriformis syndrome.

Contraindications
• Local or systemic infection.
• Coagulopathy.

Step 1. Prepare the patient before the procedure
The patient should be aware of why they are having this procedure, what to expect from it and from the team. All complications and side effects related to the procedure should be explained in detail, before the procedure.

Obtain an informed consent.

The type of analgesia or sedation needs to be ascertained before performance of the invasive procedure. Intravenous fentanyl, midazolam, and/or propofol may be used judiciously for patient comfort.

Step 2. Position and monitor the patient
1. Place the patient prone on the table. Place a pillow under the abdomen to flatten the lumbar lordosis.
2. Obtain an intravenous access.
3. Administer oxygen by nasal cannula, monitor the vital signs noninvasively.
4. Prepare and drape the area in a sterile fashion.
5. The patient should not be over-sedated. The patient should remain sufficiently conscious to provide responses to any questions.

Step 3. Drugs and equipment for piriformis injection
• 5 ml syringe for skin infiltration;
• 1½ inch, 25 gauge needle for skin infiltration;
• 5 ml syringe for contrast material;
• 10 ml syringe for the piriformis injection;
• 10 cm 22 gauge needle for piriformis injection, 1% lidocaine for skin infiltration;
• nonionic contrast material;
• 5 ml of 0.5% bupivacaine and 40 mg triamcinolone.

Step 4. Visualization
Place the C-arm in the PA position first, identify the greater trochanter and the sacrum, and draw a line between these two points (Fig. 11.50).

Step 5. Surface landmarks for the needle entry
Mark the midpoint of this line, which is the entry point.

Step 6. Direction of the needle
Infiltrate the skin with 1% lidocaine. Insert a 10 cm needle, perpendicular with the skin, advance slightly, holding the

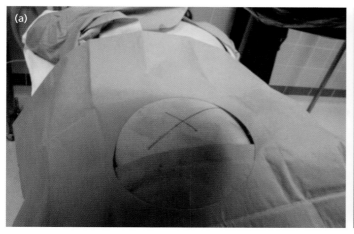
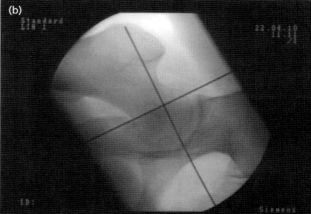

Figure 11.50 (a,b) The landmarks for piriformis injection.

needle with the thumb and index finger. Advance slightly, holding the needle with the thumb and index finger. While advancing one should feel the first resistance. Continue to advance the needle until the second layer of muscles is passed and stop immediately. Confirm the final position of the needle just above the hip joint.

Step 7. Confirm the position of the needle
Inject 2 ml of contrast material. The contrast material should delineate the contour of the piriformis muscle (Fig. 11.51).

Step 8. Piriformis block
Inject 3–5 ml of 0.5% bupivacaine with 40 mg of triamcinolone.

Step 9. Postprocedure care
After the procedure the patient should be observed for a reasonable time for the risk of hypotension. In case of hypotension, intravenous electrolyte solutions should be administered. The recovery and observation time depends on the sedation and analgesia used, which also facilitates the assessment of any impairment of intellectual function, tolerance of oral intake, assessment of the immediate results of the neural blockade, and pain response to the procedure.

The patient should be provided with all instructions, including whom to call or where to go for any postprocedure urgent or emergency care. The patient should be discharged, accompanied by a responsible adult.

Complications
Bleeding and hematoma formation.
Sciatic nerve injury due to the contact of the needle to the nerve.
Infection.

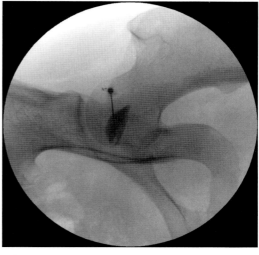

Figure 11.51 Confirm the position of the needle by contrast material.

Psoas and quadratus lumborum muscle

History
Travell and Simons (1983) identified the psoas and quadratus lumborum muscles as the cause of low-back pain and TP injections as the method of pain relief.

Anatomy
The psoas major is a long fusiform muscle located on the side of the lumbar region of the vertebral column and brim of the lesser pelvis. It joins the iliacus muscle to form the iliopsoas. In fewer than 50% of humans the psoas major is accompanied by the psoas minor. The psoas major is divided into a superficial and deep part. The deep part originates from the transverse processes of lumbar vertebrae I–V. The

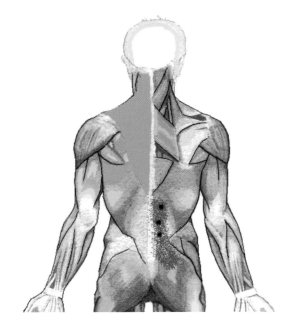

Figure 11.52 Trigger points on psoas muscle.

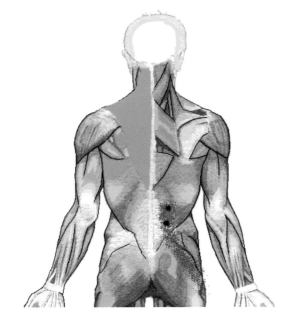

Figure 11.53 Trigger points on quadratus lumborum muscle.

superficial part originates from the lateral surfaces of the last thoracic vertebra, lumbar vertebrae I–IV, and from neighboring invertebral discs. The lumbar plexus lies between the two layers. Joined by the iliacus, the psoas major forms the iliopsoas which is surrounded by the iliac fascia. The iliopsoas runs across the iliopubic eminence through the muscular lacuna to its insertion on the lesser trochanter of the femur. The iliopectineal bursa separates the bone from the muscle at the level of the iliopubic eminence. The iliac subtendinous bursa lies between the lesser trochanter and the attachment of the iliopsoas. Innervation of the psoas major is through the anterior rami of lumbar vertebrae 1–3 (Fig. 11.52).

The iliopsoas muscle, along with the quadratus lumborum muscle, is frequently responsible for failed low back postsurgical syndrome. Pain from the psoas major muscle is often referred from the ipsilateral spine in the thoracic region to the sacroiliac area. Occasionally, this pain extends to the upper buttocks.

The quadratus lumborum muscle is irregular and quadrilateral in shape, and broader below than above. It arises by aponeurotic fibers from the iliolumbar ligament and the adjacent portion of the iliac crest for about 5 cm, and is inserted into the lower border of the last rib for about half its length, and by four small tendons into the apices of the transverse processes of the upper four lumbar vertebrae.

Occasionally a second portion of this muscle is found in front of the preceding one. It arises from the upper borders of the transverse processes of the lower three or four lumbar vertebrae, and is inserted into the lower margin of the last rib.

Anterior to the quadratus lumborum are the colon, the kidney, the psoas major and (if present) psoas minor, and the diaphragm; between the fascia and the muscle are the twelfth thoracic, ilioinguinal, and iliohypogastric nerves. The number of attachments to the vertebrae and the extent of its attachment to the last rib vary.

The quadratus lumborum can perform four actions: (1) lateral flexion of vertebral column, with ipsilateral contraction; (2) extension of lumbar vertebral column, with bilateral contraction; (3) fixes the twelfth rib during forced expiration; (4) elevates the ilium, with ipsilateral contraction.

Symptoms of quadratus lumborum spasm are low-back pain, pain with weight-bearing posture, and discomfort turning over in bed. Relief can be provided by positions or maneuvers that unload the lumbar spine of the upper body's weight. Simple coughing or sneezing can exacerbate the pain. History of irritation of pain is associated with falling, major body trauma, or any activity where one is simultaneously bending and reaching to one side to pull or lift something. Other factors that can cause persistence of this pain are leg-length discrepancies, small hemipelvis, and/or short upper arms (Fig. 11.53).

Indications
- Low back pain in the region.
- Myofascial pain syndrome.

Contraindications
- Local or systemic infection.
- Coagulopathy.

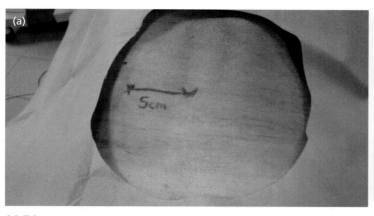
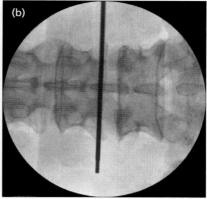

Figure 11.54 (a,b) Palpate the iliac crest and select a point 5 cm lateral to the spinous process at the level of lumbar vertebra 5. Mark this point.

Psoas muscle injection

Step 1. Prepare the patient before the procedure
The patient should be aware of why this procedure is being done, what to expect from the procedure and from the team. All complications and side effects related to the procedure should be explained in detail, before the procedure.

After informed consent has been obtained, an intravenous infusion is started and normal saline infused.

The type of analgesia or sedation needs to be ascertained before performance of the invasive procedure. Intravenous fentanyl, midazolam, and/or propofol may be used judiciously for patient comfort.

Step 2. Position and monitor the patient
1. Place the patient prone on the table. Place a pillow under the abdomen to flatten the lumbar lordosis.
2. Obtain an intravenous access.
3. Administer oxygen by nasal cannula, monitor the vital signs noninvasively.
4. Prepare and drape the area in a sterile fashion.
5. The patient should not be over-sedated. The patient should remain sufficiently conscious to provide responses to any questions.

Step 3. Drugs and equipment for psoas major injection
• 1½ inch, 25 gauge needle for skin infiltration;
• 5 ml syringe for local anesthesia;
• 10 ml syringe for muscle injection;
• 22 gauge, 10 cm needle for the block;
• 1% lidocaine for skin infiltration;
• 5 ml nonionic contrast material;
• 5 ml lidocaine;
• 40 mg methylprednisolone.

Step 4. Surface landmarks for the needle entry
1. Palpate the iliac crest and select a point 5 cm lateral to the spinous process at the level of lumbar vertebra 5. Mark this point (Fig. 11.54).
2. Infiltrate the skin with local anesthetic.

Step 5. Visualization
Position the C-arm in the PA position first.

Insert a 22 gauge needle perpendicular to the skin, and advance under "tunneled vision" (Fig. 11.55).

Step 6. Confirm the position of the needle
1. Advance the needle toward approximately anterior one-third of the vertebral body in the lateral view (Fig. 11.56).
2. Inject 2 ml of contrast material in the psoas muscle. The contrast material should spread along the psoas major muscle vertically over anterior one-third of the lumbar vertebral body. It should always be anterior to the foramen (Fig. 11.57).

Step 7. Psoas major muscle injection
After confirmation of the position of the needle, inject 8–10 ml of local anesthetic, steroid combination.

Quadratus lumborum muscle injection

Step 1. Prepare the patient before the procedure
The patient should be aware of why this procedure is being done, what to expect from the procedure and from the team. All complications and side effects related to the procedure should be explained in detail, before the procedure.

After informed consent has been obtained, an intravenous infusion is started and normal saline infused.

The type of analgesia or sedation needs to be ascertained before performance of the invasive procedure. Intravenous

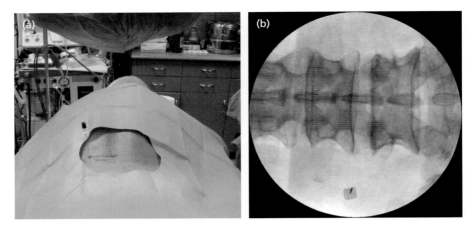

Figure 11.55 (a,b) Insert and advance the needle under "tunneled vision."

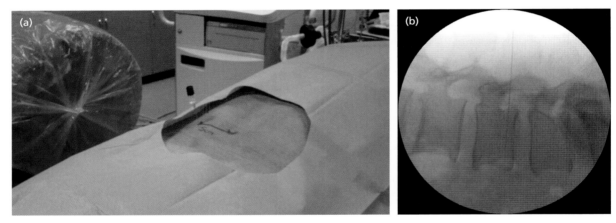

Figure 11.56 (a,b) Advance the needle under lateral view.

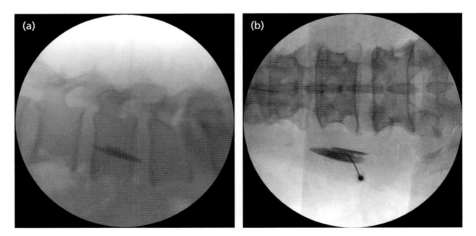

Figure 11.57 (a,b) Spread of the contrast material under lateral and PA view.

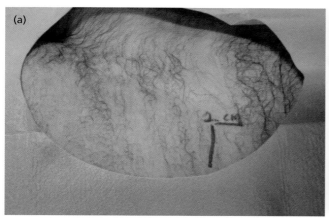
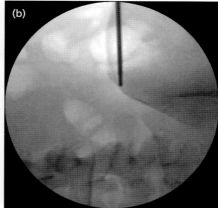

Figure 11.58 (a,b) Mark the entry point.

fentanyl, midazolam, and/or propofol may be used judiciously for patient comfort.

Step 2. Position and monitor the patient
1. Place the patient prone on the table. Place a pillow under the abdomen to flatten the lumbar lordosis.
2. Obtain an intravenous access.
3. Administer oxygen by nasal cannula, and monitor the vital signs noninvasively.
4. Prepare and drape the area in a sterile fashion.
5. The patient should not be over-sedated. The patient should remain sufficiently conscious to provide responses to any questions.

Step 3. Drugs and equipment for quadratus lumborum injection
- 1½ inch, 25 gauge needle for skin infiltration;
- 5 ml syringe for local anesthesia;
- 10 ml syringe for muscle injection;
- 10 cm 22 gauge needle for the block;
- 1% lidocaine for skin infiltration;
- 5 ml nonionic contrast material;
- 5 ml lidocaine;
- 40 mg methylprednisolone.

Step 4. Surface landmarks for the needle entry
Mark the point 2 cm above the iliac crest and posterior superior iliac spine (Fig. 11.58).

Step 5. Visualization
1. Position the C-arm in the PA position first.
2. Insert a 22 gauge needle perpendicular to the skin, and advance under "tunneled vision" (Fig. 11.58).

Step 6. Direction of the needle
Position the C-arm laterally, and advance the needle at the level of the transverse process (Fig. 11.59).

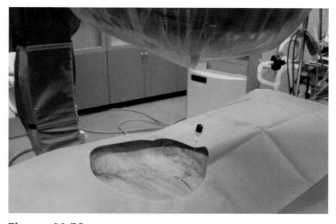

Figure 11.59 Advance the needle perpendicular to the skin.

Step 7. Confirm the position of the needle
Inject 2 ml of contrast material. The needle tip should be behind the transverse process (Fig. 11.60).

Step 8. Quadratus lumborus muscle injection
Inject 5 ml of local anesthetic, steroid combination (Fig. 11.61).

Postprocedure care
After the procedure the patient should be observed for a reasonable time for the risk of hypotension. In case of hypotension, intravenous electrolyte solutions should be administered. The recovery and observation time depends on the sedation and analgesia used, which also facilitates the assessment of any impairment of intellectual function, tolerance of oral intake, assessment of the immediate results of the neural blockade, and pain response to the procedure.

The patient should be provided with all instructions including whom to call or where to go for any postprocedure urgent or emergency care. The patient should be discharged accompanied by a responsible adult.

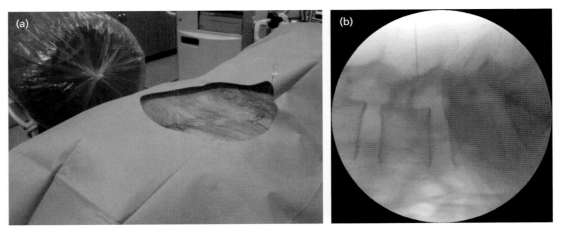

Figure 11.60 (a,b) Position of the needle in lateral view.

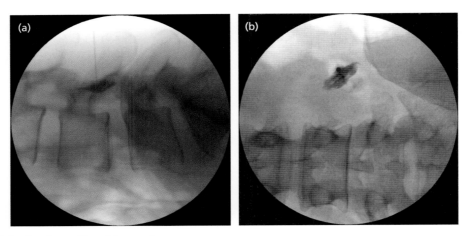

Figure 11.61 (a,b) Confirm the position of the needle.

Complications

Increased pain in area of injection.
Infection.
Hematoma in the muscles.

Helpful hints

To avoid potential damage in the quadratus lumborum muscle injection, do not use needles that are too long. Lateral views should be used to confirm the needle tip in muscular tissue. Psoas muscle injection should be at the lateral aspect of the transverse processes to avoid the nerve roots and the epidural space.

Further reading

Alvarez, D.J. & Rockwell, P.G. (2002) Trigger points: diagnosis and management. *American Family Physician* **65**(4), 653–660.

Blumenfeld, A. & Ashkenazi, A. (2010) Nerve blocks, trigger point injections and headache. *Headache* **50**(6), 953–954.

Borg-Stein, J. & Simons, D.G. (2002) Myofascial pain. *Archives of Physical Medicine and Rehabilitation* **83**, S40–S47.

Cheng, J. & Abdi, S. (2007) Complications of joint, tendon, and muscle injections. *Techniques in Regional Anesthesia and Pain Management* **11**(3), 141–147.

Cummings, T.M. & White, A.R. (2001) Needling therapies in the management of myofascial trigger point pain: a systematic review. *Archives of Physical Medicine and Rehabilitation* **82**, 986–992.

De Andrés, J., Cerda-Olmedo, G., Valía, J.C., et al. (2003) Use of botulinum toxin in the treatment of chronic myofascial pain. *Clinical Journal of Pain* **19**, 269–275.

Fishman, L.M., Dombi, G.W., Michaelsen, C., et al. (2002) Piriformis syndrome: diagnosis, treatment, and outcome – a 10-year study. *Archives of Physical Medicine and Rehabilitation* **83**(3), 295–301.

Gerwin, R.D. (1997) Myofascial pain syndromes in the upper extremity. *Journal of Hand Therapy* **10**(2), 130–136.

Gerwin, R.D. (2001) Classification, epidemiology, and natural history of myofascial pain syndrome. *Current Pain and Headache Reports* **5**, 412–420.

Harden, R.N., Bruehl, S.P., Gass, S., et al. (2000) Signs and symptoms of the myofascial pain syndrome: a national survey of pain management providers. *Clinical Journal of Pain* **16**, 64–72.

Hong, C.Z. (1996) Pathophysiology of myofascial trigger point. *Journal of the Formosan Medical Association* **95**(2), 93–104.

Hubbard, D.R. & Berkoff, G.M. (1993) Myofascial trigger points show spontaneous needle EMG activity. *Spine* **18**, 1803–1807.

Kirschner, J.S., Foye, P.M. & Cole, J.L. (2009) Piriformis syndrome, diagnosis and treatment. *Muscle & Nerve* **40**(1), 10–18.

Kuncewicz, E., Gajewska, E., Sobieska, M. & Samborski, W. (2006) Piriformis muscle syndrome. *Annales Academiae Medicae Stetinensis* **52**(3), 99–101; discussion 101.

Lavelle, E.D., Lavelle, W. & Smith, H.S. (2007) Myofascial trigger points. *Medical Clinics of North America* **91**(2), 229–239.

Harris, R.E. & Clauw, D.J. (2002) The use of complementary medical therapies in the management of myofascial pain disorders. *Current Pain and Headache Reports* **6**, 370–374.

Malanga, G.A. & Cruz Colon, E.J. (2010) Myofascial low back pain: a review. *Physical Medicine and Rehabilitation Clinics of North America* **21**(4), 711–724.

Meyer, H.P. (2002) Myofascial pain syndrome and its suggested role in the pathogenesis and treatment of fibromyalgia syndrome. *Current Pain and Headache Reports* **6**, 274–283.

Rachlin, I. (2002) Physical therapy treatment approaches for myofascial pain syndromes and fibromyalgia. In *Myofascial Pain and Fibromyalgia*, 2nd edition (ed. Rachlin, E.S. & Rachlin, I.S.), pp. 467–524. St. Louis, MO: Mosby.

Rivner, M.H. (2001) The neurophysiology of myofascial pain syndrome. *Current Pain and Headache Reports* **5**, 432–440.

Rudin, N.J. (2003) Evaluation of treatments for myofascial pain syndrome and fibromyalgia. *Current Pain and Headache Reports* **7**, 433–442.

Simons, D.G., Travell, J.G. & Simons, L.S. (1999) *Myofascial Pain and Dysfunction: The Trigger Point Manual*, volume 1, 2nd edition. Baltimore, MD: Williams & Wilkins.

Travell, J.G. & Simons, D.G. (1983) *Myofascial Pain and Dysfunction: The Trigger Point Manual*. Baltimore, MD: Williams & Wilkins.

Walsh, N.E., Ramamurty, S., Calder, T.M., et al. (2003) Nociceptive pain. In *Pain Medicine: A Comprehensive Review*, 2nd edition (ed. Raj, P.P. & Paradise, L.A.), pp. 61–76. St. Louis, MO: Mosby.

Wheeler, A.H. (2004) Myofascial pain disorders: theory to therapy. *Drugs* **64**, 45–62.

Percutaneous block and lesioning of the trigeminal ganglion

History

The trigeminal ganglion was described first by the Viennese anatomist Johann Gasser, since when it has commonly been called the Gasserian ganglion. The blocking of this ganglion was first described by Hartel in 1912. His technique is still the most commonly performed, with minor modifications.

Anatomy

The trigeminal nerve is the largest of the cranial nerves. Its ganglion is located within Meckel's cave and contains the cell bodies of incoming sensory nerve fibers. The trigeminal ganglion (Fig. 12.1) is analogous to the dorsal-root ganglia of the spinal cord. From the trigeminal ganglion, a single, large sensory root enters the brainstem at the level of the pons. Immediately adjacent to the sensory root, a smaller motor root emerges from the pons at the same level. **Motor** fibers pass through the trigeminal ganglion on their way to peripheral muscles. Their cell bodies are located in the nucleus of the fifth nerve, deep within the pons. The most significant portions of the trigeminal nerve are (1) the trigeminal nucleus and (2) the trigeminal ganglion.

The trigeminal nucleus

The trigeminal nucleus extends throughout the entire brainstem, from the midbrain to the medulla, and continues into the cervical cord (Fig. 12.2). The nucleus is divided anatomically into three parts, from caudal to rostral direction, i.e., the **spinal trigeminal** nucleus, **main trigeminal nucleus**, and **mesencephalic trigeminal nucleus.** The three parts of the trigeminal nucleus receive different types of sensory information. The spinal trigeminal nucleus receives **pain/temperature** fibers. The main trigeminal nucleus receives **touch/position** fibers. The mesencephalic nucleus receives **proprioceptor and mechanoreceptor fibers** from the jaws and teeth.

Spinal trigeminal nucleus

The spinal trigeminal nucleus represents pain/temperature sensation from the face. On entering the brainstem, sensory fibers group together and traverse to the spinal trigeminal nucleus. This bundle of incoming fibers can be identified in cross sections of the pons and medulla as the spinal tract of the trigeminal nucleus. The spinal trigeminal nucleus contains a pain/temperature sensory map of the face and mouth. The lowest levels of the nucleus represent peripheral areas of the face, scalp, ears and chin; higher levels in the upper medulla represent more central areas, such as the nose, cheeks, and lips; the highest levels in the pons represent the mouth, teeth, and pharyngeal cavity.

Main trigeminal nucleus

The main trigeminal nucleus represents touch/position sensation from the face. It is located in the pons, close to the entry site of the fifth nerve.

Mesencephalic trigeminal nucleus

The mesencephalic trigeminal nucleus is not really a nucleus. Rather, it is a sensory ganglion (like the trigeminal ganglion) that happens to be embedded in the brainstem. Only certain types of sensory fiber have cell bodies in the mesencephalic nucleus: **proprioceptor** fibers from the jaw and **mechanoreceptor** fibers from the teeth. Some of these incoming fibers go to the motor nucleus of the trigeminal nerve; thus, the mesencephalic nucleus fibers bypass entirely the pathways for conscious perception. The jaw-jerk reflex is an example. Tapping the jaw elicits a reflex closure of the jaw, in exactly the same way that tapping the knee elicits a reflex kick of the lower leg. Other incoming fibers from the teeth and jaws go to the main nucleus.

The trigeminal ganglion

The trigeminal ganglion lies within the cranium, close to the anterior surface of the petrous portion of the temporal bone. It is somewhat crescentic in shape, with its convexity directed

Pain-Relieving Procedures: The Illustrated Guide, First Edition. P. Prithvi Raj and Serdar Erdine.
© 2012 John Wiley & Sons, Ltd. Published 2012 by John Wiley & Sons, Ltd.

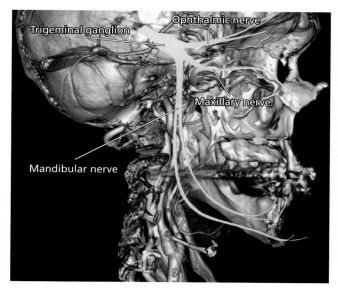

Figure 12.1 Three-dimensional computed tomography scan of the trigeminal ganglion and its branches.

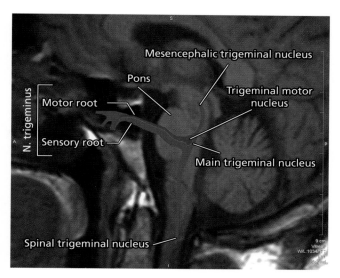

Figure 12.3 The formation of the trigeminal nucleus and trigeminal nerve, trigeminal ganglion and its branches.

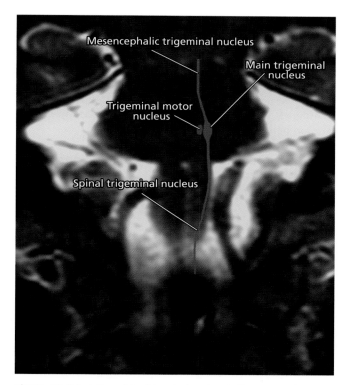

Figure 12.2 Location of the trigeminal nucleus in the pons and upper spinal-cord segments.

anteriorly. It is in close relation with the internal carotid artery and the posterior part of the cavernous sinus. The motor root runs anterior and medial to the sensory root and passes inferior to the ganglion. The motor root then leaves the skull through the foramen ovale, and immediately below this foramen the motor root joins the sensory root of the mandibular nerve. The greater superficial petrosal nerve lies underneath the ganglion.

The ganglion receives, on its medial side, filaments from the carotid plexus of the sympathetic chain. From its convex border, which is directed forward and laterally, three large nerves are formed; they are the ophthalmic, maxillary, and mandibular divisions. The ophthalmic and maxillary nerves consist exclusively of sensory fibers; the mandibular nerve is joined outside the cranium by the motor root.

Associated with the three divisions of the trigeminal nerve are four small ganglia. The ciliary ganglion is connected with the ophthalmic nerve; the sphenopalatine ganglion (SPG) is connected with the maxillary nerve; and the otic and sub-maxillary ganglia are connected with the mandibular nerve. All four receive sensory filaments from the trigeminal ganglion; in the motor and sympathetic ganglion of these divisions arise filaments from various sources.

The branches and course of the trigeminal nerve

Three main branches of the trigeminal ganglion arise from the anterior border of the ganglion, from the medial to the lateral aspect (Fig. 12.3). The ophthalmic nerve arises first (V1); the maxillary nerve arises second (V2); and, finally, the mandibular nerve (V3) arises. The origins of these nerves in the ganglion are somatotropically located in the ganglion; the ophthalmic branch is situated most medioposteriorly, the maxillary branch intermediately, and the mandibular branch occupies the ventrolateral position.

Innervation of the trigeminal ganglion

The trigeminal nerve is predominately a **sensory nerve**. It innervates the following regions of the face.

Superficial structures
- Face.
- Anterior half of the scalp.

Bony structures
- Anterior and middle cranial fossa.

Deep-tissue structures
- Oral and nasal mucosa.
- Paranasal sinuses.
- Nasopharynx.
- Part of the ear, cartilaginous region.
- External acoustic meatus.
- Part of the tympanic membrane.
- Orbits.

Visceral structures
- Conjunctiva.

Anatomy and formation of the foramen ovale

At the base of the skull, the foramen ovale (see Fig. 12.6) is one of the larger of the several foramina that transmit nerves through the skull. The foramen ovale is situated in the posterior part of the sphenoid bone, posterolateral to the foramen rotundum. Several nerves and vessels pass through the foramen ovale. The significant ones are as follows.
- Mandibular nerve.
- Accessory meningeal artery.
- Lesser petrosal nerve.

The foramen ovale differs in shape and size throughout its natural life. The average adult maximal length is about 7.48 mm, and the width is 3.7 mm (Fig. 12.7).

Indications for trigeminal ganglion block

Common indications are the following:
- idiopathic trigeminal neuralgia;
- secondary trigeminal neuralgia (multiple sclerosis (Fig. 12.4), tumor (Fig. 12.5));
- intractable headaches.

Contraindications for trigeminal ganglion block

It is important to consider the following contraindications:
- local infection;
- coagulopathy;
- vital function instability;
- psychopathologies.

Percutaneous techniques commonly performed on the trigeminal ganglion and its nerves

The following percutaneous techniques are commonly performed on the trigeminal ganglion:
- radiofrequency (RF) thermocoagulation (described by Sweet and Wepsic in 1974);
- retrogasserian glycerol injection (described by Hakanson in 1981);
- percutaneous balloon compression (described by Mullan and Lichtor in 1983);
- diagnostic (local anesthetic) or neurolytic block.

Note: all these techniques require the visualization of the foramen ovale and its confirmation with standard imaging techniques. It is important to have an expert knowledge of location before performing these procedures.

RF thermocoagulation of the trigeminal ganglion and its branches

A step-by-step approach is described to perform this procedure.

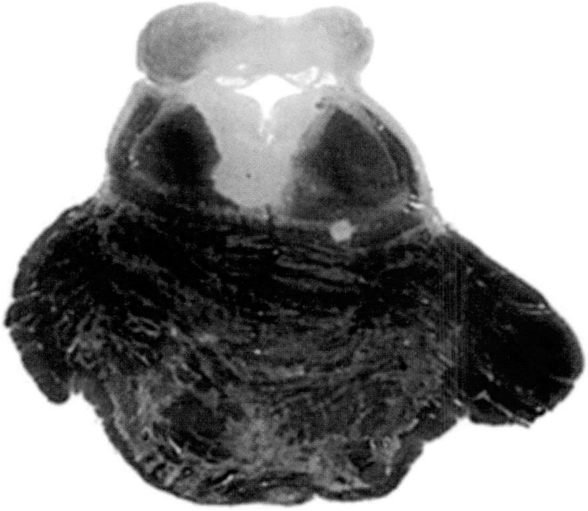

Figure 12.4 Trigeminal neuralgia caused by multiple sclerosis.

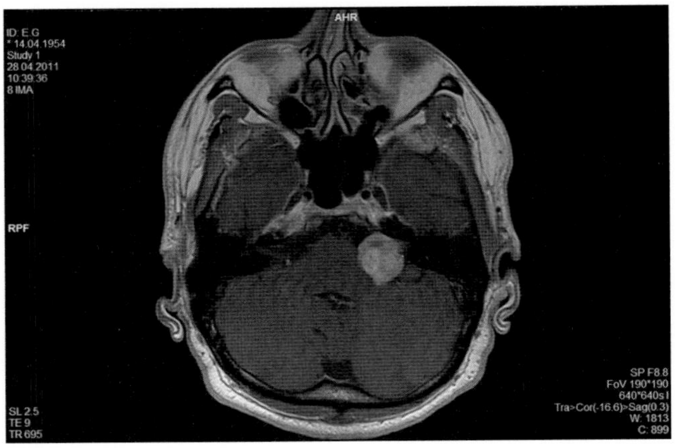

Figure 12.5 Computed tomography scan showing trigeminal neuralgia caused by a tumor growth.

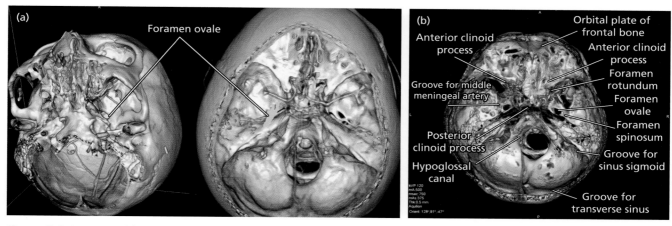

Figure 12.6 Anatomy and formation of the foramen ovale. (a) Three-dimensional computed tomography scan of the base of the skull, in an oblique view. (b) Three-dimensional computed tomography scan showing the various foramina at the base of the skull.

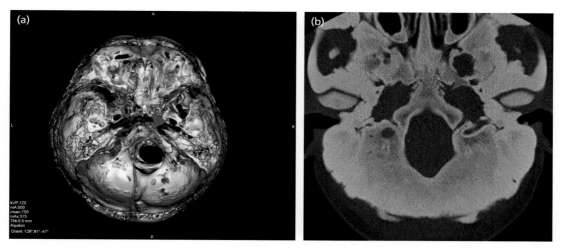

Figure 12.7 (a) Three-dimensional computed tomography scans showing, with red arrows, the location of the foramen ovale at the base of the skull. (b) Computed tomography scan of the base of the skull showing the dimensions of the foramen ovale (red arrow).

Step 1. Prepare the patient before the procedure
Ascertain the type of analgesia or sedation before performing the invasive procedure. The type of sedation varies, based on the technique being used. If a diagnostic trigeminal block with a local anesthetic or therapeutic block with a neurolytic agent is being considered or balloon compression is planned, **deep sedation and analgesia** may be appropriate for some patients. If RF thermocoagulation is planned, the patient needs to be **awake** to respond to the stimulation test. Intravenous fentanyl, midazolam, and/or propofol may be used judiciously for patient comfort.

Step 2. Position and monitor the patient
1. Place the patient in a supine position on the table.
2. Fix the head on the table with a strip of adhesive tape.
3. Insert an intravenous (IV) cannula for injecting medication.

4. Provide oxygen by nasal cannula.
5. Monitor vital signs (mandatory).
6. Prepare the area for needle entry in a sterile fashion.

Step 3. Drugs and equipment for radiofrequency thermocoagulation
Prepare and confirm that the following equipment, needles, and drugs are ready to be used for the procedure:

Common drugs and needles
- 1½ inch, 25 gauge needle (for infiltration of the skin);
- 5 ml syringe (for local anesthetic solution);
- 2 ml empty syringe (for aspiration test);
- 3½ inch, 22 gauge needle (for the nerve block);
- 1% lidocaine for skin infiltration or diagnostic injections.

Special equipment for RF
- RF machine, with cables and electrodes;
- 10 cm RF needle with 2 mm active-tip electrode.

Step 4. Visualization
All trigeminal nerve-lesioning techniques are performed with initial needle entry through the foramen ovale. Visualize the foramen ovale by aproaching it in a submental view of the fluoroscope. This is best done by first placing the C-arm in a posteroanterior (PA) view (Fig. 12.8a). Then rotate the C-arm slowly, obliquely (approximately 30°) (Fig. 12.8b), until the foramen ovale is clearly visible (Fig. 12.8c).

Note: generally the foramen ovale is close to the medial side of the mandible at the level of the maxilla (second molar tooth).

Step 5. Mark the surface landmarks for needle entry
Mark the skin for needle entry at the angle of the mouth in line with the pupil when looking at the front of the face and the midpoint of the zygomatic arch when looking from the side of the face (Fig. 12.9).

Step 6. Direction of the needle
1. When the foramen ovale is clearly visible, advance the needle through it, parallel to the axis of the C-arm in a "submental view" (Fig. 12.10).
2. Then direct the needle to the lateral edge of the foramen ovale for the mandibular branch, to the middle for the maxillary branch, and medially for the ophthalmic branch (Fig. 12.11).
3. Note: to facilitate needle entry into the foramen ovale, direct the needle toward the angle produced by the clivus and petrous ridge of the temporal bone in a lateral fluoroscopic view. Avoid advancing the needle too deeply, which could cause it to penetrate the cerebral cortex or the brainstem (Fig. 12.12).

Step 7. Confirm the position of the needle
1. Confirm the position of the needle. Perform the aspiration test (mandatory) when the needle enters the foramen

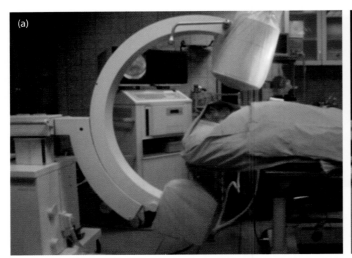
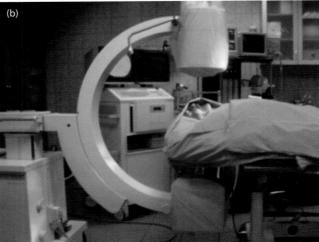
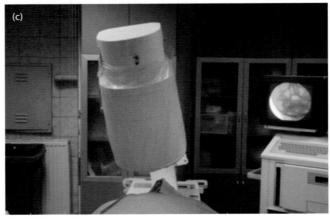

Figure 12.8 Positions of the C-arm to locate the foramen ovale. (a) Posteroanterior view. (b) Oblique view. (c) Final position for the foramen ovale to be clearly identified.

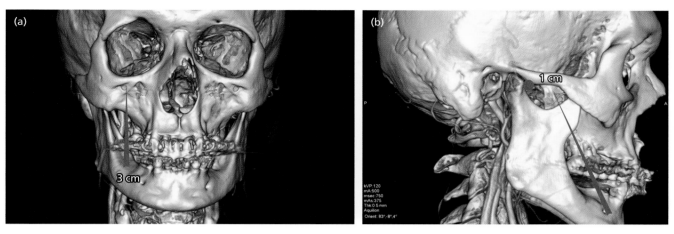

Figure 12.9 (a) Three-dimensional computed tomography scan in the AP view identifying the point of entry from the upper molar tooth. The needle needs to be toward the middle of the ipsilateral orbit (red arrow). (b) Three-dimensional computed tomography lateral scan identifying the point of entry at the mandibular notch (red dot).

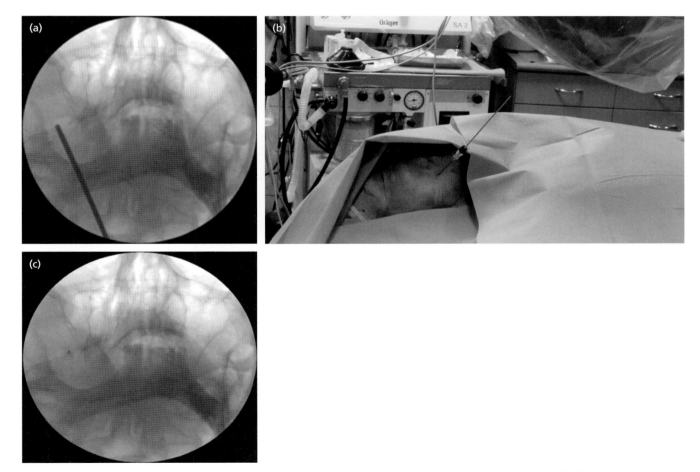

Figure 12.10 (a) Location of the foramen ovale in the submental fluoroscopic view. The tip of the marker locates the middle of the foramen ovale. (b) Red arrows show the direction of the needle from the skin towards the foramen ovale. (c) Submental fluoroscopic view showing a needle in the foramen ovale in the tunnel vision (black dot).

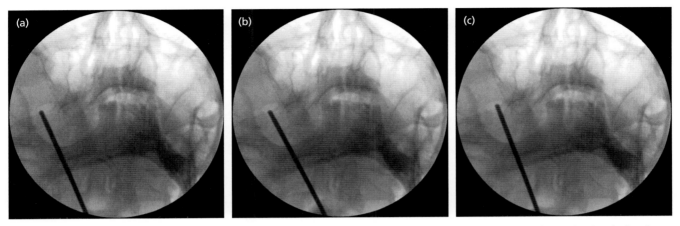

Figure 12.11 (a) Submental view showing the location of the electrode for mandibular radiofrequency site. (b) Submental view showing the location of the electrode for maxillary radiofrequency site. (c) Submental view showing the location of the electrode for ophthalmic radiofrequency site.

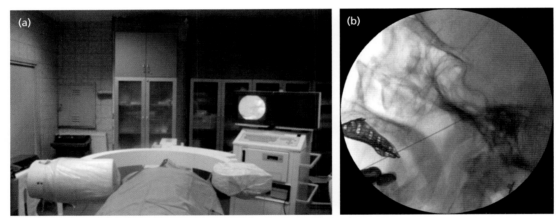

Figure 12.12 (a) The position of the fluoroscope in the lateral view to identify the foramen ovale. (b) Identification of significant structures seen in the lateral view.

ovale to avoid entering into the cerebrospinal fluid (CSF) or a blood vessel. If blood is aspirated, change the position of the needle slightly and aspirate again. If blood is still aspirated, terminate the procedure.

2. If the needle penetrates deeper than required, it can enter the dura mater in Meckel's cave. If that happens, one may see CSF during aspiration. Aspiration of CSF does not interfere with RF thermocoagulation. However, it could interfere with injection of therapeutic agents with high viscosity, such as contrast material or glycerol or phenol in glycerine; the injected solution is likely to spread to the brain stem, causing nausea and vomiting and other neurologic side effects. This should be avoided.

3. Improper positioning of the needle is diagnosable if both the lateral and PA fluoroscopic view are used. However, to prevent the needle entering through the other foramina at the base of the skull, use the submental view carefully, to detect whether the needle has penetrated the

- infraorbital fissure, or
- the foramen lacerum, or
- the jugular foramen.

Step 8. Test stimulation

1. Initiate the RF thermocoagulation procedure, beginning with a test stimulation (Fig. 12.13).

2. The aim of the test stimulation is to verify entry of the electrode through the foramen ovale, as well as to place the tip of the electrode precisely at the desired portion of the trigeminal ganglion or its branches.

3. The patient should be awake to respond to the stimulation at this stage. Start by stimulating the region at 2 Hz, with 0.1–1.5 V settings. Because the mandibular branch of

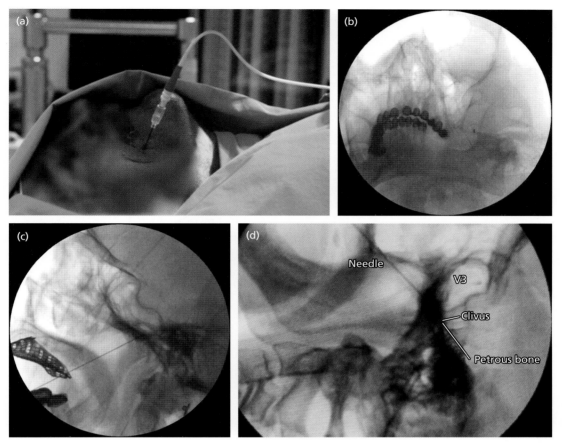

Figure 12.13 Radiofrequency techniques for trigeminal ganglion lesioning. (a) Photograph of a patient with a radiofrequency needle electrode in position during thermocoagulation. (b) Submental fluoroscopic view confirming needle position in the foramen ovale, on the right. (c) Confirmed needle electrode position for radiofrequency thermocoagulation, in the lateral view. (d) Significant structures in the lateral views.

the trigeminal nerve has motor fibers, the contraction of the mandible is observable at this setting. Next, seek paresthesia at the desired branch. Stimulate the nerve at 50–100 Hz at a 0.1–1.5 V setting. Generally, patients feel paresthesia at the 0.5 V setting. Next, confirm negative aspiration. When the electrode is confirmed to be in place for RF, then proceed with the thermocoagulation lesioning.

Step 9. RF thermocoagulation
1. After confirming that the electrode is in the proper location, sedate the patient if they are anxious, keeping them sufficiently able to respond to questions. One may inject 0.5 ml of 0.25% bupivacaine or 1% lidocaine, to provide comfort before actual thermocoagulation lesioning. Wait for a short time (30 seconds to 1 minute) before the start of the lesioning.
2. Proceed with lesioning at 70 °C for 60 seconds. After this first lesioning, stimulate the nerve again at 2 Hz, with a 0.1–1.5 V setting to compare the level of motor response with the first test stimulation. Stimulate the nerve again at

50–100 Hz with a 0.1–1.5 V setting to see if the level of paresthesia has diminished.
3. If more than one branch of the trigeminal nerve is affected, perform several lesions by repositioning the electrode on these nerve regions. Repeat the stimulation test after repositioning to seek for paresthesia at the affected branch.
4. If the ophthalmic branch of the trigeminal nerve is affected, keep the level of lesioning at 60 °C or below to preserve the corneal reflex. Evaluate the corneal reflex after each lesioning.

Step 10. Postprocedure care
Observe the patient for at least 2 hours after the procedure. Monitor vital signs (mandatory). In addition, objectively document the pain relief. After a satisfactory observation, discharge the patient with appropriate and adequate instructions given to the escort. Written instructions are preferable for emergencies and they are helpful to the patient and the family.

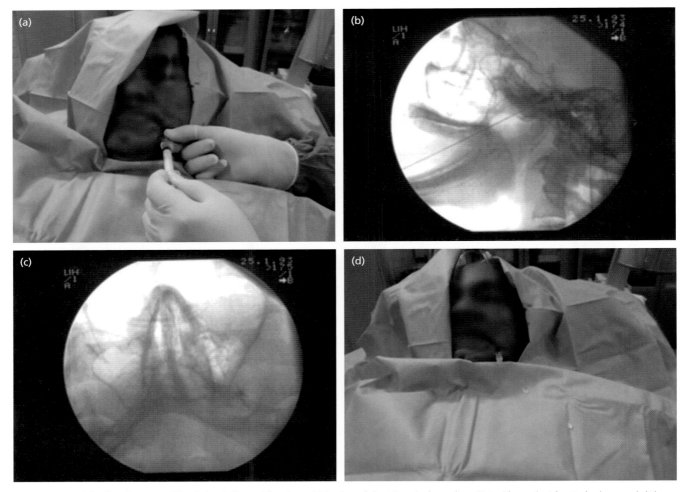

Figure 12.14 (a) Point-of-entry position being infiltrated for glycerol injection of the trigeminal ganglion. Note: The patient has to be in a semi-sitting position for the procedure. (b) Lateral fluoroscopic view showing a needle having entered the foramen ovale. (c) Oblique fluoroscopic view confirming needle placement in the foramen ovale, on the right side. (d) Position of the patient to allow the CSF to drain by gravity before glycerol is injected.

Technique of retrogasserian glycerol lesioning

If this technique is under consideration, proceed to prepare and position the patient as descibed in the section on RF thermocoagulation (see page 133). Prepare the equipment and drugs as described for the RF technique.

Step 3. Drugs and equipment

Common drugs and needles

- 1½ inch, 25 gauge needle (for infiltration of the skin);
- 5 ml syringe (for local anesthetic solution);
- 2 ml empty syringe (for aspiration test);
- 3½ inch, 22 gauge needle;
- 1% lidocaine for skin infiltration or for diagnostic injections.

Special equipment

- 3½ inch, 22 gauge needle for the glycerol injection;
- 2 ml syringe with 50% glycerol solution.

Step 4. Visualization

Again, confirm the position of the foramen ovale under the submental fluoroscopic view.

Step 5. Direction of the needle

Next, direct the needle to the foramen ovale's geometric center by rotating the C-arm laterally (Fig. 12.14).

Step 6. Confirm the position of the needle

1. In this view, advance the needle until free flow of the CSF is obtained. If blood is aspirated instead of CSF, withdraw the needle. Then advance again slightly in another

direction. If blood is still aspirated, terminate the procedure.

2. After observing the free flow of clear CSF by gravity alone, place the patient in a **semi-sitting** position, with the neck flexed and fixed in that position.

3. Then, using the lateral fluoroscopic view, inject 0.1–0.5 ml contrast solution (iohexol).

4. Visualize this solution filling the cistern. If this is not observed, reposition the needle. When the cistern is seen to be appropriately filled, allow some time for the solution to saturate the region.

5. After this period to allow the contrast solution to flow out with gravity, do not aspirate.

Step 7. Retrogasserian glycerol injection

When this is seen to be satisfactory, inject 0.5 ml of 50% glycerol into the cistern. Keep the patient in the semi-sitting position for the next 2 hours.

Note: observation of the patient is extremely important at this stage. In some patients, severe headache can occur after glycerol injection. This may last for some days. If, inadvertently, glycerol spreads away from the cistern towards the brain stem, stop the injection immediately. Nausea and vomiting for more than 1 week may be observed. Pain relief may be felt immediately, or in some patients may take 2 weeks.

Step 8. Postprocedure care

After completing the procedure, observe the patient for at least 2 hours. Monitor vital signs (mandatory). In addition, objectively document the pain relief. After a satisfactory observation, discharge the patient with appropriate and adequate instructions given to the escort. Written instructions are preferable for emergencies and are helpful to the patient and family.

Technique of percutaneous balloon compression

Prepare and position the patient as described in the section on RF thermocoagulation. Ready common equipment and drugs for use, in addition to the special equipment and drugs required for this procedure.

Step 3. Drugs and equipment

Common drugs and needles (Fig. 12.15)

- 1½ inch, 25 gauge needle (for infiltration of the skin);
- 5 ml syringe (for local anesthetic solution);
- 2 ml empty syringe (for aspiration test);
- 3½ inch, 22 gauge needle;
- 1% lidocaine for skin infiltration or for diagnostic injections.

Special equipment

- 2 ml iohexol solution;
- 14 gauge, 10 cm needle;
- Fogarty catheter (4 French).

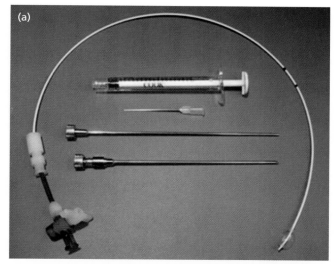

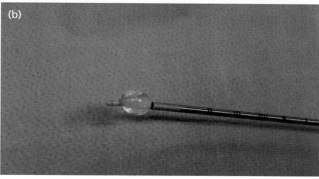

Figure 12.15 (a) Table arrangement of sterile equipment in place for trigeminal ganglion balloon lesioning. (b) Tip of the Fogarty catheter with balloon inflated.

Step 4. Visualization

Begin the Fogarty balloon placement as follows. After confirming that the submental and lateral views of the foramen ovale are visualized, advance the needle to the middle of the foramen ovale in the submental view. Do not advance beyond the entrance of the foramen ovale.

Step 5. Direction of the needle

Next, introduce and advance the tip of the Fogarty catheter (4 French) through the needle in the foramen ovale in the lateral view (Fig. 12.16).

Step 6. Confirm the position of the needle

After satisfactorily advancing the Fogarty catheter beyond the needle tip, inflate the balloon of the Fogarty catheter by injecting 1 ml of contrast material (iohexol). In the lateral fluoroscopic view, the balloon should resemble a pear. Verify this view in both lateral and anteroposterior (AP) fluoroscope images (Fig. 12.17).

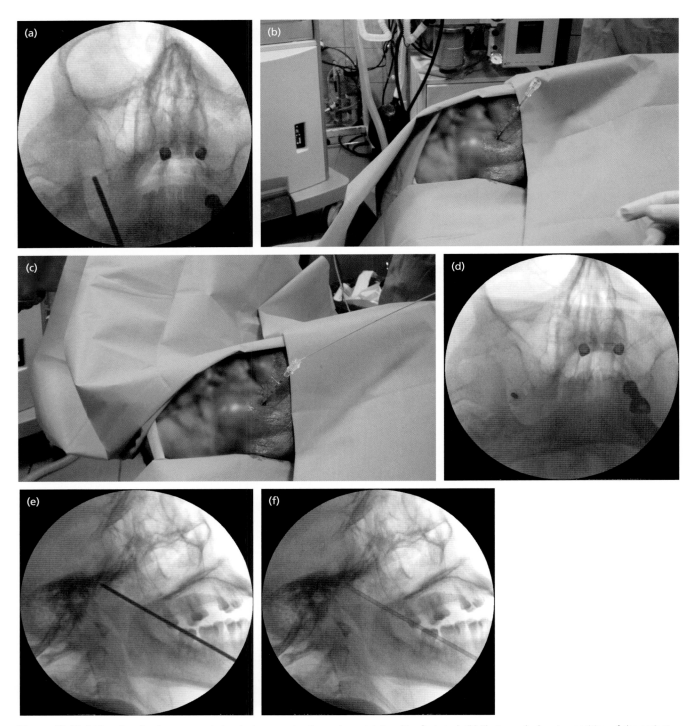

Figure 12.16 (a) Locating the foramen ovale by placing a marker in a submental view (the first step). (b) Photograph showing position of the patient with the needle in position for balloon-compression procedure. (c) Photograph of the patient with a needle in position for advancing the Fogarty catheter. (d) Submental fluoroscopic view of correct placement of the needle tip in the foramen ovale on the left side. (e) Lateral fluoroscopic view showing a catheter in place. (f) Lateral fluoroscopic view with the stylet removed.

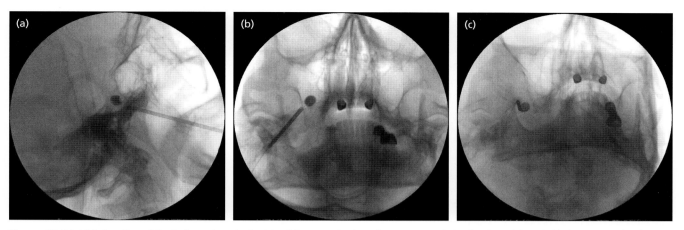

Figure 12.17 (a) Delineation of the balloon shape in the lateral fluoroscopic view after contrast solution has been injected. (b) Anteroposterior view showing the balloon in place when inflated with a contrast solution. (c) Oblique view of the balloon inflated with a contrast solution.

Step 7. Balloon compression
1. Inflate the balloon, and maintain it for 60 seconds to 6 minutes; there is no consensus about the duration of this inflation.
2. After completing the desired time for inflation, aspirate the contrast solution and confirm that the balloon appears to be deflated.
3. Then withdraw the catheter together with the needle as one unit.

Step 8. Postprocedure care
After completing the procedure, observe the patient for at least 2 hours. Monitor vital signs (mandatory). In addition, objectively document the pain relief. After a satisfactory observation, discharge the patient with appropriate and adequate instructions given to the escort. Written instructions are preferable for emergencies and they are helpful to the patient and the family.

Technique for local anesthetic or neurolytic lesioning of the trigeminal nerve
This technique is usually recommended for **diagnostic** and **therapeutic neurolysis** in cancer patients. The patient's preparation and position are similar to those described in the section on RF thermocoagulation (see page 132).

Step 3. Common drugs and equipment
Confirm that the following equipment and drugs are ready for use:
• 1½ inch, 25 gauge needle (for infiltration of the skin);
• 5 ml syringe (for local anesthetic solution);
• 2 ml empty syringe (for aspiration test);
• 3½ inch, 22 gauge needle (for the nerve block);
• 1% lidocaine for skin infiltration or diagnostic injections;
• 2 ml of absolute or 50% alcohol; or
• 2 ml of 6% phenol in saline or glycerine or iohexol.

Step 4. Visualization
Follow the same procedure as for a diagnostic or neurolytic procedure. Position the patient for entry of the needle through the foramen ovale, as described in the section on RF thermocoagulation.

Step 5. Confirm the position of the needle
After again confirming that the needle is in the correct position in both AP and lateral fluoroscopic views, slowly inject 2 ml of local anesthetic.

Step 6. Diagnostic or neurolytic block
When planning a neurolytic therapeutic lesioning, prepare 6% phenol in glycerine, or equivalent. Initially, use 6% phenol, not exceeding 1 ml slowly injected in 0.2–0.5 ml aliquots.
   If the first neurolytic (phenol) procedure is unsucessful, inject 50% alcohol at another sitting.

Step 7. Postprocedure care
After completing the procedure, observe the patient for at least 2 hours. Monitor vital signs (mandatory). In addition, objectively document the pain relief. After a satisfactory observation, discharge the patient with appropriate and adequate instructions given to the escort. Written instructions are preferable for emergencies and they are helpful to the patient and the family.

Complications observed with trigeminal ganglion and nerve lesioning
• **Hypesthesia and dysesthesia**
These are most commonly seen with RF thermocoagulation. They are less common after glycerol injection or balloon compression.
• **Anesthesia dolorosa**
Anesthesia dolorosa is one of the most serious and significant complications after RF lesioning. It is a syndrome of burning

pain, allodynia, and dysesthesia, despite the lesioning in the distribution of the affected branch of the trigeminal nerve. Patients should be informed preoperatively about the possibility of this complication. The incidence of anesthesia dolorosa is reduced if the thermocoagulation is done at below a 60–70 °C setting. Tricyclic antidepressants and gabapentin may be helpful for treating anesthesia dolorosa.

- **Corneal reflex loss and neurolytic keratitis**

The incidence of corneal reflex and keratitis varies, depending on the technique used, ranging from low for balloon compression to high for RF lesioning. In the case of corneal reflex loss, the patient may use artificial eye drops and protective spectacles with side shields to prevent the discomfort and introduction of foreign body inflammation of the eye.

- **Motor deficit and masseter weakness**

Motor deficit and masseter weakness occur during lesioning of the mandibular nerve. The incidence of masseter weakness is the highest with balloon compression, when compared to other techniques.

- **Retrobulbar hematoma and hematoma in the cheek**

Retrobulbar hematoma occurs if the needle is advanced into the infraorbital fissure. The eyeball is pushed anteriorly into the retrobulbar space, and exophthalmus develops. With compression of the orbit (in a confined space), bleeding usually stops; and the swelling subsides within a few days. If the needle passes through a vessel, hematoma in the cheek may develop. Compression over the cheek by cold pack is helpful to arrest the size of the hematoma.

- **Diplopia**

Diplopia may occur after RF lesioning and retrogasserian glycerol injection. It may be due to damage to the other cranial nerves at the base of the skull. Generally, this deficit is temporary.

- **Infection and meningitis**

Although the incidence of infection and meningitis is very low, it should be addressed aggressively when it occurs.

- **Other cranial nerve deficits**

Deficit of the other cranial nerves may occur if the procedure is performed only under lateral view and is generally due to the spread of solutions such as glycerol and phenol onto these nerves.

Helpful hints

Trigeminal neuralgia occurs very rarely in younger patients. Percutaneous interventions should not be the first choice in such patients.

Psychological assessment of the patient before the procedure is necessary. If there are concerns about his/her psychological stability, perform a prognostic block with 2 ml 0.05% bupivacaine to assess the patient's behavior. They may complain of significant sequelae when the technique is safe and simple.

In all techniques, there is a recurrence rate, which means trigeminal neuralgia will reappear after a variable period.

Because of this possibility, begin treatment for trigeminal neuralgia with medications, and, when they do not provide the required pain relief, consider percutaneous techniques.

Percutaneous interventions for trigeminal neuralgia should be performed only by fully trained pain physicians certified in interventional techniques.

It is helpful to keep the artificial dental prosthesis in situ. With edentulous patients, point of entry changes. The entry is more posterior, and the needle will strike the foramen at too acute an angle.

The patient and family should be informed about the side effects and complications of the interventions before the procedure.

Before the entry through the foramen ovale, feel the bony edge of the foramen. At this point, turn the C-arm to a lateral position, to view clearly the entry through the foramen ovale.

The advantages of RF lesioning are a high incidence of pain relief with a low relapse rate. The disadvantages are anesthesia dolorsa, paresthesia, or dysesthesia.

The advantages of balloon compression are that it causes less sensory deficit and has a moderate rate of recurrence. However, significant masseter weakness and transient otalgia are the main disadvantages.

There is less sensory deficit following local or neurolytic injection than with RF lesioning. In contrast, an expensive procedure such as RF lesioning may not be available or affordable. Shorter duration of pain relief, higher recurrence rates, and development of fibrosis at the entry of the needle tip at the foramen ovale are the disadvantages of neurolytic solution.

Percutaneous maxillary nerve block

History

Because maxillary nerve lesioning is related to trigeminal ganglion lesioning, its history will not be discussed here.

Anatomy

Origin of the maxillary nerve

The maxillary nerve is the third division of the trigeminal nerve. It arises from the trigeminal ganglion, which lies within the cranium, close to the anterior surface of the petrous portion of the temporal bone.

The branches and course of the trigeminal nerve

Three main branches of the trigeminal ganglion arise from the anterior border of the ganglion, from the medial to the lateral aspect. The ophthalmic nerve arises first (V1); the maxillary nerve (V2) arises second; and, finally, the mandibular nerve (V3) arises. The origins of these nerves in the ganglion are somatotropically located in the ganglion; the

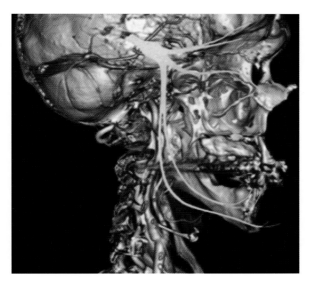

Figure 12.18 Three-dimensional computed tomography scan showing the branches of the trigeminal ganglion. Note, specifically, the second branch and its course.

ophthalmic branch is situated medioposteriorly, the maxillary branch is intermediate, and the mandibular branch occupies the ventrolateral position (Fig. 12.18).

Course of the maxillary nerve and its branches

The maxillary nerve is the second branch of the trigeminal nerve (V2). The maxillary nerve arises from the trigeminal ganglion, in between the ophthalmic and mandibulary branches, and exits through the foramen rotundum. After exiting, it continues into the superior aspect of the pterygopalatine fossa in the inferior portion of the orbit in the infraorbital fissure.

The maxillary nerve has orbital, palatinal, nasal, and pharyngeal branches and filaments to the SPG. It finally exits through the infraorbital foramen in the face.

Innervation of the maxillary nerve

Unlike the mandibular nerve, the maxillary nerve is purely sensory. It innervates the maxillary sinus, teeth of the upper jaw, gums, skin of the ipsilateral face, side of the nose, upper lip, mucosa from the lower eyelid to the upper lip, hard and soft palates, nasal cavity, pharynx, and dura mater of the medial cranial fossa.

Indications

- Idiopathic maxillary neuralgia.
- Secondary maxillary neuralgia due to cancer or compression neuropathy.

Contraindications

- Local infection or sepsis.
- Coagulopathy.

- Vital function instability.
- Psychopathologies.

Technique of maxillary nerve block

Step 1. Prepare the patient before the procedure
Ascertain the type of analgesia or sedation before performing the invasive procedure. If planning a local anesthetic or neurolytic block, mild sedation is all that is necessary. If pulsed RF is planned, the patient needs to be awake to respond to the stimulation test. Intravenous fentanyl or midazolam may be used judiciously for patient comfort.

Step 2. Position and monitor the patient
1. Place the patient in a supine position on the table.
2. Fix the head on the table with a strip of adhesive tape, appropriately away from the point of entry.
3. Prepare and drape the area in a sterile fashion.
4. Obtain an IV access if drugs need to be administered.
5. Monitor vital signs (mandatory) in unstable patients.
6. Prepare the area in a sterile fashion for needle entry.

Step 3. Drugs and equipment
Prepare and confirm that the following equipment, needles, and drugs are sterilized and ready to be used for the procedure:
- 1½ inch, 25 gauge needle for skin infiltration;
- 5 ml syringe for local anesthetic injection;
- 3½ inch, 22 gauge needle for the nerve block;
- 5 ml of 1% lidocaine.
If a neurolytic procedure is performed, use the following:
- steroid solution (decadron or equivalent);
- 2 ml alcohol, if preferred;
- 2 ml of 6% phenol in iohexol (recommended).
  The extraoral technique is commonly performed.

Step 4. Mark the surface landmarks for needle entry
1. With the patient in the supine position, turn the head a few degrees to the opposite side.
2. Identify the mandibular notch, near the external auditory meatus (Fig. 12.19).
3. Mark the entry point on the skin.

Step 5. Direction of the needle
1. After infiltration of local anesthetic in the entry site, introduce an 8 cm, 3¼ inch, 22 gauge needle perpendicularly to the skin at the posterior and inferior aspects of the notch.
2. Advance the needle towards the lateral pterygoid plate, which commonly lies at a 4–5 cm depth (Fig. 12.20).

Step 6. Confirm the position of the needle
1. When the bone (lateral pterygoid plate) is contacted, slip the needle anteriorly and superiorly toward the root of the nose.

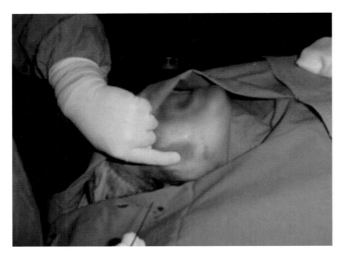

Figure 12.19 Photograph showing the patient in the supine position about to have a maxillary nerve block. The index finger identifies the point of entry of the needle at the mandibular notch.

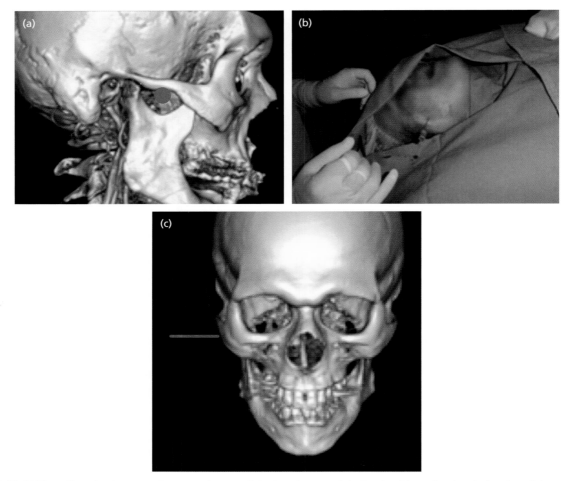

Figure 12.20 (a) Three-dimensional computed tomography scan of the lateral aspect of the head and face, showing the location of the mandibular notch in front of the temporal mandibular joint and below the zygoma. (b) Photograph showing the needle entry at the mandibular notch for the maxillary nerve block. (c) Three-dimensional computed tomography scan showing the direction of the needle in the anterioposterior view as it enters the mandibular notch and is directed toward the root of the nose.

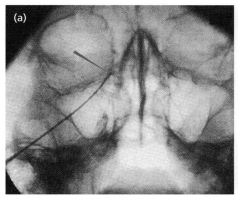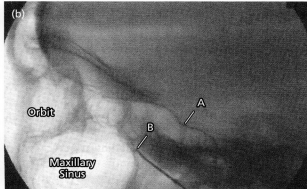

Figure 12.21 (a) Radiographic AP view showing the position of the needle tip as it enters the inverted vase, which is then entry for the pterypalatine fossa. (b) Lateral radiograph showing entry of the needle in the inverted vase.

2. At this point, check with the lateral fluoroscopic image that the pterygopalatine fossa is visualized as an inverted vase (Fig. 12.21).

Step 7. Test stimulation

When the needle tip enters the pterygopalatine fossa, seek for paresthesia in the distribution of the maxillary nerve.

Note: when advancing the needle, if it slips off at the lateral pterygoid plate more than 1 cm, it may enter the pterygomaxillary fissure. Injection of a local anesthetic may spread to the posterior aspect of the orbit.

Step 8. Maxillary nerve block

1. Because the pterygopalatine fossa has a rich blood supply, aspiration before injecting any solution is mandatory.

2. If blood is aspirated before injection, redirect the needle until blood is not aspirated.

3. After confirming the location with fluoroscopic imaging and paresthesia, inject 3 to 5 ml of 1% lidocaine.

4. For the neurolytic technique, inject 1–1.5 ml of 6% phenol in iohexol.

Note: do not advance the needle more than 5.5 cm. If the patient does not feel paresthesia, redirect the needle.

Step 9. Pulsed RF

1. Pulsed RF is performed for the maxillary nerve (Fig. 12.22) because it contains somatic large A-delta fibers and thermocoagulation is not recommended.

2. Advance a 5 cm or 5 mm active-tip electrode to the nerves, as described for a diagnostic block. Perform sensory stimulation with 50 Hz at a 0.5 V setting. When the patient confirms paresthesia in the distribution of the nerve tested, inject 1 ml of 1% lidocaine. Wait for 5 minutes. Perform pulsed RF at 42 °C, for 120 seconds, for two or three cycles.

Step 10. Postprocedure care

After the procedure is completed, observe the patient for up to 2 hours. Monitor vital signs (mandatory). In addition,

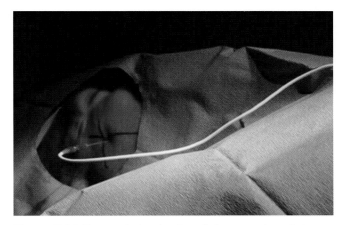

Figure 12.22 Photograph showing the radiofrequency electrode in place where it should be for the maxillary nerve radiofrequency procedure.

objectively document the pain relief. After a satisfactory observation, discharge the patient, with appropriate and adequate instructions given to the escort. Written instructions are preferable for emergencies and they are helpful to the patient and family.

Complications

• **Ophthalmic complications**

If the needle is advanced too deeply in a cephalad direction, it may enter the upper portion of the pterygomaxillary fissure. The local anesthetic agent may spread to the orbit, and the optic nerve; this may cause temporary blindness. The neurolytic agents are contraindicated if this occurs. If the needle enters the infraorbital fissure, orbital hematoma may occur, along with ophthalmoplegia, loss of visual acuity, or diplopia.

• **Inadvertent puncture of the pharynx**

If the needle is directed too posteriorly, there is a risk of inadvertent puncture of the pharynx. Air can be aspirated in the syringe during the aspiration test.

• **Toxic reaction to local anesthetics**
Toxic reaction to local anesthetics may occur due to intravascular injection, as well as due to the large amount of local anesthetic injected. The recommendation is to keep the volume of local anesthetic solution below 5 ml, injected intermittently in smaller aliquots.

Helpful hints

Aspiration is mandatory before injecting any analgesic solution when the needle tip is at the maxillary nerve. Terminate the procedure if blood is aspirated.

Do not perform the block if the patient does not confirm paresthesia.

Be careful not to be deep anteriorly, as the maxillary nerve is close to many significant neural and vascular structures.

Keep the injectate below 5 ml of local anesthetic or 1.5 ml for neurolytic agents.

Percutaneous mandibular nerve block

History

The history of mandibular nerve lesioning is related to that of trigeminal ganglion lesioning, so it will not be discussed here.

Anatomy

Origin of the mandibular nerve

The mandibular nerve is the third division of the trigeminal nerve. It arises from the trigeminal ganglion, which lies within the cranium, close to the anterior surface of the petrous portion of the temporal bone.

The course of the mandibular nerve

Three main branches of the trigeminal ganglion arise from the anterior border of the ganglion, from the medial to the lateral direction. Their orientation is, first, the sensory root of the ophthalmic nerve (V1); second, the maxillary nerve (V2); and, finally, the mandibular nerve (V3). The origins of these nerves in the ganglion are somatotropically located in the ganglion; the ophthalmic branch is situated most medioposteriorly, the maxillary branch is situated in an intermediate position, and the mandibular branch occupies the ventrolateral position.

The motor root of the mandibular nerve runs anterior and medial to the sensory root and passes inferior to the ganglion. The motor root then leaves the skull through the foramen ovale. Immediately below this foramen, the motor root joins the sensory root of the mandibular nerve (Fig. 12.23).

Innervation

The mandibular nerve innervates the temporal region; the skin of the lower face; cheek; lower lip; anterior part of the

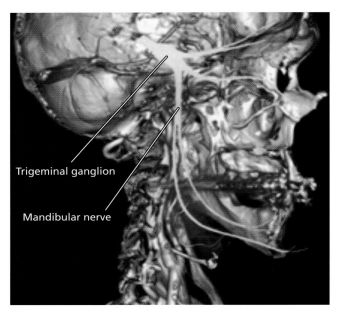

Figure 12.23 Computed tomography scan highlighting in red the course of the mandibular nerve, which originates from the trigeminal ganglion.

external ear, which is part of the external acoustic meatus; the anterior two-thirds of the tongue; the teeth of the lower jaw ipsilaterally; the mastoid air cells; the mucous membranes of the cheek; the mandible; and the dura of the middle cranial fossa. The motor fibers innervate the muscles of mastication (the temporalis, masseter, external and internal pterygoid, bucinator, digastric, mylohyoid, tensor palatini and tensor tympani muscles).

Indications
• Idiopathic trigeminal neuralgia affecting the mandibular branch of the trigeminal nerve.
• Seconary mandibular neuralgia (for example, cancer pain).
• Compressive mandibular neuropathy from miscellaneous causes.

Contraindications
• Local infection or sepsis.
• Coagulopathy.
• Instability of vital functions.
• Psychopathologies.

Technique of diagnostic and/or therapeutic mandibular nerve block

Step 1. Prepare the patient before the procedure
Ascertain the type of analgesia or sedation before performing the invasive procedure. If planning a local anesthetic or considering a neurolytic block, mild sedation is all that is

necessary. If planning pulsed RF, the patient needs to be awake to respond to the stimulation test. Intravenous fentanyl or midazolam may be used judiciously for patient comfort.

Step 2. Position and monitor the patient
1. Place the patient in a supine position on the table.
2. Fix the head on the table with a strip of adhesive tape appropriately away from the point of entry.
3. Obtain an IV access if drugs need to be administered.
4. Monitor vital signs (mandatory in unstable patients).
5. Prepare the area for needle entry in a sterile fashion.

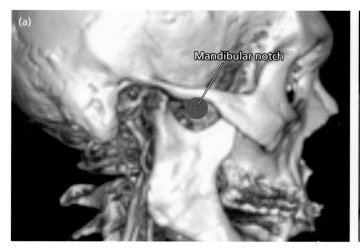

Figure 12.24 Photograph showing the patient in the supine position about to have a mandibular nerve block. The index finger identifies the point of entry of the needle at the mandibular notch.

Step 3. Drugs and equipment

Common drugs and needles
Prepare and confirm that the following equipment, needles, and drugs are ready to be used for the procedure:
• 1½ inch, 25 gauge needle for skin infiltration;
• 5 ml syringe containing local anesthetic solution;
• 3½ inch, 22 gauge needle for the nerve block;
• 5 ml of 1% lidocaine;
• preferred steroid solution (decadron or equivalent);
• 2 ml of 6% phenol (usually prepared in iohexol).
The technique usually used is the extraoral route.

Step 4. Mark the surface landmarks for needle entry
1. Initiate the procedure. Ask the patient to open and shut their mouth to allow identification of the mandibular notch.
2. Next, locate the skin entry point at the mandibular notch, which is close to the external auditory meatus (Fig. 12.24).

Step 5. Direction of the needle
Start with a 3½ inch, 22 gauge needle entering perpendicularly to the skin at the posterior and inferior aspects of the notch, and confirm radiographically (Fig. 12.25).

Step 6. Confirm the position of the needle
1. Advance the penetrating needle towards the lateral pterygoid plate, which lies at a 4–5 cm depth.
2. Walk posteriorly on the lateral pterygoid plate until the needle tip slips off the plate (Fig. 12.26).

Step 7. Test stimulation
Immediately seek for paresthesia in the mandibular nerve distribution, which needs to be sought at the lower lip, lower jaw, ipsilateral tongue, and ear.

Note: the pterygopalatine fossa has a rich blood supply.

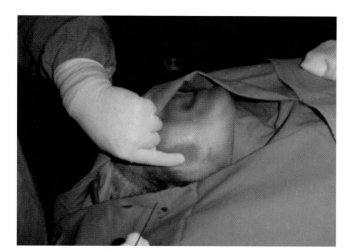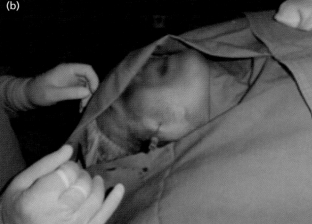

Figure 12.25 (a) Three-dimensional computed tomography scan of the lateral aspect of the head and face, showing the location of the mandibular notch in front of the temporal mandibular joint and below the zygoma. (b) Photograph showing needle entry at the mandibular notch for the mandibular nerve block.

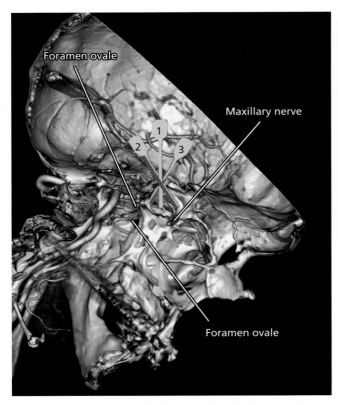

Figure 12.26 The technique for the extraoral block of the mandibular nerve is essentially the same as that for the maxillary block, except that the needle is directed upward and posteriorly; thus, the mandibular nerve is contacted as it exits from the foramen ovale.

Step 8. Mandibular nerve block
1. Aspirate before injecting any diagnostic or therapeutic solution. If blood is aspirated during the injection, redirect the needle until it is negative for any fluid.
2. After confirming correct needle placement, inject 3–5 ml of 1% lidocaine.
3. For a neurolytic block, inject 1–1.5 ml of 6% phenol with iohexol. Alcohol is not recommended.
  Note: do not advance the needle more than 5.5 cm from the point of entry. If the patient does not feel paresthesia, redirect the needle until finding the correct placement.

Step 9. Pulsed RF lesioning of the mandibular nerves
1. Pulsed RF lesioning is performed for the mandibular nerve because it contains somatic A-delta and A-alpha fibers. Thermocoagulation is not recommended, even though some physicians still practice it.
2. Advance a 5 cm or 5 mm active-tip electrode to the nerves, as described for a diagnostic block (Fig. 12.27).
3. Perform sensory stimulation with 50 Hz at a 0.5 V setting.
4. Perform pulsed radiofrequency at 42°C for 120 seconds, for two or three cycles.

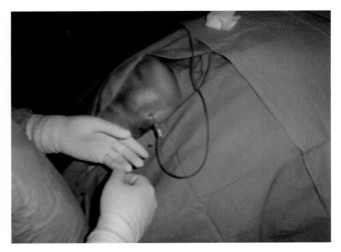

Figure 12.27 Photograph showing the needle in position for the mandibular nerve block.

Step 10. Postprocedure care
After the procedure is completed, observe the patient for up to 2 hours. Monitor vital signs (mandatory). In addition, objectively document pain relief. After a satisfactory observation, discharge the patient with appropriate and adequate instructions given to the escort. Written instructions are preferable for emergencies and they are helpful to the patient and family.

Complications
During the procedure, beware of the following.
- **Inadvertent puncture of the pharynx**
Be aware of inadvertent puncture of the pharynx. This can happen if the needle is directed too posteriorly. Air can be aspirated in the syringe during the aspiration test if the needle enters the pharynx.
- **Puncture of the blood vessels**
Puncture of the blood vessels (middle meningeal artery) can occur. The middle meningeal artery enters the cranial cavity through the foramen spinosum, in close proximity to the mandibular nerve posterolaterally.
- **Toxic reaction to local anesthetics**
Toxic reaction to local anesthetics may occur due to intravascular injection, as well as due to the large amount of local anesthetics injected in the region. Keep the volume of local anesthetic or neurolytic solution as low as possible.

Helpful hints
Aspirate before injecting any solution onto the mandibular nerve. If blood is aspirated, redirect the needle and aspirate again.

  Do not inject the diagnostic or therapeutic solution if the patient does not feel paresthesia. Redirect the needle until this is obtained.

Do not go too deep posteriorly. This will help prevent the inadvertent puncture of significant nerves and/or vessels in the pharyngeal region.

Do not inject more than 5 ml of local anesthetic or 1.5 ml of neurolytic agents.

Inject the solution in small boluses of ½ ml at a time.

Percutaneous block of the terminal branches of the trigeminal nerve

History
The history of the trigeminal ganglion and lesioning of its branch is described in the section on trigeminal ganglion lesioning (see page 130).

Supraorbital nerve block and lesioning

Anatomy
The supraorbital nerve is the terminal branch of the ophthalmic nerve. It exits the orbit through the supraorbital foramen. The supraorbital nerve innervates the forehead, upper eyelid, and anterior scalp (Fig. 12.28).

Indications for supraorbital nerve lesioning
Common indications are the following:
• idiopathic and secondary trigeminal neuralgia;
• intractable headaches.

Contraindications for supraorbital nerve lesioning
It is important to consider the following contraindications:
• local infection;
• coagulopathy;
• vital function instability;
• psychopathologies.

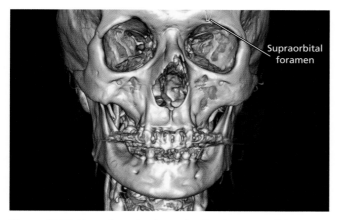
Figure 12.28 Three-dimensional scan showing the course of the supraorbital nerve as it enters the supraorbital foramen (arrow).

Technique of supraorbital nerve block

Step 1. Prepare the patient before the procedure
Ascertain the type of analgesia or sedation before performing the invasive procedure. If considering a local anesthetic or planning a neurolytic block, mild sedation is all that is necessary. If planning pulsed RF, the patient needs to be awake to respond to the stimulation test. Intravenous fentanyl or midazolam may be used judiciously for patient comfort.

Step 2. Position and monitor the patient
1. Obtain an IV access if drugs need to be administered.
2. Place the patient in a supine position on the table.
3. Fix the head on the table with a strip of adhesive tape, appropriately away from the point of entry.
4. Monitor vital signs (mandatory) in unstable patients.
5. Prepare the area for needle entry in a sterile fashion.

Step 3. Drugs and equipment
Prepare and confirm that the following equipment, needles, and drugs are ready to be used for block of the peripheral branches of the trigeminal nerve:
• 1½ inch, 25 gauge needle (for infiltration of the skin);
• 5 ml syringe (for local anesthetic solution).
For neurolytic solution and diagnostic block, use the following:
• 1% lidocaine solution;
• 1 ml of 6% phenol in saline or glycerine or iohexol;
• 2 mm tip with a 5 cm electrode and required cables (for a pulsed RF procedure).

Step 4. Mark the surface landmarks for needle entry
Identify the surface landmarks by palpating to locate the supraorbital notch, then infiltrating the skin with 1 ml of 1% lidocaine.

Step 5. Direction of the needle
Direct the needle, as follows.
1. Insert the needle first perpendicularly to the supraorbital notch and then redirect medially (15°).
2. When the needle touches the periosteum, avoid entering the supraorbital foramen. If the needle enters the foramen, withdraw it and redirect it slightly more medially.

Step 6. Confirm the position of the needle
Confirm the position of the needle, and aspirate for negative blood.

Step 7. Supraorbital nerve block
Perform a supraorbital nerve block, as follows.
1. After the negative aspiration test, inject 2 ml of 1% lidocaine.

2. If a neurolytic block is contemplated, use alcohol or phenol. This is recommended for advanced cancer patients only.

3. Because the surrounding tissue is loose, apply gentle pressure after the procedure to prevent swelling or hematoma.

Step 8. Pulsed RF

To administer pulsed RF, advance a 5 cm with 5 mm active-tip electrode to the nerves, as described for diagnostic block. Perform sensory stimulation with 50 Hz at a 0.5 V setting. When the patient confirms paresthesia in the distribution of the nerve tested, inject 1 ml of 1% lidocaine. Wait for 5 minutes. Perform pulsed RF at 42 °C for 120 seconds for two or three cycles.

Step 9. Postprocedure care

After completing the procedure, observe the patient for up to 2 hours. Monitor vital signs (mandatory). In addition, objectively document the pain relief. After a satisfactory observation, discharge the patient with appropriate and adequate instructions given to the escort. Written instructions are preferable for emergencies, and they are helpful to the patient and the family.

Infraorbital nerve block and lesioning

Anatomy

The infraorbital nerve is the terminal branch of the maxillary nerve. It exits the orbit through the infraorbital foramen. The infraorbital foramen is located 0.5–1 cm below the lower border of the orbit. The infraorbital nerve innervates the lower eyelid, lateral part of the nose and upper lip.

Step 1. Prepare the patient before the procedure

Ascertain the type of analgesia or sedation before performing the invasive procedure. If considering a local anesthetic or planning a neurolytic block, mild sedation is all that is necessary. If planning pulsed RF, the patient needs to be awake to respond to the stimulation test. Intravenous fentanyl or midazolam may be used judiciously for patient comfort.

Step 2. Position and monitor the patient

1. Obtain an IV access if drugs need to be administered.

2. Place the patient in a supine position on the table.

3. Fix the head on the table with a strip of adhesive tape, appropriately away from the point of entry.

4. Monitor vital signs (mandatory) in unstable patients.

5. Prepare the area for needle entry in a sterile fashion.

Step 3. Drugs and equipment

Prepare and confirm that the following equipment, needles, and drugs are ready to be used for the procedure:

- 1½ inch, 25 gauge needle (for infiltration of the skin);
- 5 ml syringe (for local anesthetic solution).

For neurolytic solution and diagnostic block, use the following:

- 1% lidocaine solution;
- 1 ml of 6% phenol in saline or glycerine or iohexol;
- 2 mm tip with 5 cm electrode and required cables (for pulsed RF).

Step 4. Mark the surface landmarks for needle entry

Identify the surface landmarks by palpating the infraorbital notch with the index finger.

Step 5. Direction of the needle

Insert the needle, as follows.

1. Infiltrate the skin 0.5–1 cm lateral to the midportion of the ala of the nose, with 1% lidocaine.

2. Insert the needle, first perpendicular to the infraorbital notch, then advancing upward and backward, 15° perpendicularly, until the needle touches the periosteum near the infraorbital notch (Fig. 12.29).

Step 6. Confirm the position of the needle

Confirm the position. Aspirate. If blood is aspirated, redirect the needle.

Note: avoid entering the foramen. If the needle enters the foramen, withdraw it and redirect slightly more medially.

Step 7. Infraorbital nerve block

1. After the negative aspiration test, inject 0.5 ml of 1% lidocaine.

2. For neurolytic procedures, use phenol only for cancer patients.

3. Do not inject more than 0.5 ml inside the foramen; larger doses may cause compression neuropathy.

4. Because the surrounding tissue is loose, apply gentle pressure after the procedure to prevent swelling or hematoma.

Step 8. Postprocedure care

After completing the procedure, observe the patient for up to 2 hours. Monitor vital signs (mandatory). In addition, objectively document the pain relief. After a satisfactory observation, discharge the patient with appropriate and adequate instructions given to the escort. Written instructions are preferable for emergencies and they are helpful to the patient and the family.

Auriculotemporal nerve block and lesioning

Anatomy

The auriculotemporal nerve is one of the terminal branches of the mandibular nerve. It is located between the temporomandibular joint and the external auditory meatus. The

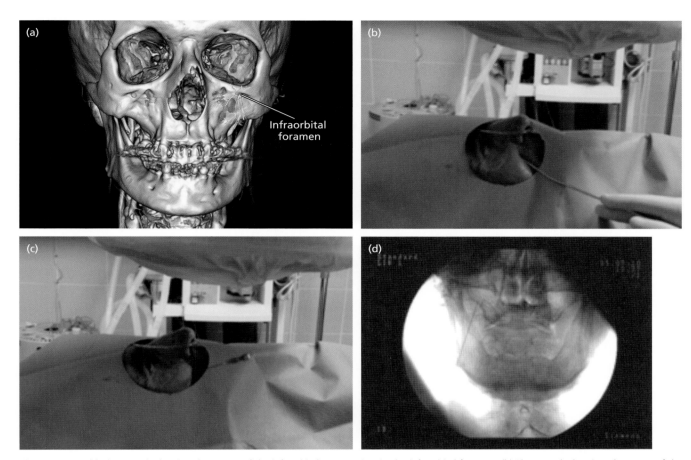

Figure 12.29 (a) Photograph showing the course of the infraorbital nerve as it exits the infraorbital foramen. (b) Photograph showing placement of the marker for needle entry into the infraorbital foramen. (c) The position of the patient and the needle for the infraorbital nerve block. (d) Posteroanterior view of the face showing the direction of the needle in the infraorbital foramen.

nerve innervates the temporomandibular joint, pinna of the ear and external auditory meatus, as well as the temporal region and the lateral scalp. The auriculotemporal nerve courses along with the temporal artery, which is a landmark to use when performing the auriculotemporal block (Fig. 12.30).

Step 1. Prepare the patient before the procedure
Ascertain the type of analgesia or sedation before performing the invasive procedure. If considering a local anesthetic or planning a neurolytic block, mild sedation is all that is necessary. If planning pulsed RF, the patient needs to be awake to respond to the stimulation test. Intravenous fentanyl or midazolam may be used judiciously for patient comfort.

Step 2. Position and monitor the patient
1. Obtain an IV access if drugs need to be administered.
2. Place the patient in a supine position on the table.
3. Fix the head on the table with a strip of adhesive tape appropriately away from the point of entry.

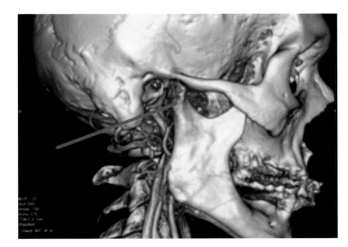

Figure 12.30 Three-dimensional computed tomography scan showing the temporomandibular joint in the vicinity of the auriculotemporal nerve.

4. Monitor vital signs (mandatory) in unstable patients.
5. Prepare the area for needle entry in a sterile fashion.

Step 3. Drugs and equipment
Prepare and confirm that the following equipment, needles, and drugs are ready to be used for the procedure:
- 1½ inch, 25 gauge needle (for infiltration of the skin);
- 5 ml syringe (for local anesthetic solution).
    For neurolytic solution and diagnostic block, use the following:
- 1% lidocaine solution;
- 1 ml of 6% phenol in saline or glycerine or iohexol;
- 2 mm tip with 5 cm electrode and required cables (for pulsed RF procedure).

Step 4. Mark the surface landmarks for needle entry
Identify the surface landmarks by turning the head slightly to the contralateral side and palpating and feeling the pulsation of the temporal artery.

Step 5. Direction of the needle
Introduce a 1½ inch, 25 gauge needle on the zygoma and advance it until the needle contacts the bone (Fig. 12.31).

Step 6. Confirm the position of the needle
Confirm the position of the needle. The needle tip should rest on the bony surface.

Step 7. Auriculotemporal nerve block
To perform the auriculotemporal nerve block, carry out the following steps.
1. After the negative aspiration test, inject 0.5 ml of 1% lidocaine.
2. For a neurolytic procedure, use alcohol or phenol only for cancer patients.

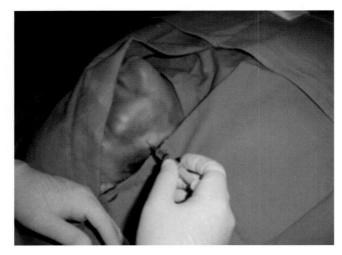

Figure 12.31 The procedure for blocking the auriculotemporal nerve.

3. Apply gentle pressure with a cold pack after the nerve block.

Step 8. Postprocedure care
After completing the procedure, observe the patient for up to 2 hours. Monitor vital signs (mandatory). In addition, objectively document the pain relief. After a satisfactory observation, discharge the patient with appropriate and adequate instructions given to the escort. Written instructions are preferable for emergencies and they are helpful to the patient and the family.

Mental nerve block and lesioning

Anatomy
The mental nerve is one of the terminal branches of the inferior alveolar nerve, which is also a branch of the mandibular nerve. The mental nerve exits the mandible through the mental foramen. It innervates the lower lip, chin and oral mucosa of that region. The mental foramen is approximately at the level of the second premolar tooth in the mandible.

Step 1. Prepare the patient before the procedure
Ascertain the type of analgesia or sedation before performing the invasive procedure. If considering a local anesthetic or planning a neurolytic block, mild sedation is all that is necessary. If pulsed RF is planned, the patient needs to be awake to respond to the stimulation test. Intravenous fentanyl or midazolam may be used judiciously for patient comfort.

Step 2. Position and monitor the patient
1. Obtain an IV access if drugs need to be administered.
2. Place the patient in a supine position on the table.
3. Fix the head on the table with a strip of adhesive tape appropriately away from the point of entry.
4. Monitor vital signs (mandatory in unstable patients).
5. Prepare the area for needle entry in a sterile fashion.

Step 3. Drugs and equipment
Prepare and confirm that the following equipment, needles, and drugs are ready to be used for the procedure:
- 1½ inch, 25 gauge needle (for infiltration of the skin);
- 5 ml syringe (for local anesthetic solution).
For neurolytic solution and diagnostic block, use the following:
- 1% lidocaine solution;
- 1 ml of 6% phenol in saline or glycerine or iohexol;
- 2 mm tip with 5 cm electrode and required cables for pulsed RF procedure.

Step 4. Mark the surface landmarks for needle entry
Identify the surface landmarks by palpating the mental notch. Prepare the area with antiseptic solution (Fig. 12.32).

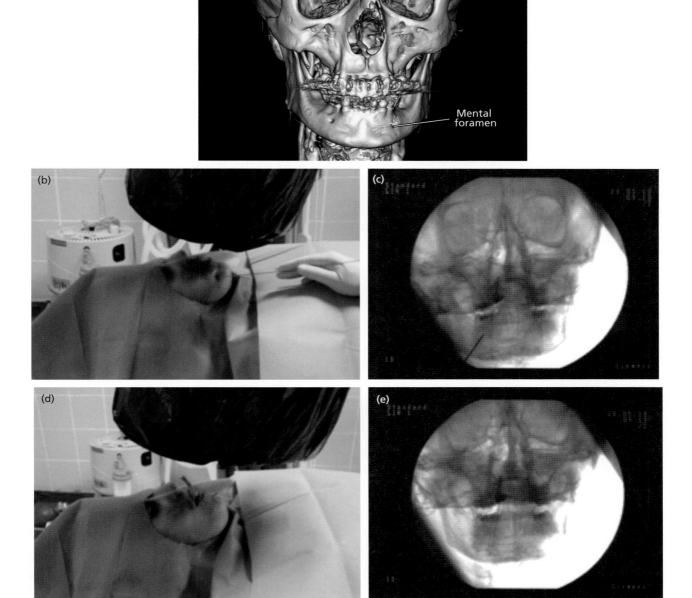

Figure 12.32 (a) Computed tomography scan showing the mental foramen and the mental nerve. (b) Photograph showing the location of the mental nerve, with the patient in the supine position. (c) The marker in this radiograph points to the mental foramen. (d) Photograph showing the patient in the supine position, having a mental nerve block being done. (e) Radiograph showing the needle in position for a mental nerve block.

Step 5. Direction of the needle
Insert a 1½ inch, 25 gauge needle perpendicular to the mental notch. Then advance it medially (15° perpendicularly), until the needle contacts the periosteum near the mental notch.

Step 6. Confirm the position of the needle
1. Avoid entering the foramen itself. If the needle enters the foramen, withdraw it, and redirect it slightly more medially.
2. Aspirate for blood and redirect the needle.

Step 7. Mental nerve block
Perform the mental nerve block.
1. After the negative aspiration, inject 0.5 ml of 1% lido-caine. Do not inject more than 0.5 ml inside the mental foramen; larger doses may cause compression neuropathy. For neurolytic procedures, use alcohol or phenol.
2. Apply gentle pressure with a cold pack after the nerve block.

Step 8. Postprocedure care
After completing the procedure observe the patient for up to 2 hours. Monitor vital signs (mandatory). In addition, objectively document the pain relief. After a satisfactory observation, discharge the patient with appropriate and adequate instructions given to the escort. Written instructions are preferable for emergencies, and they are helpful to the patient and the family.

Complications
• Hematoma
The subcutaneous tissue at the peripheric branches of the trigeminal nerve is highly vascular and loose. Owing to this vascularity, ecchymosis and hematoma may develop after the block. Gentle pressure with a cold pack may decrease the incidence of these complications, especially during the supraorbital and infraorbital nerve blocks. A hematoma may lead to swelling of the eyelids.
• Compression neuropathy
The volume of the foramina where the peripheric branches of the trigeminal nerve are located is considerably smaller than elsewhere. Injection of even very small amounts of solution inside the foramina may cause damage to the nerve, resulting in a compression neuropathy. Permenant paresthe-sia and burning pain may develop. To prevent this complica-tion, do not advance the needle inside the foramina but, instead, keep it outside.
• Permanent paresthesia
Permenant paresthesia may occur owing to the use of neu-rolytic agents for blocking the peripheral branches of the trigeminal nerve.
• Anesthesia dolorosa
The risk of anesthesia dolorosa is present if neurolytic agents are used for the block.

Helpful hints
• Block of the peripheral branches of the trigeminal nerve should be performed if neuralgia is confined to the innerva-tion of these nerves or if the patient has cancer pain.
• Neurolytic agents are preferred in cancer patients. In the treatment of idiopathic trigeminal neuralgia confined to these branches, the first step should be use of a combination of a 2 ml local anesthetic–steroid solution.
• Pulsed RF may also be applied. Because there are not ade-quate efficacy data on this procedure, it is not described here.

Percutaneous block and lesioning of the sphenopalatine ganglion

History
The SPG has been involved in the pathogenesis of pain since Sluder first described sphenopalatine neuralgia in 1908 and treated it with an SPG block. Over the past century, physi-cians have performed SPG block for pain syndromes ranging from headaches and facial pain to sciatica and dysmenor-rhea. Currently this procedure is recommended mainly for head and facial pain.

Anatomy of the SPG (Figs 12.33 and 12.34)

Location
The SPG (also known as Meckel's ganglion) is located in the pterygopalatine fossa. It lies posterior to the middle tur-binate of the nose.

Structure
The SPG, the largest of the parasympathetic ganglia, is deeply placed in the pterygopalatine fossa, close to the sphe-nopalatine foramen. It is triangular shaped and is situated just below the maxillary nerve as it crosses the fossa.

Functionally, it is one of four parasympathetic ganglia of the head and neck. The flow of blood to the nasal mucosa, particularly the venous plexus of the conchae, is regulated by the SPG and maintains the body temperature of the air in the nose.

Innervation
The SPG supplies the lacrimal gland, paranasal sinuses, glands of the mucosa of the nasal cavity and pharynx, gingiva, and mucous membrane and glands of the hard palate. It communicates anteriorly with the nasopalatine nerve.

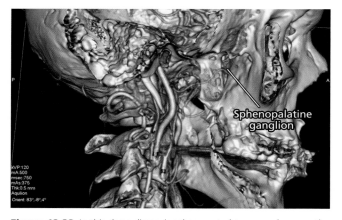

Figure 12.33 In this three-dimensional computed tomography scan, the location of the SPG is shown.

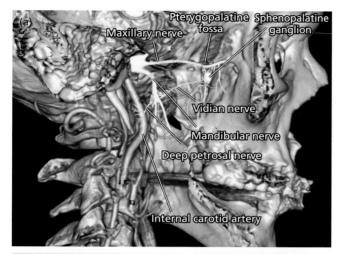

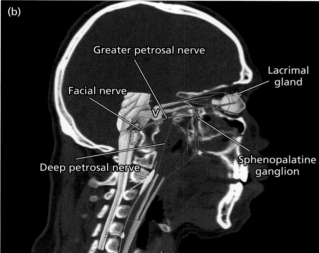

Figure 12.34 (a) Three-dimensional computed tomography scan showing the location of the SPG and its relationship to the surrounding structures. (b) The location of the SPG as shown in MRI.

Composition of the ganglion
The SPG is composed of fibers received from sensory, motor, and sympathetic origins.

Sensory origins
The sensory fibers are derived from two sphenopalatine branches of the maxillary nerve; they, for the most part, pass directly into the palatine nerves. A few, however, enter the ganglion, constituting its sensory root.

Parasympathetic origins
Its parasympathetic origin is derived from the nervus intermedius (a part of the facial nerve) through the greater petrosal nerve. In the SPG, the preganglionic parasympathetic fibers from the greater petrosal branch of the facial nerve synapse with neurons having postganglionic axons, vasodilator and secretory fibers distributed with the deep branches

of the trigeminal nerve, to the mucous membrane of the nose, soft palate, tonsils, uvula, roof of the mouth, upper lip and gums, and to the upper part of the pharynx. It also sends postganglionic parasympathetic fibers to the lacrimal gland through the zygomatic nerve, a branch of the maxillary nerve, which then connects with the lacrimal nerve to arrive at the lacrimal gland. The nasal glands are innervated with secretomotor fibers from the nasopalatine and greater palatine nerve. Similarly, the palatine glands are innervated by the nasopalatine, greater palatine, and lesser palatine nerves. The pharyngeal nerve innervates pharyngeal glands. These are all branches of the maxillary nerve.

Sympathetic origins
The ganglion also consists of sympathetic efferent (postganglionic) fibers from the superior cervical ganglion. These fibers, from the superior cervical ganglion, travel through the carotid plexus and then through the deep petrosal nerve. The deep petrosal nerve joins with the greater petrosal nerve to form the nerve of the pterygoid canal, which enters the ganglion. Branches of the SPG are the following:
- orbital branches;
- nasopalatine nerve;
- greater palatine nerve;
- lesser palatine nerve;
- posterior superior nasal branch;
- pharyngeal branch of maxillary nerve.

Anatomy and formation of pterygopalatine fossa
The pterygopalatine fossa is formed by three bony structures: the palatine, maxilla, and sphenoid bones. The borders of the pterygopalatine fossa are the posterior surface of the maxilla anteriorly, lateral surface of the palatine bone medially, and the anterosuperior surface of the pterygoid process of the sphenoid bone posteriorly and on the roof. Several structures enter and leave the pterygopalatine fossa through several foramina and fissures. The maxillary nerve enters the pterygopalatine fossa through the foramen rotundum. It courses anteriorly and exits as the infraorbital nerve through the inferior orbital fissure (Fig. 12.35).

Indications for SPG lesioning
- Sphenopalatine neuralgia.
- Idiopathic trigeminal neuralgia in combination with Gasserian ganglion block.
- Headache.
- Cluster headache.
- Migraine.
- Postherpetic neuralgia.
- Atypical facial neuralgia.

Contraindications for SPG lesioning
It is important to consider the following contraindications:
- local infection;
- coagulopathy;

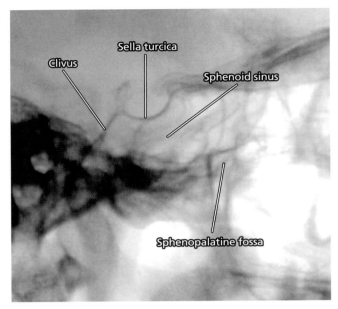

Figure 12.35 Bony structures surrounding the pterygopalatine fossa, as seen in the lateral fluoroscopic view.

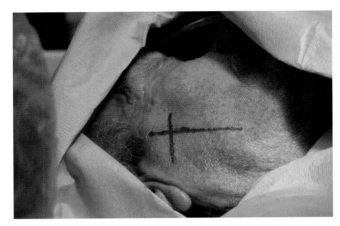

Figure 12.36 Superficial landmarks for the entry point of the SPG.

- vital function instability;
- psychopathologies.

Percutaneous techniques commonly performed on the SPG

- RF thermocoagulation.
- Pulsed RF.
- Diagnostic and therapeutic local anesthetic and/or steroid injections.

For all techniques, it is mandatory that these procedures are performed under radiographic imaging. It is essential that the pterygopalatine fossa is clearly visualized and confirmed before starting the procedure.

RF thermocoagulation of the SPG

A step-by-step approach is described to perform this procedure.

Step 1. Prepare the patient before the procedure
Ascertain the type of analgesia or sedation before performing the invasive procedure. The type of sedation varies, based on the technique being used. If considering a diagnostic trigeminal block with a local anesthetic or planning to use a neurolytic agent, deep sedation and analgesia may be appropriate for some patients. If planning RF thermocoagulation or pulsed RF, the patient needs to be awake to respond to the stimulation test. Intravenous fentanyl, midazolam, and/or propofol may be used judiciously for patient comfort.

Step 2. Position and monitor the patient
1. Place the patient in a supine position on the table.
2. Fix the head on the table with a strip of adhesive tape.
3. Insert an IV cannula for medication injections.
4. Provide oxygen by nasal cannula.
5. Monitor vital signs (mandatory).
6. Prepare the area for needle entry in a sterile fashion.

Step 3. Common drugs and needles
Prepare and confirm that the following equipment, needles, and drugs are ready to be used for the RF thermocoagulation or pulsed RF:
- 1½ inch, 25 gauge needle (for infiltration of the skin);
- 5 ml syringe (for local anesthetic solution);
- 2 ml empty syringe (for aspiration test);
- 3½ inch, 22 gauge needle (for the nerve block);
- 1% lidocaine for skin infiltration.

Special equipment for RF
- RF machine, with cables and electrodes;
- 10 cm RF needle with 5 mm active-tip electrode.

Step 4. Visualize the pterygopalatine fossa
1. Rotate the C-arm laterally until the rami of the mandible are superimposed one on each other.
2. Rotate the C-arm slightly cephalad until the pterygopalatine fossa is visualized. It should be seen as an inverted vase when two pterygopalatine plates are superimposed just posterior to the posterior wall of the maxillary sinus.
3. The lower border of the zygomatic arch, mandibular notch, anterior clinoid process, and orbits should also be visualized for confirmation.

Step 5. Identify the surface landmarks for needle entry (Fig. 12.36)
1. The entry point is identified by feeling on the surface of the skin the coronoid (mandibular) notch just anterior

to the temporomandibular joint. It is best identified by asking the patient to open and close their mouth and feeling the notch anterior to the temporomandibular joint movement.

2. The second method is to view the pterygopalatine fossa in the lateral fluoroscopic view. Place an opaque marker at the fossa. Draw a line from that position toward the arch of the zygomatic bone; mark that point as the entry point.

Step 6. Direction of the needle
Direct the needle as follows:
1. Infiltrate the skin with 2 ml of 1% lidocaine.
2. Insert and advance a 10 cm, 22 gauge needle toward the pterygopalatine fossa where the SPG is visualized in the lateral view (Fig. 12.37).

Step 7. Confirm the position of the needle
1. As soon as the needle enters the fossa and touches the maxillary nerve, the patient will report a sharp, shooting pain in the middle of the face.

2. Rotate the C-arm to the AP position at this time, and advance the needle until it is in line with the lateral aspect of the ala of the nose.
3. Take care to avoid advancing the needle through the lateral nasal wall. When the needle is properly positioned, inject 1 ml of contrast material. The contrast material should fill the pterygopalatine fossa.
4. Confirm this with AP and lateral imaging. Remove the stylet and aspirate. If blood is aspirated, redirect the needle (Figs 12.38 and 12.39).

Step 8. Stimulation test
Perform the stimulation test of the SPG as follows:
1. Stimulate at 50 Hz, between 0.2 and 1 V. This should result in paresthesia in the nose. Paresthesia of the cheek and/or upper lip indicates that the maxillary nerve has been stimulated. Redirect the electrode caudally and medially, as shown in Table 12.1 (Fig. 12.40). Paresthesia at the hard palate indicates the stimulation of major and minor palatinal nerves.
2. Redirect the electrode posteriorly and medially.

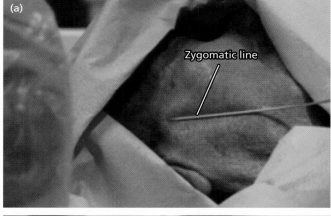
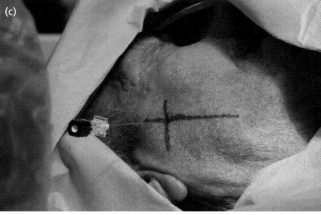
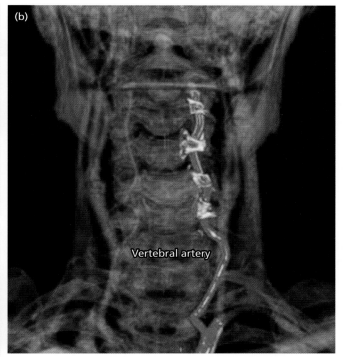

Figure 12.37 (a) First, an opaque marker is placed on the lateral side of the face at the mandibular notch. (b) A line is drawn at the mandibular notch, and a perpendicular line is drawn from there towards the pterygopalatine fossa. (c) The needle needs to be directed toward that from the entry point.

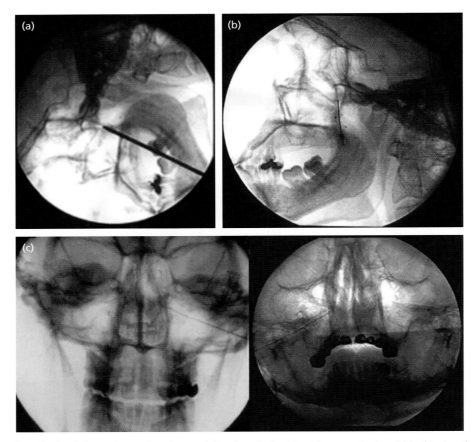

Figure 12.38 (a) First place the tip of the marker on the pterygopalatine fossa in the lateral fluoroscopic view. (b) In this view the needle is shown to be in the pterygopalatine fossa. Note the inverted flower vase. (c) Needle at the lateral wall of the nose in the AP fluoroscopic view.

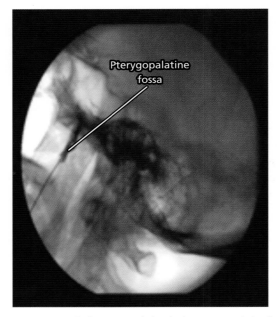

Figure 12.39 Spread of contrast solution in the pterygopalatine fossa, traversing cephalad to caudad behind the posterior wall of the maxillary sinus.

Step 9. RF lesioning

Perform SPG RF lesioning as follows.

1. After confirming that the electrode is in the proper location, sedate the patient if they are anxious, keeping them sufficiently able to respond to questions.

2. Inject 0.5 ml of 0.25% bupivacaine or 1% lidocaine, to provide comfort before actual thermocoagulation lesioning.

3. Wait a short time (30 seconds to 1 minute) before starting the lesioning. Proceed with lesioning at 70 °C for 60 seconds.

Step 10. Pulsed RF

Proceed with the pulsed RF procedure as follows.

1. When the ganglion is correctly located through sensory stimulation at 50 Hz with a 1 ms pulse duration, increase the voltage in 0.1 V increments until sensory stimulation is felt in the maxillary distribution. Sensory stimulation is noted at 0.6 V.

2. The duration of the pulsed RF treatment is 300 s, using a duration of 20 ms at 42 °C at a rate of 2 pulses per second. Complete two cycles on auto-pulse mode. Following the pulsed RF treatment, administer 4 ml of 0.125% bupivacaine with 16 mg dexamethasone. Then remove the needle.

Table 12.1 Sites of paresthesia and nerves stimulated for verification of needle placement

Location of paresthesia	Nerves stimulated	Location of the electrode tip	Action needed
Upper teeth and gums	Maxillary nerve	Superolateral	Redirect the needle caudally and medially
Hard palate	Greater and lesser palatine nerves	Anterior, lateral caudal	Redirect the needle posteromedially and cephalad
Root of the nose	PPG efferents, posterior lateral nasal nerves	Correct placement	None

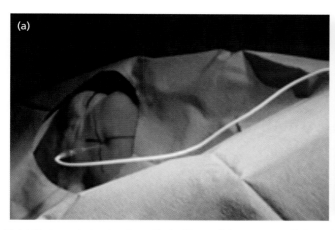 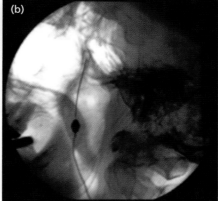

Figure 12.40 (a) Photograph showing the patient with a radiofrequency needle in position for SPG lesioning. (b) Lateral fluoroscopic view showing the needle tip in the inverted vase in the pterygopalatine fossa.

Step 11. Postprocedure care

After completing the procedure observe the patient for at least 2 hours. Monitor vital signs (mandatory). In addition, objectively document the pain relief. After a satisfactory observation, discharge the patient with appropriate and adequate instructions given to the escort. Written instructions are preferable for emergencies and they are helpful to the patient and family.

Technique for local anesthetic or neurolytic lesioning of the SPG

Diagnostic local anesthetic block of the SPG can be performed as described below. This technique is usually recommended for diagnostic and therapeutic management or neurolysis in cancer patients.

Steps 1 and 2

Prepare and position the patient similarly to the manner described in the section on RF thermocoagulation (see page 133).

Step 3. Drugs and equipment

Confirm that the following equipment and drugs are ready for use:

- 1½ inch, 25 gauge needle (for infiltration of the skin);
- 5 ml syringe (for local anesthetic solution);
- 2 ml empty syringe (for aspiration test);
- 3½ inch, 22 gauge needle (for the nerve block).

Drugs for diagnostic or therapeutic blocks

- 1% lidocaine for skin infiltration or diagnostic injections.
- Decadron solution.

Drugs for neurolysis

- 2 ml of absolute or 50% alcohol (not recommended).
- 2 ml of 6% phenol in saline or glycerine (preferred).

Step 4. Local anesthetic or neurolytic lesioning of SPG

Perform the procedure (Fig. 12.41) as follows.

1. Follow the same procedure as for a diagnostic or neurolytic procedure. The position of the patient for entry of the needle through the pterygopalatine fossa is as described in the section on RF thermocoagulation.

2. After confirming that the needle is in the correct position in both AP and lateral fluoroscopic views, slowly inject 2 ml of local anesthetic.

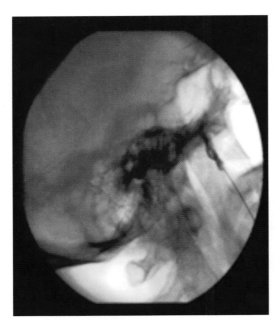

Figure 12.41 Needle in the pterygopalatine fossa. Note the spread of the contrast solution posterior to the maxillary sinus.

3. When planning a neurolytic therapeutic lesioning, prepare alcohol or 6% phenol in glycerine. Initially, use 6% phenol. Do not exceed 1 ml, slowly injected in 0.2–0.5 ml aliquots.

4. If the first neurolytic (phenol) procedure is unsuccessful, the next drug to be injected is alcohol, at another sitting.

Intranasal procedure

Another common diagnostic SPG block is performed intranasally. Because that is not an invasive procedure, it will not be described here.

Complications

During the procedure.

• **Epistaxis**

If the needle or electrode is pushed hard, it will enter the nose and may cause epistaxis. Ala nasi is a soft tissue, and the needle may easily enter the nose.

• **Direct injury or lesioning of the maxillary nerve**

If the needle is directed superolaterally, it will contact the maxillary nerve. This may be understood by sensory stimulation. If neurolytics are injected or conventional RF is performed without sensory stimulation, permanent paresthesia will develop.

• **Injury of the major and minor palatinal nerves**

Injury of the major and minor palatinal nerves may occur if the needle is directed anterolaterally and caudally.

• **Inadvertent puncture of the maxillary artery**

The terminal part of the maxillary artery is located in the pterygopalatine fossa. Inadvertent puncture of the maxillary artery may cause hematoma in the fossa. Local anesthetics injected to the maxillary artery may cause convulsions. An aspiration test is mandatory before any injection to the fossa.

• **Reflex bradycardia during RF lesioning**

A reflex bradycardia may occur during RF lesioning. When the lesioning is halted, bradycardia resolves.

• **Inadvertent puncture of the parotid gland**

If the needle is misdirected, inadvertent puncture of the parotis is possible. Palpation of the parotid gland before the procedure may be helpful.

After the procedure.

• **Hematoma at the cheek**

Inadvertent puncture of the venous plexus or the maxillary artery may cauce hematoma at the cheek. As soon as the needle is withdrawn, apply a cold pack at the cheek.

• **Hypesthesia**

Hypesthesia of the palate maxilla or the posterior pharynx may occur due to RF lesioning.

• **Diplopia**

Spread of the local anesthetic may cause transient diplopia.

• **Infection**

The incidence of infection is the same as for other procedures.

Helpful hints

Although the anatomical landmarks are easy to recognise fluoroscopically, performance of the SPG block is complex owing to superimposed bony structures and anatomic variations encountered during entry of the needle.

When a bony structure is encountered, be careful advancing the needle. Withdraw it slightly and redirect. After each redirection, control the needle tip, visualize both anteroposteriorly and laterally under fluoroscopic views to confirm location of the needle.

The two pterygopalatine plates should be superimposed in the lateral view to visualize the pterygopalatine fossa, as this may be difficult under lateral vision. Move the C-arm slightly until the pterygopalatine fossa is visualized.

Do not begin the procedure before the inverted vase is properly and clearly visualized.

Do not perform the procedure before local sensory testing to show that the tip of the electrode is correctly placed. The maxillary and palatinal nerves are in close proximity with the SPG. Test with electrical stimulation to locate the electrode properly.

Stop when the needle reaches the edge of the ala nasi under an AP view. If you advance the needle, there is a risk of local bleeding and epistaxis. The subcutaneous tissues of the face are loose, and there is a risk of ecchymosis after the procedure. Apply a cold pack to the face immediately after withdrawing the needle.

Percutaneous block and lesioning of the glossopharyngeal nerve

History

In the late 1950s, clinical use of the glossopharyngeal nerve block as an adjunct to awake endotracheal intubation was documented. Weisenburg first described pain in the distribution of the glossopharyngeal nerve in a patient with a cerebellopontine angle tumor in 1910. In 1921, Harris reported the first idiopathic case and coined the term **glossopharyngeal neuralgia**. He suggested that blockade of the glossopharyngeal nerve might be useful in palliating this painful condition.

Early attempts at permanent treatment of glossopharyngeal neuralgia and cancer pain in the distribution of the glossopharyngeal nerve consisted principally of extracranial surgical section or alcohol neurolysis of the glossopharyngeal nerve. These approaches met with limited success in treating glossopharyngeal neuralgia but were useful in some patients suffering from cancer pain mediated by the glossopharyngeal nerve. Recently, interest in extracranial destruction of the glossopharyngeal nerve by glycerol or creation of an RF lesion has been renewed.

Anatomy

Origin and course

From the medulla oblongata, the glossopharyngeal nerve passes lateralward across the flocculus and leaves the skull through the central part of the jugular foramen, in a separate sheath of the dura mater, lateral to and in front of the vagus and accessory nerves. In its passage through the jugular foramen, it grooves the lower border of the petrous part of the temporal bone, and, at its exit from the skull, passes forward between the internal jugular vein and internal carotid artery; it descends in front of the internal carotid, and beneath the styloid process and the muscles connected with it, to the lower border of the stylopharyngeus. It then curves forward, forming an arch on the side of the neck and lying upon the sylopharyngeus and constrictor pharyngis medius. From there it passes under cover of the hyoglossus and is finally distributed to the palatine tonsil, the mucous membrane of the fauces and base of the tongue, and the mucous glands of the mouth (Fig. 12.42).

The composition of the nerve

Sensory

Sympathetic afferent sensory fibers of the glossopharyngeal nerve arise from the cells of the superior and inferior ganglia, which are situated on the trunk of the nerve. Originating in the medulla, the sensory fibers, the sympathetic afferent, arborize around the cells of the upper part of a nucleus.

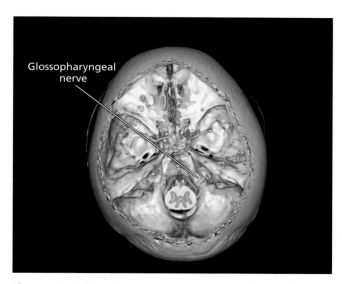

Figure 12.42 Three-dimensional computed tomography scan showing the course of the glossopharyngeal nerve exiting the jugular foramen. Note the close relationship to the vagus nerve, internal carotid artery, and internal jugular vein.

Many of the fibers, probably the taste fibers, form a strand, the fasciculus solitarius, which descends in the medulla oblongata. The **somatic sensory fibers** (few in number) join the spinal tract of the trigeminal nerve.

Motor

The somatic motor fibers spring from the cells of the **nucleus ambiguus**, which lies in the lateral part of the medulla, and are continuous below with the anterior gray column of the medulla spinalis. From this nucleus, the fibers join the fibers of the sensory root. The nucleus ambiguus gives origin to the motor branches of the glossopharyngeal and vagus nerves and to the cranial part of the accessory nerve.

The **sympathetic efferent fibers** from the dorsal nucleus are probably both preganglionic motor fibers and preganglionic secretory fibers of the sympathetic system. The secretory fibers pass to the otic ganglion, and from it secondary neurons are distributed to the parotid gland.

Ganglia formation of the glossopharyngeal nerve

In passing through the jugular foramen, the nerve presents two ganglia, the superior and the inferior (petrous) ganglia.

The superior ganglion is situated in the upper part of the groove in which the nerve is lodged during its passage through the jugular foramen. It is very small and is usually regarded as a detached portion of the petrous ganglion.

The inferior ganglion (petrous ganglion) is larger than the superior ganglion and is situated in a depression in the lower border of the petrous portion of the temporal bone.

Branches of the glossopharyngeal nerve

Branches of the glossopharyngeal nerve communicate with the vagus, sympathetic and facial nerves. The distal branches of the glossopharyngeal are the tympanic, carotid, pharyngeal, muscular, tonsillar, and lingual. The carotid branches descend along the trunk of the internal carotid artery with the pharyngeal branch of the vagus and with branches of the sympathetic nerves. The muscular branch is distributed to the stylopharyngeus. The tonsillar branches supply the palatine tonsil, forming around it a plexus from which filaments are distributed to the soft palate and fauces, where they communicate with the palatine nerves. The lingual branches (rami linguales) are two in number; one supplies the papillae vallatae and the mucous membrane covering the base of the tongue; the other supplies the mucous membrane and follicular glands of the posterior part of the tongue and communicates with the lingual nerve.

Indications for glossopharyngeal nerve block

Common indications are the following:
- diagnostic nerve block for pain in the glossopharyngeal nerve distribution;
- glossopharyngeal neuralgia.

Contraindications for glossopharyngeal nerve block

It is important to consider the following contraindications:
- local infection;
- coagulopathy;
- vital function instability;
- psychopathologies.

Pulsed RF of the glossopharyngeal nerve

Because the glossopharyngeal nerve is composed of both sensory and motor fibers, RF thermocoagulation is not wise, not recommended, and will not be discussed. A step-by-step approach is described to perform the glossopharyngeal nerve block procedure.

Step 1. Prepare the patient before the procedure
Ascertain the type of analgesia or sedation before performing this invasive procedure. The type of sedation varies, based on the technique being used. If considering a diagnostic glossopharyngeal block with a local anesthetic or planning a neurolytic agent or balloon compression, deep sedation and analgesia may be appropriate for some patients. If pulsed radiofrequency is planned, the patient needs to be awake to respond to the stimulation test. Intravenous fentanyl, midazolam, and/or propofol may be used judiciously for patient comfort.

Step 2. Position and monitor the patient
Position and monitor the patient as follows (Fig. 12.43).

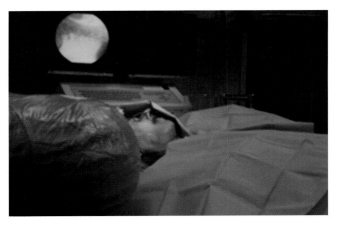

Figure 12.43 Photograph showing the position of the patient in a supine position with the head turned slightly to the opposite side in preparation for a glossopharyngeal nerve block.

1. Place the patient in a supine position on the table.
2. Fix the head on the table with a strip of adhesive tape.
3. Insert an IV cannula for medication injections.
4. Provide oxygen by nasal cannula.
5. Monitor vital signs (mandatory).
6. Prepare the area for needle entry in a sterile fashion.

Step 3. Equipment and drugs for glossopharyngeal nerve block

Common drugs and needles
- 1½ inch, 25 gauge needle (for infiltration of the skin);
- 5 ml syringe (for local anesthetic solution);
- 2 ml empty syringe (for aspiration test);
- 3½ inch, 22 gauge needle (for the nerve block);
- 1% lidocaine for skin infiltration or diagnostic injections.

Special equipment for pulsed RF lesioning
- RF machine, with cables and electrodes;
- 5 cm RF needle with 2 mm, active-tip electrode.

Step 4. Identify the surface landmarks (Fig. 12.44)
1. Mark the mastoid process and the angle of the mandible on the skin.
2. Draw a line between these two landmarks, or place a marker under fluoroscopy. The styloid process lies below the midpoint of this line.

Step 5. Visualization
Visualize by rotating the C-arm laterally; try to view the styloid process laterally or in a slightly oblique position.

Step 6. Direction of the needle
Advance the needle as follows (Fig. 12.45).
1. Infiltrate the skin with 1% lidocaine.
2. Advance a 3½ inch, 22 gauge needle over the landmark, between the mastoid process and the angle of the mandible

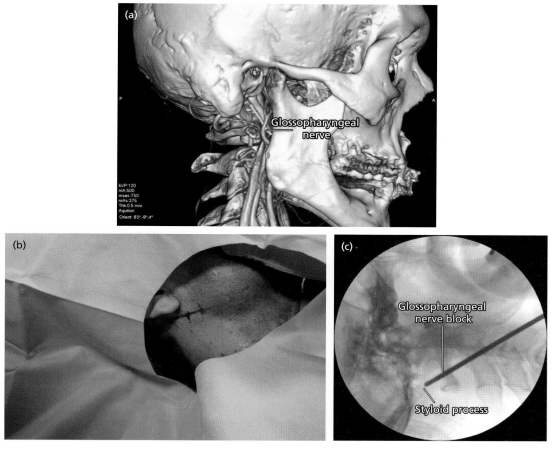

Figure 12.44 (a) Three-dimensional computed tomography scan showing the course of the glossopharyngeal nerve and its relationship to the vagus nerve, internal carotid vessel, and internal jugular vein as it exits from the jugular foramen and courses toward the angle of the mandible and mastoid process. (b) Mark the mastoid process and the angle of the mandible on the skin. Draw a line between these two landmarks, place a marker under fluoroscopy. The styloid process lies below the midpoint of this line. (c) Lateral fluoroscopic view showing the marker being placed at the site of needle entry for the glossopharyngeal nerve block.

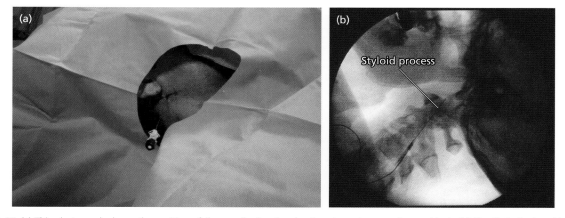

Figure 12.45 (a) This photograph shows the position of the needle direction for the glossopharyngeal nerve block. (b) Needle in final position as it touches the styloid process for the glossopharyngeal nerve block.

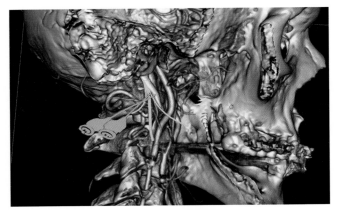

Figure 12.46 This three-dimensional computed tomography scan shows how to walk off the styloid process posteriorly.

perpendicularly. Try to contact the styloid process at a depth of 3 cm.

3. Do not advance more than 3 cm. If you do not contact the bone, redirect the needle, if needed.

Step 7. Confirm the position of the needle (Fig. 12.46)

1. After the contact is made, walk off the styloid process posteriorly.

2. As soon as contact is lost, aspirate for blood or CSF. If negative for either proceed to the next step.

Step 8. Test stimulation

Apply stimulation as follows. The technique for RF is the same as for diagnostic block except an RF needle is used instead of a 3½ inch needle.

1. When the electrode tip reaches the nerve, stimulate the nerve with 50 Hz, at 0.5–1 V. The sensory stimulation should reproduce a concordant pain at the base of the tongue, pharynx and tonsils if appropriately placed.

2. Then stimulate with 2 Hz, at 0.5–2 V motor stimulation; this should cause contractions of the stylopharyngeus muscle.

Step 9. RF lesioning

Perform therapeutic lesioning, using pulsed RF in three cycles of 120 s with a rate of 2 Hz, at a constant temperature of 42 °C.

Step 10. Postprocedure care

After completing the procedure, observe the patient for at least 2 hours. Monitor vital signs (mandatory). In addition, objectively document the pain relief. After a satisfactory observation, discharge the patient with appropriate and adequate instructions given to the escort. Written instructions are preferable for emergencies and they are helpful to the patient and the family.

Technique for local anesthetic or neurolytic lesioning of the glossopharyngeal nerve

This technique is usually recommended for **diagnostic** and **therapeutic neurolysis** in cancer patients.

Steps 1 and 2

Prepare and position the patient similarly to the technique described in the section on pulsed RF (see page 162).

Step 3. Drugs and equipment

Confirm that the following equipment and drugs are ready for use:

- 1½ inch, 25 gauge needle (for infiltration of the skin);
- 5 ml syringe (for local anesthetic solution);
- 2 ml empty syringe (for aspiration test);
- 3½ inch, 22 gauge needle (for the nerve block);
- 1% lidocaine for skin infiltration or for diagnostic injections;
- 2 ml of absolute or 50% alcohol; or
- 2 ml of 6% phenol in saline or glycerine.

Step 4. Position the needle

For the diagnostic block and neurolytic block, a 3½ inch, 22 gauge needle is inserted, as described earlier, through the entry point until the styloid process is contacted and the tip of the needle is on the glossopharyngeal nerve as confirmed by fluoroscopy.

Step 5. Perform the glossopharyngeal block

After negative aspiration, up to 3 ml of local anesthetic with steroid is commonly injected. For the neurolytic procedure, 1–2 ml of 6% phenol and glycerine or a contrast solution is recommended.

Complications

During the procedure:

- Inadvertent puncture of the surrounding vessels.
- Puncture of the carotid artery.

The carotid artery is in very close proximity to the glossopharyngeal nerve. Even very small amounts of local anesthetic injected into the carotid artery may cause symptoms of local anesthetic toxicity. Thus, a negative aspiration test is mandatory. This procedure should be performed under fluoroscopy. If the carotid artery is injected with solution, sudden vasospasm of the artery may occur.

- Inadvertent puncture of the internal jugular vein (may cause hematoma).

After the procedure:

- Trauma or inadvertent block of the nerves in proximity.
- Trauma to the glossopharyngeal nerve.

Trauma to the glossopharyngeal nerve may result in dysphagia secondary to the weakness of the stylopharyngeus muscle.

• Trauma to the vagus nerve

Trauma to the vagus nerve may result in dysphonia secondary to the paralysis of the ipsilateral vocal cord. Reflex tachycardia secondary to vagal nerve block may also be observed.

• Trauma to hypoglossal and spinal accessory nerves

Trauma to hypoglossal and spinal accessory nerves may result in weakness of the tongue and trapezius muscle.

• Permanent paresthesia and dysesthesia

Permanent paresthesia and dysesthesia with symptoms of burning pain and discomfort: possible results of neurolytic blocks or neurodestructive procedures.

• Anesthesia dolorosa

This is a significant complication; severe burning pain and difficulty in swallowing develop.

Helpful hints

Even though the skin entry point for the glossopharyngeal nerve is easy to locate, the actual technique is hazardous to perform in clinical practice, owing to very significant vital structures that lie very close to the nerve (vagus, spinal accessory nerves, vessels such as the internal carotid artery and the internal jugular vein).

It should be performed only by skilled pain physicians using fluoroscopy.

Further reading

Apfelbaum, R.I. (1997) Trigeminal nerve and ganglion procedures. In *Neurosurgical Management of Pain* (ed. North, R.B. & Levy, R.M.), pp. 221–242. New York: Springer.

Apfelbaum, R.I. (1999) Glycerol trigeminal neurolysis. In: *Techniques in Neurosurgery*, volume 5 (ed. Burchiel, K.J.), pp. 225–231. Philadelphia: Lippincott Williams & Wilkins.

Bayer, E., Racz, G.B., Miles, D. & Heavner, J. (2005) Sphenopalatine ganglion pulsed radiofrequency treatment in 30 patients suffering from chronic face and head pain. *Pain Practice* **5**(3), 223–227.

Benzon, H.T., Rathmell, J.P., Wu, C.L., Turk, D.C. & Argoff, C.E. (eds) (2008) *Raj's Practical Management of Pain*, 4th edition. Philadelphia: Saunders-Elsevier.

Brisman, R. (1993) Analgesia and sedation during percutaneous radiofrequency electrocoagulation for trigeminal neuralgia. *Neurosurgery* **32**(3), 400–405.

Day, M. (2001) Neurolysis of the trigeminal and sphenopalatine ganglions. *Pain Practice* **1**, 171–182.

Erdine, S. (2007) Targets and optimal imaging for cervical spine and head blocks. *Techniques in Regional Anesthesia and Pain Management* **11**(2), 63–72.

Erdine, S. (2008) Sympathetic blocks of the head and neck. In *Interventional Pain Management, Image Guided Procedures*, 2nd edition (ed. Raj, P.P., et al.), pp. 108–127. Philadelphia: Saunders-Elsevier.

Erdine, S., Racz, G.B. & Noe, C.E. (2008) Somatic blocks of the head and neck. In *Interventional Pain Management, Image Guided Procedures* (ed. Raj, P.P., et al.), pp. 77–108. Philadelphia: Saunders-Elsevier.

Gauci, C. (2004) *Manual of RF Techniques*. Switzerland: Flivo Press.

Hakanson, S. (1981) Trigeminal neuralgia treated by the injection of glycerol into the trigeminal cistern. *Neurosurgery* **9**, 638–646.

Lopez, B.C., Hamlyn, P.J. & Zakrzewska, J.M. (2004) Systemic review of ablative neurosurgical techniques for the treatment of trigeminal neuralgia. *Neurosurgery* **54**, 973–983.

Mullan, S. & Lichtor, T. (1983) Percutaneous microcompression of the trigeminal ganglion for trigeminal neuralgia. *Journal of Neurosurgery* **59**, 1007–1012.

Narouze, S. (2007) Complications of head and neck procedures. *Techniques in Regional Anesthesia and Pain Management* **1**, 171–177.

Narouze, S., Kapural, L. & Casanova, J. (2009) Sphenopalatine ganglion radiofrequency ablation for the management of chronic cluster headache. *Headache* **49**(4), 571–577.

Raj, P.P., Lou, L., Erdine, S., Staats, P.S. & Racz, G., Infusion Nurses Society (2002) *Interventional Pain Management: Image-Guided Procedures*, 2nd edition. Philadelphia: Saunders-Elsevier.

Raj, P.P., Lou, L., Erdine, S., Staats, P.S. & Waldman, S.D. (2003) *Radiological Imaging for Regional Anesthesia and Pain Management*, pp. 37–49. Philadelphia: Churchill Livingstone.

Raj, P.P., Rauck, R. & Racz, G. (1996) Autonomic nerve blocks. In *Pain Medicine, A Comprehensive Review* (ed. Raj, P.P.), pp. 227–256. St. Louis, MO: Mosby.

Ruiz-Lopez, R. & Erdine, S. (2002) Treatment of cranio-facial pain with radiofrequency procedures. *Pain Practice* **2**(3), 206–213.

Salar, G., Ori, C. & Iob, I. (1987) Percutaneous thermocoagulation for sphenopalatine ganglion neuralgia. *Acta Neurochirurgica* **84**, 24–28.

Sanders, M. & Zuurmond, W.A. (1997) Efficacy of sphenopalatine ganglion blockade in 66 patients suffering from cluster headache: a 12- to 70-month follow-up evaluation. *Journal of Neurosurgery* **87**, 876–880.

Sist, T. (1997) Head and neck nerve blocks for cancer pain management. *Techniques in Regional Anesthesia and Pain Management* **1**(1), 3–10.

Slujter, M. (2003) *Radiofrequency, Part 2: Thoracic and Cervical Region, Headache and Facial Pain*. Switzerland: Flivo Press.

Sweet, W.H. & Wepsic, S.G. (1974) Controlled thermocoagulation of trigeminal ganglion and rootlets for differential destruction of pain fibers. Part 1: Trigeminal neuralgia. *Journal of Neurosurgery* **40**, 143–156.

Van Kleef, M., Lataster, A., Naouze, S., Mekhail, N., Geurts, J.W. & Van Zundert, J. (2009) Cluster headache. *Pain Practice* **9**(6), 435–442.

Van Kleef, M., Van Genderen, W.E., Narouze, S., et al. (2009) Trigeminal neuralgia. *Pain Practice* **9**(4), 252–259.

Van Zundert, J., Mekhail, N. & Van Kleef, M. (2012) *Evidence-Based Interventional Pain Procedures*. Hoboken, NJ: Wiley-Blackwell, Hoboken. In the press.

Waldman, S. (1993) Sphenopalatine ganglion block: 80 years later. *Regional Anesthesia* **18**, 274–276.

Yin, W. (2004) Radiofrequency gasserian rhizotomy: the role of RF lesioning in the management of facial pain. *Techniques in Regional Anesthesia and Pain Management* **8**(1), 30–34.

Yin, W. (2004) Sphenopalatine ganglion radiofrequency lesions in the treatment of facial pain. *Techniques in Regional Anesthesia Pain Management* **8**, 25–29.

Percutaneous block and lesioning of greater and lesser occipital nerves

History
The term "occipital neuralgia" was first used in 1821, when Beruta y Lentijo and Ramos made reference to an occipital neuralgic syndrome. The technique of occipital nerve block seems to have been first described by Bonica in 1953.

Anatomy

The greater occipital nerve, formation and course
The medial branch (ramus medialis; internal branch), called from its size and distribution the greater occipital nerve (nervus occipitalis major; great occipital nerve), ascends obliquely between the obliquus inferior and the semispinalis capitis, and pierces the latter muscle and the trapezius near their attachments to the occipital bone. It is then joined by a filament from the medial branch of the posterior division of the third cervical, and, ascending on the back of the head with the occipital artery, divides into branches that communicate with the lesser occipital nerve and supply the skin of the scalp as far forward as the vertex of the skull. It gives off muscular branches to the semispinalis capitis, and occasionally a twig to the back of the auricula. The lateral branch (ramus lateralis; external branch) supplies filaments to the splenius, longus capitis, and semispinalis capitis, and is often joined by the corresponding branch of the third cervical nerve.

The lesser occipital nerve: formation and course
The lesser occipital nerve is derived from the cervical plexus arising from the anterior ramus of the second spinal nerve and, to a lesser extent, it receives fibers from the third cervical nerve. It ascends superiorly on the posterior border of the sternocleidomastoid muscle. It innervates an area of the scalp anterior and superior to the ear (Figs 13.1, 13.2, and 13.3).

Indications
- Primary occipital neuralgia.
- Secondary occipital neuralgia.
- Generalized muscle tension headache.
- Cervicogenic headache.

Contraindications
- Local or systemic infection.
- Coagulopathies.
- Vital function instability.

Greater and lesser occipital nerve block

Step 1. Prepare the patient before the procedure
The type of analgesia or sedation needs to be ascertained before performance of the invasive procedure. If a diagnostic greater and lesser occipital nerve block is planned, deep sedation and analgesia is not necessary. If a local anesthetic is considered or neurolytic block is planned, mild sedation is all that is necessary. If pulsed radiofrequency (RF) lesioning is planned, the patient needs to be awake to respond to the stimulation test. Intravenous fentanyl or midazolam may be used judiciously for the patient's comfort.

Step 2. Position and monitor the patient
Obtain an intravenous access if drugs need to be administered.
1. The patient is placed either in a supine or sitting position on the table, with the head flexed forwards (Fig. 13.4).
2. One can also place the patient in a prone position, with a pillow under the thorax, to maintain the forward flexion of the head.
3. The portion of the head where the entry point is located should be shaved and sterilized.
4. An intravenous cannula is inserted for medication injection for an anxious patient.
5. Oxygen is provided by nasal cannula if indicated.
6. Monitoring of vital signs is minimal.

Pain-Relieving Procedures: The Illustrated Guide, First Edition. P. Prithvi Raj and Serdar Erdine.
© 2012 John Wiley & Sons, Ltd. Published 2012 by John Wiley & Sons, Ltd.

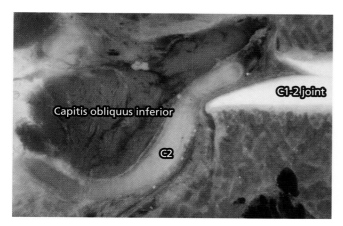

Figure 13.1 The anatomy of the C2 nerve as it exits the C1–2 joint foramen. Note the relationship of the muscle capitis and obliquus inferior. (Courtesy of J Taylor.)

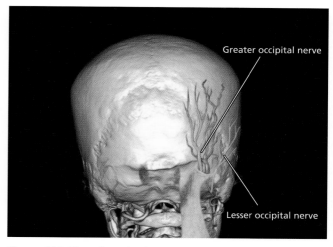

Figure 13.3 Three-dimensional CT scan identifying the course of the greater and lesser occipital nerves as they traverse toward the occiput.

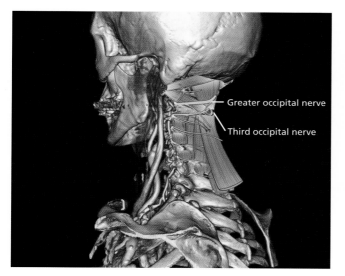

Figure 13.2 Three-dimensional CT scan of the occipital region showing the course of the greater occipital nerve and the third occipital nerve near the intervertebral foramen. Note the course of these nerves and their branches.

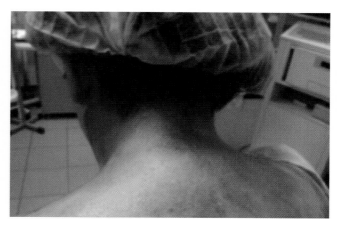

Figure 13.4 Photograph of a patient readied for greater and lesser occipital nerve block in a sitting position.

Step 3. Equipment and drugs for greater and lesser occipital nerve blocks and lesioning
Prepare and confirm that the following equipment, needles, and drugs are ready to be used for the procedure:
- 25 gauge, 1½ inch needle for the skin infiltration;
- 22 gauge, 1½ inch needle for the block;
- 2 ml syringe for the skin infiltration;
- 5 ml syringe for the block;
- 5 mm active-tip electrode (for RF lesioning);
- 1% lidocaine for skin infiltration;
- 0.5% bupivacaine for the nerve block;
- 40 mg triamcinolone or equivalent.

Step 4. Mark the surface landmarks for needle entry
1. Mark on the skin landmarks for the greater occipital and lesser occipital nerve blocks.
2. To do that one should palpate the mastoid process, identify the greater occipital protuberance, palpate the superior nuchal line, if possible feel the medial border of the sterno-cleidomastoid muscle and the occipital artery.
3. Next, draw a line through these landmarks. The greater occipital nerve is located at a point one-third distance from the occipital protuberance on the superior nuchal line together with the occipital artery (Fig. 13.5).
4. The lesser occipital nerve is located at a two-thirds distance from the occipital protuberance on the superior nuchal line.
5. Next, palpate the occipital artery with the index finger.

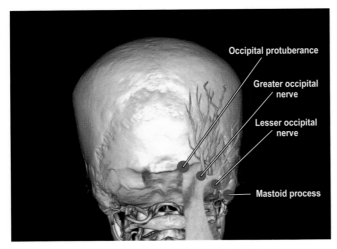

Figure 13.5 This three-dimensional CT scan of the skull shows the location of two important landmarks in pink showing the occipital protuberance and mastoid process. The areas marked in green represent the location of the greater and lesser occipital nerves, as one palpates the bony skull.

Step 5. Direction of the needle
1. Infiltrate the skin over the artery with 1% lidocaine.
2. Insert a 22 gauge 1½ inch needle perpendicular to the skin, medial to the occipital artery.
3. Advance the needle until it contacts the bone; seek for paresthesia.

Step 6. Confirm the position of the needle
After the patient describes the paresthesia (in the greater occipital nerve distribution) withdraw the needle slightly (2 mm).

Step 7. Greater and lesser occipital nerve block
1. After a negative aspiration, inject 2–5 ml of 0.5% lidocaine or bupivacaine together with a steroid solution if preferred.
2. If paresthesia is not felt after a few attempts, inject 5 ml of the solution in a fan-like fashion around the occipital artery (Fig. 13.6). Note: for a diagnostic block, do not inject more than 1–2 ml of local anesthetic, to prevent a false-positive diagnosis.
3. For lesser occipital nerve block or lesioning, introduce the needle medial to the origin of the sternocleidomastoid muscle at the mastoid process. Advance the needle cephalad and medially until it contacts the bone. Seek for paresthesia.
4. After contacting the bone, withdraw the needle 2 mm, aspirate, and then inject 5 ml of local anesthetic together with a steroid solution. When neurolytic block is contemplated (only in cancer patients) use 1 or 2 ml of 6% phenol in glycerine.

Pulsed RF lesioning of the occipital nerves
Pulsed RF lesioning is performed for greater and lesser occipital nerves because they contain somatic fibers and thermocoagulation is not recommended.
1. Advance a 5 cm or 5 mm active-tip electrode to the nerves as described for diagnostic block.
2. Perform sensory stimulation with 50 Hz at 0.5 V setting. When the patient confirms paresthesia in the distribution of the nerve tested, inject 1%, 1 ml lidocaine. Wait for 5 minutes. Perform pulsed RF at 42 °C, for 120 seconds, for two or three cycles.

Step 8. Postprocedure care
After the procedure is completed, the patient needs to be observed for up to 2 hours. Monitoring of vital signs is mandatory. In addition the pain relief should be objectively documented. After a satisfactory observation, the patient should be discharged with appropriate and adequate instructions given to the escort. Written instructions are preferable for emergencies and are helpful to the patient and their family.

Complications
- **Hematoma and ecchymosis**
The scalp is rich with vascular supply. Ecchymosis and hematoma formation can occur. Apply cold pack to the region as soon as you withdraw the needle.
- **Intravascular injection of a local anesthetic**
Intravascular injection of local anesthetics to the occipital artery is possible, although it is very rare. CNS toxicity may develop.
- **Transient or permanent paresthesia**
When the patient feels paresthesia, withdraw the needle immediately to prevent injury of the nerve.
- **Inadvertent needle placement into the foramen magnum**
The most serious complication is the inadvertent needle placement into the foramen magnum, while advancing the needle to seek for paresthesia. Injecting a local anesthetic into the foramen magnum will result in a total spinal block and respiratory depression. In some cases, local anesthetic may spread into the foramen magnum, even if the needle is not placed deep. To prevent this complication, do not inject more than 2–3 ml of local anesthetic to the region and a neurolytic block is not recommended.

Helpful hints
Prepare the patient's entry point in a sterile fashion. Here, hair growth usually gets in the way; we recommend shaving this region before performing the procedure.

The sitting position is easier for identifying the landmarks and marking them on the skin. Radiographic imaging of the bony landmarks is not helpful here.

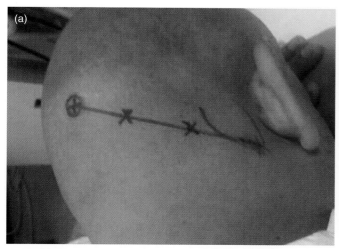

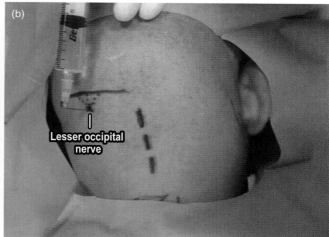

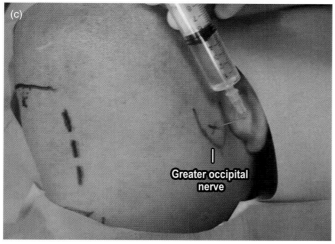

Figure 13.6 The landmarks for greater and lesser occipital nerve blocking. (a) Location of the occipital protuberance and mastoid process. (b) The injection in progress for the lesser occipital nerve. (c) The injection in progress for the greater occipital nerve.

Treat the transient paresthesia (post-block) as soon as possible so it does not become permanent.

Percutaneous block and lesioning of third occipital nerve

Anatomy of the third occipital nerve

The third occipital nerve is a large nerve of about 1.5 mm in diameter. It runs slightly horizontally in a posterocaudal direction. The third occipital nerve is the only nerve to cross the facet joint and gives off articular branches to the C2–C3 facet joint from its deeper surface.

Formation of third occipital nerve and its course

The C3 spinal nerve divides into an anterior ramus and a posterior ramus. The posterior ramus divides into two medial branches and a lateral branch. The larger, superior medial branch is the third occipital nerve. The third occipital nerve courses posteriorly and medially around the superior articular process of the C3 vertebra. It crosses the C2–C3 facet joint either just below or across the joint margin. The innervation of the C2–C3 facet joint primarily is from the large, superior medial branch of the C3 spinal nerve, the third occipital nerve. The deep medial branch of the C3 dorsal ramus is parallel but caudal (Fig. 13.7).

Innervation of the third occipital nerve

The third occipital nerve provides cutaneous neural supplies to the suboccipital region. The third occipital nerve significantly innervates the C2–C3 joint and produces cutaneous anesthesia in the distribution of the nerve.

Indications

For a diagnostic and therapeutic block for occipital headache.
• For RF neurotomy of the third occipital nerve.

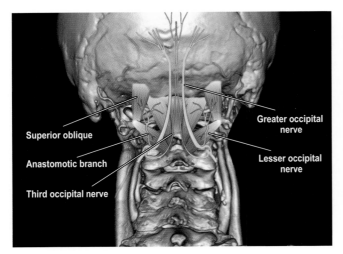

Figure 13.7 Three-dimensional CT scan showing the course of the third occipital nerve formation and the course of the greater occipital nerve in relation to it. Note the superior and inferior oblique muscles close to the origins of these nerves.

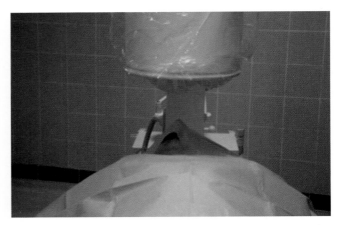

Figure 13.8 The third occipital nerve procedure is about to begin with the area sterilized and appropriate drapes in place.

Contraindications
- Local infection or sepsis.
- Coagulopathy.
- Vital functions instability.
- Psychopathologies.

Technique of local anesthetic injection of third occipital nerve
- Commonly performed technique is for diagnostic local anesthetic block.
- RF technique for therapeutic lesioning.

Step 1. Prepare the patient before the procedure

The patient should be aware of why this procedure is being done and what to expect from it. All complications and side effects related to the procedure should be explained in detail, before it is performed. Valid, written consent should be obtained.

The type of analgesia or sedation needs to be ascertained before performance of the procedure. Intravenous fentanyl or midazolam may be used judiciously for the patient's comfort. If RF thermocoagulation or pulsed RF lesioning is planned, the patient needs to be awake to respond to the stimulation test.

Step 2. Position and monitor the patient (Fig. 13.8)
1. Place the patient in supine position.
2. Ensure that the patient is in a comfortable position by placing a small pillow under their head. Position the arms of the patient on both sides.
3. Fasten their head on the table using a strip of adhesive tape.

4. The area for needle entry is prepared in a sterile fashion. Note: the patient should not be over-sedated. They should remain sufficiently conscious to provide response to any questions or stimulation.

Step 3. Drugs and equipment for the third occipital nerve block

Prepare and confirm that the following equipment, needles, and drugs are ready to be used for the procedure:
- 1½ inch, 25 gauge needle for skin infiltration;
- 5 ml syringe for local anesthetic solution;
- 5 ml syringe for the block;
- 22 gauge, 3½ inch needle with extension line for the cervical facet block;
- 1% lidocaine for skin infiltration;
- steroid solution of choice (decadron or equivalent).

Special drugs and equipment for the RF lesioning
- RF machine.
- 5–10 cm, with 2 mm active-tip, electrode with cables.

Technique for local anesthetic and/or steroid injection of the third occipital nerve

Step 4. Visualization
1. The C-arm should be placed in posteroanterior, lateral, and oblique views as necessary.
2. First place the C-arm in the posteroanterior position to identify the vertebral bodies of C2, C3.
3. Then position the C-arm laterally and check whether all cervical vertebrae are on the same plane. Slightly move the C-arm cephalad or caudally until one gets the best view of the articular pillars at C2–C3 joint is superimposed perfectly (Fig. 13.9).

Step 5. Mark the surface landmarks for the needle entry
1. Mark the lateral edge of the sternocleidomastoid muscle at this vertebral level. The point of entry should be located behind the lateral edge of the muscle (Fig. 13.10).
2. Infiltrate the skin with local anesthetic solution. The patient may feel pain when the needle is inserted into lateral cervical muscles after penetrating the skin. The pain may be felt both in this area and in the shoulder region.
3. Infiltrate with a small amount of local anesthetic to make the patient comfortable.
Note: anatomically, the third occipital nerve lies in the peri-capsular fascia of the C2–C3 joint. To achieve an adequate block, it should be blocked at three target areas: (1) opposite

the apex of the C3 superior articular process; (2) opposite the base of the C2–C3 foramen; (3) at a point midway between them both (Fig. 13.11).

Step 6. Direction of the needle (Fig. 13.12)
1. Insert the needle under lateral fluoroscopic guidance toward the target area.
2. Advance the needle or electrode toward the anterior third of the superior articular process or the upper process of the C2–C3 foramen.

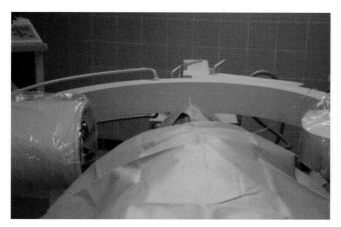

Figure 13.9 This is the lateral C-arm position for the third occipital nerve block.

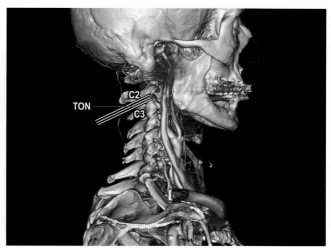

Figure 13.11 Three-dimensional CT scan showing the direction of the needle for performing the third occipital nerve block. The target is the superior articular process and the vertebral foramen.

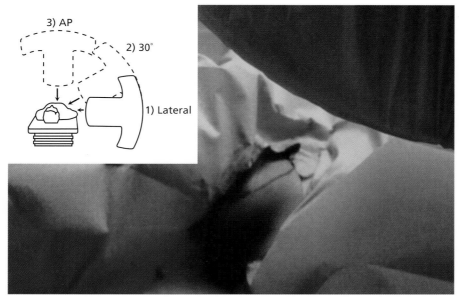

Figure 13.10 The landmark of the skin for the third occipital nerve block and the inset shows the positions of C-arms (posteroanterior lateral and oblique) for performing this procedure.

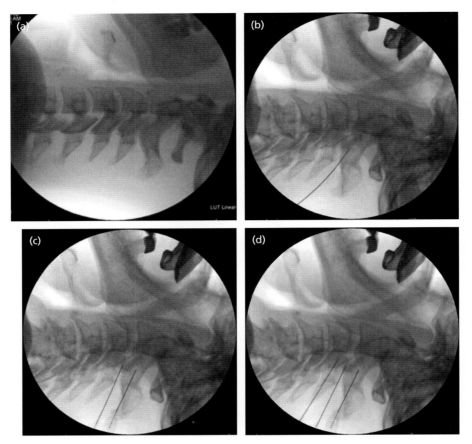

Figure 13.12 (a) Lateral photograph of the cervical spine identifying the upper cervical vertebrate and the foramina. (b) Lateral radiographic image showing the direction of the needle for the third occipital nerve block. (c) Lateral radiographic image showing the direction of two needles for the third occipital nerve block. (d) Lateral radiographic image showing the direction of three needles for the third occipital nerve block.

Step 7. Confirm the position of the needle (Fig. 13.13)
1. The final position of the tip of the needle should lie at the anterior border of the superior articular process.
2. Then place the C-arm in the posteroanterior position, to confirm the position of the needle tip. It should lie medial to the C2–C3 facet joint in the lateral view.

Step 8. Nerve block technique of the third occipital nerve (Fig. 13.14)
1. Inject 0.5 ml contrast material to verify the correct position of the needle and absence of inadvertent puncture of a vessel or dural puncture.
2. Inject 0.4–0.6 ml of local anesthetic for the third occipital nerve block if satisfactory.

Thermocoagulation RF lesioning

After the needle electrode tip is confirmed to be located at the target site, follow the procedure with a stimulation test.

Step 9. Stimulation test
1. Sensory testing. Test with a frequency at 50 Hz, pulse width 1 ms, voltage up to 0.5 V. There should be paresthesia

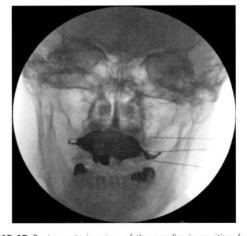

Figure 13.13 Posteroanterior view of the needles in position for the third occipital nerve block.

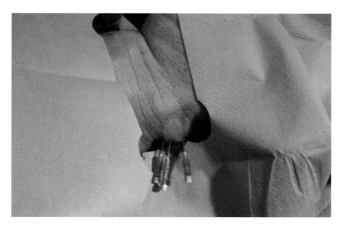

Figure 13.14 The three needless in position in a patient undergoing a third occipital nerve block.

only in the occipital region, not radiating to the upper extremity.

2. Motor testing. Test with a frequency at 2 Hz, pulse width 1 ms, voltage up to 1 V. There should not be motor contraction.

Step 10. RF thermocoagulation
1. Thermocoagulation RF. The lesioning is done for 60 seconds at 60 °C. Some prefer to do this twice.

Pulsed RF
2. Advance a 5 cm or 5 mm active-tip electrode to the nerves as described for diagnostic block.
3. Perform sensory stimulation with 50 Hz at 0.5 V setting. When the patient confirms paresthesia in the distribution of the nerve tested, inject 1%, 1 ml lidocaine. Wait for 5 minutes. Perform pulsed RF at 42 °C for 120 seconds, for two or three cycles.

Step 11. Postprocedure care
After any of these procedures, the patient should be observed for a reasonable time, up to 2 hours. The recovery and observation time depends on the sedation and analgesia used, as the type of quality assessment depends upon any impairment of intellectual function, tolerance of oral intake, assessment of the immediate results of the neural blockade, and pain response to the procedure.

The patient should be provided with all instructions, including whom to call or where to go for any postprocedure urgent/emergency care. The patient should be discharged accompanied by a responsible adult. The patient should not be allowed to drive themselves. The patient should be informed that there may be slight sensory changes in the upper extremity which may be transient. However, if sensory changes last more than one day, the patient should return to the pain clinic immediately. They should also be informed

that if they develop a fever or there is an increase in pain, then they should make an appointment at the pain clinic.

Complications
• **Transient numbness**
There may be numbness in the cutaneous distribution of the third occipital nerve after the nerve block; this should be expected for a successful block.
• **Transient ataxia**
Ataxia may be due to the block of the proprioceptors in the cervical nerves. Generally, ataxia is transient and the patient should be informed before the procedure about the possibility of ataxia, which may last for several weeks.
• **Dysesthesia**
Dysesthesia may develop, especially after RF lesioning, and may last for several weeks.
• **Inadvertent arterial puncture**
The region is rich in arteries and veins and one should be very careful while advancing the needle to the target. Injection of contrast material before lesioning is mandatory to prevent entering a blood vessel.
• **Inadvertent dural puncure**
One should be aware while advancing the needle that the needle should touch the lateral aspect of the vertebral surface. One should be careful not to pass the lateral vertebral surface, confirmed by anteroposterior and lateral fluoroscopic views. Injection of the contrast solution is essential to verify the correct position of the needle.

Helpful hints
The area of the nerve block or lesioning should be infiltrated with small aliquots of 0.5% lidocaine to keep the patient comfortable.

Carefully identify the movement of the needle tip toward the target area and stop short of entering the cervical epidural space.

Do not inject a local anesthetic if contrast solution is instantly removed from the area (owing to entering a blood vessel). In this case, remove the needle and reinsert or abandon the procedure for another time.

Percutaneous interlaminar block of the cervical epidural space

History
Although Pagés' description of the paramedian approach to the lumbar epidural space in 1921 is considered the first clinically relevant report of the technique of lumbar epidural nerve block, it appears that Dogliotti was the first to describe the technique of epidural block in the cervical region.

Epidural steroids have been introduced for the treatment of acute radiculopathy. The initial numbers of procedures performed by physicians were relatively small and the complexity of the procedure failed to reveal the serious hazards associated with the technique. With better understanding of the anatomy, the consensus seems to be heading in the direction of injecting into the site-specific area.

Lumbar epidural corticosteroid injections have been used for over 30 years.

Anatomy of the epidural space and its boundaries

The cervical epidural space starts at the foramen magnum superiorly and descends into the thoracic epidural space at the C8–T1 vertebral level. The superior border of the cervical epidural space is the fusion of the periosteal and spinal layers of the dura mater at the foramen magnum. The boundaries of the cervical epidural space at each particular vertebral level are the posterior longitudinal ligament anteriorly and lamina and ligamentum flavum posteriorly. The lateral border of the cervical epidural space is formed by the pedicles and the intervertebral foramina. The intervertebral foramen is formed by these superior and inferior vertebral notches in the upper and lower pedicles. The cervical pedicle extends from the vertebral body posteriorly and laterally to form the edge of intervertebral foramen anterolaterally. The transverse process extends from the pedicle to surround the foramen transversum posterolaterally (Fig. 13.15).

Contents of the cervical epidural space

The cervical epidural space is occupied by fat, arteries, venous and lymphatic plexuses, and connective fibrous tissue.

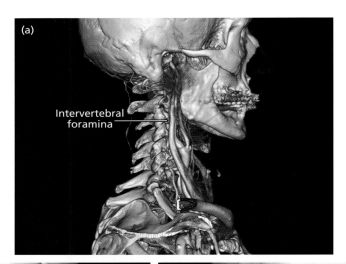

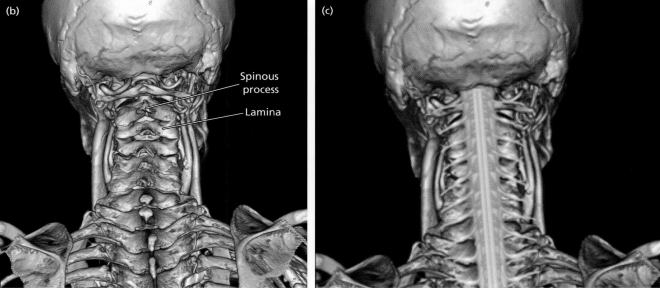

Figure 13.15 (a) Three-dimensional CT scan showing the anatomy of the cervical spine and the contents of the spinal canal. (b) Three-dimensional CT scan of the posterior cervical spine showing the alignment of the vertebral bodies and the intervertebral spaces. (c) Three-dimensional CT scan of the cervical spine with a cartoon showing the spinal cord and its adjacent nerves as they leave the spinal canal.

The measurement of the cervical epidural space

The distance between the ligamentum flavum and dura mater is 1.5–2.0 mm at the C5 level, and 4 mm at the T1 level horizontally. During the flexion of the neck, the cervical epidural space widens to 3.0–4.0 mm. This widening of the epidural space is the primary reason for approaching the interlaminar cervical epidural space at the C7–T1 level (Figs 13.16 and 13.17).

Vasculature of the cervical epidural space

Arterial structure of the cervical epidural space

Arterial branches arise from the vertebral and costocervical arteries. The anterior and posterior spinal arteries surround the cord circumferentially, commonly known as the vasa corona. The arteries of the vasa corona supply the deeper layers of the spinal cord. The aortic arterial branches traverse to the intervertebral foramen and are called segmental arteries. Entering into the spinal cord from intervertebral foramina, segmental arteries are called anterior or posterior branches based on the anterior or posterior branches of the spinal roots. Radicular arteries arise from them at the intervertebral foramen and traverse toward the epidural space and along the nerve roots. The branches of the radicular arteries extend to the spinal cord and are called spinal medullar arteries (Figs 13.18, 13.19, and 13.20).

Venous structure of the cervical epidural space

The venous system of the spinal column is considerably variable. It originates at the center of spinal cord as the anterior central vein, posterior central vein, and peripheral veins. Such venous vessels then traverse to anterior and posterior radicular veins. The radicular veins are combined with vertebral venous plexuses after passing through the dura mater. This venous plexus in the epidural space is called "Batson's venous plexus." Describing this plexus vertically,

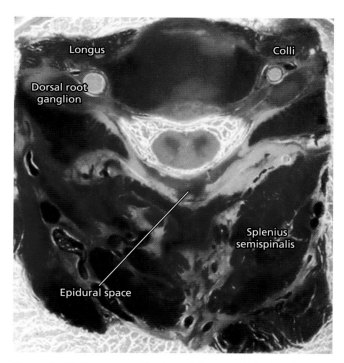

Figure 13.16 Transverse section through lower cervical spine of 72-year-old woman showing muscles and nerve roots. Note the disparity in size between the small anterior longus colli and the large posterior muscles, including trapezius, splenius semispinalis, and the smaller deep muscles. Note also the oblique course of the nerve roots (arrow) and the asymmetry of the vertebral arteries. (Courtesy of J Taylor.)

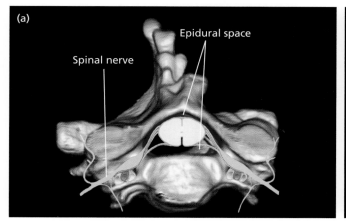
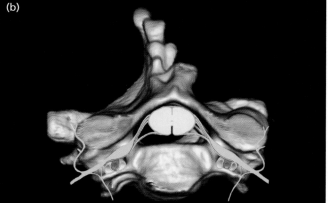

Figure 13.17 (a) The transverse section at the cervical vertebral lateral showing the boundaries and contents of the epidural space. (b) The cervical epidural space showing the location of the vertebral artery in relationship to the spinal nerve roots as they exit the intervertebral foramina.

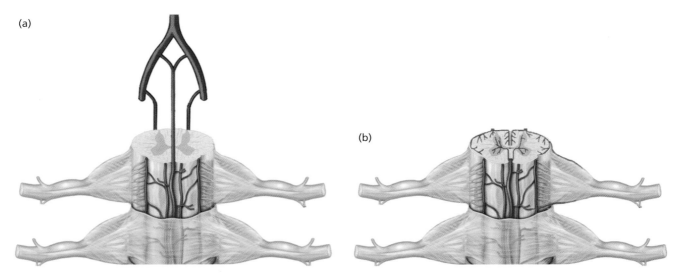

Figure 13.18 (a) Three spinal arteries are derived from the vertebral arteries (VA), one anterior and two posterior. The larger anterior spinal artery supplies the gray matter; the smaller posterior spinal arteries supply the white matter. (b) At several cervical levels, "feeders" from the vertebral arteries pass as radicular branches along the nerve roots to reinforce the spinal arteries.

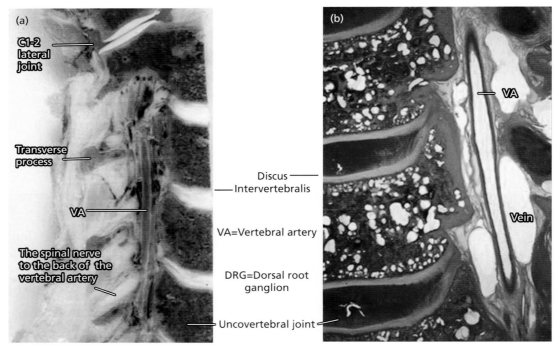

Figure 13.19 Coronal sections of sub-axial spine. VA, vertebral artery. (Courtesy of J.Taylor.) (a) Thick, unstained section. (b) 100 μm stained section.

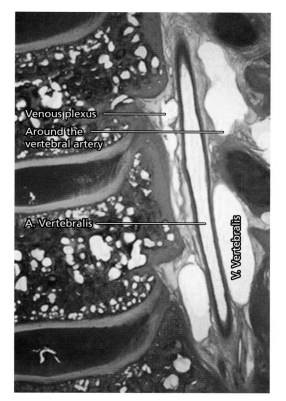

Figure 13.20 Vertebral arteries: they are frequently asymmetrical; branches provide blood supply to the cervical spine. (Courtesy of J Taylor.)

it is located within the anterolateral epidural space, and extends along the entire spinal column.

Indications for cervical interlaminar epidural block (Figs 13.21 and 13.22)

Common indications are the following:

- acute disc herniation causing radiculopathy;
- cervicalgia;
- complex regional pain syndrome of the upper extremity;
- acute and postherpetic neuralgia in the cervical and upper extremity region;
- shoulder–hand syndrome;
- postlaminectomy syndrome due to cervical discectomy;
- cervical spondylosis causing cervical and upper arm pain syndrome;
- spinal stenosis in the cervical region, causing regional and/or radicular pain.

Contraindications for cervical interlaminar epidural block

These contraindications should be taken most seriously because of the importance of deleterious effects due to injury to any or all cervical epidural structures:

- local infection;
- coagulopathy;
- vital function instability;
- psychopathologies.

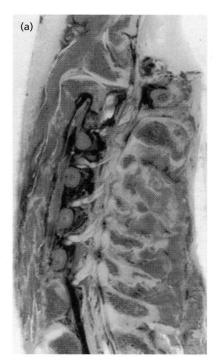

(TP=Tranverse process
VA=Vertebral artery)

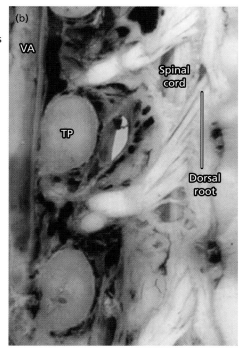

Figure 13.21 (a, b) Cervical nerve roots: oblique exit from spinal canal, they pass forwards as well as laterally. (Courtesy of J Taylor.)

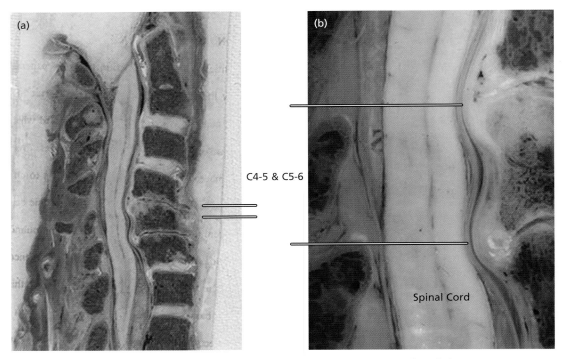

Figure 13.22 (a,b) These photomicrographs show disc protrusions indenting the spinal cord. (Courtesy of J Taylor.)

Technique of approaches to the cervical epidural block

Techniques to identify the epidural space have included the hanging drop, loss of resistance, and test dose of local anesthetic techniques. Fluoroscopic guidance with anterior, posterior, and lateral views plus radiopaque contrast is now commonly used to confirm placement in conjunction with the loss of resistance technique.

There are two approaches to the technique of the cervical epidural block: (1) cervical interlaminar approach; (2) cervical transforaminal approach.

Cervical interlaminar epidural block approach

The procedure of the cervical interlaminar epidural block can be performed in three positions: sitting, lateral, and prone. The sitting position technique is usually blind with loss of resistance technique parameters. We do not recommend this and hence it will not be described here.

Technique for epidural interlaminar lateral approach

A step-by-step approach is described to perform this procedure.

Step 1. Prepare the patient before the procedure
The type of analgesia or sedation needs to be ascertained before performance of the procedure. The type of sedation varies, based on the technique being used. If a diagnostic epidural block with a local anesthetic is considered, some

form of sedation and analgesia may be appropriate for some patients. If placement of an epidural catheter for cervical neuroplasty or similar long-term technique is planned, the patient needs to be able to respond to the stimulation test. Intravenous fentanyl, midazolam, and/or propofol may be used judiciously for the patient's comfort.

Step 2. Position and monitor the patient
1. Place the patient in the lateral decubitus position on the table. Support the abdomen and thorax with pillows, to make the patient comfortable.
2. Pull the shoulders down to obtain a better view of the cervical vertebra. In the lateral position, care must be taken that there is no rotation of patient's spine and the head should be flexed to enlarge the width of the cervical epidural space.
3. An intravenous cannula is inserted for medication injections.
4. Monitoring of vital signs is mandatory.
5. Oxygen is provided by nasal cannula.
6. The area for needle entry is prepared in a sterile fashion.
7. The position of the head and neck is stabilized on the table.

Step 3. Equipment and drugs for the technique
• 1½ inch, 25 gauge needle (for the infiltration of the skin);
• 5 ml syringe (for local anesthetic solution);
• 2 ml empty syringe (for aspiration test);

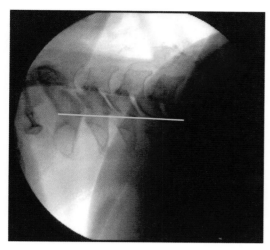

Figure 13.23 The virtual line under lateral view, at the base of the spinal process.

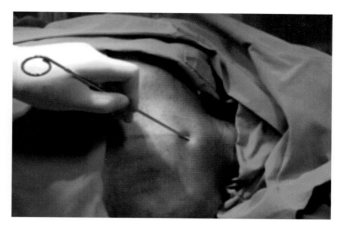

Figure 13.24 This photograph shows the marker pointing to the side of entry at C-71 for the cervical interlaminar approach.

- 28 or 20 gauge, 3½ inch Tuohy or equivalent needle (for the nerve block);
- 1% lidocaine for skin infiltration and for diagnostic injections.

Special equipment
Nerve stimulation equipment for catheter placement.

Step 4. Visualization
1. Place the C-arm in the posteroanterior position. As the patient lies in the lateral decubitus position, the image on the fluoroscopy will be the lateral view of the cervical vertebra.
2. Identify the vertebral body, intervertebral space, and spinous process in the lateral view.
Note: the base of the spinal process appears as a virtual line on the lateral view. Anterior to this virtual line lies the ligamentum flavum. The target of the needle is to direct the needle toward the virtual line (Fig. 13.23).

Step 5. Mark the surface landmarks for needle entry (Fig. 13.24)
Palpate the spinous process of the C7 vertebra and the intervertebral space between the C7–T1 vertebrae.
Note: the C7–T1 intervertebral space is preferred for the cervical interlaminar block.

Step 6. Direction of the needle (Figs 13.25 and 13.26)
1. Infiltrate the skin with local anesthetic.
2. The needle is gently pushed toward the entrance to the cervical epidural space in the lateral fluoroscopic view. The "loss of resistance technique" or "hanging drop technique" is used to identify the epidural space.

Step 7. Confirm the position of the needle (Fig. 13.27)
Confirm the loss of resistance as the needle enters the epidural space as follows.
1. Advance the needle through the supraspinous and interspinous ligament under fluoroscopy. Stop at the level of the "virtual line," the line drawn at the base of the spinous process.
2. Remove the stylet of the needle. Attach a well-lubricated 5 ml syringe filled with saline (some prefer air).
3. Hold the hub of the epidural needle firmly with the left thumb and index finger.
4. Place the wrist of the left hand against the neck of the patient to prevent uncontrolled advance of the needle.
5. Hold the syringe with the right hand; advance the needle under fluoroscopy with the thumb applying pressure on the plunger.
6. As soon as the needle bevel passes through the ligamentum flavum, there will be a "loss of resistance" and the plunger will slide forward without resistance.
7. After negative aspiration of blood or cerebrospinal fluid, inject 2 ml of contrast material; some prefer steroid mixed with a low concentration of local anesthetic. Look for a "straight" line view in lateral vision (Fig. 13.28).

Step 8. Cervical interlaminar epidural block
Once the needle is placed correctly in the cervical epidural space one can inject 2–5 ml of either 1% lidocaine for diagnostic block or decadron or equivalent with or without a low concentration of local anesthetic.

Technique for interlaminar cervical epidural prone approach
Follow steps 1, 2, and 3 (Figs 13.29, 13.30, and 13.31).
Note: interventionists prefer the prone position owing to better delineation of the interlaminar space and because the epidural catheter may be more easily placed on the preferred side. The sitting and lateral position seems easier for the pain physician.

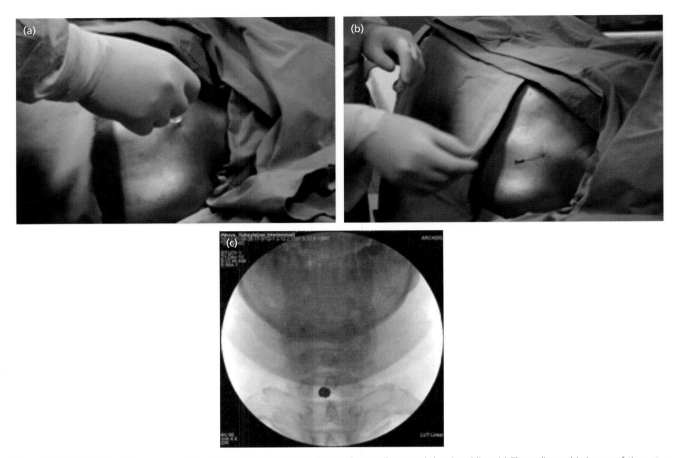

Figure 13.25 (a) Infiltrate the entry point with local anesthetic. (b) Advance the needle toward the virtual line. (c) The radiographic image of the entry point on posteroanterior view for cervical interlaminar approach.

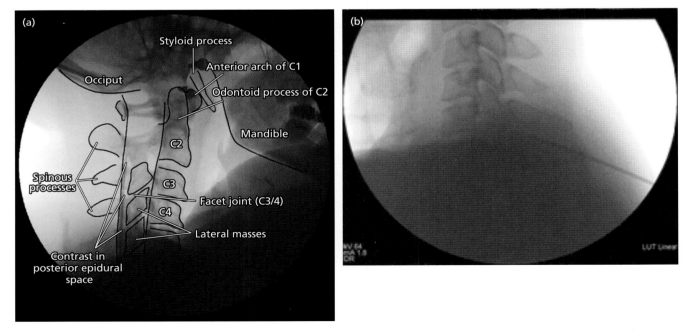

Figure 13.26 (a) See the line drawings of the significant structures of the cervical spine to recognize the direction of the needle into the epidural space. (b) Lateral radiographic image showing the direction of the needle as it approaches the laminar to enter the cervical epidural space.

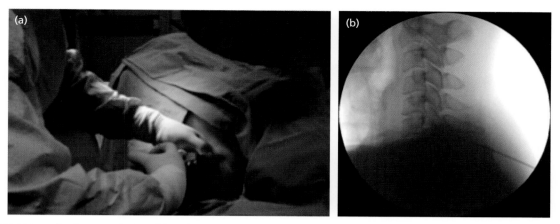

Figure 13.27 (a) Loss of resistance technique. (b) Further progression of the epidural needle in the epidural space as identified by the loss of resistance technique.

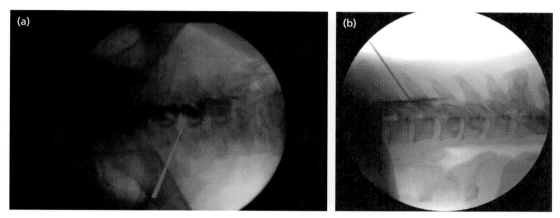

Figure 13.28 (a) Position of the needle and spread of the contrast material in the epidural space. (b) Note the straight line of contrast solution in the epidural space as 2 ml of iohexol has been injected. This confirms the needle is in the epidural space.

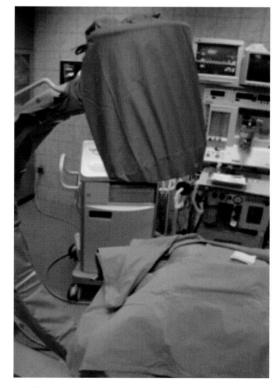

Figure 13.29 The patient in the prone position with the C-arm in posteroanterior view for the cervical interlaminar approach.

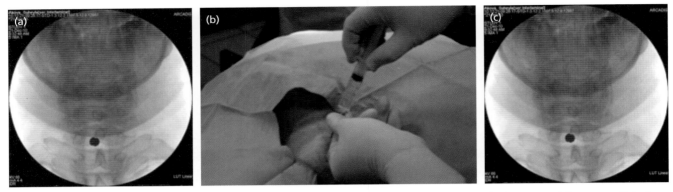

Figure 13.30 (a) Injection of the local anesthetic at the entry side to start the procedure. (b) The cervical interlaminar approach in progress. Note the loss of resistance technique. (c) Note the location of the needle in the cervical intervertebral space for the interlaminar approach in posteroanterior view.

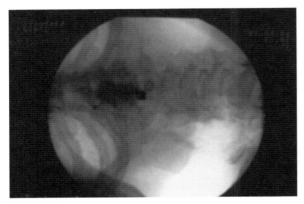

Figure 13.31 Spread of the contrast material in prone position.

Step 4. Visualization
Place the C-arm in a posteroanterior position. Identify the midpoint of the intervertebral space at the C7–T1 level.

Step 5. Direction of the needle
1. Infiltrate the skin with local anesthetic.
2. Advance the needle toward the intervertebral space.

Step 6. Confirm the position of the needle
Position the C-arm laterally and advance the needle with the loss of resistance technique toward and through the vertical line as described in the lateral approach.

Step 7. Cervical interlaminar block
Once entering the epidural space and confirming the correct needle position, follow the same steps as described for the lateral technique to inject the steroid solution (see step 8 in Percutaneous transforaminal block of the cervical epidural space on page 190).

Catheter placement in the cervical epidural space (Fig. 13.32)
1. Enter the cervical epidural space as explained in prone approach.
2. Verify that the bevel of the needle is in the cervical epidural space by injecting contrast solution in both posteroanterior and lateral views, noting that the contrast solution is spreading correctly in the epidural space.
3. Fill the epidural catheter with saline before inserting through the needle.
4. Insert and advance the catheter through the needle under fluoroscopy in lateral view.
5. Aspirate for blood or fluid. If negative for both, inject contrast material through the catheter to verify the tip of the catheter in the epidural space both in posteroanterior and lateral views.
6. Withdraw the Tuohy needle gently; be careful that the catheter is not withdrawn together with the Tuohy needle.
7. Anchor the catheter on the skin firmly in a sterile fashion with a special anchoring technique if you prefer.
8. Once the catheter is correctly placed and anchored, the next procedure will be determined based on the purpose of the cervical catheter placement.
Note: if the catheter was inserted to inject drug infusions intermittently, then that protocol should be observed.
9. If the catheter was placed for cervical epidural adhesiolysis, then that protocol should be followed strictly.
10. If the catheter was inserted for continuous infusions, then that protocol should be followed rigidly.

Step 8. Postprocedure care
After the procedure is completed, the patient needs to be observed for at least 2 hours. Monitoring of vital signs is mandatory. In addition to monitoring the pain relief, one should document it. After a satisfactory observation in the recovery room, the patient should be discharged to the in-patient floor to continue with the protocol for the procedure or to home with appropriate and adequate instructions

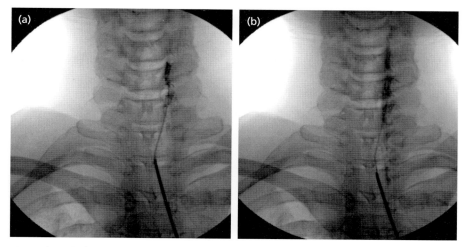

Figure 13.32 (a) Advancing catheter in the cervical epidural space. (b) Spread of the contrast material through the catheter.

given to the escort. Written instructions are preferable for emergencies and are helpful to the patient and their family.

Complications
• Inadvertent dural puncture
The risk of inadvertent dural puncture is possible, even in the most experienced hands. During the dural puncture, cerebrospinal fluid may not be aspirated. Rapid clearance of the contrast material can signify that the needle is in the subarachnoid space.

• Inadvertent subdural puncture
The subdural space is a potential space between the subarachnoid and epidural spaces. Injection of a very small amount of contrast material will appear like a thin straight line at multiple levels. Unlike in the subarachnoid space, contrast material does not disappear. Administration of local anesthetic solution in the subdural space may result in a total spinal block but may take a long time, i.e. as long as 20 minutes.

• Spinal cord injury
The disadvantage of the interlaminar cervical epidural block is there is a greater risk of causing immediate injury to the spinal cord by advancing the epidural needle too far and a greater risk of delayed injury by causing an epidural hematoma or abscess. In some patients there may be inconsistencies in the ligamentum flavum, especially in the midline at the upper cervical levels. This, interestingly, may not provide the loss of resistance sensation sufficient to assess firmness of the ligamentum flavum. To prevent this complication, intermittent lateral fluoroscopic views should be used while advancing the needle and approach the epidural space with a confirmatory radiological marker.

The patient may not feel pain or paresthesia when the needle contacts the spinal cord. They may feel pain only if the needle contacts the sensory fibers within the meninges. Permanent damage within the spinal cord may also develop owing to the injection of local anesthetics or other solutions. Quadriplegia may develop owing to the spinal cord injury.

• Epidural hematoma
Bleeding within the epidural space is a major complication if hematoma develops. The most important cause of epidural hematoma is the bleeding of venous plexuses within the cervical epidural space. Bleeding of the vessels within the epidural space may give rise to signs and symptoms of epidural compression but may be delayed by hours, days, and/or weeks.

If severe pain, paresthesia, and loss of strength in the upper extremities develop within hours or days, one should use the protocol for epidural hematoma.

• Inadvertent puncture of vertebral artery
Normally the vertebral artery is not encountered during the interlaminar cervical epidural block unless the needle is directed more paramedially.

• Infarct due to particulate steroid
A particulate steroid suspension (e.g. triamcinolone) injected into a vertebral or radicular artery may cause an infarct in the brain stem or spinal cord.

Helpful hints
• The advantage of the interlaminar route is that the risk of injecting into a vertebral or radicular artery is minimal. The disadvantages are the risk of causing immediate injury to the spinal cord by advancing the epidural needle too far and the risk of delayed injury by causing an epidural hematoma or abscess.

• Patient selection is a critical part of the procedure in the cervical region. If the patient has bilateral or multilevel symptoms, cervical interlaminar epidural block is more favorable.

The following guidelines are important for the success of the cervical interlaminar epidural block.

• Be sure that the patient is not receiving anticoagulants. If the patient is receiving anticoagulants, instruct them to cease taking them, according to the drug. Withdrawal protocol is agreed upon in consultation with the neurologist.

• Confirming radiological documentation such as a recent magnetic resonance image (MRI) or computed tomography (CT), myelogram, or a comprehensive radiologic report of such scans, should be available and reviewed.

• The patient should be awake enough to respond to arm or leg pain during the procedure.

• Do not perform an interlaminar cervical epidural block if a disc protrusion or spondylosis causes significant narrowing of the midline spinal canal diameter, which should be determined by CT myelography or MRI.

• Use an epidural needle blunt enough to feel the ligamentum flavum when the epidural space is entered.

• Monitor the direction of the needle under lateral view while advancing it toward the cervical epidural space. Attach a T-line to the needle after the loss of resistance, and inject a nonionic contrast medium to confirm epidural placement under direct fluoroscopic visualization.

• If the contrast material disappears, it is probably in the subarachnoid space; stop the procedure at this point.

• In the case of intravenous injection, reposition the needle. If most of the contrast material remains, proceed carefully using a nonparticulate steroid solution.

• Inject corticosteroid slowly. The venous system surrounding the spinal cord is valveless; rapid or forceful administration of the injectate might force the mixture retrograde into the arterial system toward the craniospinal structure.

• Use nonparticulate corticosteroid.

• Catheters can potentially cause bleeding; if used, pass the catheter laterally.

Percutaneous transforaminal block of the cervical epidural space

History

The history of cervical transforaminal injections cannot be ascertained with any accuracy. The first report of the use of cervical transforaminal injections was that of Morvan et al. in 1988. This was followed by another descriptive study by Bush and Hillier in 1996.

Anatomy of the epidural space and its boundaries

The cervical epidural space starts at the foramen magnum superiorly and descends into the thoracic epidural space at the C8–T1 vertebral level. The superior border of the cervical epidural space is the fusion of the periosteal and spinal layers of the dura mater at the foramen magnum. The boundary of the cervical epidural space at each particular vertebral level is the posterior longitudinal ligament anteriorly and the lamina and ligamentum flavum posteriorly. The lateral border of the cervical epidural space is formed by the pedicles and the intervertebral foramina. The intervertebral foramen is formed by these superior and inferior vertebral notches in the upper and lower pedicles. The cervical pedicle extends from the vertebral body posteriorly and laterally to form the edge of the intervertebral foramen anterolaterally. The transverse process extends from the pedicle to surround the foramen transversum posterolaterally (Figs 13.33, 13.34, 13.35, and 13.36).

Contents of the cervical epidural space

The cervical epidural space is occupied by fat, arteries, venous and lymphatic plexuses, and connective fibrous tissue.

The measurement of the cervical epidural space

The distance between the ligamentum flavum and dura mater is 1.5–2.0 mm at the C5 level, and 4 mm at the T1 level horizontally. During the flexion of the neck, the cervical epidural space widens to 3.0–4.0 mm. This widening of the epidural space is the primary reason why approaching the interlaminar cervical epidural should be done at the C7–T1 level.

Vasculature of the cervical epidural space

Arterial structure to the cervical epidural space

Arterial branches arise from the vertebral and costocervical arteries. The anterior and posterior spinal arteries surround the cord circumferentially, commonly known as the vasa corona. The vasa corona supplies the deeper layers of the spinal cord. The aortic arterial branches traverse to the intervertebral foramen and are called segmental arteries. Entering the spinal cord from the intervertebral foramina, segmental arteries are called anterior or posterior branches based on the anterior or posterior branches of the spinal roots. Radicular arteries arise from them at the intervertebral foramen and traverse toward the epidural space and along the nerve roots, and are called spinal radicular arteries. The branches of the radicular arteries extend to the spinal cord and are called spinal medullar arteries (Figs 13.37 and 13.38).

Venous structure of the cervical epidural space

The venous system of the spinal column is considerably variable. It originates at the center of spinal cord as the anterior central vein, posterior central vein, and peripheral veins. Such venous vessels then traverse to anterior and posterior radicular veins. The radicular veins are combined with vertebral venous plexuses after passing through the dura mater. This venous plexus in the epidural space is called "Batson's venous plexus." Describing this plexus vertically,

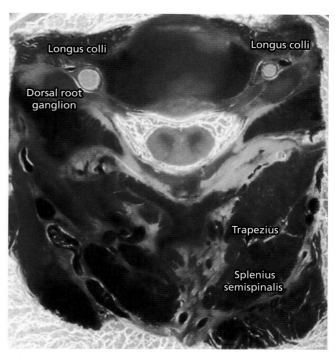

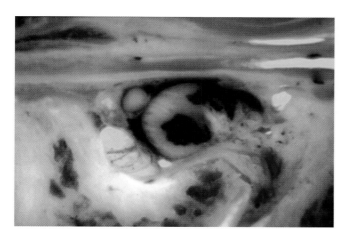

Figures 13.33 and 13.34 Transverse section through lower cervical spine showing muscles and nerve roots. Note the disparity in size between the small anterior longus colli and the large posterior muscles, including trapezius, splenius semispinalis, and the smaller deep muscles. Note the oblique course of the nerve roots and the asymmetry of the vertebral arteries. (Courtesy of J Taylor.)

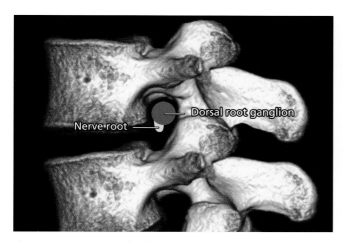

Figure 13.35 Diagram of oblique view of cervical vertebrae showing position of nerve roots in intravenous foramen. (Courtesy of J Taylor.)

it is located within the anterolateral epidural space, and extends along the entire spinal column.

The spinal nerve roots exit from the lower half of the foramen. The spinal artery is located next to the spinal nerve. The specified anatomic characteristics should be carefully considered during the cervical transforaminal injection.

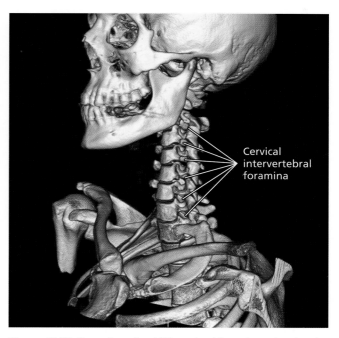

Figure 13.36 Three-dimensional CT scan in oblique view enhancing the cervical intervertebral foramina.

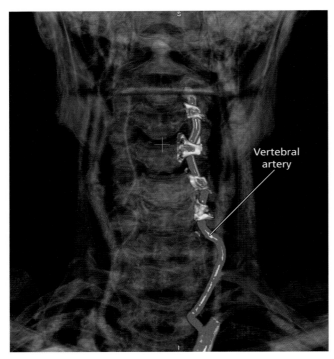

Figure 13.37 The course of the vertebral artery as it ascends from its origin cephalad through the transverse processes.

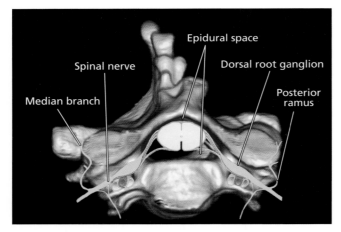

Figure 13.38 The anatomy of the cervical epidural space and the structures which traverse the intervertebral foramina. Note the location of the vertebral artery and the other vascular structures at the level of the nerve root in the foramina.

Indications for transforaminal cervical epidural block

Common indications are the following:
- acute disc herniation causing radiculopathy;
- cervicalgia;
- complex regional pain syndrome of the upper extremity;

- acute and postherpetic neuralgia in the cervical and upper extremity region;
- shoulder–hand syndrome;
- postlaminectomy syndrome due to cervical discectomy;
- cervical spondylosis causing cervical and upper arm pain syndrome;
- spinal stenosis in the cervical region, causing regional and/or radicular pain.

Contraindications for transforaminal cervical epidural block

These contraindications should be taken most seriously because of the importance of deleterious effects due to injury to any or all cervical epidural structures:
- local infection;
- coagulopathy;
- vital function instability;
- psychopathologies.

Technique of transforaminal cervical epidural block

Step 1. Prepare the patient before the procedure

The type of analgesia or sedation needs to be ascertained before performance of the procedure. The type of sedation varies, based on the technique being used. If a diagnostic epidural block with a local anesthetic is considered, some form of sedation and analgesia may be appropriate for some patients. Intravenous fentanyl, midazolam, and/or propofol may be used judiciously for the patient's comfort.

Step 2. Position and monitor the patient

1. Place the patient in the supine position. Ensure that the patient is in a comfortable position by placing a small pillow under their head. Fasten their head on the table using a strip of adhesive bandage.

2. Position the arms of the patient on both sides. Position the C-arm laterally and check whether all cervical vertebrae are on the same plane.

3. Obtain an intravenous access. Administer oxygen by nasal cannula; monitor the vital signs noninvasively.

4. Prepare and drape the area in a sterile fashion.

5. The patient should not be over-sedated. The patient should remain sufficiently conscious to provide response to any questions.

Step 3. Equipment and drugs for the cervical transforaminal block
- 1½ inch, 25 gauge needle for skin infiltration;
- 5 ml syringe for local anesthetic solution;
- 22 gauge, 3½ inch needle with extension line for the cervical transforaminal block;
- 2 ml syringe for the contrast material;
- 1% lidocaine for skin infiltration;

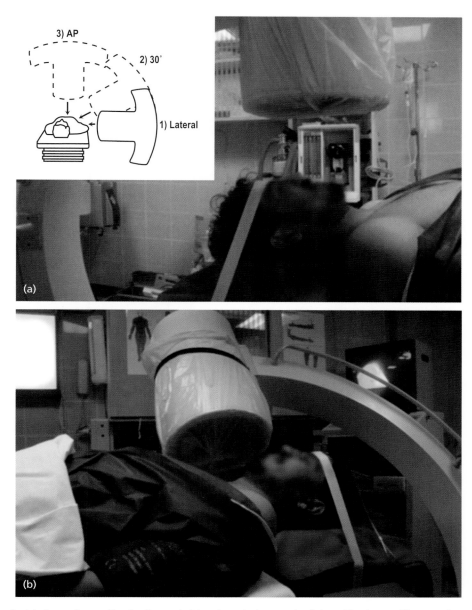

Figure 13.39 (a) A patient in the supine position for the cervical transforaminal approach of the epidural space. The procedure starts with the C-arm in the posteroanterior position. (b) A patient with the C-arm in the oblique position.

- contrast material, e.g. iohexol;
- saline;
- nonparticulate steroid solution.

Step 4. Visualization (Figs 13.39 and 13.40)
1. Place the C-arm in the anteroposterior position, so that cervical vertebrae can be visualized.
2. Then rotate the C-arm laterally slowly to the oblique position to view the widest intervertebral foramina. Sometimes this image cannot be obtained in the anterior oblique position. In this case, the C-arm should be guided to cephalad or caudal in direction for the optimal view.

3. The first intervertebral foramen to be viewed under fluoroscopy is C3. Other intervertebral foramina should be counted, based on this first one.
4. The physician performing the procedure should stand on the opposite side of the patient. Standing allows easier placement of the needle.

Step 5. Mark the surface landmarks for the needle entry Extendable and stimulatable needles must be used for the cervical transforaminal block. The extension should be filled with saline to avoid any air bubble formation before the procedure (Fig. 13.41).

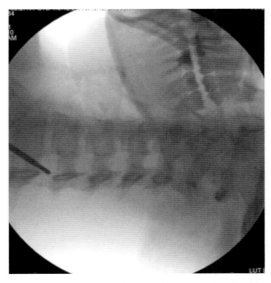

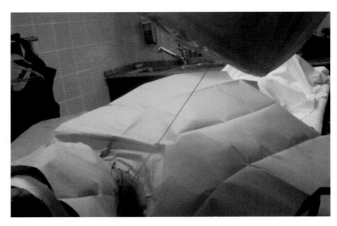

Figure 13.42 The axis of the needle and C-arm should be aligned with each other.

Figure 13.40 The physician performing the intervention should cross to the opposite side of the patient. Standing in this position allows easier placement of the needle. Extendable and stimulatable needles must be used for the cervical transforaminal block. The extension should be filled with saline to avoid formation of any air bubbles before the procedure.

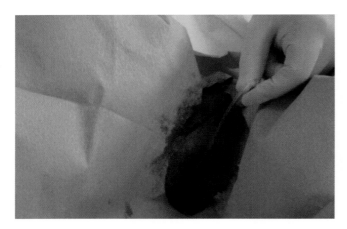

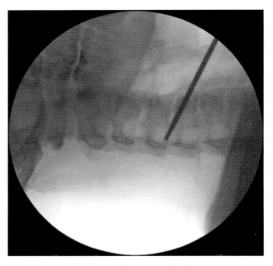

Figure 13.43 The target point of the needle placement is the 6 o'clock position.

Figure 13.41 Mark the lateral edge of the sternocleidomastoid muscle.

1. Mark the lateral edge of the sternocleidomastoid muscle. The point of entry should be located behind the lateral edge of the muscle.

2. Infiltrate the skin with local anesthetic solution. The patient may feel pain when the needle is inserted into lateral cervical muscles after penetrating the skin. The pain may be felt both in this area and in the shoulder region. As the area is rich in veins, aspirate before infiltration.

Step 6. Direction of the needle
Determination of the target point (Fig. 13.42).
1. Guide the needle into the identified point of the intervertebral foramen using "tunneled vision." The axes of the needle and C-arm should be aligned with each other.

2. After inserting the needle to 2 cm deep, return the C-arm to the posteroanterior position for the oblique position to determine the depth of the needle. The distance between the skin and intervertebral foramen varies greatly. Therefore special care should be taken to insert the needle at a safe depth.

Step 7. Confirm the position of the needle (Figs 13.43, 13.44, and 13.45)
1. Upon determination of the depth, relocate the C-arm to the previous oblique position, then continue to push the needle forward. Move needle forward until the needle tip contacts the superior articular process on the cervical facet joint below. Considering the intervertebral foramen as a dial, the penetration point of the needle is to be at 6 o'clock. This position is considered safe because it is the most distant to both the vertebral artery and the nerve root.

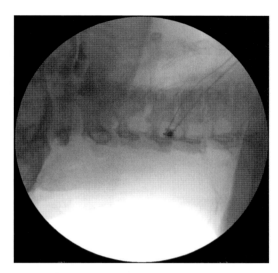

Figure 13.44 The needle is confirmed at the 6 o'clock position with a small amount of contrast material injected.

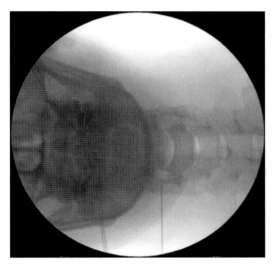

Figure 13.45 Correct placement of needle in the anteroposterior position.

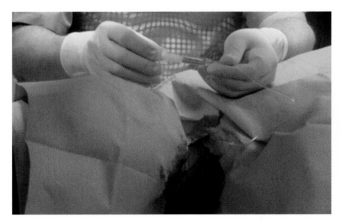

Figure 13.46 Injection of contrast material with continuous imaging.

2. Then turn the C-arm to the posteroanterior position, and slowly push the needle through the intervertebral foramen. The needle should not penetrate beyond the vertical line drawn on the uncinate process. This is the approximate middle line of the facet joint, where the lateral edge of the dura is closest. If the needle is inserted deeper, this may result in dura puncture and spinal cord injury.

3. As soon as the needle tip enters through the intervertebral foramen, check for any air bubbles in the extension catheter; unlike other interventions, the contrast material is given under uninterrupted live imaging. Any potential venous spread should be observed carefully (Figs 13.46, 13.47, and 13.48).

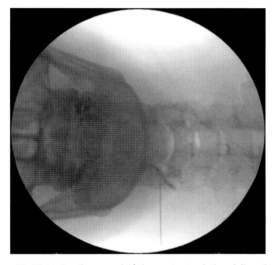

Figure 13.47 Notice the spread of the contrast solution delineating the cervical nerve root with this transforaminal approach.

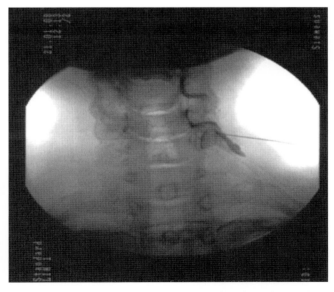

Figure 13.48 Two to three cubic centimetres of local anesthetic with contrast is injected because of the very small capacities in this region. Note the radicular appearance of this contrast solution.

4. If the needle is inside the vein, the procedure should be discontinued.

5. If the contrast material spreads safely within the foramen and surrounding the nerve root sheath proceed with the transforaminal epidural steroid injection.

Step 8. Transforaminal epidural steroid injection

1. For patients with pathologies for more than one level, injection from a single level will be sufficient, if the contrast matter is spread at those levels. Reposition the C-arm in the oblique position to determine at which levels the contrast solution is spread.

2. Cervical periradicular and epidural spaces have limited volume capacity. A volume of only 2–3 ml of solution will be sufficient. Nonparticulate steroid solution (3.0–6.0 mg) – dexamethasone – should be given if a single root is injected. A maximum 12.0 mg should be used at one sitting.

3. Some physicians do not inject local anesthetics into the solution in the cervical area.

Step 9. Postprocedure care

After the procedure is completed, the patient needs to be observed for at least 2 hours. Monitoring of vital signs is mandatory. In addition to monitoring the pain relief, one should document it. After a satisfactory observation in the recovery room, the patient should be discharged to the in-patient floor to continue with the protocol for the procedure or to home with appropriate and adequate instructions given to the escort. Written instructions are preferable for emergencies and are helpful to the patient and their family.

Complications

• Inadvertent puncture of the dura (Fig. 13.49)

The needle should not penetrate beyond the vertical line drawn on the uncinate process. This is the approximate middle line of the facet colon, where the lateral edge of the dura exists. If the needle is extended excessively, this may result in dura puncture and spinal cord injury. If there is a lateral dilatation of the dural root sleeve into the intervertebral foramen, dural puncture is also possible. Rapid dilution of the contrast material implies subarachnoid spread. In the event of dural puncture, the needle must be withdrawn and the procedure should be interrupted.

• Inadvertent puncture of vertebral artery or vertebral vein

Injury of the spinal segmental arteries during cervical transforaminal injection does not always necessarily cause spinal cord ischemia. Embolism may occur owing to the use of particulate steroids, which in turn induces ischemia. The needle should never be directed to the anterior aspect of the intervertebral foramen. During the aspiration test, blood may not be aspirated. The contrast material should be given slowly under uninterrupted live imaging. If the needle is within the vertebral artery the contrast material spreads vertically. If the needle is within the segmental artery it will spread medially toward the spinal cord. The spread of the contrast material within the epidural or paraspinous veins is slower (Fig. 13.50).

During the puncture of anterior or posterior segmental arteries, if nonparticulate steroid solutions are injected, serious complications may not occur. If particulate solutions only are used, the risks of emboli or infarct increase.

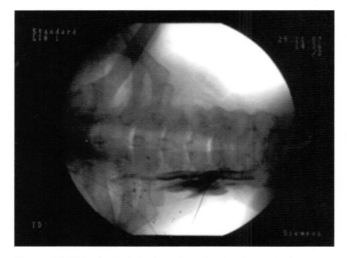

Figure 13.49 Inadvertent dural puncture showing the contrast appearing in the subarachnoid space.

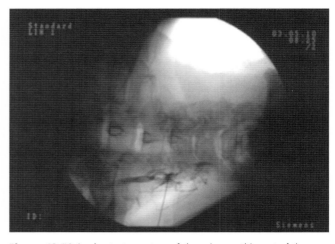

Figure 13.50 Inadvertent puncture of the vein; see this part of the contrast in continuous imaging in the vein.

• **Epidural hematoma**

The epidural space is narrowest in the cervical region. Thus, either for transforaminal or interlaminar cervical injections, if bleeding occurs during the procedure, the procedure should be terminated and the patient followed up for at least 12 hours. If epidural hematoma develops, paresthesia and loss of strength of the upper extremities may develop. In such cases, surgical consultation is mandatory.

• **Spinal cord injury**

In cases where the needle is advanced beyond the middle line of the facet joint, spinal cord injury may occur. There are cases of quadriplegia developing from this spinal cord injury.

• **Neurological complications**

The needle may contact the spinal segmental nerve or its ventral ramus while advanced through the intervertebral foramen. Immediate severe pain and paresthesia develop at that instant. The patient should remain sufficiently conscious to provide a response to such a complication. The needle is to be replaced if this paresthesia occurs. If the same symptoms reoccur after multiple attempts, the procedure should be interrupted.

Helpful hints

A cervical transforaminal block is technically and potentially a dangerous procedure. It should be performed only by physicians having extensive experience in fluoroscopically guided procedures. The experience and skill should necessarily be gained by performance of procedures such as transforaminal injections in the lumbar spine, lumbar or cervical facet injections, and medial branch blocks.

The following principles are important while performing the cervical transforaminal block.

• Position the C-arm in the posteroanterior, oblique, and lateral projections to identify the relevant anatomy.

• Try to access the intervertebral foramen with small movements using fluoroscopy in posteroanterior, oblique, and lateral positions.

• Place the needle with fine manipulation. Use a needle with an extended line.

• Correctly interpret the spread of contrast material in the epidural space.

• Correctly interpret the spread of the contrast material in the subarachnoid space.

• Correctly interpret intravascular injections.

• The volume of the cervical epidural space is quite small; use small volumes of solutions to cover the target nerves.

• Use a short acting local anesthetic in small volumes to prevent unintended vascular or subarachnoid injections.

• In the case of monoradicular pathology use betamethasone at doses of 3.0–6.0 mg; for multilevel pathology the dose may be increased to 12.0 mg.

• Follow up the patient for a reasonable time for any intravenous conscious sedation used, until the intellectual function and tolerance to oral intake become normal.

• Discharge the patient into the care of a responsible escort from their family.

Percutaneous block and lesioning of the cervical facet joint

History

Cervical facet joints have gained the attention of clinicians owing to the implications of a cervical origin for headache. Explanation of the cervical facet joints in headache can, in part, be attributed to Pawl in 1971. Similar publications can be found dating as far back as 1940 with Hadden (1948), Raney and Raney (1962), Taren and Kahn (1962), and finally with Brain and Wilkinson (1967), McNab (1973) and Mehta (1973).

Anatomy

Formation of the cervical joint

The cervical facet (zygapophyseal) joints are formed by the superior and inferior articular process of two adjacent vertebrae. The cervical facets, from C3 to C4 to C7 to T1, are lined by an articular cartilage with synovium and possess joint capsules.

The articular facets are flat and oval in form: the superior aspect of the facet joint faces backward, upward, and slightly medially; the inferior aspect faces forward, downward, and slightly lateral.

The transverse processes are each pierced by the foramen transversorium, which, in the upper six vertebrae, gives passage to the vertebral artery and vein, as well as a plexus of sympathetic nerves. Each process consists of an anterior and a posterior part. These two parts are joined, outside the foramen, by a bar of bone, which exhibits a deep sulcus on its upper surface for the passage of the corresponding spinal nerve (Figs 13.51, 13.52, and 13.53).

Innervation of the zygapophyseal joints (Figs 13.54, 13.55, and 13.56)

The cervical zygapophyseal joints (from C3 to C4 to C7 to T1) are innervated by the medial branches of the cervical dorsal rami.

Every medial branch from the dorsal rami of the C3–C8 spinal nerves passes through an anatomic tunnel dorsolateral to the facet joint. The nerve then passes laterally around the articular pillar to form C3–C6 medial branches; the nerve always passes through the centroid of the bisecting lines created by the trapezoidal shape of the articular pillar.

Because the nerve innervates the facet joint from above and below, it is necessary to block the medial branch of the named nerves at that spinal level.

Although this holds true for the C3–C6 medial branches, there are differences in both the upper and the lower

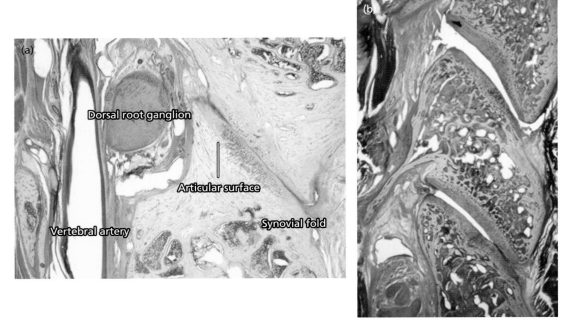

Figure 13.51 (a,b) Cervical facet joints: 100 μm sagittal sections. Note the fine synovial folds which project between the articular surfaces. (Courtesy of J Taylor.)

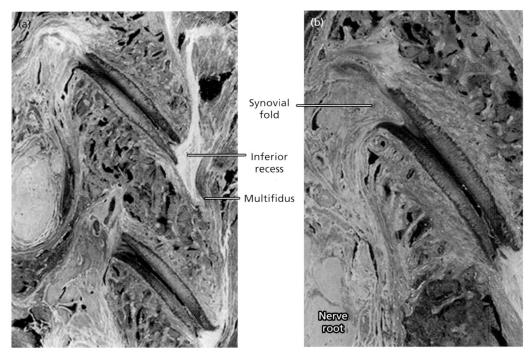

Figure 13.52 (a,b) Facet joints: sagittal sections of; C5–7; C6–7. (Courtesy of J Taylor.)

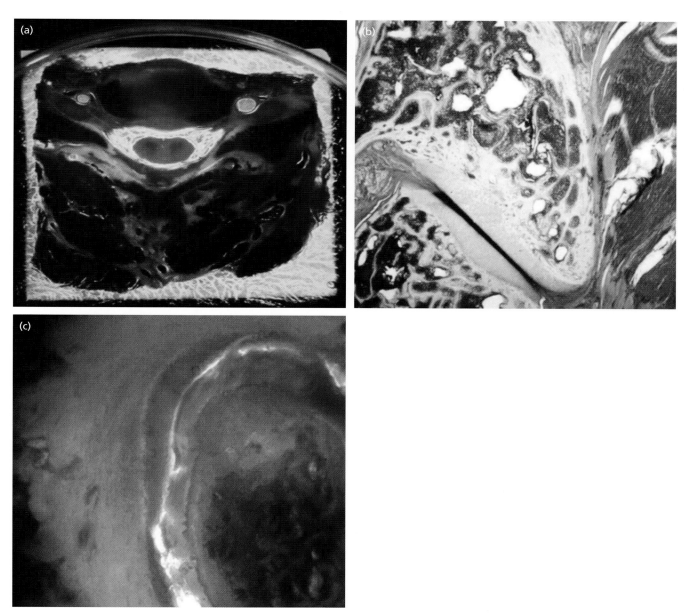

Figure 13.53 (a–c) Sagittal sections of the facet joints. (Courtesy of J Taylor.)

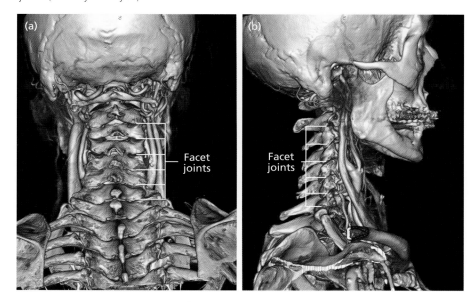

Facet joints

Facet joints

Figure 13.54 (a,b) Lateral and posterior views of the facet joints.

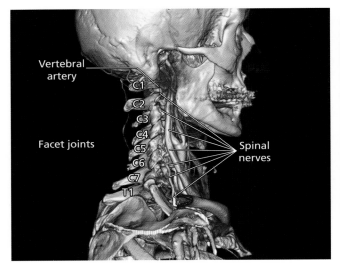

Figure 13.55 Medial branches of the cervical facet joints.

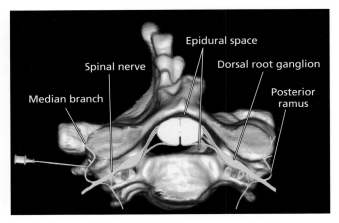

Figure 13.56 Cervical facet joint medial branch block.

cervical spine. The C2–C3 joint is supplied by a large third occipital nerve (which later becomes cutaneous just below the nuchal line) as well as afferents from C2, the position of which may be variable.

The lower cervical medial branches also have a nerve course that differs from the midcervical spine. The target for the C7 medial branch lies on the superior–medial tip of the C7 transverse process, whereas the target for the C8 medial branch lies on the superior lateral aspect of the T1 transverse process. Therefore, to block the C7–T1 joint, the C7 and C8 medial branches must be injected. It should also be noted that the medial branch innervates far more than the cervical facet joint.

The medial nerve receives sprouts from the bony lamina and spinous process as well innervating the surrounding musculature. This includes the deep segmental stabilizers of the spine (multifidus) as well as the semispinalis capitis and semispinalis cervices.

Unique to the cervical spine is the presence of the vertebral artery, which passes though the transverse foramen of the transverse processes of the C1–C6 vertebrae.

Indications
- Whiplash injury.
- Arthritis and inflammation in the cervical facet joints.
- Suboccipital headache.
- Cervicogenic headache.

Contraindications
- Local infection or sepsis.
- Coagulopathy.
- Vital functions instability.
- Psychopathologies.

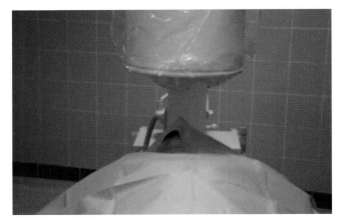

Figure 13.57 C-arm in the posteroanterior position.

C3–C7 medial branch block and RF lesioning

Step 1. Prepare the patient before the procedure
The type of analgesia or sedation needs to be ascertained before performance of the invasive procedure. If a local anesthetic is considered or neurolytic block is planned, mild sedation is all that is necessary. If pulsed RF is planned, the patient needs to be awake to respond to the stimulation test. Intravenous fentanyl or midazolam may be used judiciously for the patient's comfort.

Step 2. Position and monitor the patient (Figs 13.57, 13.58, and 13.59).
1. Place the patient in the supine position on the table.
2. The position of the head is stabilized on the table.
3. Ensure that the patient is in a comfortable position by placing a small pillow under their head. Position the arms of the patient on both sides.
4. Position the C-arm laterally and check whether all cervical vertebrae are on the same plane.

5. Place the C-arm through the table on the head side to view cervical vertebrae.
6. An intravenous cannula is inserted for medication injections.
7. Monitoring of vital signs is mandatory.
8. Oxygen is provided by nasal cannula.
9. The area for needle entry is prepared in a sterile fashion.

Step 3. Drugs and equipment for the facet joint block
- 1½ inch, 25 gauge needle for skin infiltration;
- 5 ml syringe for local anesthetic solution;
- 5 ml syringe for the block;
- 22 gauge, 3½ inch needle with extension line for the cervical facet block;
- 1% lidocaine for skin infiltration;
- saline;
- nonparticulate steroid solution.

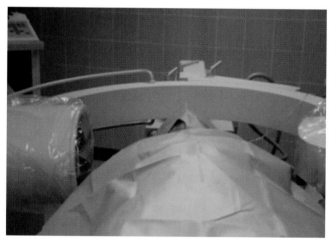

Figure 13.58 C-arm in the lateral position.

Special equipment for the medial branch RF lesioning
- RF machine.
- 5–10 cm, 2 mm active tip electrode with extension line.

Step 4. Visualization
1. Place the C-arm in the posteroanterior position, and identify the vertebral body of the targeted medial branch.
2. Then turn the C-arm to the lateral position, for C3–C6 medial branches.
Note: the nerve passes through the centroid of the bisecting lines created by the trapezoidal shape of the articular pillar.

Step 5. Mark the surface landmarks for the needle entry
1. Infiltrate the skin with local anesthetic solution. The patient may feel pain when the needle is inserted into lateral cervical muscles after penetrating the skin. The pain may be felt both in this area and in the shoulder region. As the area is rich in veins, aspirate before infiltration.
2. Slightly move the C-arm cephalad or caudally until each segmental level is perfectly superimposed and the best view of the articular pillars is seen.
3. This is not a "tunneled vision" procedure. Mark the lateral edge of the sternocleidomastoid muscle. The point of entry is approximately 1 cm below the posterior border of the sternocleidomastoid muscle (Fig. 13.60).

Step 6. Direction of the needle
1. Insert the needle under lateral fluoroscopic guidance.
2. Advance the needle toward the center of the trapezoid until a bony contact is made (Fig. 13.61).

Step 7. Important considerations (Figs 13.62, 13.63, and 13.64)
1. After contact with the body of the vertebra is made, rotate the C-arm to the oblique view, until the neural

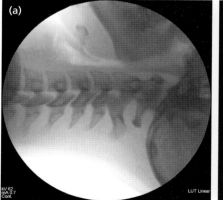
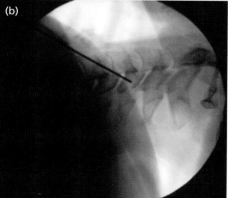

Figure 13.59 (a) Lateral view of the cervical spine. (b) Position of the medial branch of the cervical facet.

foramina come into view. To get a perfect view, a cauda-cephalad arrangement of the C-arm may be necessary.

2. The articular pillars will appear as an elliptical shape or "beads" on each level. The needle should rest at a point between the most superior third and middle superior third of the articular pillar.

3. Rotate the C-arm again laterally to confirm that the tip of the needle rests at the midpoint of the trapezoid.

4. Then rotate the C-arm to the posteroanterior position. The tip of the needle should be in the waist of the articular pillar.

Step 8. Stimulation test

After confirming the tip of the needle or electrode, aspirate, if the aspiration test is negative proceed with the stimulation test.

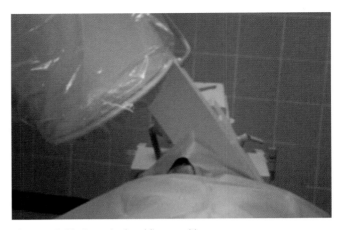

Figure 13.62 C-arm in the oblique position.

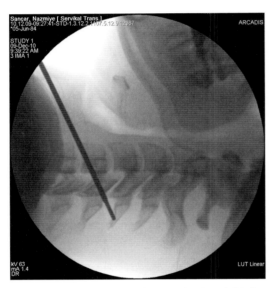

Figure 13.60 Point of entry for the facet median branch block.

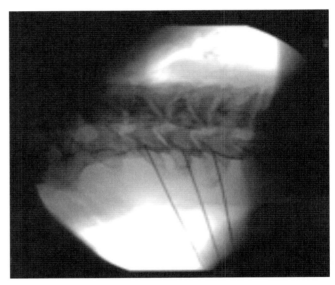

Figure 13.63 Needles in oblique view directed to the targeted site.

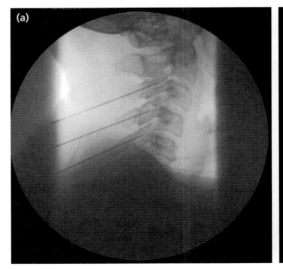
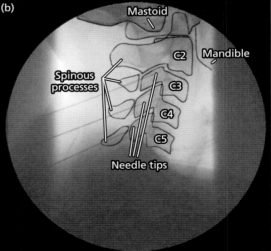

Figure 13.61 (a) Initial direction of the needles. (b) Anatomical landmarks for medial branch block.

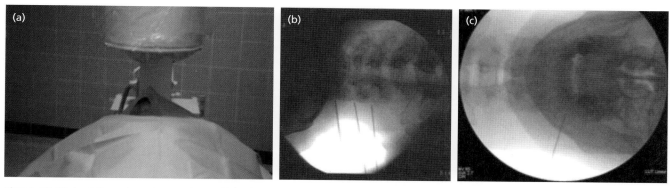

Figure 13.64 (a–c) C-arm in posteroanterior position, the needle position on the waist of the articular pillar.

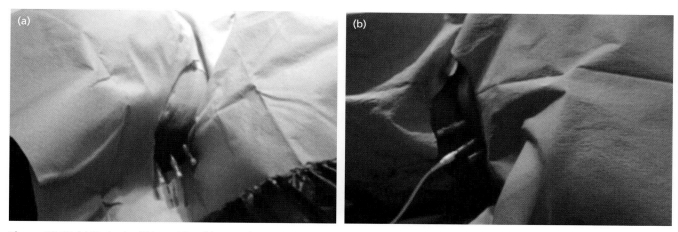

Figure 13.65 (a) Electrodes (3) in position. (b) Cervical medial branch RF procedure in progress.

Step 9. RF technique of cervical facet medial branches (Fig. 13.65)

1. One should stimulate the nerve at 50–100 Hz with 0.1–1.5 V settings. Generally, patients feel paresthesia at a setting of 0.5 V. No stimulation should be felt in a radicular manner, from the nerve roots.

2. Then start stimulating the region at 2 Hz, with 0.1–1.5 V settings. Slight motor contraction may occur in the paraspinous muscles of the neck, but there should be no motor contraction down the upper extremity or the shoulder (Fig. 13.65).

3. After confirming the correct placement of the electrode, inject 0.3 ml of 1% lidocaine for each level.

4. Wait for a short time (30 seconds to 1 minute) before the start of the lesioning. Proceed with lesioning at 70 °C, for 60 seconds.

5. Pulsed RF at 45 V for two cycles of 120 seconds with a temperature not exceeding 42 °C is possible.

Block of the C2 medial branch

The C2 medial branch block is slightly different from the lower levels. The needle tip should be at the tip of the center

of the C2–C3 facet joint, the second on the subcondral plate of the C2 inferior articular process, and the third needle on the subcondral plate of the C3 superior articular process.

Block of the medial branch of C7 and C8

1. The needle is directed first toward the back of the C7 superior articular process under anteroposterior view, until a bony contact is made, then redirected slipping on the lateral surface of the superior articular process under lateral view. The position of the needle tip should be confirmed under anteroposterior, lateral, and oblique views.

2. The C8 medial branch lies on the superior lateral aspect of the T1 transverse process.

Prone technique (Figs 13.66 and 13.67)

1. The patient is placed prone on the table. The posterior aspect of the neck is prepared and draped in a sterile fashion.

2. The posterior aspects of the waists of the articular pillars are identified under posteroanterior view.

3. It may be difficult to identify the articular pillars of the upper levels: place a pillow under the chest and slightly

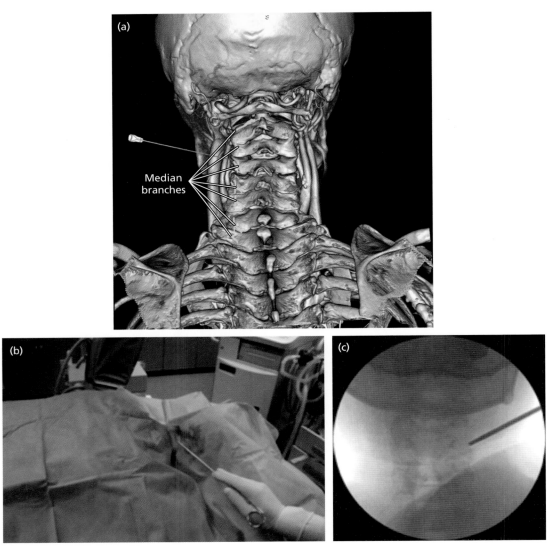

Figure 13.66 (a) The patient is placed prone on the table. The posterior aspect of the neck is prepped and draped in a sterile fashion. (b,c) Identify the articular pillars.

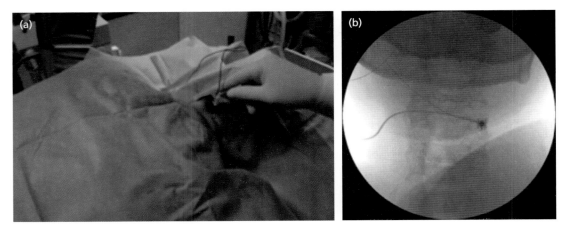

Figure 13.67 (a,b) Position of the needle under posteroanterior view.

hyperextend the head or ask the patient to open their mouth.

4. Infiltrate the skin; advance the needle under posteroanterior view in a tunneled vision toward the articular pillar.

5. As soon as the bony contact is made, rotate the C-arm laterally. The tip of the needle should rest on the posterior aspect of the articular pillar.

6. Proceed with the procedure as described above.

Technique for cervical facet joint block

1. Prepare and position the patient as described earlier for medial branch block.

2. Position the C-arm laterally. Slightly move the C-arm cephalad or caudal until each segmental level is perfectly superimposed and the best view of the articular pillars is seen.

3. Advance a 22 gauge, 10 cm needle toward the facet joint from a posterior or posterolateral angle under lateral view. As soon as the needle arrives at the facet joint walk off the needle into the facet joint.

4. Confirm radiographically in anteroposterior and lateral views.

5. Inject 0.2 ml of contrast material into the joint. The contrast material will fill the joint.

Note: one should not inject a greater amount of contrast material.

6. For each joint, inject 0.5 ml of a combination of local anesthetic and steroid solution if the contrast solution confirms the needle tip in the targeted facet joint (Figs 13.68 and 13.69).

Step 10. Postprocedure care

After the procedure is completed, the patient needs to be observed for up to 2 hours. Monitoring of vital signs is man-datory. In addition the pain relief should be objectively documented. After a satisfactory observation, the patient should be discharged with appropriate and adequate instructions given to the escort. Written instructions are preferable for emergencies and are helpful to the patient and their family.

Complications

• **Transient increase in pain**

Transient increase in pain immediately after the procedure owing to the irritation of the facet joint or RF lesioning may be experienced. In most of the cases it recovers within days.

• **Neuritis**

Although it is not common, neuritis may develop after RF lesioning. It is manifested by a new-onset radicular-type burning pain.

• **Dysesthesia and numbness**

Dysesthesia and numbness in the cutaneous branches of the medial branch may develop.

• **Inadvertent dural puncture**

Incorrect placement of the needle may cause inadvertent dural puncture. The needle should not be advanced deeper than the facet joint under fluoroscopic imaging. Injection of local anesthetic may cause respiratory depression, sensorial and motor block.

• **Incorrect placement of the needle transforaminally**

If the needle is directed deeper than the level of the facet joint, it may enter the intervertebral foramen. The correct placement of the needle has to be confirmed under lateral, oblique, and posteroanterior views. The needle should lie in

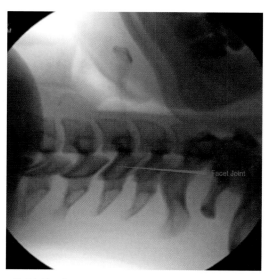

Figure 13.68 The facet joint.

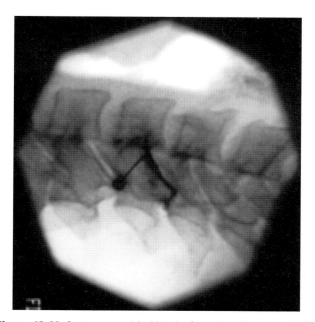

Figure 13.69 Contrast material within the facet joint. (Courtesy of P Finch.)

the midpoint of the waist formed by the articular pillar in contact with the bone.

- **Chemical meningism**

Chemical meningism may occur owing to inadvertent dural puncture and injection of particulate steroids into the subarachnoid space.

- **Inadvertent injection into vertebral artery**

If the needle tip during a supine approach median branch block is too far anterior, this could result in vertebral artery puncture. However, inadvertent injection of local anesthetic or nonwater-soluble steroid into the vertebral artery is more likely to occur during intraarticular injections than median branch blocks.

- **Spinal cord injury**

Incorrect placement of the needle may cause inadvertent puncture of the spinal cord, which will be a devastating complication.

- **Vasovagal syncope**

The procedure should be explained in detail to the patient before it is performed. Otherwise, vasovagal syncope may develop in some patients.

- **Transient ataxia**

Transient ataxia may occur due to the partial block of the upper cervical proprioceptive afferent fibers during the third occipital nerve block. It is more significant if conventional RF lesioning is performed. Otherwise it recovers within a couple of weeks.

- **Koebner's phenomenon**

Koebner's phenomenon, also called the "Koebner response" or the "isomorphic response," refers to skin lesions appearing on lines of the injection. Koebner's phenomenon may result from either a linear exposure or irritation. Causes of Koebner's phenomenon are secondary to scratching rather than an infective or chemical cause.

Helpful hints

The clinical criteria for facet syndrome are nonspecific and still unreliable. Intraarticular facet injections or median branch blocks should be reserved for patients with no neurologic deficit, when no other cause for their chronic pain can be identified. Also, the pain should be unresponsive to simpler therapies such as rest during acute exacerbations and oral medications, including nonsteroidal anti-inflammatory drugs. The facets to be blocked can be identified by physical examination and analysis of the patient's symptoms. If the patient has marked tenderness to palpation over a particular facet joint or if pain increases with motion or loading of the joint, trial blockade of the joint should be considered.

Before a medial branch RF denervation in the cervical region is performed, a differential diagnosis between radicular, segmental, and localized pain limited to the cervical area should be made.

Pain radiating to the maxillary area may be due to a problem on the C3 cervical joint.

Differential diagnosis for atypical facial pain, cluster headache, tension headache, or classical migraine is also essential.

Diagnostic or prognostic block before medial branch denervation may be performed to verify the diagnosis. However, excessive amounts of local anesthetic will produce a false-positive response.

If medial block is to be performed for several levels, it is more appropriate to begin from the lower levels up to upper levels (C6–C5–C4–C3–C2).

It is difficult to reach the medial branches on C7–C8 levels in the supine position. It will be more appropriate to use the prone approach for these levels.

The posterior approach offers the advantage that the vertebral artery, the spinal nerves, and the radicular arteries lie anterior to the final anterior location of the needle.

Percutaneous discography of the cervical discs

History

In 1948, Hirsch first described the procedure for injecting procaine in the herniated disc. In 1940 Roofe investigated the annulus fibrosus innervation, which provided an incentive for conceptualizing the disc as a painful source independent of a neurocompressive component of the disc herniation. In 1944 following Roofe's studies, Lindblom first demonstrated the presence of radial annular fissures in a cadaveric disc.

Hirsch followed this demonstration with a clinical study to determine if the course of the ruptures or tears in the annulus would lead to pathologic processes causing pain. He hypothesized that putting pressure on a ruptured or degenerated disc could cause a patient's pain. He demonstrated that if one injected saline to pressurize the disc, it will cause pain. In addition, injection of a local anesthetic like procaine will relieve this pain. In 1964, Crock advanced the theory of internal disc disruption, and showed that patients have abnormal discograms and that pain is reproduced by a small volume (0.3 ml) of solution injected, owing to hypersensitivity of pain fibers in the disc. Discographic patterns on radiographs were shown to be abnormal. In 1987 Sachs demonstrated pathological disruption and classified it as what is known as the Dallas discogram scale. Bogduk later modified this Dallas Scale.

Anatomy of cervical discs

Cervical discs have characteristics that are distinct from lumbar discs. The cervical disc is contained by anterior and posterior longitudinal ligaments and periosteofascial tissue.

Anteriorly, the annulus fibrosus has a concentric thick collagen fiber, which thins out as the annulus approaches the uncinate process. The annulus fibrosus in the anterior segment of the disc is frequently subject to stress and strain and has, consequently, adapted to being thicker.

The anterior portion of the cervical disc space is larger than the posterior portion, which makes it difficult for the nuclear material to move anteriorly unless great force is applied to the disc. The tough outer annulus is also thicker in the anterior portion of the cervical disc; this makes for increased load on the disc and is likely to cause a posterior bulge (Figs 13.70, 13.71, 13.72, 13.73, and 13.74).

Innervation of cervical discs

Nerve fibers enter the disc from the posterolateral direction and traverse perpendicular to the fibrocartilaginous bundles in the deep layers of the annulus fibrosus.

Posteriorly, the annulus receives fibers from the sinuvertebral nerves. Laterally, fibers from the exiting spinal nerve roots provide sensory innervation and the anterior portion of the disc receives fibers from the sympathetic chain.

Indications

- Neck pain lasting greater than 3 months with failure to achieve adequate improvement with a multidisciplinary program.

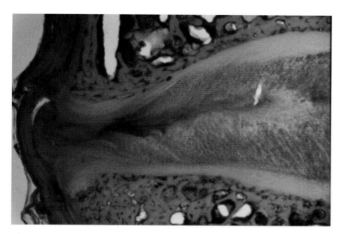

Figure 13.70 A 22-year-old man: fissure through posterior third of the disc (sagittal section). (Courtesy of J Taylor.)

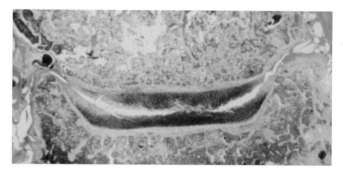

Figure 13.72 Coronal section across the posterior part of a lower cervical disc showing the complete fissure extending across between uncovertebral clefts.

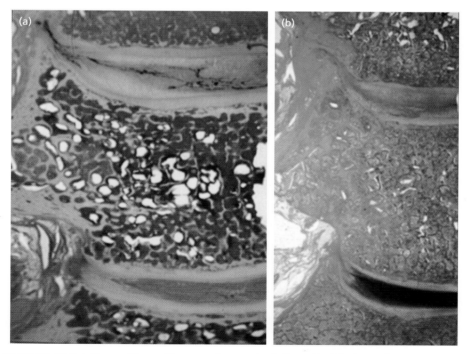

Figure 13.71 (a) C5–C6 and C6–C7 in a 36-year-old man. The upper discs are clearly fissured but the lower discs are not, except for a few fine fissures in C6–C7 on the left. (b) C6–C7 and C7–T1 in a 43-year-old man. C7–T1 is generally spared from the fissures, which are almost universal in the other adult cervical discs.

- Nondiagnostic MRI scan with cervical pathology.
- Diagnostic measure before surgical planning for cervical fusion.
- For delineating a painful disc among multiple degenerated discs.
- To evaluate an intervertebral disc adjacent to a structural abnormality such as spondylolisthesis or fusion.
- Evaluating suspected lateral or recurrent disc herniation.
- To access the pathology of cervical laminectomy.

- To determine the appropriate percutaneous technique for the disc pathology.

Contraindications
- Local infection or sepsis.
- Coagulopathy.
- Vital functions instability.
- Psychopathologies.

Technique of cervical discography

Step 1. Prepare the patient before the procedure
The patient should be told why the procedure is being done and what to expect. All complications and side effects related to the procedure should be explained in detail, before it is performed. Valid, written consent should be obtained.

The type of analgesia or sedation needs to be ascertained before performance of the invasive procedure. Intravenous fentanyl, midazolam, and/or propofol may be used judiciously for the patient's comfort. Patient response should be monitored and the dosage titrated to establish a level of sedation allowing the patient to be conversant and responsive after needle placements. Because the disc is avascular, there is an increased risk of disc space infection and most discographers use prophylactic antibiotics: prophylactic intravenous antibiotics 20 minutes before the procedure are recommended.

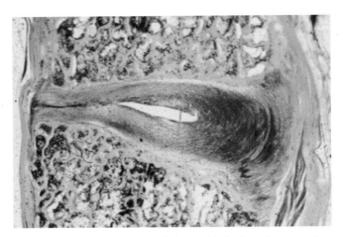

Figure 13.73 A sagittal section of the C2–C3 disc from the same spine shows that there is no nucleus or posterior annulus; only the anterior annulus and the longitudinal ligaments are preserved.

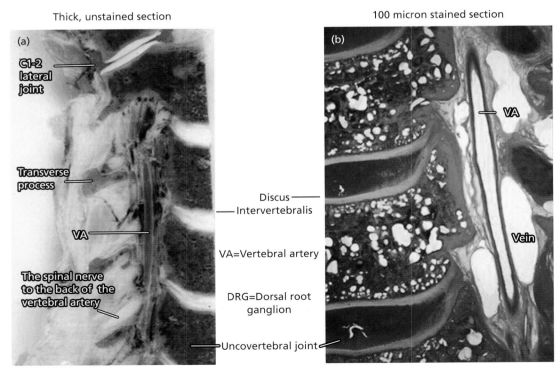

Figure 13.74 Coronal sections of sub-axial spine. (a) A thick unstained slice. (b) A 100 μm stained section.

Step 2. Position and monitor the patient
1. Place the patient in the supine position.
2. Turn the head slightly to the contralateral side.
3. Ensure that the patient is in a comfortable position by placing a small pillow under their head.
4. Fasten their head on the table using adhesive tape.
5. Position the arms of the patient on both sides. Position the C-arm laterally and check whether all cervical vertebrae are on the same plane.
6. Obtain an intravenous access. Administer oxygen by nasal cannula, and monitor the vital signs.
7. The right anterior side is chosen to prevent the puncture of the esophagus, which descends on the left side. Prepare and drape the area in a sterile fashion.
8. The patient should not be over-sedated. The patient should remain sufficiently conscious to provide responses to the physician's questions.

Step 3. Drugs and equipment for discography
- 5 ml syringe for skin infiltration;
- 25 gauge, 2½ inch needle for local anesthesia;
- 18 gauge, 10 cm needle for discography;
- 10 ml syringe for discography;
- manometry;
- 1% lidocaine for skin infiltration;
- nonionic contrast material for discography;
- antibiotic of choice for administration.

Step 4. Visualization
1. Place the C-arm across the table laterally at the level of the head to visualize the cervical vertebrae. Then the C-arm is rotated in a cephalad–caudal direction to bring the endplates of the cervical vertebral discs parallel to the beam (Figs 13.75 and 13.76).
2. Then rotate the C-arm 20–30° until the anterior margin of the uncinate process is moved approximately one-quarter

of the distance between the anterior and posterior lateral vertebral margins (Fig. 13.77).

Step 5. Mark the surface landmarks for the needle entry
1. Pressure is applied with the index finger in the space between the trachea and the medial border of the sternocleidomastoid muscle. Firm but careful effort needs to be taken to displace the vascular structures laterally and the laryngeal structures and trachea medially.
2. Below C4, the right common carotid artery and the internal carotid artery above C4 are palpated. The needle entry point should be medial to the medial border of the sternocleidomastoid muscle. The delineation of the sternocleidomastoid ensures that at C3–C4 the point of entry lies more laterally and will avoid the pharynx, whereas at C7–T1 it will be more medial and avoid the apex of the lung.
3. The entry point of the needle is 1–2 mm medial to the anterior margin of the uncinate process (Figs 13.78 and 13.79).

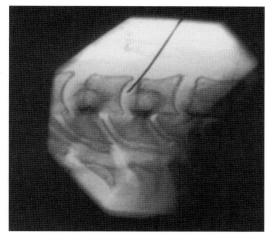

Figure 13.76 The cervical vertebral discs parallel to the beam.

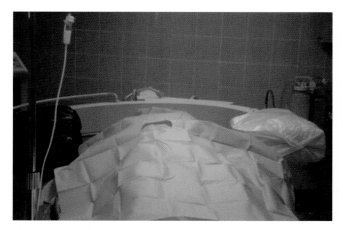

Figure 13.75 The C-arm in the lateral position.

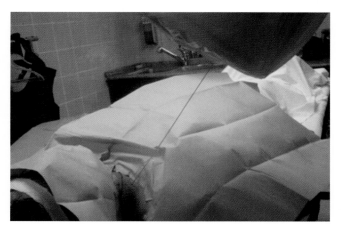

Figure 13.77 Rotate the C-arm 20–30°.

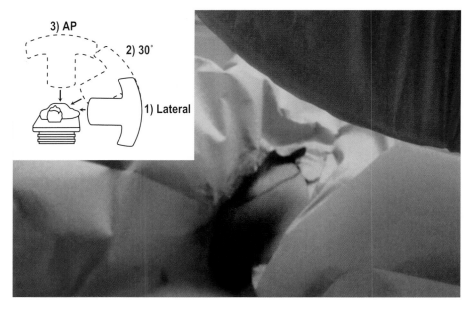

Figure 13.78 The needle entry point should be medial to the medial border of the sternocleidomastoid muscle.

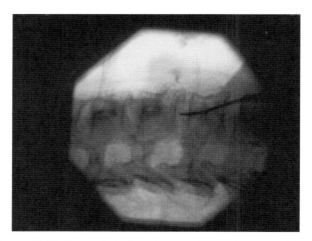

Figure 13.79 The needle is directed toward the anterior aspect of the uncinate process.

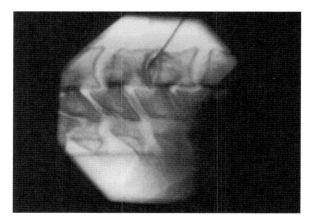

Figure 13.80 Spread of contrast material in lateral view.

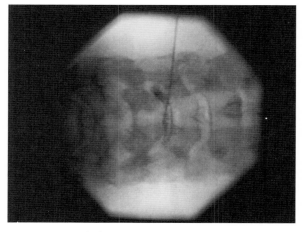

Figure 13.81 Spread of contrast material in posteroanterior view.

Step 6. Direction of the needle
A 25 gauge, 2½ inch spinal needle is directed toward the anterior aspect of the uncinate process and should enter the disc 1–2 mm anterior to the process, then is slowly advanced to the center of the disc (Fig. 13.79).

Step 7. Confirm the position of the needle
The needle position should be confirmed by injecting 1 ml of contrast solution into the disc, and should be confirmed both by posteroanterior and lateral views (Figs 13.80 and 13.81).

Step 8. Discography
1. Normal cervical discs commonly allow only small volumes (0.25–0.5 ml) in their intradiscal space; injection of normal

discs is not painful. A 1 or 3 ml syringe containing contrast medium is attached to the needle. Manual syringe pressure is increased slowly until the intrinsic disc pressure is exceeded. Concordant pain intensity is recorded at 0.2 ml increments.

2. A positive response requires provocation of significant (6/10) concordant pain during a confirmatory repeat injection of another 0.1–0.2 ml of contrast medium. One should also consider retesting adjacent levels to compare pain intensities and concordance of pain. It is not uncommon to provoke concordant pain at multiple levels. In addition, one will often cause separation of the endplates during pressurization, and this movement may cause pain secondary to injection of the facet joint.

3. This cervical region is highly vascular and one should carefully observe patients for signs of hematoma during and after the procedure. At C7–T1 the medial approach is preferred to avoid puncturing the apex of the lung.

4. The procedure should be stopped if the contrast material escapes into the epidural space, or the patient experiences nonconcordant pain.

Step 9. Postprocedure monitoring
After the procedure is complete, the patient should be observed for 30 minutes before discharge. The patient should be told to expect minor postprocedure discomfort, which may include some difficulty swallowing. Icepacks placed on the injection site for 20 minute periods help to decrease these untoward effects. The patient should be instructed to call immediately if any fever or other systemic symptoms suggestive of infection develop.

Patients are asked to report any unusual pain or pain not relieved by the prescribed medications. Severe or unusual pain may be a symptom of discitis. The incidence of this complication is extremely low, but the symptoms of discitis can present as late as 6 weeks after the procedure.

Complications
Discitis.
Spinal cord injury.
Vertebral osteomyelitis.
Epidural abscess.
Hematoma or vascular injury.
Nerve root irritation.
Drug-related allergic reactions.
Inadvertent puncture of the thecal sac (which rarely results in arachnoiditis).
Headache.
Superior laryngeal nerve damage.
Laryngeal damage or penetration, particularly at the C2–C3 level.
Pneumothorax, particularly when operating at the C7–T1 level.

Vasovagal response due to compression of the carotid body when manually displacing the carotid artery.

Helpful hints
The usefulness of cervical discography has not been proven. It should be performed only when other procedures have been tried and failed. Only experienced physicians competent in performing this technique should perform it.

Percutaneous block of the phrenic nerve

History
The phrenic nerve has been blocked for intractable severe hiccups historically. Interestingly, it has been stimulated on a long-term basis by neurosurgeons for diaphragmatic paresis.

Anatomy

Origin and course of the phrenic nerve
The phrenic nerve contains motor and sensory fibers in a proportion of about two to one. It arises chiefly from the anterior division of the fourth cervical nerve, but also receives a branch from the third and another from the fifth cervical nerve.

Course in the neck
The phrenic nerve descends to the root of the neck, traversing obliquely across the front of the scalenus anterior, and beneath the sternocleidomastoid, the inferior belly of the omohyoid muscles, and the transverse cervical and transverse scapular vessels.

Course in the thorax
From the root of the neck, the phrenic nerve next passes in front of the first part of the subclavian artery, between this artery and the subclavian vein, and, as it enters the thorax, crosses the internal mammary artery near its origin.

Within the thorax, it descends nearly vertically in front of the root of the lung, and then between the pericardium and the mediastinal pleura, to the diaphragm. It is accompanied by the pericardiacophrenic branch of the internal mammary artery. The two inferior phrenic nerves differ in their length, and in their relations at the upper part of the thorax. The right nerve is situated deeper, and is shorter and descends more vertically in direction than the left. The right phrenic nerve lies lateral to the right innominate vein and superior vena cava. The left phrenic nerve is rather longer than the right, from the inclination of the heart to the left side, and from the diaphragm being lower on this than on the right side (Fig. 13.82).

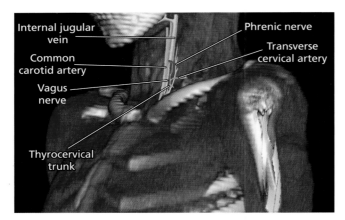

Figure 13.82 Three-dimensional CT scan showing the course of the phrenic nerve.

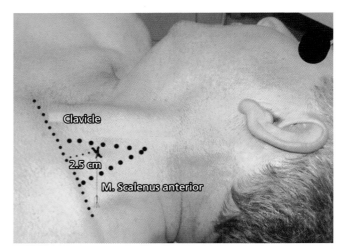

Figure 13.83 The anatomical landmarks for phrenic nerve block.

Significant relations of the phrenic nerve at the root of the neck

At the root of the neck it is crossed by the thoracic duct; in the superior mediastinal cavity it lies between the left common carotid and left subclavian arteries, and crosses superficial to the vagus on the left side of the arch of the aorta.

Innervation of the phrenic nerve

Each nerve supplies filaments to the pericardium and pleura, and at the root of the neck is joined by a filament from the sympathetic, and, occasionally, by one from the ansa hypoglossi. Branches have been described as passing to the peritoneum. From the right nerve, one or two filaments pass to join in a small phrenic ganglion with phrenic branches of the celiac plexus; branches from this ganglion are distributed to the falciform and coronary ligaments of the liver, the suprarenal gland, inferior vena cava, and right atrium. From the left nerve, filaments pass to join the phrenic branches of the celiac plexus, but without any ganglionic enlargement; a twig is distributed to the left suprarenal gland.

Indications

For intractable hiccups.

Contraindications

It is important to consider the following contraindications:
- local infection;
- coagulopathy;
- vital function instability;
- psychopathologies.

Technique of phrenic nerve block

Step 1. Prepare the patient before the procedure
The patient should be aware of the reason why this procedure is being done and what to expect from it. All complica-

tions and side effects related to the procedure should be explained. Written consent is mandatory.

The type of analgesia or sedation needs to be ascertained before the procedure is started. Intravenous fentanyl, midazolam, or equivalent may be used judiciously for the patient's comfort.

Step 2. Position and monitor the patient
1. Turn the head to the opposite side to be blocked in a supine position.
2. The head is fixed on the table by adhesive tape appropriately away from the point of entry.
3. Obtain an intravenous access if drugs need to be administered.
4. Monitoring of vital signs is mandatory in unstable patients.
5. The area for needle entry is prepared in a sterile fashion.

Step 3. Equipment and drugs for the phrenic nerve block
Prepare and confirm that the following equipment, needles, and drugs are ready to be used for the procedure:
- 1½ inch, 25 gauge needle for skin infiltration;
- 5 ml syringe containing local anesthetic solution;
- 22 gauge, 3½ inch needle for the nerve block;
- 5 ml of 1% lidocaine and 40 mg of methylprednisolone for the phrenic nerve block;
- preferred steroid solution (decadron or equivalent);
- equipment assembly for nerve stimulation if desired.

Step 4. Mark the surface landmarks for the needle entry
1. Raise the head of the patient to identify the posterior border of the sternocleidomastoid muscle.
2. Identify the groove between the posterior border of the sternocleidomastoid muscle and the anterior scalene muscle.
3. The entry point is 1 inch above the clavicle at the posterior border of the sternocleidomastoid muscle (Fig. 13.83).

Step 5. Direction of the needle
1. Insert the needle slightly anteriorly and advance to a depth of about 1 inch. Feel the tip of the needle with your index finger.
2. The tip of the needle can be confirmed as correctly placed by palpation of the ipsilateral contractions of the diaphragm with a nerve stimulator test.
Note: one needs to keep a hand on the skin near the diaphragm to feel it contract. The contractions are not visible to the eye.

Step 6. Phrenic nerve block
1. Once the needle is confirmed to be in the correct position, aspirate. If the aspiration test is negative, check if there is negative paresthesia in the branches of the brachial plexus.
2. If there is no paresthesia, inject a small amount of contrast solution to see the spread of the solution is not on the brachial plexus.
3. Then inject 5 ml of local anesthetic and/or steroid solution in a fanlike manner.
Note: do not perform phrenic nerve block bilaterally at the same session to prevent the paralysis of the diaphragm in patients with respiratory compromise.

One may place a cold pack for 10 minutes after the procedure.

There is no common indication for the RF technique for phrenic nerve lesioning.

Step 7. Postprocedure care
After the procedure is completed, the patient needs to be observed for up to 2 hours. Monitoring of vital signs is mandatory. In addition, the pain relief should be objectively documented. After a satisfactory observation, the patient should be discharged with appropriate and adequate instructions given to the escort. Written instructions are preferable for emergencies and are helpful to the patient and their family.

Complications
• Inadvertent puncture of the external jugular vein
The external jugular vein is in proximity with the phrenic nerve at the root of the neck. An aspiration test is mandatory; if blood is aspirated interrupt the procedure. Any small amount of injection of local anesthetic in the vein may cause local anesthetic toxicity.
• Block of the recurrent laryngeal nerve
If excessive amounts of local anesthetics are injected, one may block the recurrent laryngeal nerve, which may cause vocal cord paralysis.
• Inadvertent injection to the epidural, subdural or subarachnoid space
If the needle is placed too deep, there is a potential for inadvertent epidural, subdural or subarachnoid injection, which may cause fatal complications.

• Paralysis of the diaphragm
The phrenic nerve innervates the diaphragm bilaterally. Bilateral block of the phrenic nerve may cause paralysis of the diaphragm, which may lead to severely compromised respiratory depression.

Helpful hints
The phrenic nerve block is used for the diagnosis and treatment of intractable hiccups when pharmacological treatments have failed.

The cause of intractable hiccups should be diagnosed before the phrenic nerve block; MRI of the region would be helpful.

Percutaneous block and lesioning of the stellate ganglion

History
Selective block of the sympathetic trunk was first reported by Sellheim and, shortly thereafter, by Kappis in 1923 and Brumm and Mandl in 1924. After 1930, the technique and indications were established by White and Sweet in the United States, and Leriche and Fontaine in Europe.

Anatomy

Location, formation, and size of the stellate ganglion
The inferior cervical ganglion joins with the first thoracic ganglion to form the stellate ganglion. The stellate ganglion is 2.5 cm long, 1 cm wide, and 0.5 cm thick; it lies in front of the interspace between the C7 and T1 vertebral bodies (Figs 13.84 and 13.85).

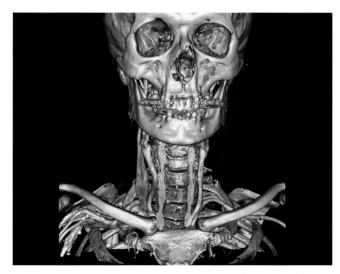

Figure 13.84 Three-dimensional CT scan showing the course of the stellate ganglion.

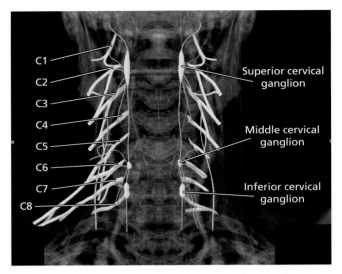

Figure 13.85 The superior, middle, and inferior cervical ganglia.

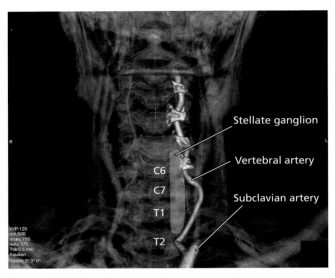

Figure 13.86 Three-dimensional CT scan showing the close relation of the vertebral artery with the stellate ganglion.

Origin of stellate ganglion sympathetic fibers

Preganglionic sympathetic fibers originate from cell bodies in the anterolateral column of the spinal cord. Nerves supplying the head and neck arise from the first and second thoracic spinal segments. Fibers destined to the upper extremities are traceable from the second through the ninth thoracic segments (T2–T9). The preganglionic axons leave the T1 and T2 ventral roots, pass through the white communicating rami, join the sympathetic chain, and ultimately synapse at the inferior (stellate), middle, or superior cervical ganglion. Postganglionic sympathetic fibers pass the gray rami and then join the cervical or upper cervical plexus. Most of the sympathetic fibers for the head and neck travel along the common and the internal or external carotid artery. However, some of the fibers leave the stellate ganglion and form the vertebral plexus, which innervates the cranial structures. Consequently, blockade of the sympathetic innervations of the head and neck must incorporate blockade of the stellate ganglion.

Close relations of the stellate ganglion

The stellate ganglion is intimately related to the transverse processes and the prevertebral fascia anteriorly, the subclavian artery superiorly, the posterior aspect of the pleura posteriorly, and the initial portion of the vertebral artery anteriorly.

Anatomically, the stellate ganglion is medial to the scalene muscles and lateral to the longus colli muscle. Other significant structures in close proximity to the stellate ganglion are the subclavian artery, inferior thyroid artery, intercostal arteries, and recurrent laryngeal nerve.

The vertebral artery traverses over the stellate ganglion and enters the vertebral foramen, and is located posterior to the anterior tubercle of C6. The nerve roots of the brachial

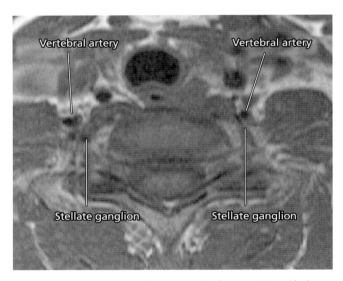

Figure 13.87 MRI showing the structures in close proximity with the stellate ganglion.

plexus, including C6, C7, C8, and T1, lie posterior to the respective tubercles (Figs 13.86 and 13.87).

Indications

Vascular insufficiency
- Raynaud's disease.
- Raynaud's phenomenon.
- Frost bite.
- Vasospasm.
- Occlusive vascular disease.
- Embolic vascular disease.
- Scleroderma.

Pain syndromes

- Complex regional pain syndrome type I.
- Complex regional pain syndrome type II.
- Vascular headaches.
- Acute herpes zoster (shingles).
- Postherpetic neuralgia.
- Phantom limb pain.
- Paget's disease.
- Neoplastic disorders.
- Postradiation neuritis.
- Intractable angina pectoris.
- Diabetic neuropathy.
- Pain from cranial nerve disorders (tic douloureux, Bell's palsy).

Other

- Hyperhidrosis.

Contraindications

- Local or systemic infection.
- Coagulopathy.
- Asthma.
- Pneumothorax and pneumonectomy on the contralateral side (against the risk of pneumothorax).
- Recent myocardial infarction.

Techniques of block or lesioning of the sympathetic ganglion

There are multiple approaches for stellate ganglion block or lesioning. The most commonly described are (1) the C6 or C7 paravertebral approach, (2) the oblique or lateral approach, and (3) the RF technique.

C6 or C7 paravertebral approach

Step 1. Prepare the patient before the procedure
The patient should be made aware of the reasons for this procedure. They should be told what to expect from it. All complications and side effects related to the procedure should be explained in detail, before it is performed. Valid, written consent should be obtained.

The type of analgesia or sedation needs to be ascertained before performing the procedure. Intravenous fentanyl, midazolam, and/or propofol may be used judiciously for the patient's comfort. If RF thermocoagulation or pulsed RF lesioning is planned, the patient needs to be awake to respond to the stimulation test.

Step 2. Position and monitor the patient
1. Place the patient in the supine position on the table; one may fix the head of the patient by adhesive tape. Obtain an intravenous access. Administer oxygen by nasal cannula. Monitor the vital signs noninvasively.

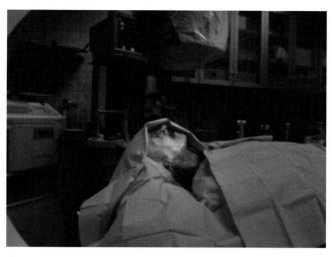

Figure 13.88 The position of the patient, prepared in a sterile fashion.

2. Place a pillow under the shoulders to further facilitate extension of the neck and make palpation of the thyroid cartilage easier.
3. Prepare and drape the area in a sterile fashion (Fig. 13.88).
4. Warn the patient not to talk, cough, or swallow during the procedure.
5. Instruct the patient to respond either by blinking the eyes or moving a finger in a meaningful manner, when the procedure is ongoing with the needle in the neck.

Step 3. Equipment and drugs for the stellate ganglion block
Prepare and confirm that the following equipment, needles, and drugs are ready to be used for the procedure:

- 25 gauge needle for skin infiltration;
- 5–10 cm needle with extended line for the block;
- 5–10 cm electrode with 2–5 mm active tip;
- 5 ml syringe for skin infiltration;
- 5 ml syringe for the nerve block;
- 1% lidocaine for skin infiltration;
- 0.5% bupivacaine for the block;
- nonparticulate steroid;
- contrast material, e.g. iohexol;
- 3–6% phenol in saline or iohexol (only for cancer patients).
  Special equipment for RF is the following:
- RF lesion generator and appropriate needle;
- ultrasound machine and appropriate needle.

Step 4. Mark the surface landmarks for the needle entry

C6–C7 anterior approach

Diagnostic and therapeutic local anesthetic block
1. The stellate ganglion block is performed by blind technique at many centers. The authors recommend the use of

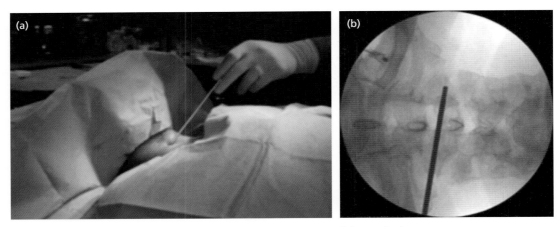

Figure 13.89 (a) Identify the vertebral body of C6 or C7. (b) The target is the junction of the vertebral transverse process.

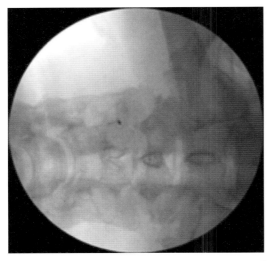

Figure 13.90 The needle should stay on the ventrolateral side of the vertebral body.

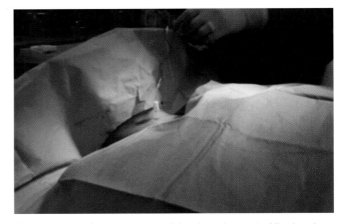

Figure 13.91 Inject contrast material under uninterrupted live imaging.

fluoroscopy to prevent serious complications by the blind technique.
2. The physician should stay at the ipsilateral side of the patient.
3. Palpate the C6 tubercle (Chassaignac's tubercle) with the index finger on the other hand near the cricoid cartilage at the medial border of the sternocleidomastoid muscle, 1.5 cm lateral to the midline.

Step 5. Visualization (Fig. 13.89)
1. Place the C-arm in the posteroanterior view first.
2. Identify the vertebral body of C6 or C7. The target is the junction of the vertebral transverse process.
3. Infiltrate the skin over the entry point with local anesthetic.

Step 6. Direction of the needle (Fig. 13.90)
1. Direct a 5–10 cm needle with an extension line to the target point until a bony contact is made. (Identify this to

be either at a transverse process or the anterior surface of the vertebral body.)
2. The needle should stay on the ventrolateral side of the vertebral body.
Note: the longus colli muscle is located over the lateral aspect of the vertebral body and is on the medial aspect of the tranverse process.
3. Take care to stay on the bone, to avoid injection into the longus colli muscle.
Note: if a paresthesia of the upper extremity is elicited during needle placement, one must assume the needle has penetrated too deeply and encountered a nerve root of the brachial plexus. The needle should be withdrawn and repositioned.

Step 7. Confirm the position of the needle (Figs 13.91, 13.92, and 13.93)
1. Aspirate; if blood is aspirated reposition the needle. If the aspiration test is negative, inject 3–5 ml of contrast material under uninterrupted live imaging at the C6–T1 level.

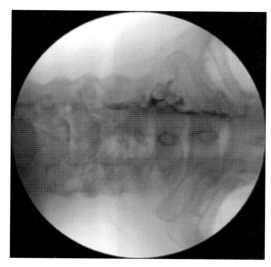

Figure 13.92 Spread of the contrast material in posteroanterior view.

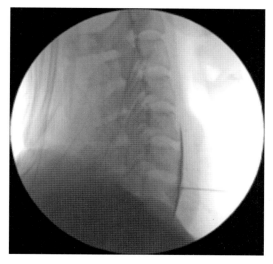

Figure 13.93 Spread of the contrast material in lateral view.

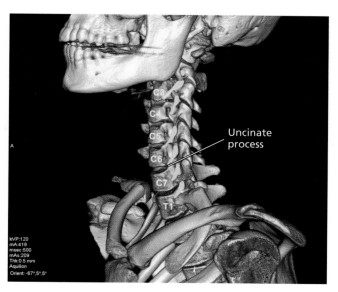

Figure 13.94 Identify the uncinate process.

40 mg of methylprednisolone if preferred. Some authors advise injection of higher volumes, up to 10 ml; however, if the stellate ganglion is properly localized, 5 ml of solution is sufficient.

2. Monitor the effect continuously. Within minutes one should expect the presence of Horner syndrome: myosis (pinpoint pupil), ptosis (drooping of the upper eyelid), and enophthalmos (sinking of the eyeball). Associated findings include conjunctival injection, facial anhidrosis, and nasal congestion.

Neurolysis of the stellate ganglion
• Avoid using neurolytic solutions in noncancer pain.
• For neurolysis use the same technique described above with 2–3 ml of 6% phenol in saline or glycerine (iohexol).
• Be extremely cautious not to produce brachial plexus block or allow drug injection into the epidural or subarachnoid space.

Oblique or lateral approach for stellate ganglion block (Figs 13.94, 13.95, 13.96, and 13.97)
Steps 1–3 are as vide supra.

Step 4. Visualization
1. Place the C-arm in a posteroanterior position.
2. Rotate the C-arm in oblique view until the neural foramina are clearly visualized.
3. Move the C-arm caudally 30–60° until the disc between the sixth and seventh cervical vertebra is visualized as a flattened disc.

Step 5. Direction of the needle
1. Identify the disc, the foramina, and the uncinate process.
2. Direct a 22 gauge spinal needle onto the vertebral body at the base of the uncinate process, just anterior to the foramina.

2. Then turn the C-arm laterally. The contrast material should spread in the retropharyngeal space anterior to the longus colli and anterior scalene muscles.
Note: an irregular image will appear if the contrast material is injected into the muscle. If there is a resistance to injection, one should suspect that the needle is within the periosteum of the bone.

If the needle is advanced medially or deeper there is a risk of entering the epidural or subarachnoid space. The contrast material should be checked for appearance in the epidural or subarachnoid space.

Step 8. Injection of local anesthetic and/or steroid
1. After confirming the correct placement of the needle, inject 5 ml of 0.5% bupivacaine or 1% lidocaine together with

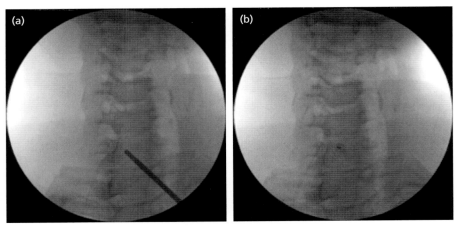

Figure 13.95 (a) Direct a 22-gauge spinal needle onto the vertebral body at the base of the uncinate process, just anterior to the foramina. (b) Inject 1–2 ml contrast material with real-time imaging. A direct line will appear along the longus colli muscle.

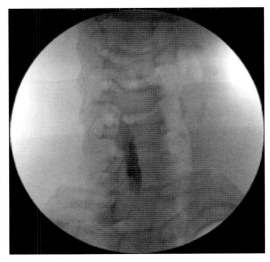

Figure 13.96 Inject 1–2 ml contrast material with real-time imaging. A direct line will appear along the longus colli muscle.

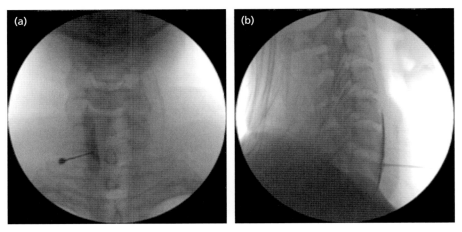

Figure 13.97 (a,b) Spread of the contrast material in posteroanterior and lateral views.

Step 6. Confirm the position of the needle
Inject 1–2 ml contrast material with real-time imaging. A direct line will appear along the longus colli muscle.

Note: with this technique the chance of intravascular injection, esophageal perforation, or recurrent laryngeal nerve paralysis is minimal.

Step 7. Oblique or lateral approach.
Injection of local anesthetic or neurolytic solution are as vide supra.

RF lesioning of the stellate ganglion
Steps 1–4 are as vide supra.

Step 5. Direction of the electrode
1. Insert a 5 mm active-tip electrode at a posteroanterior view, similar to the technique described in the anterolateral approach, at the junction of the vertebral body with the transverse process (Fig. 13.98).
2. Place the electrode tip at the target location under fluoroscopy.

Step 6. Confirm the position of the electrode
Then confirm the electrode placement under posteroanterior and lateral view.

Step 7. Stimulation test
1. Then stimulate the region at 2 Hz, with 0.1–1.5 V, to locate or identify the phrenic nerve laterally and the recurrent laryngeal nerve anteriorly and medially. The patient should be able to say "ee" to preserve the motor function. There should be no motor response on proper localization.
2. Second, seek paresthesia for localization. For that, stimulate the nerve at 50–100 Hz with 0.1–1.5 V. Generally, a patient feels paresthesia at a setting of 0.5 V. The patient should be awake to respond to the stimulation at this stage (Fig. 13.98).

Step 8. RF lesioning of the stellate ganglion
1. Inject a small volume of local anesthetic before lesioning.
2. Apply RF for 60 seconds at 70 °C.
3. Redirect the electrode to the most medial part of the transverse process in the same plane. Apply RF again.
4. Redirect the electrode in the ventral aspect. Apply RF to this point.
Note: at each point, one needs to repeat sensory and motor stimulation before lesioning.

Ultrasound technique of stellate ganglion block
We now describe the technique of Narouze et al. (2007) for an ultrasound-guided stellate ganglion block (Figs 13.99, 13.100, and 13.101).

Step 1. Prepare the patient before the procedure
The patient should be made aware of the reasons for this procedure. They should be told what to expect from it. All complications and side effects related to the procedure should be explained in detail, before it is performed. Valid, written consent should be obtained.

The type of analgesia or sedation needs to be ascertained before performing the procedure. Intravenous fentanyl, midazolam, and/or propofol may be used judiciously for the patient's comfort. If RF thermocoagulation or pulsed RF lesioning is planned, the patient needs to be awake to respond to the stimulation test.

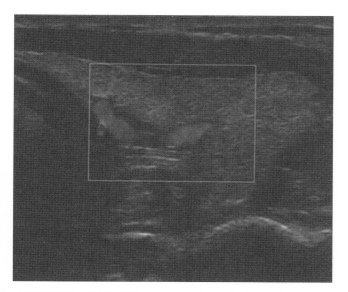

Figure 13.99 Ultrasound image showing that with the anterior paratracheal approach the needle may inadvertently injure the thyroid vessels, with the potential for hematoma formation. (From Narouze et al. 2007. Reproduced with permission from Cleveland Clinic Center for Medical Art & Photography. Copyright 2007–2011. All rights reserved.)

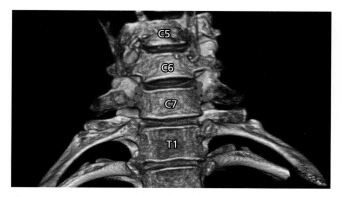

Figure 13.98 Targets for RF lesioning of the stellate ganglion.

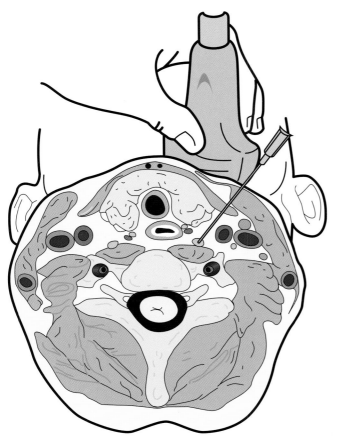

Figure 13.100 The position of the ultrasound probe and the needle in the oblique path. (From Narouze et al. 2007. Reproduced with permission from Cleveland Clinic Center for Medical Art & Photography. Copyright 2007–2011. All rights reserved.)

Step 2. Position the patient

The patient is positioned in the supine position with the neck extended by placement of a pillow under the shoulder to stretch the esophagus and make it move medially under the trachea.

Step 3. Equipment and drugs

Necessary equipment includes the following.
- 25 gauge local infiltration needle.
- 22 gauge, 1–2 inch block needle.
- 5 or 10 cm (2 or 5 mm tip) sharp Sluijter Mehta or Racz, Finch, Kit needle.
- RF machine.
- Ultrasound-guided procedures typically require high-resolution, multiple-beam imaging to allow visualization of small nerves and the interface between soft tissue and bone.
- 43 color Doppler is a standard feature that helps to identify neighboring blood vessels.
- The choice of transducer is primarily related to the anticipated target depth and size. As a rule of thumb, a broadband, high-frequency linear transducer is used for superficial targets. Needle choice depends on both target depth and

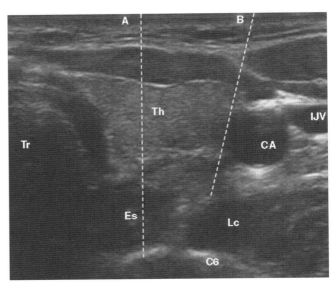

Figure 13.101 Ultrasound imaging of the left stellate ganglion. (a) The needle path with the anterior paratracheal approach. (b) The needle path with ultrasound guidance. CA, carotid artery; Es, esophagus; IJV, internal jugular vein; Lc, longus colli muscle; Th, thyroid; Tr, trachea. (From Narouze et al. 2007. Reproduced with permission from Cleveland Clinic Center for Medical Art & Photography. Copyright 2007–2011. All rights reserved.)

operator preference. For instance, one operator may favor a B-beveled stimulating needle, whereas others would feel comfortable using a Quincke-type spinal needle. Various needle types with improved ultrasound visibility are now available.

Step 4. Visualization

1. Under fluoroscopic guidance, the bony target is identified at the junction of the anterolateral vertebral body with the transverse process at the C6 level in the anteroposterior view.
2. The skin is marked with complete aseptic technique.
3. A 22 gauge blunt needle is used, aimed toward the identified bony target under fluoroscopic guidance.

Step 5. Direction of the needle

1. After the skin and subcutaneous tissue are penetrated and the needle is stabilized, a 3–12 MHz linear-array probe (HD11-XL, Philips, Bothell, Wash) is used to verify the position of the needle.
2. The needle may be shown to be aiming toward the thyroid tissue anteriorly and the esophagus posteriorly.

Step 6. Confirm the position of the needle

1. At this point, the needle is withdrawn and reinserted obliquely; it should then be advanced with real-time ultrasound imaging so that the needle tip will lie anterior to the longus colli muscle (anterior to the C6 transverse process).
2. After negative aspiration, 1 ml of contrast agent is injected which should show adequate spread without vascular escape.

Step 7. Stellate ganglion block under ultrasonography
1. Then, 5 ml of bupivacaine 0.25% can be injected in divided doses with real-time ultrasound imaging, which should show extensive spread of the local anesthetic agent at the area of the lower cervical sympathetic chain with both cephalad and caudal spread (approximately two segments each).
2. Five minutes later, the patient should develop Horner syndrome as well as vasodilatation of the ipsilateral upper extremity.

Helpful hints for ultrasonographic techniques

Nerve localization
The cervical sympathetic nerve trunk is within the prevertebral fascia. However, it is impossible to distinguish the sympathetic nerve trunk from the prevertebral fascia. In some patients, the middle cervical ganglion is clearly visualized within the prevertebral fascia.

Needle insertion approach
In ultrasound-guided stellate ganglion block, the needle is not directed toward the stellate ganglion; rather, it is directed to the cervical sympathetic nerve trunk and its gray rami communicating branches at the C6 level.

It is possible to perform a C6 stellate ganglion block by penetrating the prevertebral fascia with the needle and injecting local anesthetic into the compartment of the longus colli muscle.

In-plane approach
• A 25 gauge, 1 inch bevel needle is used for stellate ganglion block.
• A fine extension tube is connected between the needle and the syringe.
• The needle is inserted between the transducer and the trachea using an in-plane approach.
• The needle is advanced while avoiding the thyroid gland.
• The prevertebral fascia is penetrated, and the operator stops when the tip of the needle reaches inside the longus colli muscle. The tip of the needle does not need to contact the transverse process of C6.
• Negative aspiration for blood is confirmed.
• The operator injects 0.5 ml of local anesthetic and checks whether the injectate has reached the longus colli muscle deep to the prevertebral fascia.
• If the spread is above the prevertebral fascia, the needle is advanced further.
• Once the needle is inside the longus colli muscle, a total of 5–8 ml of local anesthetic is injected.
• The extent of local anesthetic spread inside the longus colli muscle and bulging of the prevertebral fascia is observed. In addition, scanning is performed cephalad and caudal to assess local anesthetic spread in the sagittal plane.

Caution
• One must pay particular attention to the location of the vertebral artery and the superior and inferior thyroid arteries. Color Doppler imaging is used to visualize these vascular structures.
• The vertebral artery does not always enter the C6 transverse foramen. It may bypass the C6 transverse foramen and enter the neural foramen at a higher cervical level.
• The superior thyroid artery is usually visualized on the lateral edge of the thyroid gland at the C6 level.
• The inferior thyroid artery ascends directly upward and cuts across the anterior surface of the longus colli muscle.
• These arteries are located in the path of the needle in some patients.

Step 8. Postprocedure care
After the procedure is completed, the patient needs to be observed for up to 2 hours. Monitoring of vital signs is mandatory. In addition, the pain relief should be objectively documented. After a satisfactory observation, the patient should be discharged with appropriate and adequate instructions given to the escort. Written instructions are preferable for emergencies and are helpful to the patient and their family.

Complications

Frequent complications
• Transient Horner syndrome (this denotes a successful block and is to be expected).
• Recurrent laryngeal nerve block.
• Phrenic nerve block.
• Block of the branches of the brachial plexus.

Serious complications
• Pneuthorax.
• Inadvertent puncture of the vertebral artery and vein.
• Inadvertent puncture of the carotid artery.
• Inadvertent epidural or subarachnoid puncture and injection.
• Cardiac emergency (severe hypotension or cardiac arrhythmias).

Rare complications
• Paratracheal hematoma.
• Inadvertent puncture of the esophagus.
• Osteitis of the transverse process.

Frequent complications

Horner syndrome
Horner syndrome: myosis (pinpoint pupil), ptosis (drooping of the upper eyelid), and enophthalmos (sinking of the eyeball) is in a way a documentation of the stellate ganglion

block. Associated findings include conjunctival injection, facial anhidrosis, and nasal congestion. If the stellate ganglion block is performed using a local anesthetic, these symptoms will disappear within hours. If a neurolytic agent is used, the symptoms may become permanent.

Block of the recurrent laryngeal nerve
The block of the recurrent laryngeal nerve is due to the diffusion of the local anesthetic solution onto the nerve. Hoarseness, a lump in the throat, and sometimes subjective shortness of breath may be seen.

Block of the phrenic nerve
Block of the phrenic nerve nearby may cause temporary paralysis of the diaphragm and possible respiratory embarrassment. Thus, the stellate ganglion block should not be performed bilaterally at the same session.

Block of the branches of the brachial plexus
Branches of the brachial plexus also can be blocked secondary to spread along the prevertebral fascia or when needle location is too posterior.

Serious complications

Pneumothorax
There is a risk of pneumothorax with all approaches to the stellate ganglion. The pleural dome extends variably. It is closer in the anterior C7 approach. The risk is higher in the blind technique. Under the guidance of fluoroscopy and with close contact to the bone, the risk of pneumothorax is minimal. If there is a doubt of pneumothorax, the patient has to be followed up for a day in the hospital.

Inadvertent puncture of vertebral artery or vein
The vertebral artery and vein are in close proximity to the anterior tubercle of C6 or C7. Inadvertent puncture of the vertebral artery may occur if the needle is inserted too medially and posteriorly. There may be a bony contact with the posterior tubercle instead of the anterior tubercle. Slight withdrawal of the needle from the posterior tubercle medially may puncture the vertebral artery. Injection into a vein may not cause serious complications if the amount of local anesthetic is small. However, even small amounts of local anesthetic injected into the vertebral artery may produce unconsciousness, respiratory paralysis, seizures, and hypotension (Fig. 13.102).

Inadvertent puncture of carotid artery
The carotid artery is also in close proximity to the stellate ganglion. There is a risk of inadvertent puncture of the carotid artery. Palpate the carotid artery and retract laterally before the injection. Injection of local anesthetics into the carotid artery may produce similar effects to those of verte-

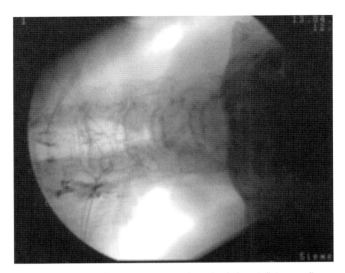

Figure 13.102 Inadvertent puncture of a vein during stellate ganglion block.

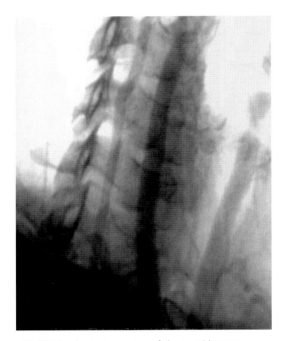

Figure 13.103 Inadvertent puncture of the carotid artery.

bral artery injection. To avoid air embolism, be sure that there is no air in the syringe (Fig. 13.103).

Epidural or intrathecal injection
If the needle is placed posterior to the anterior tubercle, there is a risk of inserting the needle inside the epidural space or dural sleeve of a cervical spinal nerve. If the needle is in the subarachnoid space, cerebrospinal fluid may be aspirated. It is always better to inject contrast material before the local anesthetic to see the spread of the contrast material

along the stellate ganglion. If you have any doubt about the correct positioning of the needle after the injection of the contrast material, do not inject local anesthetics.

Epidural injection may produce sensory or motor block.

Intrathecal injection will produce a total spinal block, which is a catastrophic complication.

Cardiac arrest

Cardiac arrest may occur owing to the spread of the local anesthetic to the cardiac acceleratory nerve.

Rare complications

Hematoma

The vascular supply around the stellate ganglion is rich. There is always a risk of puncturing the vessels while advancing the needle toward the ganglion. Thus hematoma is always possible. Apply icepack over the entry point.

Inadvertent puncture of the esophagus

The esophagus lies on the left side of the neck. Be more careful while performing a stellate ganglion block on the left side of the patient (Fig. 13.104).

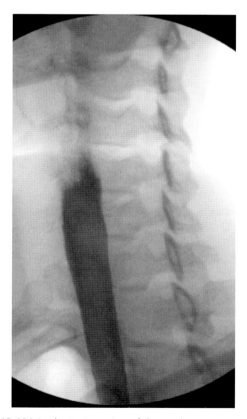

Figure 13.104 Inadvertent puncture of the esophagus.

Osteitis of the transverse process

Cease to advance the needle as soon as it contacts the bone. If you insist on advancing the needle, osteitis may occur at the transverse process.

Helpful hints

Block of the stellate ganglion is one the very first procedures taught to practitioners in the earlier stages of their education. This is not free of complications and should be performed under fluoroscopy, not with a blind technique. Practitioners should be familiar with the technique and be able to handle all complications efficiently and in a timely fashion.

Further reading

Abdi, S., Zhou, Y., Doshi, R. & Patel, N. (2005) Stellate ganglion block: emphasis on the new oblique fluoroscopic approach. *Techniques in Regional Anesthesia and Pain Management* **9**(2), 73–80.

Abdi, S., Zhou, Y., Patel, N., et al. (2004) A new and easy technique to block the stellate ganglion. *Pain Physician* **7**, 327–331.

Abram, S. & O'Connor, T. (1996) Complications associated with epidural steroid injections. *Regional Anesthesia* **21**, 149–162.

Baker, R., Dreyfuss, P. & Bogduk, N. (2002) Cervical transforaminal injection of corticosteroids into a radicular artery: a possible mechanism for spinal cord injury. *Pain* **103**, 211–215.

Bogduk, N. (1997) International Spinal Injection Society guidelines for the performance of spinal injection procedures. Part 1: zygapophyseal joint blocks. *Clinical Journal of Pain* **13**(4), 285–302.

Bogduk, N., Aprill, C. & Derby, R. (1995) Epidural steroid injections. In: *Spine Care Operative Treatment* (ed. White, A.H.), pp. 322–342. St. Louis, MO: Mosby.

Botwin, K., Castellanos, R. & Rao, S. (2003) Complications of fluoroscopically guided interlaminar cervical epidural injections. *Archives of Physical Medicine and Rehabilitation* **84**, 627–633.

Brain, L. & Wilkinson, M. (eds) (1967) *Cervical Spondylosis and Other Disorders of the Cervical Spine*. London: Heinemann Medical.

Cicala, R.S., Westbrook, L. & Angel, J.J. (1989) Side effects and complications of cervical epidural steroid injections. *Journal of Pain and Symptom Management* **4**, 64–66.

Cousins, M.J. (1998) Sympathetic neural blockade of upper and lower extremity. In: *Neural Blockade in Clinical Anesthesia and Management of Pain*, 3rd edition (ed. Cousins M.J. & Bridenbaugh P.O.), pp. 423–430. Philadelphia: Lippincott.

Derby, R. (1998) Discussion of cervical epidural steroid injection with intrinsic spinal cord damage. Two case reports. *Spine* **23**, 2141–2142.

Derby, R. (2004) Cervical radicular pain: transforaminal vs. interlaminar steroid injections. *SpineLine* **5**, 16–21.

Derby, R., Kim, B.J. & Lee, S.Y. (2004) Cervical interlaminar epidural injection. In: International Spinal Injection Society 12th Annual Scientific Meeting, Maui, Hawaii.

Derby, R., Lee, S.H., Kim, B.J., et al. (2004) Complications following cervical epidural steroid injections by expert interventionalists in 2003. *Pain Physician* **7**(4), 445–449.

Dreyfuss, P., Baker, R. & Bogduk, N. (2006) Comparative effectiveness of cervical transforaminal injections with particulate and nonparticulate corticosteroid preparations for cervical radicular pain. *Pain Medicine* **7**, 237–242.

Elias, M. (2000) Cervical sympathetic and stellate ganglion blocks. *Pain Physician* **3**(3), 294–304.

Ferrante, F., Wilson, S. & Evans, P. (1993) Clinical classification as a predictor of therapeutic outcome after cervical epidural steroid injection. *Spine* **18**, 730–736.

Gawel, M.J. & Rothbart, P.J. (1992) Occipital nerve blocks in the management of headache and cervical pain. *Cephalalgia* **12**, 9–13.

Geurts, J.W. & Stolker, R.J. (1993) Percutaneous radiofrequency lesion of the stellate ganglion in the treatment of pain in upper extremity reflex sympathetic dystrophy. *Pain Clinic* **6**, 17–25.

Govind, J. & Bogduk, N. (2002) International Spinal Injection Society practice guidelines and protocol: percutaneous radiofrequency cervical medial branch neurotomy. In *Proceedings of the ISIS 10th Annual Scientific Meeting*, 2002, pp. 51–75.

Hadden, S.B. (1940) Neurologic headache and facial pain. *Archives of Neurology* **43**, 405.

Hogan, Q.H., Erickson, S.J. & Haddox, J.D. (1992) The spread of solution during stellate ganglion block. *Regional Anesthesia* **17**(2), 78–83.

Kaplan, M. & Derby, R. (1998) Epidural corticosteroid injections: when, why, and how. *Journal of Musculoskeletal Medicine* **15**, 39–46.

Kline, M. (1996) Radiofrequency lesion of the stellate ganglion. Stereotactic radiofrequency lesion as part of the management of pain. Boston: St. Lucie Press, Radionics.

Lord, S.M., Barnsley, L., Wallis, B.J., et al. (1996) Percutaneous radio-frequency neurotomy for chronic cervical zygapophyseal-joint pain. *New England Journal of Medicine* **335**(23), 1721–1726.

Manchikanti, L. (1999) Neural blockade in cervical pain syndromes. *Pain Physician* **2**(3), 65–84.

McNab, I. (1973) The whiplash syndrome. *Clinical Neurosurgery* **20**, 232.

Mehta, M. (1973) *Intractable Pain*. Philadelphia: W.B. Saunders.

Narouze, S., Vydyanathan, A. & Patel, N. (2007) Ultrasound-guided stellate ganglion block successfully prevented esophageal puncture. *Pain Physician* **10**, 747–752.

Pawl, R.P. (1971) Headache, cervical spondylosis, and anterior cervical fusion. *Surgery Annual* **9**, 391.

Racz, G.B. & Hulubec, I.T. (1989) Stellate ganglion neurolysis. In *Techniques of Neurolysis* (ed. Racz, G.), pp. 133–144. Boston: Kluwer Academic.

Raj, P.P. (1996) Stellate ganglion block. In: *Interventional Pain Management* (ed. Waldman, S. & Winner, A.), pp. 267–274. Philadelphia: W.B. Saunders.

Raj, P.P. (2000) *Practical Management of Pain*, 3rd edition. St. Louis, MO: Mosby.

Raney, A. & Raney, R.B. (1948) Headache: a common symptom of cervical disc lesions. *Archives of Neurology* **59**, 603.

Rathmell, J.P., April, C. & Bogduk, N. (2004) Cervical transforaminal injection of steroids. *Anesthesiology* **100**, 1595–1600.

Rauck, R.L. (1990) Sympathetic nerve blocks: head, neck and trunk. In *Practical Management of Pain*, 3rd edition (ed. Raj, P.P.), pp. 651–682. St. Louis, MO: Mosby.

Rauck, R.L. (2001) Stellate ganglion block. *Techniques in Regional Anesthesia and Pain Management* **5**(3), 88–93.

Rosenberg, S.K. (2005) Cervical epidural steroid injections. *Techniques in Regional Anesthesia and Pain Management* **9**(2), 58–61.

Rowlingson, J.C. & Kirschenbaum, L.P. (1986) Epidural analgesic techniques in the management of cervical pain. *Anesthesia & Analgesia* **65**, 938–942.

Slipman, C.W. & Chow, D.W. (2002) Therapeutic spinal corticosteroid injections for the management of radiculopathies. *Physical Medicine and Rehabilitation Clinics of North America* **13**(3), 697–711.

Slipman, C.W., Lipetz, J.S., Jackson, H.B., et al. (2000) Therapeutic selective nerve root block in the nonsurgical treatment of atraumatic cervical spondylotic radicular pain: a retrospective analysis with independent clinical review. *Archives of Physical Medicine and Rehabilitation* **81**(6), 741–746.

Sluijter, M.E. (1981) Percutaneous facet denervation and partial posterior rhizotomy. *Acta Anaesthesiologica Belgica* **32**(1), 63–79.

Sluijter, M.E. (1990) *Radiofrequency Lesions in the Treatment of Cervical Pain Syndromes*. Burlington: Radionics.

Sluijter, M.E. (2003) Cervicobraquialgia. In *Radiofrequency (Part 2)* (ed. Sluijter, M.E.), pp. 9–22. Switzerland: Flivo Press.

Stanton-Hicks, M. (2007) Complications of sympathetic blocks for extremity pain. *Techniques in Regional Anesthesia and Pain Management* **11**(3), 148–151.

Stevens, R.A. & Ruesch, S. (1998) Sympathetic blocks of the upper extremity and their complications. *Techniques in Regional Anesthesia and Pain Management* **2**(3), 130–136.

Stojanovic, M.P., Vu, T.N. & Caneris, O. (2002) The role of fluoroscopy in cervical epidural steroid injections: an analysis of contrast dispersal patterns. *Spine* **27**, 509–514.

Taren, J.A. & Kahn, E.A. (1962) Anatomic pathways related to pain in face and neck. *Journal of Neurosurgery* **19**, 116.

Van Kleef, M., Spaans, F. & Dingemans, W. (1993) Effects and side effects of a percutaneous thermal lesion of the dorsal root ganglion in patients with cervical pain syndrome. *Pain* **52**, 49–53.

Vervest, A.C.M. & Stolker, R.J. (1991) The treatment of cervical pain syndromes with radiofrequency procedures. *Pain Clinic* **4**, 103–112.

Waldman, S. (1989) Complications of cervical epidural nerve blocks with steroids: a prospective study of 790 consecutive blocks. *Regional Anesthesia* **14**, 149–151.

Windsor, R.E., Storm, S., Sugar, R. & Nagula, D. (2003) Cervical transforaminal injection: review of the literature, complications, and a suggested technique. *Pain Physician* **6**, 457–465.

Yin, W. (2004) Stereotactic dorsal root ganglion lesioning techniques in the treatment of cervicogenic headache. *Techniques in Regional Anesthesia and Pain Management* **1**, 17–24.

Zhang, J., Tsuzuki, N. & Hirabayashi, S. (2003) Surgical anatomy of the nerves and muscles in the posterior cervical spine: a guide for avoiding inadvertent nerve injuries during the posterior approach. *Spine* **28**, 1379–1384.

14 Interventional Pain Procedures in the Thoracic Region

Percutaneous interlaminar block of the thoracic epidural space

History

Corning has been accepted as the first author describing epidural anesthesia. In a case report he published in the *New York Medical Journal* in 1885, he mentioned administering cocaine into the spinal canal in a dog and in man. The first two authors documenting epidural anesthesia were Cathelin and Sicard. In 1942 Edwards and Hingston described continuous caudal anesthesia. Epidural anesthesia and analgesia have been widely used since Tuohy modified the epidural needle in 1949. Tuohy recognized that the directional point might facilitate placement of spinal catheters. As a further embellishment, Tuohy added a stylet, thereby hoping to decrease further the risk of skin plugging. However, it was Curbelo, not Tuohy, who realized how the directional needle might facilitate the placement of epidural catheters. In 1949, 2 years after his visit to the Mayo Clinic, Curbelo published an article describing how he had used a 16 gauge Tuohy needle with 3.5F silk ureteral catheter for continuous segmental lumbar peridural anesthesia.

Anatomy

The thoracic epidural space continues from the cervical region, extending from the lower margin of the C7 vertebra to the upper margin of L1 vertebral space. The spinous processes in the thoracic region are longer and more acutely angled. The most acute angle is between the T4 and T5 vertebrae. Thoracic vertebral laminae are wider and broader than in other parts of the spine. At this level, in addition to the facet joints, there are articular segments between the ribs and the vertebrae. They form the costovertebral as well as costotransverse joints. The intervertebral foramina are narrower than at the lumbar spine. The level of the tip of the spinous process corresponds to lower levels of the adjacent vertebrae in the upper, middle, and lower thoracic spine. Especially at the midthoracic level, these posterior ends of the spinous process may actually overlie the inferior vertebral body.

The epidural space is 3–4 mm wide in the thoracic area. The thoracic epidural space, just like in the rest of the spinal region, contains loose areolar tissue, fat, and vertebral venous plexus (Figs 14.1–14.5).

Indications

- Thoracic trauma.
- Acute herpes zoster and postherpetic neuralgia.
- Cancer pain.
- Bulging or protrusion of the disc at the thoracic level.

Contraindications

- Local or systemic infection.
- Coagulopathy.
- Hypotension.
- Anatomic distortion.

Technique of thoracic interlaminar epidural approach

Thoracic interlaminar epidural block is commonly performed in the prone or lateral position. There are some who perform the block in the sitting position, but we do not recommend this approach.

Prone position

Step 1. Prepare the patient before the procedure
The patient should be told why the procedure is being done and what to expect. All complications and side effects related to the procedure should be explained in detail, before the procedure. Valid, written consent should be obtained.

The type of analgesia or sedation needs to be ascertained before performance of the invasive procedure. Intravenous fentanyl, midazolam, and/or propofol may be used judiciously for the patient's comfort. Patient response should be

Pain-Relieving Procedures: The Illustrated Guide, First Edition. P. Prithvi Raj and Serdar Erdine.
© 2012 John Wiley & Sons, Ltd. Published 2012 by John Wiley & Sons, Ltd.

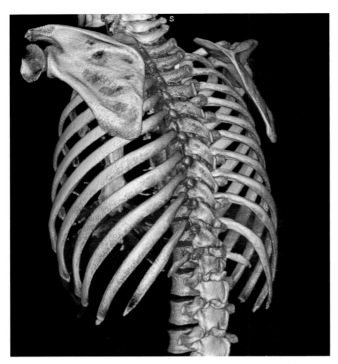

Figure 14.1 Three-dimensional CT scan showing the thoracic vertebrae and the spinous processes.

monitored and the dosage titrated to establish a level of sedation allowing the patient to be conversant and responsive after needle placements.

Step 2. Position and monitor the patient
1. Place the patient prone on the table. Place a pillow under the chest to flex the thoracolumbar spine. The patient's head is turned to the side, with the arms either raised above the head and crossed or at the side. Obtain an intravenous access through a large vein.
2. Administer oxygen by nasal cannula.
3. Monitor the vital signs noninvasively throughout the procedure.
4. Prep and drape the area in a sterile fashion.
5. Sedation may be used to relax the patient; however, the patient should be awake enough to respond to the physician's questions.

Step 3. Drugs and equipment for thoracic interlaminar block
• 1½ inch needle for skin infiltration;
• 5 ml syringe for local anesthesia;
• 5 ml syringe for contrast material;
• special loss of resistance syringe;
• 5–10 ml syringe for epidural block;
• 18–20 gauge Tuohy needle;
• 5 ml of 1% lidocaine for skin infiltration;
• 5–10 ml of 0.5% bupivacaine;
• contrast solution (iohexol);
• nonparticulate steroid;
• preservative-free normal saline.

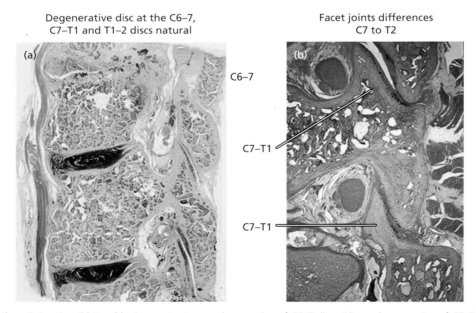

Figure 14.2 Cervicothoracic junction. (a) An old spine contrasts gross degeneration of C6–7 disc with good preservation of C7–T1 and T1–2 discs. (b) C7–T2 in a 22-year-old man; upper thoracic facets show a laminar "step" below them. (Courtesy of J. Taylor.)

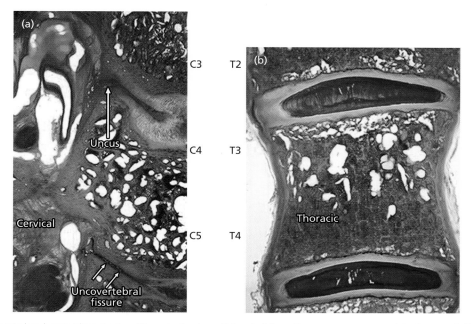

Figure 14.3 Lower cervical and upper thoracic discs. Thoracic discs have flat end-plates with no uncus or uncovertebral segment. (Courtesy of J. Taylor.)

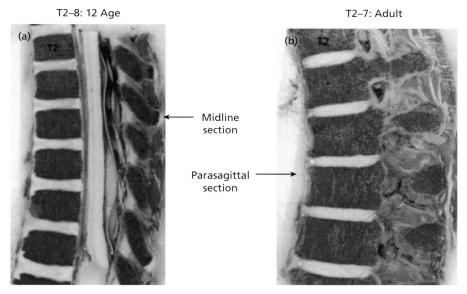

Figure 14.4 Sagittal sections of upper thoracic spine, showing normal kyphosis increase with age. (Courtesy of J. Taylor.)

Step 4. Visualization

Place the C-arm in the posteroanterior (PA) position first at the chosen thoracic level. Identify the midpoint of the intervertebral space at the target point. Adjust the lower endplate of the target vertebral body so that the disc borders are aligned and open the disc space in a cephalocaudal direction (Fig. 14.6).

Step 5. Mark the entry site

The entry site is about 1 to 1½ levels more caudal than the target site at the vertebral level. Infiltrate the skin over the entry point with lidocaine with a short 25 gauge needle down to the lamina.

Step 6. Direction of the needle

1. Introduce the needle about 1 cm paramedian at the level of the tip of the spinous process. The needle is then angled slightly superior and medial and advanced to make contact with the lamina. Once the bony contact is made, redirect the needle with an angle of 45° with the parasagittal and 15° axial plane medial and cephalad (Fig. 14.7).

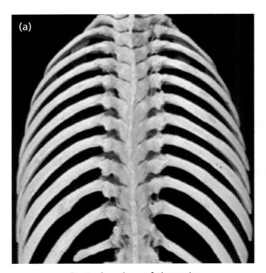

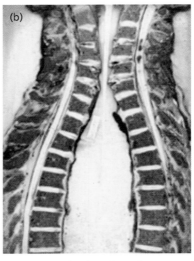

Posterior view of thoracic
vertebrae and ribs

Sagittal section of
thoracic vertebrae

Figure 14.5 (a,b) Thoracic spine: central axis of the thoracic skeleton. This contains the thoracic spinal cord and most of the lumbar spinal cord; the rib cage contains and protects the heart and lungs. (Courtesy of J. Taylor.)

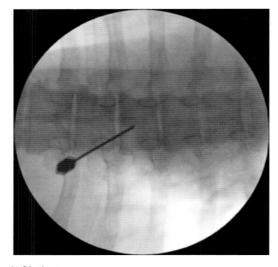

Figure 14.6 Identify the intervertebral space in PA view.

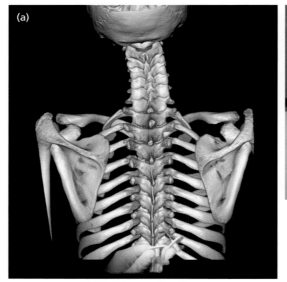

Needle position under PA view

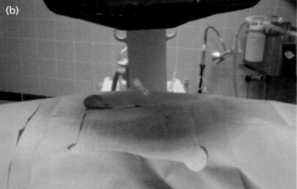

Figure 14.7 (a) Three-dimensional CT scan showing the direction of the epidural needle. (b) The needle about 1 cm paramedian at the level of the tip of the spinous process. Once the bony contact is made, redirect the needle with an angle of 45° with the parasagittal and 15° axial plane medial and cephalad.

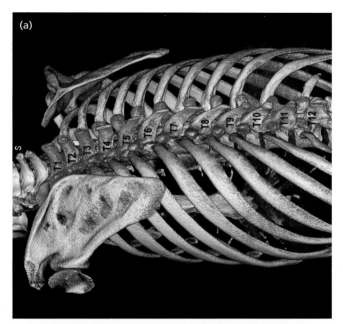

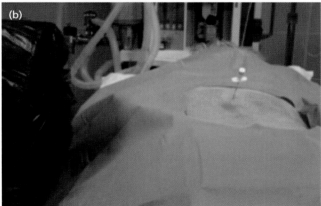

Figure 14.8 (a) Three-dimensional CT scan showing the thoracic vertebra in lateral view. (b) The direction of the needle in lateral view.

2. Then position the C-arm laterally. The needle should be placed between the spinous processes of the upper and lower vertebral bodies (Fig. 14.8).

Step 7. Loss of resistance technique
1. Advance the needle through the supraspinous and interspinous ligament under fluoroscopy. Stop at the level of the "virtual line," the line drawn at the base of the spinous processes (Fig. 14.9).
2. Remove the stylet of the needle. Attach a well-lubricated 5 ml syringe filled with saline.
3. Hold the hub of the epidural needle firmly with the left thumb and index finger.
4. Place the wrist of the left hand against the neck of the patient to prevent the advance of the needle due to unexpected movement of the patient.

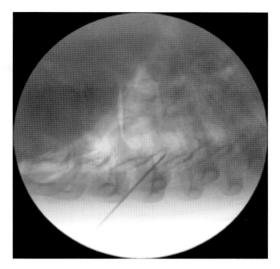

Figure 14.9 Stop at the level of the "virtual line," the line drawn at the base of the spinous processes.

5. Hold the syringe with the right hand and advance the needle under fluoroscopy with the thumb applying pressure on the plunger.
6. As soon as the needle bevel passes through the ligamentum flavum, there will be a "loss of resistance" and the plunger will slide freely.

Step 8. Confirm the position of the needle
1. Aspiration test is mandatory. If blood or cerebrospinal fluid is aspirated cease the procedure.
2. Injection of the contrast material will reveal a linear image in the posterior border of the epidural space.
3. Then turn the C-arm to the PA position. Verify the spread of the contrast solution in this view. If both views confirm the correct position of the needle tip in the epidural space, proceed to the next step (Fig. 14.10).

Step 9. Interlaminar epidural block
1. Inject 5 ml of 6–12 mg of nonparticulate steroid (dexamethasone) in saline or with a low concentration of local anesthetic.
2. Remove the needle and cover the entry site with a sterile gauze.

Lateral approach
Step 1 is as described above.

Step 2. Position and monitor the patient
1. Place the patient in the lateral decubitus position on the table. Support the abdomen and thorax with pillows, so the patient feels comfortable. Flex the neck as much as possible.
2. Between T1–T4 and T9–T12, the median approach and between T5–T8 the paramedian approach is preferable.

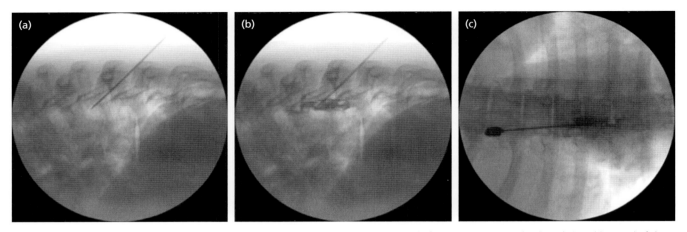

Figure 14.10 (a) The tip of the needle is within the epidural space in lateral view. (b) Spread of the contrast material in lateral view. (c) Spread of the contrast material in PA view.

Step 3. Drugs and equipment are as described above.

Step 4. Visualization
1. First position the C-arm laterally. As the patient lies in a lateral decubitus position, the vertebral column will appear in anteroposterior view. The entry point is just below the spinous process of the upper vertebral body between the intervertebral spaces.
2. Then move the C-arm to the PA position where the lateral view of the vertebral bodies will appear. The needle should be placed between the spinous processes of the upper and lower vertebral bodies.
3. Advance the needle as described above in the prone paraspinal approach with the loss of resistance technique.

Note: the rest of the steps are the same as those described for the prone approach.

Step 10. Postprocedure care
After the procedure, the patient should be observed for a reasonable time. The recovery and observation time depends on the sedation and analgesia used, as well as facilitating the assessment of any impairment of intellectual function, tolerance of oral intake, assessment of the immediate results of the neural blockade, and pain response to the procedure.

If pneumothorax is suspected, then a plain radiography is necessary.

The patient should be provided with all necessary instructions, including who to call or where to go for any postprocedure urgent/emergency care. The patient should be discharged accompanied by a responsible adult. The patient should not be allowed to drive themselves. They should also be informed that if changes like an increase in body temperature, fever, or pain occurs, they should return to the hospital immediately.

Complications
- **Inadvertent dural puncture**

The risk of inadvertent dural puncture is possible even in the most experienced hands. During the dural puncture, cerebrospinal fluid may not be aspirated. Rapid clearance of the contrast material can signify that the needle is in the subarachnoid space.
- **Inadvertent subdural puncture**

Subdural space is a potential space between the subarachnoid and epidural space. Injection of a very small amount of contrast material will appear like a thin straight line in multiple levels. Unlike injection of the contrast material in the subarachnoid space, the contrast material does not disappear in the subdural space. Administration of local anesthetic solution to the subdural space will end with total spinal block.
- **Spinal cord injury**

The disadvantage of the interlaminar thoracic epidural block is that there is a greater risk of causing immediate injury to the spinal cord by advancing the epidural needle too far and a greater risk of delayed injury by causing an epidural hematoma or abscess. To prevent this complication, an intermittent lateral fluoroscopic view should be used while advancing the needle. The patient may not feel pain or paresthesia when the needle contacts the spinal cord. They may feel pain only if the needle contacts the sensory fibers within the meninges. If local anesthetics are injected around the meninges they may not feel this sensation. Permanent damage within the spinal cord may also develop due to the injection of local anesthetics or other solutions. Quadriplegia may develop due to spinal cord injury.
- **Nerve injury**

If the tip of the needle contacts a spinal segmental nerve, the patient will complain of sudden severe pain. The needle has to be redirected.

• **Epidural hematoma**

Bleeding within the epidural space is a major complication if hematoma develops. The most important cause of epidural hematoma is the bleeding of the venous plexus within the thoracic epidural space. Bleeding due to the mechanical damage of the arteries within the epidural space gives rise to early findings, whereas bleeding in the venous plexus may give rise to findings in later stages, even some days after. Hematoma in the thoracic epidural space can have a mass effect on arterial or venous blood flow, which results in spinal cord ischemia. If neurological signs appear, urgent surgery may be necessary.

• **Respiratory depression**

If large amounts of local anesthetics are administered to the epidural space, the tidal volume will decrease over 50% and respiratory depression may develop.

• **Pneumothorax**

Pneumothorax may develop if the needle is misdirected. This complication may occur if the epidural block is performed by a blind technique.

• **Hypotension and bradycardia**

Thoracic epidural block at the midthoracic levels may cause the inhibition of the cardiac accelerator nerve, which may cause hypotension and bradycardia.

• **Infection**

The risk of infection is higher in the thoracic epidural space than in the lumbar epidural space.

Helpful hints

The advantage of the interlaminar route is that the risk of injecting into a vertebral or radicular artery is minimal. The disadvantages are the risk of causing immediate injury to the spinal cord by advancing the epidural needle too far and a risk of delayed injury by causing an epidural hematoma or abscess.

Patient selection is a critical part of the procedure in the thoracic region. If the patient has bilateral or multilevel symptoms, usually a thoracic interlaminar epidural block is more favorable.

Thoracic transforaminal steroid injection is different from thoracic interlaminar epidural steroid injection because, with the thoracic transforaminal injection, the steroid is delivered directly on the spinal nerve and close to the site of pathology; whereas, in the interlaminar technique, the steroid injection may travel away from the pathology.

To place a catheter across a tight area of stenosis is difficult and may increase the risk of epidural hematoma or spinal cord injury.

Positioning of the patient and the needle is very important for the thoracic interlaminar epidural approach. If the needle is misdirected the needle may pass the supraspinous ligament and the physician will feel a loss of resistance. Thus the position of the needle should always be confirmed under fluoroscopy and confirmed with injection of the contrast solution.

The thoracic epidural space is rich with sympathetic innervation. Use of high doses of local anesthetics will cause hypotension and bradycardia.

Again, use of higher concentrations of local anesthetics will, if they block T1–T4, cause motor loss in intercostal muscles, which may cause respiratory insufficiency, especially in obese patients.

Percutaneous transforaminal block of the thoracic epidural space

The history and anatomy of the thoracic epidural space is described earlier (vide supra) so will not be discussed here (Fig. 14.11).

Indications
• Thoracic trauma.
• Acute herpes zoster and postherpetic neuralgia.
• Cancer pain.
• Bulging or protrusion of the disc at the thoracic level.

Contraindications
• Local or systemic infection.
• Coagulopathy.
• Hypotension.
• Anatomic distortion.

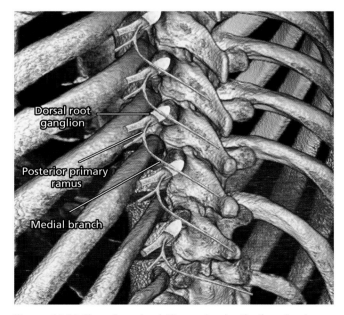

Figure 14.11 Three-dimensional CT scan showing the thoracic spine and the nerve roots coming out of the foramina.

Technique of thoracic epidural block, transforaminal approach

Step 1. Prepare the patient before the procedure
The patient should be told why the procedure is being done and what to expect. All complications and side effects related to the procedure should be explained in detail, before the procedure. Valid, written consent should be obtained.

The type of analgesia or sedation needs to be ascertained before performance of the invasive procedure. Intravenous fentanyl, midazolam, and/or propofol may be used judiciously for the patient's comfort. Patient response should be monitored and the dosage titrated to establish a level of sedation allowing the patient to be conversant and responsive after needle placements. Because the disc is avascular, there is an increased risk of disc space infection, and most discographers use prophylactic antibiotics: prophylactic intravenous antibiotics 20 minutes before the procedure are recommended.

Step 2. Position and monitor the patient
1. Place the patient prone on the table. Place a pillow under the chest, to flex the thoracolumbar spine. The patient's head is turned to the side, with the arms either raised above the head or crossed at the side.
2. Obtain an intravenous access through a large vein.
3. Administer oxygen by nasal cannula.
4. Monitor the vital signs noninvasively throughout the procedure.
5. Prep and drape the area in a sterile fashion.
6. Sedation may be used to relax the patient; however, the patient should be awake enough to respond to the physician's questions.

Step 3. Drugs and equipment for thoracic transforaminal epidural block
• 1½ inch needle for skin infiltration;
• 5 ml syringe for local anesthesia;

• 5 ml syringe for contrast material;
• special loss of resistance syringe;
• 5–10 ml syringe for epidural block;
• 18–20 gauge Tuohy needle;
• 5 ml of 1% lidocaine for skin infiltration;
• 5–10 ml of 0.5% bupivacaine;
• contrast solution (iohexol);
• nonparticulate steroid;
• preservative-free normal saline.

Step 4. Visualization
1. Place the C-arm in a PA position first. Identify the midpoint of the intervertebral space at the targeted site. Adjust the lower endplate of the targeted vertebral body to be aligned by moving the C-arm in a cephalocaudal direction (Fig. 14.12).
2. Rotate the C-arm obliquely 25–30° to the ipsilateral side until the neuroforamen under the pedicle is visualized as an oblong image. The ribs and the costovertebral articulations can also be seen in the background in this view (Fig. 14.13).

Step 5. Site of entry and direction of the needle
1. Inject local anesthetic at the skin entry site just inferior to the pedicle.
2. Advance a 22 gauge, 10 cm needle in "tunnel vision" toward the most superior aspect of the foramen just under the pedicle but always medial to the rib, costovertebral joint, and lateral to the border of the lamina (Fig. 14.14).

Step 6. Confirm the position of the needle
1. On reaching the appropriate depth, rotate the C-arm laterally. The needle should rest above the nerve root at the superior border of the foramen and in the posterior to midportion of the foramen in the lateral fluoroscopic view (Fig. 14.15).
2. Rotate the C-arm again to the PA position. The needle should not be more medial than the 6 o'clock position

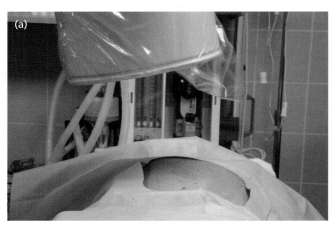

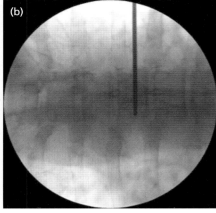

Figure 14.12 (a,b) Identify the level under PA view first.

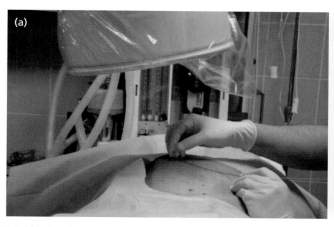
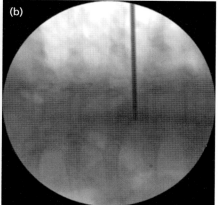

Figure 14.13 (a,b) Point of entry under oblique view.

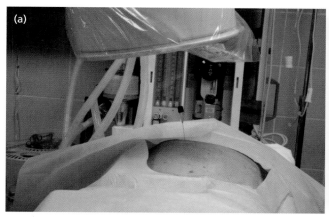
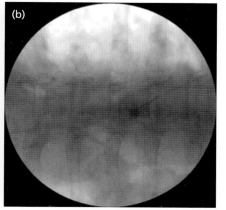

Figure 14.14 (a,b) Direction of the needle under "tunneled vision."

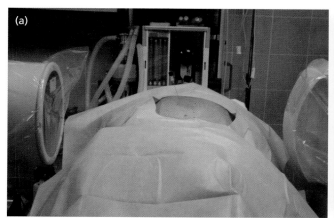
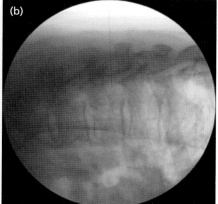

Figure 14.15 (a,b) The needle under lateral view.

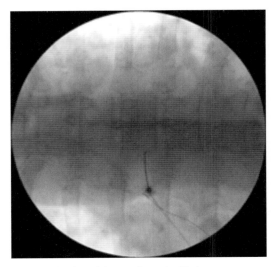

Figure 14.16 Direction of the needle under PA view.

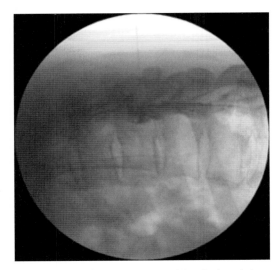

Figure 14.18 Spread of the contrast material under lateral view.

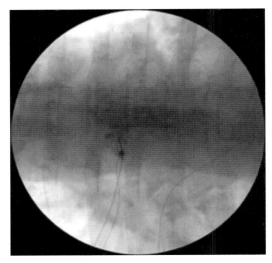

Figure 14.17 Spread of the contrast material under PA view.

of the pedicle as seen as a clock face on anteroposterior imaging. Inject 1–2 ml of contrast solution to confirm this (Fig. 14.16).

3. After negative aspiration, inject 2 ml of an ionic contrast solution, which should flow under the pedicle, around the nerve root, and into the epidural space in the PA view (Fig. 14.17).

4. In the lateral view, the intervertebral foramen should be seen to be filled with contrast, and a cross section of the nerve root may be identified (Fig. 14.18).

Step 7. Thoracic transforaminal block
After a satisfactory pattern is observed and there is no evidence of subdural, subarachnoid, or intravascular spread of contrast, 3–6 mg of betamethasone solution, or 20–40 mg of

methylprednisolone, or equivalent drug, is slowly injected. Local anesthetic at low concentration is also injected by some physicians.

Step 8. Postprocedure care
Observe the patient for at least 2 hours after the procedure. Monitoring of vital signs is mandatory. In addition, objectively document the pain relief. If pneumothorax is suspected, then a plain radiography is necessary.

After a satisfactory observation, discharge the patient with appropriate and adequate instructions given to their escort. Written instructions are preferable for emergencies and they are helpful to the patient and their family.

Complications
• Inadvertent dural puncture
The risk of inadvertent dural puncture is possible even in the most experienced hands. During the dural puncture, cerebrospinal fluid may not be aspirated. Rapid clearance of the contrast material under fluoroscopy can signify that the needle is in the subarachnoid space. Failure to recognize unintentional dural puncture can result in immediate total spinal anesthesia with associated loss of consciousness, hypotension, and apnea. If epidural doses of opioids are accidentally placed into the subarachnoid space, significant respiratory and central nervous system depression will result.

• Inadvertent subdural puncture
Subdural space is a potential space between the subarachnoid and epidural space. Injection of a very small amount of contrast material will appear like a thin straight line in multiple levels. Unlike injection of the contrast material to the subarachnoid space, contrast material does not disappear. If subdural placement is unrecognized and epidural

doses of local anesthetics are administered, the signs and symptoms are similar to those of massive subarachnoid injection, although the resulting motor and sensory block may be delayed and spotty. Administration of local anesthetic solution to the subdural space will end with total spinal block.

• **Spinal cord injury**

The disadvantage of the transforaminal thoracic epidural block is that there is a greater risk of causing immediate injury to the spinal cord by advancing the epidural needle too far and a greater risk of delayed injury by causing an epidural hematoma or abscess. To prevent this complication, an intermittent lateral fluoroscopic view should be used while advancing the needle. The patient may not feel pain or paresthesia when the needle contacts the spinal cord. They may feel pain only if the needle contacts the sensory fibers within the meninges. If local anesthetics are injected around the meninges they may not feel this sensation. Permanent damage within the spinal cord may also develop due to the injection of local anesthetics or other solutions. Quadriplegia may develop due to the spinal cord injury.

• **Nerve injury**

If the tip of the needle contacts a spinal segmental nerve, the patient will complain of sudden severe pain. The needle has to be redirected.

• **Intravascular injection**

If the misplacement is unrecognized, injection of local anesthetic directly into an epidural vein will result in significant local anesthetic toxicity. Damage or injection to the segmental artery can occur with increased incidence when performing the transforaminal approach to the T7–L4 neural foramen on the left.

• **Epidural hematoma**

Bleeding within the epidural space is a major complication if hematoma develops. The most important cause of epidural hematoma is the bleeding of the venous plexus within the thoracic epidural space. Bleeding due to the mechanical damage of the arteries within the epidural space gives rise to early findings, whereas bleeding in the venous plexus may give rise to findings in later stages, even some days after. Hematoma in the thoracic epidural space can have a mass effect on arterial or venous blood flow, which results in spinal cord ischemia. If neurological signs appear, urgent surgery may be necessary.

• **Respiratory depression**

If high amounts of local anesthetics are administered to the epidural space, tidal volume will decrease over 50% and respiratory depression may develop.

• **Pneumothorax**

Pneumothorax may develop if the needle is misdirected too laterally and too deep. Pneumothorax may not be diagnosed immediately. Shortness of breath and pain on the lateral side of the chest are the first signs of pneumothorax. Chest radiography should be ordered to rule out pneumothorax.

• **Hypotension and bradycardia**

Thoracic epidural block in the midthoracic levels may cause the inhibition of the cardiac accelerator nerve, which may cause hypotension and bradycardia.

• **Infection**

The risk of infection is higher in the thoracic epidural space than in the lumbar space. Because of the potential for hematogenous spread through Batson's plexus, local infection and sepsis represent absolute contraindications to the thoracic approach to the epidural space.

Percutaneous block and lesioning of the thoracic facet joint and medial branch

History

The facet joints of the spine are also known as the apophyseal joints. The Greek word apophysis means "an offshoot," and the anatomical definition of the word is a natural outgrowth or process on a vertebra on another bone. The degenerative changes and associated muscle spasm that develop when a facet joint is involved in a sprain from a forceful or violent twisting motion was termed the "facet syndrome" by Ghormley in 1933. The intraarticular facet joints at all levels are subject to trauma. Pain emanating from various structures of the spine is a major cause of chronic pain problems. Linton et al. estimated the prevalence of spinal pain in the general population as 66%, with 44% of patients reporting pain in the cervical region, 56% in the lumbar region, and 15% in the thoracic region. Manchikanti et al. reported similar results. Despite the high prevalence of spinal pain, it has been suggested that a specific etiology of back pain can be diagnosed in only about 15% of patients with certainty.

Bogduk identified four factors necessary for any structure to be deemed a cause of spinal pain: a nerve supply to the structure; the ability of the structure to cause pain similar to that seen clinically in normal volunteers; the structure's susceptibility to painful diseases or injuries; and demonstration that the structure can be a source of pain in patients using diagnostic techniques of known reliability and validity.

The facet or zygapophyseal joints of the spine are well innervated by the medial branches of the posterior primary rami. Facet joints have been shown to be capable of causing pain in the neck, upper and mid-back, and low back with pain referred to the head or upper extremity, chest wall, and lower extremity in normal volunteers. They also have been shown to be a source of pain in patients with chronic spinal pain using diagnostic techniques of known reliability and validity. Conversely, the reliability of physical examination in diagnosing the specific cause of back pain has been questioned.

Anatomy

The thoracic facet (zygapophyseal) joints are located between the superior and inferior articular pillars of adjacent vertebrae. The joint's articular surface is inclined 60° from the horizontal to the frontal plane and rotated 20° from the frontal to the sagittal plane in a medial direction. Thus, the lateral aspect of the joint is placed anterior and the medial aspect of the joint posterior. The superior articular facet from the inferior vertebrae is almost flat and faces posterior, superior, and slightly lateral. The inferior articular facet is oriented in a reciprocal manner. There is some variation in the inclination of the joints by region with the midthoracic level approximately 60° off the horizontal plane whereas the upper segments achieve a more vertical orientation. The lower thoracic segments show some characteristics of the lumbar segments as their angle approaches the sagittal plane.

The articular capsules of the thoracic facet joints are attached to the lateral margins of the articular processes. The anterior capsule is reinforced by the capsular fibers of the ligamentum flavum, and the posterior ligamentous complex reinforces the posterior capsule. The interspinous and supraspinous ligaments blend with the superior articular capsule.

The thoracic posterior rami arise from spinal nerves and traverse posteriorly through an osseoligamentous tunnel bound by the transverse process, the neck of the rib below, the medial border to the superior costotransverse ligament, and the lateral border of a zygapophyseal joint.

The nerve then runs laterally through the space formed between the anterior lamella of the superior costotransverse ligament anteriorly, the costolamellar ligament, and the posterior lamella of the superior costotransverse ligament posteriorly. At the distal lateral end of this space the nerve divides into lateral and medial branches. The medial branch wraps around the posterior lamella of the superior costotransverse ligament's lateral border to lie a short distance above the next lower transverse process. The medial branch then crosses the transverse process obliquely and runs caudomedially between the semispinalis and the multifidus muscles. Here it divides into three branches. A short branch enters each of the last two muscles and a longer branch continues caudally and medially along the lateral surface of the multifidus muscle. Articular branches are believed to arise from the medial branch of the dorsal rami running above and below each joint (Figs 14.19–14.22).

Indications
- Thoracic trauma.
- Acute herpes zoster and postherpetic neuralgia.
- Cancer pain.
- Bulging or protrusion of the disc at the thoracic level.

Contraindications
- Local or systemic infection.
- Coagulopathy.

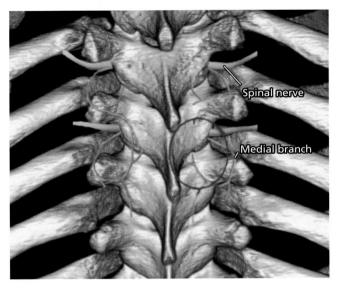

Figure 14.19 Medial branch of the thoracic facet joint.

- Vital function instability.
- Anatomic distortion.

Technique of thoracic facet medial branch lesioning

Step 1. Prepare the patient before the procedure
Ascertain the type of analgesia or sedation before performing the invasive procedure. If a local anesthetic or neurolytic block is planned, mild sedation is all that is necessary. If pulsed radiofrequency (RF) is planned, the patient needs to be awake to respond to the stimulation test. Intravenous fentanyl or midazolam may be used judiciously for the patient's comfort.

Step 2. Position and monitor the patient
1. Place the patient prone on the table.
2. Place a pillow under the chest to flex the thoracolumbar spine. The patient's head is turned to the side, with the arms either raised above the head or crossed or at the side.
3. Insert an intravenous cannula for injecting medication.
4. Provide oxygen by nasal cannula.
5. Monitor vital signs (mandatory).
6. Prepare the area for needle entry in a sterile fashion.

Step 3. Drugs and equipment for thoracic facet joint and median branch block
Prepare and confirm that the following equipment, needles, and drugs are ready to be used for the procedure.

Common drugs and needles
- 1½ inch, 25 gauge needle (for infiltration of the skin);
- 5 ml syringe (for local anesthetic solution);

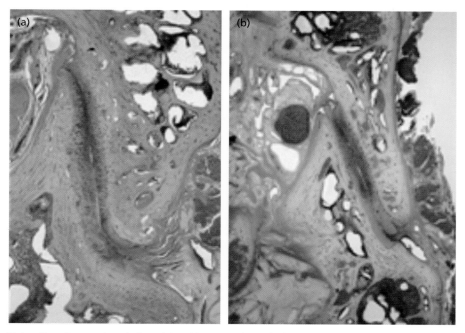

Figure 14.20 (a,b) Sagittal section of upper thoracic facet joints. (Courtesy of J. Taylor.)

Degenerative disc at the C6–7,
C7–T1 and T1–2 discs natural

Facet joints differences
C7–T2

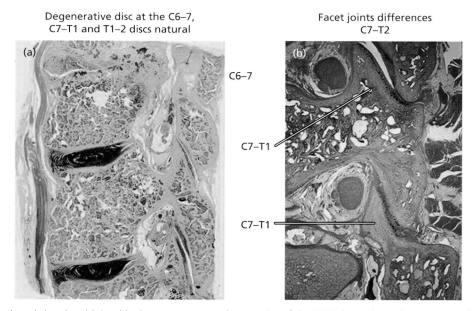

C6–7

C7–T1

C7–T1

Figure 14.21 Cervicothoracic junction. (a) An old spine contrasts gross degeneration of the C6–7 disc with good preservation of the C7–T1 and T1–2 discs. (b) C7–T2 in a 22-year-old man; upper thoracic facets show a laminar "step" below them. (Courtesy of J. Taylor.)

- 2 ml empty syringe (for aspiration test);
- 22 gauge, 3½ inch needle (for the nerve block);
- 1% lidocaine for skin infiltration or diagnostic injections.

Special equipment for RF
- RF machine, with cables and electrodes;
- 10 cm RF needle with 2 mm active-tip electrode.

Step 4. Visualization

1. Place the C-arm in a PA position. Identify the midpoint of the intervertebral space at the target level. Adjust the lower endplate of the target vertebral body to be aligned by moving the C-arm in a cephalocaudal direction (Fig. 14.23).
2. Move the C-arm 5–10° to the contralateral side to distinguish the transverse process from the ribs, lamina, and the lung.

231

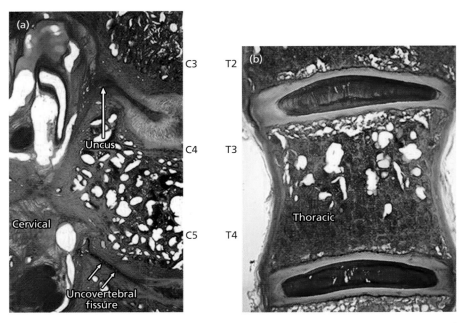

Figure 14.22 (a,b) Lower cervical and upper thoracic disc. Thoracic discs have flat end-plates with no uncus and no uncovertebral clefts. (Courtesy of J. Taylor.)

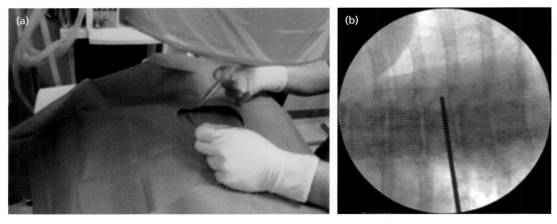

Figure 14.23 (a,b) Identify the entry point.

Step 5. Direction of the needle
1. Infiltrate the skin with local anesthetic. Advance a 22 gauge needle to the midportion at the lateral ⅓ of the transverse process until a bony contact is made. The superolateral corner of the transverse process at the inflection point is the target (Figs 14.24 and 14.25).
2. An aspiration test is mandatory to verify that the needle or electrode tip is not in a vessel.
3. Position the C-arm laterally to view the depth of the needles or electrodes. The needle should not go deeper toward the intervertebral foramina (Fig. 14.26).

Step 6. Stimulation test
Apply motor stimulation at 2 Hz, with 1 ms pulse width at or below 1 V. There may be slight contractions in the paravertebral muscles. Then apply sensory stimulation at 50 Hz, at 1 ms pulse width at 0.5 V. Seek for paresthesia.

Step 7. RF lesioning
3. Inject 0.5–1 ml of local anesthetic, depot steroid combination.
4. Radiofrequency lesioning should be performed at 70 °C for 60 seconds twice at two adjacent points (Fig. 14.27).

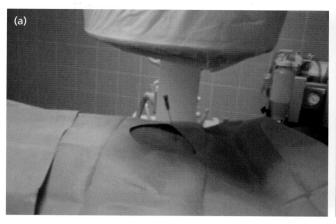

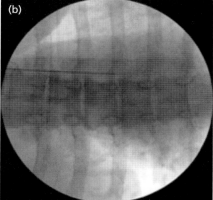

Figure 14.24 (a,b) Target of the needle tip.

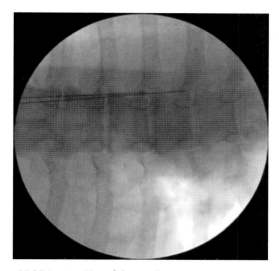

Figure 14.25 Last position of the needles.

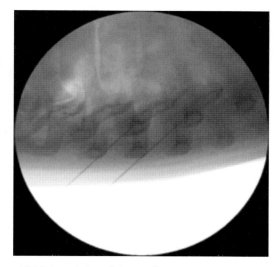

Figure 14.26 Lateral view of the needles.

Technique of thoracic facet joint block

Follow steps 1, 2, and 3 as previously described to start this procedure.

Step 4. Visualization
1. The C-arm is placed in the anteroposterior position first to visualize the thoracic vertebral bodies.
2. Slightly move the C-arm in a cephalocaudal direction until the lower endplate of the vertebral body is aligned and visualized as a straight line. Identify the transverse process at this level.

Step 5. Mark the site of entry
1. For T1–T5 facet joints, the inferior margin of the same vertebra and for T6–T10 facet joints, just superior to the pedicle below, is marked.
2. Insert a 3½ inch, 22 gauge needle through the skin angling approximately 60° of the skin toward the target joint.

Step 6. Direction of the needle
1. Advance the needle cephalad toward the superior articular process. The needle should remain on an imaginary vertical line connecting the midportion of the upper and lower pedicles always on the bone.
2. To prevent inadvertent entry to the epidural or subarachnoid spaces, the needle should not stay medial to the medial aspect of the pedicle on the PA view.
3. Rotate the C-arm away from the side being injected approximately 20–30° until the outline of the joint is clearly visible.

Step 7. Confirm the position of the needle
1. The needle tip should be positioned at or near the inferior aspect of the joint to enter the capsule of the joint.
2. Inject 0.1–0.2 ml of contrast material. The contrast material should fill the joint space and the inferior or superior capsular recesses on both PA and lateral views.

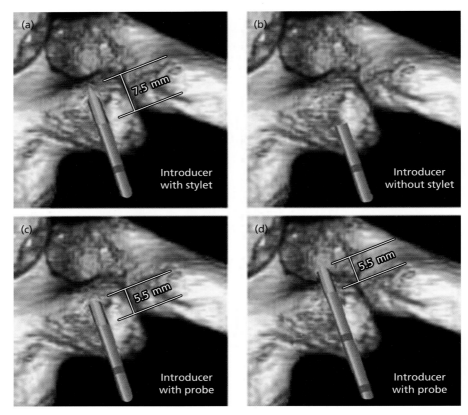

Radiofrequency lesioning

Figure 14.27 (a–d) Three-dimensional CT scan showing the final position of the tip of the electrodes for RF lesioning.

Step 8. Thoracic facet joint block
The thoracic facet joints are very small. Do not inject more than 0.5–0.7 ml of 5% bupivacaine and steroid combination (Fig. 14.28).

Step 9. Postprocedure care
After completing the procedure, observe the patient for at least 2 hours. Monitoring vital signs is mandatory. In addition, objectively document the pain relief. If pneumothorax is suspected, then a plain radiograph is necessary. After a satisfactory observation, discharge the patient with appropriate and adequate instructions given to their escort. Written instructions are preferable for emergencies and are helpful to the patient and their family.

Complications
• **Transient increase in pain**
Pain may increase after facet joint block or RF lesioning. The pain may be due to injury of the facet joint or irritation due to the injected solutions. Generally, it is transient.
• **Neuritis**
Neuritis may develop after RF lesioning. It is transient.
• **Dysesthesia and sensorial loss**

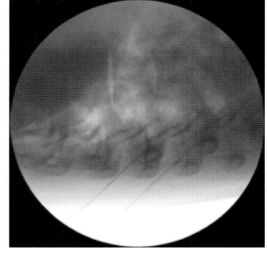

Figure 14.28 Lateral view of the needles for facet joint block.

Dysesthesia and sensorial loss may develop at the trajectory of the median branch after RF lesioning.

Helpful hints

Differential diagnosis of pain in the thorax is important. Pain in the thorax may be due to referred pain outside the thorax and pain originating from the thoracic spine.

Referred pain can be as follows.
- Cervical discs or facet joints.
- Pain from the cervical ligaments and musculature.
- Shoulder pain.
- Cardiovascular, pulmonary, and mediastinal sources.
- Hepatobiliary and gastrointestinal pain

Pain originating from the thoracic spine can be as follows.
- Bulging, protrusion, or extruded discs in the thoracic spine.
- Pain from the paravertebral muscles and ligaments.
- Costovertebral joints.
- Injury of the vertebral bodies or compression fracture.

Procedures in the thorax are performed less often than for the other parts of the spine.

Percutaneous thoracic discography

History

In 1948, Hirsch first described the procedure for injecting procaine in the herniated disc. In 1940 Roofe investigated the annulus fibrosus innervation, which provided an incentive for conceptualizing the disc as a painful source independent of a neurocompressive component of disc herniation. In 1944, following Roofe's studies, Lindblom first demonstrated the presence of radial annular fissures in a cadaveric disc.

Hirsch followed this demonstration with a clinical study to determine the course of the ruptures or tears in the annulus which would lead to pathologic processes, causing pain. He hypothesized that putting pressure on a ruptured or degenerated disc could cause a unique set of signs and symptoms of pain. He demonstrated that if one injected saline to pressurize the disc it will cause pain. In addition, injection of a local anesthetic (e.g., procaine) will relieve this pain. In 1964, Crock advanced the theory of internal disc disruption, and showed that patients with discogenic pain have abnormal discograms and that this may be the reason pain is reproduced by a small volume (0.3 ml) of solution injected, owing to hypersensitivity of pain fibers in the disc. Discographic patterns on radiographs were shown to be abnormal. In 1987 Sachs demonstrated the pathological disruption and classified them as what is now known as the Dallas Discogram Scale. Bogduk later modified this Dallas Scale.

Anatomy of the intervertebral discs

The intervertebral discs are complex structures that consist of a thick outer ring of fibrous cartilage termed the annulus fibrosus, which surrounds a more gelatinous core known as the nucleus pulposus; the nucleus pulposus is sandwiched inferiorly and superiorly by cartilage endplates. (Note that the anatomy of the structure of the vertebral disc is described in Chapter 16. It will not be described here.)

Structure of the nucleus pulposus

The central nucleus pulposus contains collagen fibers, which are organized randomly, and elastin fibers (sometimes up to 150 μm in length), which are arranged radially. These fibers are embedded in a highly hydrated aggrecan-containing gel. Interspersed at a low density (approximately 5000/mm) are chondrocyte-like cells, sometimes sitting in a capsule within the matrix. Outside the nucleus is the annulus fibrosus, with the boundary between the two regions being very distinct in young individuals (less than 10 years).

Structure of the annulus

This is made up of a series of 15–25 concentric rings, or lamellae, with the collagen fibers lying parallel within each lamella. The fibers are oriented at approximately 60° to the vertical axis, alternating to the left and right of it in adjacent lamellae. Elastin fibers lie between the lamellae, possibly helping the disc to return to its original arrangement following bending, such as flexion or extension. They may also bind the lamellae together as elastin fibers pass radially from one lamella to the next. The cells of the annulus, particularly in the outer region, tend to be fibroblast-like, elongated, thin, and aligned parallel to the collagen fibers. Toward the inner annulus the cells can be more oval. Cells of the disc, both in the annulus and nucleus, can have several long, thin cytoplasmic projections, which may be more than 30 μm long. Such features are not seen in cells of articular cartilage (knee). Their function in the disc is unknown but it has been suggested that they may act as sensors and communicators of mechanical strain within the tissue.

The structure of the endplate

The third morphologically distinct region is the cartilage endplate, a thin horizontal layer, usually less than 1 mm thick, of hyaline cartilage. This interfaces the disc and the vertebral body. The collagen fibers within it run horizontal and parallel to the vertebral bodies, with the fibers continuing into the disc. The appearance of the intervertebral disc at young (10 months old) and adult ages are quite distinct.

Blood vessels and nerve supply of the disc

Vascular architecture

The healthy adult disc has few (if any) blood vessels, but it has some nerves, mainly restricted to the outer lamellae,

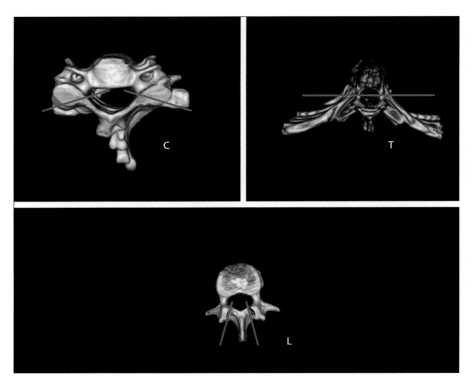

Figure 14.29 Orientation of facet joints, cervical, thoracic, and lumbar regions, seen from transverse plane 2. Orientation of the facet joints, cervical thoracic, and lumbar, seen in sagittal plane. Axial rotation in thoracic spine is restricted by facet joint orientation.

some of which carry the proprioceptor function. The cartilaginous endplate, like other hyaline cartilages, is normally totally avascular and aneural in the healthy adult. Blood vessels present in the longitudinal ligaments adjacent to the disc and in young cartilage endplates (less than about 12 months old) are branches of the spinal artery.

Nerve supply

Nerves in the disc have been demonstrated, often accompanying the vessels, but they can also occur independently, as branches of the sinuvertebral nerve which are derived from the ventral rami or gray rami communicantes. A meningeal branch of the spinal nerve, known as the recurrent sinovertebral nerve, originates near the disc space. This nerve exits from the dorsal root ganglion and enters the foramen. It then divides into a major ascending and a lesser descending branch. It has been shown in animal studies that further afferent contributions to the sinuvertebral nerve arise through the rami communicantes from multiple superior and inferior dorsal root ganglia. In addition, the anterior longitudinal ligament also receives afferent innervation from branches that originate in the dorsal root ganglion. The posterior longitudinal ligament is richly innervated by nociceptive fibers from the ascending branch of the sinuvertebral nerve. These nerves also innervate the adjacent outer layers of the annulus fibrosus. Some of the nerves in the discs also have glial support cells, or Schwann cells, alongside them.

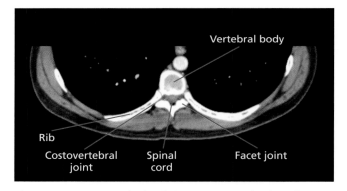

Figure 14.30 Important landmarks in cross section of cadaver thoracic cavity.

Morphological differences between different regions of thoracic vertebrae

When viewed in transverse section (anterior–posterior plane), the morphology of the thoracic vertebral structures may roughly be grouped into three regions: upper, middle, and lower. The upper region vertebrae (T1–T4) exhibit general similarities to the lower cervical vertebrae, but possess prominent transverse processes articulating with acutely angled costotransverse joints, and prominent laminae (Figs 14.29 and 14.30).

In the middle region (T5–T8), the transverse processes become more club-like, with a wider laminar component and a distinct "notch" present at the inferior-medial confluence of the transverse process and lamina.

In the lower region (T9–T12), the transverse processes become progressively less prominent, difficult to visualize at T11, and nearly vestigial at T12. The inferior vertebral arch, and thus the intervertebral neural foramen (containing the exiting nerve root and dorsal root ganglion), lies directly ventral and slightly medial to the inferior-medial border of the transverse process at its junction with the lamina.

Articulation of the vertebra

The thoracic vertebral interspaces between T3 and T9 are functionally unique because of the acute downward angle of the spinous processes. This downward slope means that the spinous process of any given midthoracic vertebra is in fact inferior to the interlaminar space of its adjacent vertebra.

The thoracic vertebra articulates with the ribs. The head of the rib articulates with the demi-facets, which are located on the posterolateral vertebral body. The tubercle of the rib articulates with a small concavity known as the transverse articular facet located at the lateral border of the transverse process (Fig. 14.31).

The thoracic intervertebral foramen lies ventral to the superior costotransverse ligament and both above and below the demi-facets of the ribs articulating at the vertebral body. The nerve leaves the foramen from the anterior and superior portion and travels obliquely posteriorly and slightly inferiorly until it may travel slightly upwards reaching its position under the segmental rib.

Indications

- Thoracic radicular pain, where radiographic imaging fails to identify the cause of thoracic pain.
- To determine the levels to be fused in patients who are candidates for instrumentation and fusion of the thoracic spine.

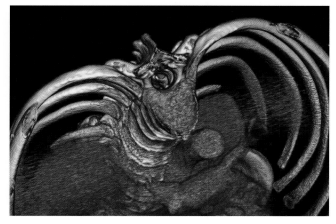

Figure 14.31 Articulations of the thoracic vertebra with the ribs.

- Failure to achieve adequate improvement with comprehensive nonoperative treatment.
- To help select an appropriate interventional technique, to treat the persistent pain.

Contraindications

- Local infection or sepsis.
- Pregnancy.
- Coagulopathy.
- Vital functions instability.
- Psychopathologies.

Technique of thoracic discography

Step 1. Prepare the patient before the procedure
The patient should be told why the procedure is being done and what to expect. All complications and side effects related to the procedure should be explained in detail, before the procedure. Valid, written consent should be obtained.

The type of analgesia or sedation needs to be ascertained before performance of the invasive procedure. Intravenous fentanyl, midazolam, and/or propofol may be used judiciously for the patient's comfort. Patient response should be monitored and the dosage titrated to establish a level of sedation allowing the patient to be conversant and responsive after needle placements. Because the disc is avascular, there is an increased risk of disc space infection and most discographers use prophylactic antibiotics. Prophylactic intravenous antibiotics 20 minutes before the procedure are recommended.

Step 2. Position and monitor the patient
1. Place the patient prone on the table. Place a pillow under the chest to flex the thoracolumbar spine. The patient's head is turned to the side, with the arms either raised above the head or crossed or at the side.
2. Obtain an intravenous access through a large vein.
3. Administer oxygen by nasal cannula.
4. Monitor the vital signs noninvasively throughout the procedure.
5. Prep and drape the area in a sterile fashion.
6. Sedation may be used to relax the patient; however, the patient should be awake enough to answer reliably.

Step 3. Drugs and equipment for discography
- 5 ml syringe for skin infiltration;
- 25 gauge, 1½ inch needle for local anesthesia;
- 22 gauge, 10 cm needle for discography;
- 10 ml syringe for discography;
- manometry;
- 1% lidocaine for skin infiltration;
- nonionic contrast solution for discography;
- appropriate antibiotic, both for intradiscal and intravenous administration.

Step 4. Visualization

1. The C-arm is placed in the anteroposterior position first to visualize the thoracic vertebral bodies. Then slightly move the C-arm in a cephalocaudal direction until the lower endplate of the vertebral body is aligned and visualized as flat and as open as possible.

2. Rotate the C-arm obliquely on the ipsilateral side until the corner of the intervertebral disc space is visualized between the superior articular process and the costovertebral joint.

Note: the tip of the spinous process will superimpose on the edge of the contralateral vertebral body.

Step 5. Mark the surface landmarks for the needle entry

1. The entry point is lateral to the interpedicular line. Infiltrate the skin and subcutaneous tissue with 1% lidocaine.

2. A 22 gauge, 10 cm needle should be directed parallel to and behind the rib as it passes anterior toward the spine at the costovertebral joints.

Step 6. Direction of the needle

When the needle passes anterior to the superior articular process in the lateral fluoroscopic view, the needle is turned posteriorly to facilitate advancing the needle in a more posterior direction, into the center of the disc (Fig. 14.32).

Step 7. Confirm the position of the needle

Nonionic contrast medium is slowly injected into each disc in 0.2–0.5 ml increments under direct fluoroscopic observation. If firm resistance to injection is encountered at this point, the needle may be embedded in the annulus or in the cartilage of a vertebral endplate.

Step 8. Discography

1. At 0.2–0.3 ml increments, observe pain response and document the intensity.

2. A positive discogram requires concordant pain (the same as the patient's clinical symptoms), with similar location and character, and a pain response of 6/10 on a numeric scale of 1–10.

3. The nucleogram of a normal thoracic disc appears as a lobulated mass with occasional posterolateral clefts, which develop as part of the normal aging process of the disc. In a damaged disc, the contrast solution may flow into tears of the inner annulus, producing a characteristic transverse pattern. If the tears in the annulus extend to the outer layer, a radial pattern is produced.

4. Contrast solution may also flow between the layers of annulus, producing a circumferential pattern. Complete disruption of the annulus allows contrast material to flow into the epidural space or into the cartilaginous endplate of the vertebra itself. Although the damage to the annulus is directly proportional to the likelihood that the disc is the source of the patient's pain, the specialist must evaluate all information obtained from discography in the context of the patient's symptoms (Figs 14.33–14.37).

5. After evaluation of the nucleogram, a decision must be made to proceed with discography of adjacent discs or to inject local anesthetic into the disc currently being imaged.

6. Analgesic discography is useful in patients whose clinical pain pattern is reproduced or provoked during the injection of contrast medium. If the pain that was provoked during the injection is relieved by a subsequent injection of local anesthetic into the disc, the inference can be drawn that the disc is the likely source of the patient's pain. It must be remembered that, if the annulus is disrupted, the injected local anesthetic may spread into the epidural space and anesthetize somatic and sympathetic nerves. If this occurs,

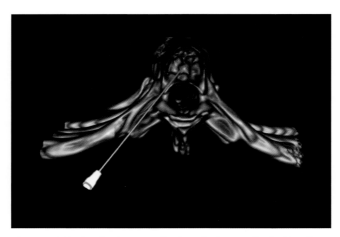

Figure 14.32 Needle placement for thoracic discography. Position for needle advancement is medial to the costotransverse junction along the lateral aspect of the superior articulating process.

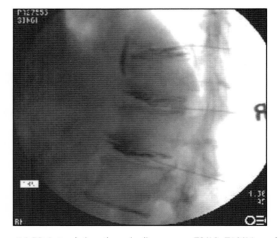

Figure 14.33 Lateral view thoracic discograms. T9/10, T10/11, and T11/12. Note contrast leaking anteriorly at T9/10. Severe degeneration at T10/11 and T11/12, with contrast highlighting posterior bulge at T11/12. (Reproduced with permission from the American Society of Interventional Pain Physicians.)

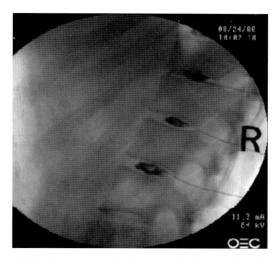

Figure 14.34 Example of wider disc spaces in the lower thoracic and upper lumbar spine. Contrast visible at four levels: T10–T11, T11–T12, T12–L1, and L1–L2. (Reproduced with permission from the American Society of Interventional Pain Physicians.)

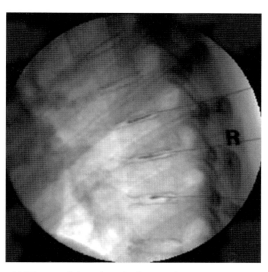

Figure 14.36 Lateral view thoracic discography. T6–T7, T7–T8, and T8–T9, showing quite narrow disc spaces at these levels. (Reproduced with permission from the American Society of Interventional Pain Physicians.)

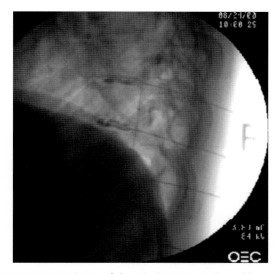

Figure 14.35 Lateral view of thoracic discogram in the midthoracic region. Disc spaces are slightly narrower in this region. (Reproduced with permission from the American Society of Interventional Pain Physicians.)

erroneous information may be obtained if discography is then performed on adjacent discs.

Step 9. Postprocedure care

After the sequence of injection procedures is completed, the patient is observed for 30 minutes before discharge from the outpatient facility. The patient should be warned to expect minor postprocedure discomfort, including some soreness of the paraspinous musculature. Icepacks placed on the

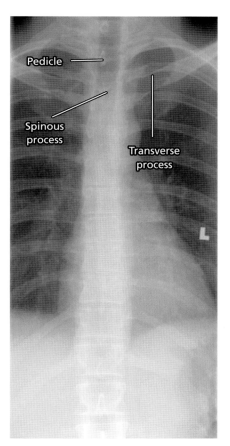

Figure 14.37 Anteroposterior view of narrow disc spaces at T6–T7, T7–T8, and T8–T9.

injection site for 20 minute periods help to decrease these untoward effects. The patient should be instructed to call immediately if any fever or other systemic symptoms occur that might suggest infection.

Complications

Discitis. With the use of prophylactic antibiotics, the incidence is 6.4/1000 cases.

Spinal cord trauma. Prolapse in patients with spinal stenosis or bulging discs may result in impingement.

Vertebral osteomyelitis.

Epidural abscess.

Hematoma or vascular injury.

Nerve root irritation.

Drug-related allergic reactions.

Inadvertent puncture of the thecal sac (which rarely results in arachnoiditis).

Headache.

Superior laryngeal nerve damage.

Laryngeal damage or penetration, particularly at the C2–C3 level.

Pneumothorax, particularly when operating at the C7–T1 level.

Vasovagal response due to compression of the carotid body when manually displacing the carotid artery. (Atropine should be available.)

Helpful hints

Although thoracic discography is performed less frequently than cervical or lumbar discography, it probably provides the most clinically useful information of the three. There are three reasons for this paradox: (1) less is known about the thoracic disc in health and disease; (2) thoracic disc herniation is less common than lumbar or cervical disc herniation; and (3) clinicians are less comfortable attributing pain symptoms to thoracic discogenic disease. For these reasons, thoracic discography can help the clinician to determine whether a damaged thoracic disc is, in fact, the true source of the patient's pain. This information is extremely valuable, given the difficulty and risks associated with surgery on the thoracic discs.

Percutaneous block and lesioning of the suprascapular nerve

History

Suprascapular nerve block was used to assist in conditions that limit the initiation of the range of motion of the shoulder, such as adhesive capsulitis, calcific tendinitis and bursitis. The advent of corticosteroids allowed suprascapular nerve blocking with local anesthetic and steroids. Consequently, the use of a suprascapular nerve block as a diagnostic block for shoulder lesions continued. Recently, there

has been renewed interest in suprascapular nerve block to allow early range of motion and rehabilitation after shoulder reconstruction or joint replacement, especially with newer techniques available such as RF.

Anatomy

Origin of the suprascapular nerve

The suprascapular nerve arises from the upper trunk, which is formed by the union of the fifth and sixth cervical nerves as it constitutes the brachial plexus.

The course of the suprascapular nerve

From its origin, the nerve runs laterally beneath the trapezius and the omohyoid muscle, and enters the supraspinatus fossa through the suprascapular notch. Then it runs below the superior transverse scapular ligament; it then passes beneath the supraspinatus muscle, and curves around the lateral border of the spine of the scapula into the infraspinatus fossa (Fig. 14.38).

Branches and innervation of the suprascapular nerve

In the supraspinatus fossa it gives off two branches to the supraspinatus muscle, and an articular filament to the shoulder joint. In the infraspinatus fossa it gives off two branches to the infraspinatus muscle, in addition to filaments to the shoulder joint and the scapula.

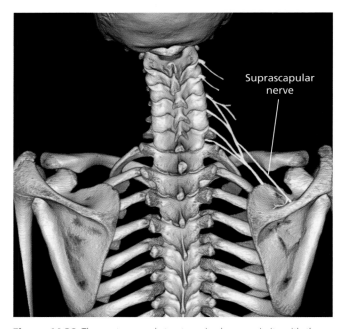

Figure 14.38 The anatomy and structures in close proximity with the suprascapular nerve.

Indications
- Frozen shoulder pain syndrome.
- Adhesive capsulitis of the shoulder.
- Calcific tendinitis involving the shoulder joint.
- Bursitis around the shoulder joint.
- Suprascapular nerve compression neuropathy.

Contraindications
- Local infection or sepsis.
- Coagulopathy.
- Vital functions instability.
- Psychopathologies.

Techniques of suprascapular nerve block and lesioning
Commonly performed techniques are as follows:
- diagnostic and therapeutic local anesthetic injections and/or steroids;
- pulsed RF.

Diagnostic and therapeutic local anesthetic injections and/or steroids
The suprascapular nerve block can be performed either by nonfluoroscopic or fluoroscopic techniques.

Nonfluoroscopic technique

Step 1. Prepare the patient before the procedure
The type of analgesia or sedation needs to be ascertained before performance of the invasive procedure. If a local anesthetic is planned, mild sedation is all that is necessary. If pulsed RF is planned, the patient needs to be awake to respond to the stimulation test. Intravenous fentanyl or midazolam may be used judiciously for the patient's comfort.

Step 2. Position and monitor the patient
1. The patient sits in an upright position on the table, if a (blind) nonfluoroscopic or ultrasound technique is performed.
2. Obtain an intravenous access if drugs need to be administered.
3. Vital signs monitoring is mandatory in unstable patients.
4. The area for needle entry is prepared in a sterile fashion.

Step 3. Equipment and drugs for suprascapular nerve block
Prepare and confirm that the following equipment, needles, and drugs are ready to be used for the procedure:
- 1½ inch, 25 gauge needle for skin infiltration;
- 5 ml syringe containing local anesthetic solution;
- 10 cm, 22 gauge needle for the nerve block (if preferred);
- 5 ml of 1% lidocaine;
- 5 ml syringe for the contrast solution;
- 3 ml of 5% bupivacaine for the nerve block;

- 40–80 mg depomedrol (methylprednisolone acetate or equivalent).

Step 4. Mark the surface landmarks for needle entry
1. Draw a line along the upper border of the spine of the scapula and mark the midpoint on that line.
2. Draw another line at this midpoint parallel to the spinous processes of the vertebral bodies.
3. Bisect the angle between these midpoint and parallel lines. Mark the point 2.5 cm superolaterally. This will be the entry point to approach to the suprascapular notch in a nonfluoroscopic technique (Fig. 14.39).

Step 5. Direction of the needle
Infiltrate the entry point with local anesthetic and insert a 10 cm 22 gauge needle perpendicularly and advance gently about 2.5 cm until a bony contact is made.
Note: do not advance deeper than that if bone is not contacted.

Step 6. Confirm the position of the needle
Gently "walk" superiorly and medially until the tip slips off the scapular body into the suprascapular notch. At this point, seek paresthesia in the suprascapular nerve distribution. If the paresthesia in the suprascapular nerve distribution is not identified, repeat the same maneuver directing the needle superiorly and laterally until the needle tip is positioned on the suprascapular nerve (Fig. 14.40).
Note: As the suprascapular nerve travels with the suprascapular artery and vein, an aspiration test is mandatory.

Step 7. Suprascapular nerve block
If the aspiration test is negative inject a combination of 3–5 ml of a local anesthetic and steroid solution after a small amount of contrast solution confirms the position.

Fluoroscopic technique
Follow the steps described above until the patient is put in the correct position for the fluoroscopic technique.

Step 1. Position the patient
Position the patient in the prone position with the ipsilateral arm hanging loosely off the side of the table.

Step 2. Visualization
1. Place the fluoroscope in PA and oblique views to identify the upper border of the scapula and the suprascapular notch (Fig. 14.41).
2. Identify the spine of the scapula and the acromion under fluoroscopy. Mark the point where the thicker acromion fuses with the thinner scapular spine.

Step 3. Mark the surface landmark for the point of entry
After identifying the suprascapular notch under fluoroscopy, infiltrate the entry point with local anesthetic.

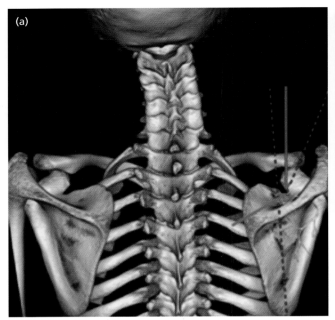
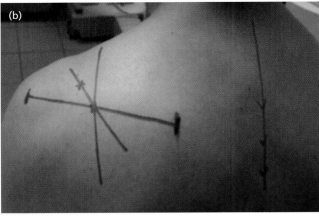

Figure 14.39 (a,b) The surface landmarks for suprascapular nerve block.

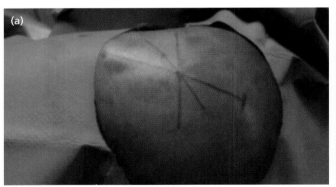
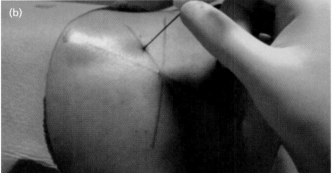

Figure 14.40 (a,b) Direction of the needle for suprascapular nerve block.

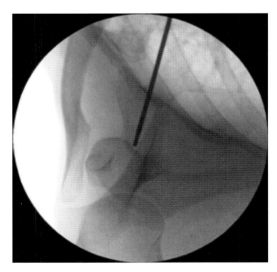

Figure 14.41 Identify the suprascapular notch.

Step 4. Direction of the needle
1. Insert a 5–10 cm needle in an inferior trajectory toward the body of the scapula and advance until a bony contact with the scapula is made at a depth of approximately 1 inch.
2. Gently "walk" superiorly and medially until the tip walks off the scapular body into the suprascapular notch. A paresthesia is often encountered as the needle tip enters the notch (Fig. 14.42).

Step 5. Confirm the position of the needle
After paresthesia confirms the correct location of the suprascapular nerve, aspirate for blood or air. If the aspiration test is negative, inject contrast solution (1–2 ml) to confirm the spread of the contrast solution in the suprascapular notch and fossa (Fig. 14.43).

Step 6. Injection of local anesthetic
If the needle tip is correctly placed, inject 5 ml of a combination of local anesthetic and/or steroid solution.

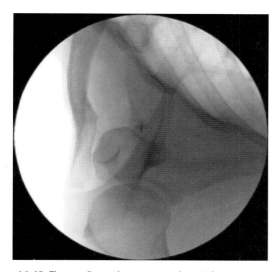

Figure 14.42 The needle on the suprascapular notch.

Technique for pulsed RF

The suprascapular nerve is a mixed nerve, thus both motor and sensory stimulation tests will provide a correct placement of the electrode tip.

Initiation of the procedure. Steps 1–5 are as described above.

Step 6. Stimulation test
1. First, stimulate the nerve at 2 Hz, with 0.1–1.5 V. This should produce local muscle contractions in the supraspinous and infraspinous muscles. These can be felt with palpation quite easily when compared to observation alone.
2. Then seek paresthesia in the distribution at the suprascapular nerve. To do that, one needs to stimulate the nerve at 50–100 Hz with 0.1–1.5 V. Generally the patient feels paresthesia at the 0.5 V setting. The patient should be awake to respond to the stimulation at this stage.

Step 7. Pulsed RF
1. Next, when the patient confirms paresthesia in the distribution of the nerve tested, inject 1%, 1 ml lidocaine. Wait for 5 minutes.
2. Perform pulsed RF at 45 V for 4 cycles of 120 seconds, at a temperature not to exceed 42 °C (Fig. 14.44).

Ultrasound technique

The ultrasound technique is based on the description by Harmon and Hearty (2007).

Step 1. Position the patient
The patient is placed in a sitting position.

Step 2. Choice of equipment
Use the ultrasound transducer (high-frequency linear, 6–13 MHz, 38 mm broadband linear-array transducer). Insert this into a sterile sheath containing ultrasound gel. A thin layer of sterile gel is placed between the draped ultrasound transducer and the skin.

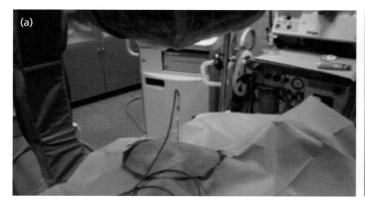
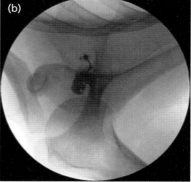

Figure 14.43 Spread of the contrast material around the suprascapular nerve.

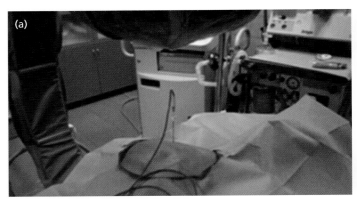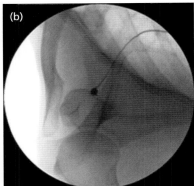

Figure 14.44 (a,b) The electrode in position under fluoroscopy.

Step 3. Visualization
1. An initial scan is performed in the sagittal orientation at the superior medial border of the scapula to identify the pleura (4 cm depth). Then proceed laterally scanning with this orientation. The ultrasound transducer is then moved around to visualize the scapular spine.
Note: this is done by moving the transducer cephalad. The suprascapular fossa then is identified.
2. The supraspinatus muscle and the bony fossa underneath the ultrasound transducer should be identified and the transducer slowly moved laterally (to maintain a transverse orientation) to locate the suprascapular notch. The suprascapular nerve is commonly seen as a round, hyperechoic structure 4 cm beneath the transverse scapular ligament in the scapular notch. The nerve has a diameter of 200 mm.

Step 4. Direction of the needle
A 21 gauge, 50 mm B-bevel needle is inserted along the longitudinal axis of the ultrasound beam. The needle should be visualized in its full course. The end point for injection is an ultrasound image demonstrating the needle tip in proximity to the suprascapular nerve in the suprascapular notch.

Step 5. Confirm the position of the needle
Electrical stimulation may or may not be used to identify the nerve.

Step 6. Injection of local anesthetic
A mixture of local anesthetic (4 ml) and triamcinolone (80 mg) is injected at this point. The injection and spread of local anesthetic need to be visualized.

Step 7. Postprocedure care
After any one of the above procedures is completed, the patient needs to be observed for up to 2 hours. Monitoring of vital signs is mandatory. In addition, the pain relief should be objectively documented. After a satisfactory observation, the patient should be discharged with appropriate and adequate instructions given to their escort. Written instructions are preferable for emergencies and are helpful to the patient and their family.

Complications
• **Pneumothorax**
The most common complication of the suprascapular block is pneumothorax. It occurs especially if the block is performed by a nonfluoroscopic technique. There is also a lesser risk of producing pneumothorax under fluoroscopy.
• **Inadvertent puncture of the suprascapular artery or vein**
There is a potential for the inadvertent puncture of the suprascapular artery or vein, which are in close proximity with the nerve. An aspiration test is mandatory. Local anesthetic toxicity may develop.

Helpful hints
Fluoroscopic guidance is preferred for suprascapular nerve block.

For patients with pulmonary pathologies, one needs to be extremely careful.

Do not perform this procedure if pulmonary infection is suspected.

Percutaneous block and lesioning of the thoracic sympathetic chain

History
In 1925, Leriche and Fontaine first used a paravertebral approach for sympathetic block with procaine on patients with severe pain due to angina pectoris, causalgia, and reflex sympathetic dystrophy. In 1926, Mandl described paravertebral blocks for diagnosis and treatment of visceral pain and anginal pain. That same year, Swetlow used 85% alcohol with the same technique. In 1954, Kux devised a transthoracic approach in which an endoscope was used for electrocoagulation. In 1996, Wilkinson devised a technique for RF thermocoagulation through percutaneous needle placement

for ablation of the T2 and T3 blocks with minimal complications. In 2001, M. Stanton-Hicks described a modified approach described as the costotransverse approach.

Anatomy

Origin of the sympathetic fibers of the thoracic region

Sympathetic nerves originate inside the vertebral column, toward the middle of the spinal cord in the intermediolateral cell column (or lateral horn), beginning at the first thoracic segment of the spinal cord, and are thought to extend to the second or third lumbar segments. Because its cells begin in the thoracic and lumbar regions of the spinal cord, the sympathetic nervous system is said to have a thoracolumbar outflow. Axons of these nerves leave the spinal cord through the anterior rootlet/root. They pass near the spinal (sensory) ganglion, where they enter the anterior rami of the spinal nerves. However, unlike somatic innervation, they quickly separate out through white rami connectors (so called from the shiny white sheaths of myelin around each axon) that connect to either the paravertebral (which lie near the vertebral column) or prevertebral (which lie near the aortic bifurcation) ganglia extending alongside the spinal column.

Course of the sympathetic fibers

The preganglionic fibers of the thoracic sympathetics exit the intervertebral foramen along with respective thoracic paravertebral nerves. After exiting the intervertebral foramen, the thoracic paravertebral nerve gives off a recurrent branch that loops back through the foramen to provide innervation to the spinal ligaments, meninges, and its corresponding vertebra. The thoracic paravertebral nerve also interfaces with the thoracic sympathetic chain through the myelinated preganglionic fibers of the white rami communicantes and the unmyelinated postganglionic fibers of the gray rami communicantes. At the level of the thoracic sympathetic ganglia, preganglionic and postganglionic fibers synapse, and some of the postganglionic fibers return to their respective somatic nerves via the gray rami communicantes. These fibers provide sympathetic innervations to the vasculature, sweat glands, and pilomotor muscles of the skin. Other thoracic sympathetic postganglionic fibers travel to the cardiac plexus and course up and down the sympathetic trunk to terminate in distant ganglia.

The first thoracic ganglion is fused with the lower cervical ganglion to help make up the stellate ganglion. As the chain moves caudad, it changes its position, the upper thoracic ganglia lying just beneath the rib and the lower thoracic ganglia moving farther anterior, to rest along the posterolateral surface of the vertebral body. The pleural space lies lateral and anterior to the thoracic sympathetic chain. Given the proximity of the thoracic somatic nerves to the thoracic sympathetic chain, the potential exists for both neural pathways to be blocked during blockade of the thoracic sympathetic ganglion. The median location of the T2 ganglia is 2 mm rostral to the midpoint of the T2 vertebral body on the right side (range 1–7 mm), between the head of the ribs. The left T2 ganglion's location is 1.5 mm (range 1–2 mm) rostral to the midpoint of the vertebral body. The T3 ganglia are located 2 mm (range 2–3 mm) rostral to the midpoint of the T3 vertebral body bilaterally (Fig. 14.45).

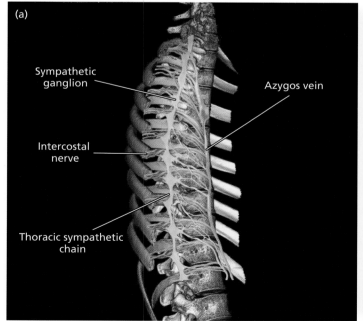
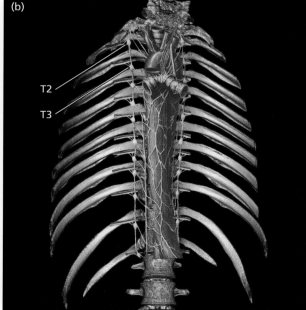

Figure 14.45 (a,b) The thoracic sympathetic chain and the structures in close proximity.

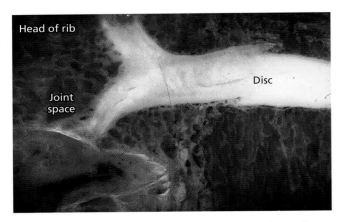

Figure 14.46 Each typical rib articulates with the disc and two adjacent vertebral body margins in the costovertebral joint. (Courtesy of J. Taylor.)

Anatomical relationship of ribs and their articulation

The most medial parts of the ribs include the head, neck, tubercle (articular eminence and a nonarticular eminence), and curved body of the shaft and the initial part of the costal groove.

The costal articulations should be noted because these, together with the tubercle and head of each rib, comprise the radiologic landmarks used in this technique. It also should be noted that a line drawn from the tubercle to the head of each rib is almost parallel with the neck of each rib (Fig. 14.46).

Indications
- Complex regional pain syndrome type 1 and 2.
- Postamputation pain syndrome of upper extremity.
- Neuropathic pain syndromes of upper extremity.
- Hyperhidrosis.
- Periperal vascular disease.
    (a) Arteriosclerotic disorders.
    (b) Raynaud's disease or phenomenon.
- Acute vascular disorders.
    (a) Posttraumatic vasospasm.
    (b) Acute arterial occlusion.
    (c) Acute venous thrombosis.
    (d) Frostbite of the upper extremities.
- Acute herpes zoster and postherpetic neuralgia.
- Visceral pain in the thoracic and upper abdominal region.
- Angina pectoris.
- Cancer pain associated with sympathetically mediated pain.

Contraindications
- Local or systemic infection.
- Coagulopathy.
- Hypotension.

- Anatomic distortion.
- Thoracic aortic aneurysm.
- Respiratory insufficiency.

Step 1. Prepare the patient before the procedure
The patient should be told why the procedure is being done and what to expect. All complications and side effects related to the procedure should be explained in detail, before the procedure. Valid, written consent should be obtained.

The type of analgesia or sedation needs to be ascertained before performance of the invasive procedure. Intravenous fentanyl, midazolam, and/or propofol may be used judiciously for the patient's comfort. Patient response should be monitored and the dosage titrated to establish a level of sedation allowing the patient to be conversant and responsive after needle placements. Because the disc is avascular, there is an increased risk of disc space infection and most discographers use prophylactic antibiotics. Prophylactic intravenous antibiotics 20 minutes before the procedure are recommended.

Step 2. Position and monitor the patient
1. Place the patient prone on the table. Place a pillow under the chest to flex the thoracolumbar spine. The patient's head is turned to the side, with the arms resting adjacent to the body.
2. Obtain an intravenous access through a large vein. Before the procedure 500–1000 ml of electrolyte solution should be administered.
3. Administer oxygen by nasal cannula.
4. Monitor the vital signs noninvasively throughout the procedure.
5. Prep and drape the area in a sterile fashion.
6. Sedation may be used to relax the patient; however, the patient should be awake enough to respond to the physician's questions.

Step 3. Drugs and equipment for thoracic sympathetic block
- 25 gauge, 1½ inch needle for local infiltration;
- 5 ml syringe for local anesthesia;
- 5–10 cm, 22 gauge needle for the thoracic sympathetic block;
- 5 ml syringe for the block;
- 1% lidocaine for skin infiltration;
- 0.5% bupivacaine for the block;
- nonparticulate steroid solution;
- contrast solution, such as iohexol;
- 3–6% phenol in saline or glycerine for the neurolytic block.
For RF lesioning:
- 5–10 cm 2 mm active-tip electrode;
- RF machine with cables.

Step 4. Visualization

1. The C-arm is placed in the anteroposterior position first to visualize the C7–T1, T2, T3 vertebral bodies (Fig. 14.47).
2. Rotate the C-arm oblique about 20° toward the ipsilateral side, then move in a cephalocaudal direction approximately 20° to open the intervertebral space of the T2 vertebral body. The tip of the triangle formed by the T2 vertebral body and the third rib is the target point (Fig. 14.48).

Step 5. Direction of the needle

1. Infiltrate the skin with 1% lidocaine at the entry point on the skin at the lateral edge of the T2 vertebral body just cephalad to the third rib.
2. Advance the needle under tunneled vision through the entry point toward the target until it has bony contact with the vertebral body. The needle should always stay in close contact with the lateral edge of the T2 vertebral body (Fig. 14.49).
3. Position the C-arm laterally and advance the needle until the posterior half of the T2 vertebral body (Fig. 14.50).
4. Position the C-arm again to the PA position to confirm that the needle is hugging the T2 vertebral body (Fig. 14.51).

Step 6. Confirm the position of the needle

1. After confirming the needle position, inject 2 ml of contrast solution. The contrast solution should not spread into the pleural space and illuminate the dome of the lung. If this happens, remove the needle and redirect (Fig. 14.52).
2. If the contrast solution spreads into the lung, the procedure has to be stopped immediately and the patient should be followed for at least 24 hours for evidence of pneumothorax. If the needle tip is on the pleura or inside

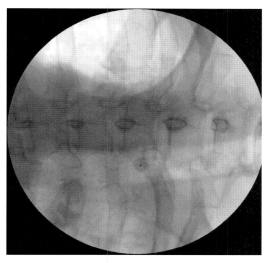

Figure 14.47 Posteroanterior view of the region.

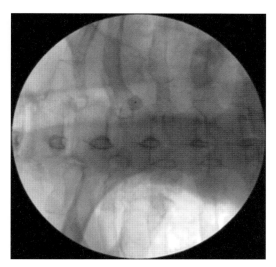

Figure 14.49 Needle under tunneled vision.

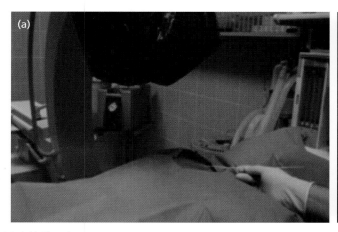

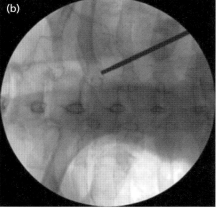

Figure 14.48 (a,b) Site of entry.

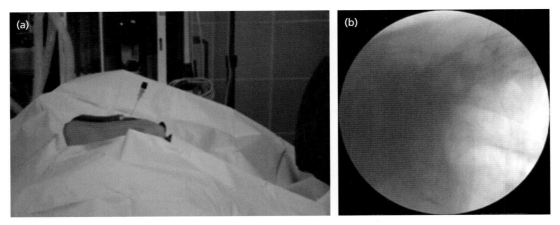

Figure 14.50 (a,b) Needle under lateral view.

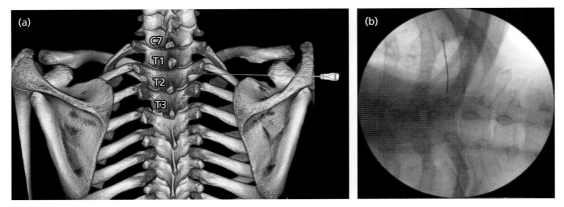

Figure 14.51 (a,b) The needle hugging the T2 vertebra under PA view.

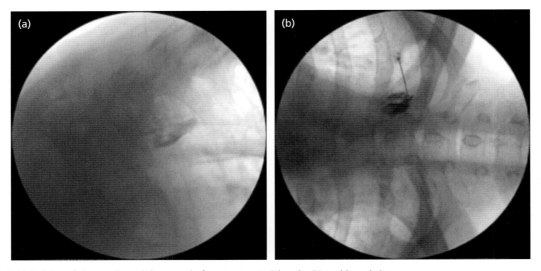

Figure 14.52 (a,b) Position of the needle and the spread of contrast material under PA and lateral views.

the lung, the patient will cough. The procedure should be halted.

Step 7. Thoracic sympathetic block
1. For a diagnostic or prognostic block inject 5 ml of a mixture of 40 mg/ml triamcinolone and 0.5% bupivacaine.
2. In cancer patients, 5 ml of 6% phenol in glycerine for neurolysis can be injected. We do not recommend this.

RF lesioning of the thoracic sympathetic chain

Step 8. Confirm the position of the electrode
1. If the diagnostic or prognostic block is beneficial, RF lesioning of the thoracic sympathetic chain is the appropriate next step.
2. The electrode tip is placed at the target site similar to the description given above for diagnostic T2–T3 block.

Step 9. Stimulation test
Apply sensory stimulation at 50 Hz and 2 V to confirm that there is no stimulation of the intercostal nerves. If paresthesia occurs in the intercostal nerves, the electrode should be redirected.

Step 10. RF lesioning
After confirming the appropriate position of the tip of the electrode, lesioning is performed at 80°C for 60–90 seconds.

Note: a curved electrode is preferred by many because the electrode tip is directed in a medial and caudal direction about 15° to make a second lesion (Fig. 14.53).

Step 11. Postprocedure care
After completing the procedure, observe the patient for at least 2 hours. The recovery and observation time depends on the sedation and analgesia used, as well as facilitating the assessment of any impairment of intellectual function, toler-

ance of oral intake, assessment of the immediate results of the neural blockade, and pain response to the procedure.

If pneumothorax is suspected, then a plain radiography is necessary.

The patient should be provided with all necessary instructions, including who to call or where to go for any postprocedure urgent/emergency care. The patient should be discharged accompanied by a responsible adult. The patient should not be allowed to drive themselves. They should also be informed that if changes like increases in body temperature, fever, and pain occur, they should again apply immediately.

Complications
• **Pneumothorax**
Pneumothorax is the most important complication. The location of the parietal pleura varies from patient. To prevent pneumothorax, the needle should always be in contact with the vertebral body, and should not be advanced more than the posterior half of the T2 vertebral body. Pneumothorax may not be diagnosed immediately. Shortness of breath and pain on the lateral side of the chest are the first signs of pneumothorax. A chest radiography should be ordered to rule out pneumothorax.
• **Inadvertent puncture of intercostal artery and veins**
The thoracic sympathetic pain is in close proximity to the intercostal artery and veins. An aspiration test is mandatory before injecting any solution.
• **Neuritis of the intercostal nerve**
Neurolytic agents may cause neuritis of the intercostal nerves. Neuritis may also occur after RF lesioning. Sensory and motor stimulation before lesioning is necessary to minimize the risk of neuritis. There should be no paresthesia or muscle contraction during the stimulation.
• **Other complications**
Inadverdent puncture of the thoracic ductus, thyroid gland, trachea, or esophagus are very rare complications that should not occur with the appropriate use of fluoroscopy.

Helpful hints
RF lesioning should not be the first choice for thoracic sympathetic block. First, a diagnostic and prognostic block using a combination of local anesthetic and steroid should be performed.

Thoracic sympathetic block should only be performed by experienced physicians.

Percutaneous block of the intercostal nerve

History
The intercostal nerves supply the major parts of the skin and musculature of the chest and abdominal wall. The block of

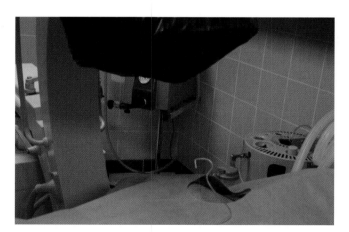
Figure 14.53 RF lesioning of the thoracic sympathetic chain.

these nerves was first described by Braun in 1907. By the 1940s, clinicians noticed that intercostal nerve blocks could favorably effect a reduction in pulmonary complications and in narcotic requirements after upper abdominal surgery. In 1981, continuous intercostal nerve block was introduced to overcome the problems associated with repeated multiple injections.

Anatomy

The intercostal nerves are formed from the anterior divisions of the thoracic spinal nerves from T1 to T11. Each intercostal nerve is connected with the adjoining ganglion of the sympathetic trunk by a gray and a white ramus communicans. The intercostal nerves are distributed chiefly to the thoracic somatic and visceral structures and abdominal peritoneum. They differ from the anterior divisions of the spinal nerves in that they pursue an independent course without forming a plexus.

The first upper two intercostal nerves supply fibers to the upper limb in addition to the upper thoracic structure; the next four, T3, T4, T5, and T6, are limited in their distribution to the parietal structures of the thorax; the lower five, T7, T8, T9, T10, and T11, supply the somatic structures of the thorax and abdomen. The seventh intercostal nerve is located at the xyphoid process, at the lower end of the sternum. The tenth intercostal nerve terminates at the umbilicus. The twelfth (subcostal) thoracic is distributed to the abdominal wall and groin.

Formation of the intercostal nerve and its relations

The anterior division of the first thoracic nerve divides into two branches. The larger branch, which leaves the thorax in front of the neck of the first rib, and enters the brachial plexus. The other smaller branch (of the first intercostal nerve) runs along the first intercostal space, and ends in the front of the chest as the first anterior cutaneous branch of the thorax.

The first intercostal nerve rarely gives off a lateral cutaneous branch; but sometimes it sends a small branch to communicate with the intercostobrachial nerve.

The second thoracic nerve frequently receives a connecting branch, which ascends over the neck of the second rib. They pass forward in the intercostal spaces below the intercostal vessels. At the back of the chest, they lie between the pleura and the posterior intercostal membranes, but soon pierce the latter and run between the two planes of intercostal muscles as far as the middle of the rib.

They then enter the substance of the internal intercostal muscle, and run as far as the costal cartilages. They remain in the inner surfaces of the muscles and lie between the innermost intercostal muscles and the pleura.

Near the sternum, they cross in front of the internal mammary artery and transverse thoracic muscle, pierce the internal intercostal muscles, the anterior intercostal membranes, and pectoralis major, and supply the integument of the front of the thorax and over the breast, forming the anterior cutaneous branches of the thorax; the branch from the second nerve unites with the anterior supraclavicular nerves of the cervical plexus.

Numerous slender muscular filaments supply the intercostals, the subcostals, the levatores costarum, the serratus posterior superior, and the transversus thoracis. At the front of the thorax, some of these branches cross the costal cartilages from each intercostal space to the contralateral side.

Lateral cutaneous branches are derived from the intercostal nerves, about midway between the vertebrae and sternum; they pierce the external intercostal muscle and serratus anterior, and divide into anterior and posterior branches.

The anterior branches run forward to the side and the front of the chest, supplying the skin and the breast; those of the fifth and sixth nerves supply the upper digitations of the external oblique muscle.

The posterior branches run backward, and supply the skin over the scapula and latissimus dorsi.

The lateral cutaneous branch of the second intercostal nerve does not divide, like the others, into an anterior and a posterior branch; it is named the intercostobrachial nerve.

The anterior divisions of the seventh, eighth, ninth, tenth, and eleventh thoracic intercostal nerves are continued anteriorly from the intercostal spaces into the abdominal wall; hence they are named thoraco-abdominal nerves.

They have the same arrangement as the upper ones as far as the anterior ends of the intercostal spaces, where they pass behind the costal cartilages, and between the internal oblique and transversus abdominis muscle, into the sheath of the rectus abdominis, which they perforate.

They supply the rectus abdominis and end as the anterior cutaneous branches of the abdomen; they supply the skin of the front of the abdomen.

The lower intercostal nerves supply the intercostales and abdominal muscles; the last three send branches to the serratus posterior inferior.

These pierce the intercostales externi and the obliquus externus abdominis muscles, in the same line as the lateral cutaneous branches of the upper thoracic nerves, and divide into anterior and posterior branches, which are distributed to the skin of the abdomen and back; the anterior branches supply the digitations of the obliquus externus abdominis, and extend downward and forward nearly as far as the margin of the rectus abdominis; the posterior branches pass backward to supply the skin over the latissimus dorsi.

The anterior division of the twelfth thoracic nerve (subcostal nerve) is larger than the others; it runs along the lower border of the twelfth rib, often giving a communicat-

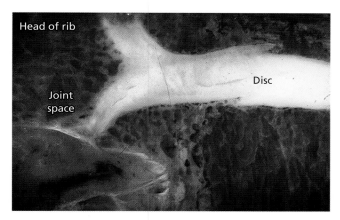

Figure 14.54 Each typical rib articulates with the disc and two adjacent vertebral body margins in the costovertebral joint. (Courtesy of J. Taylor.)

ing branch to the first lumbar nerve, and passes under the lateral lumbocostal arch.

It then runs in front of the quadratus lumborum, perforates the transversus, and passes forward between it and the obliquus internus to be distributed in the same manner as the lower intercostal nerves.

It communicates with the iliohypogastric nerve of the lumbar plexus, and gives a branch to the pyramidalis. It also gives off a lateral cutaneous branch that supplies sensory innervation to the skin over the hip (Figs 14.54–14.58).

The composition of the costovertebral joint in the thoracic region

Each typical rib articulates with the disc and two adjacent vertebral bodies at the costovertebral joint. The heads of

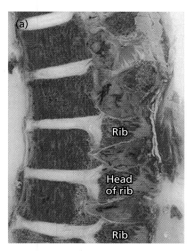
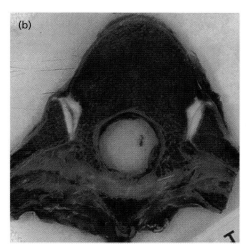

Figure 14.55 (a,b) Costovertebral joints in sagittal and transverse sections. (Courtesy of J. Taylor.)

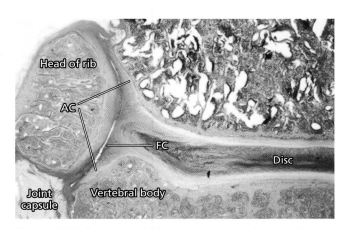

Figure 14.56 Costovertebral joint histology in coronal section. The synovial joint in a 100 μm stained section showing that hyaline articular cartilages (AC) line the head of the rib and the vertebral margins but (green-staining) fibrocartilage (FC) lines the disc surface. (Courtesy of J. Taylor.)

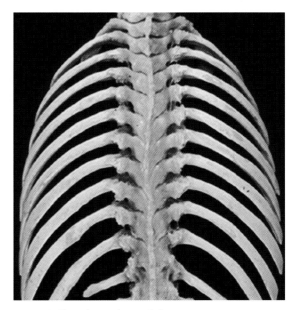

Figure 14.57 Thoracic vertebra and ribs.

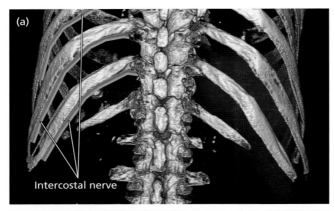

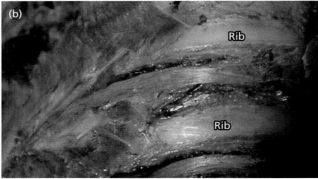

Figure 14.58 (a,b) Three-dimensional CT scan of the intercostal nerves and the nerves on the cadaver.

the second to tenth ribs each articulate with two vertebral bodies; the tubercles of these ribs articulate with the tips of transverse processes, supported by costotransverse ligaments. The heads of the first, eleventh and twelfth ribs each articulate with only one vertebra and the lowest two ribs have no costotransverse joints.

The sternocostal joint

The costal cartilages of the first seven pairs of ribs attach directly to the sternum; the costal cartilages of ribs 8–10 attach to the cartilages; the eleventh and twelfth pairs do not attach to any structures and are called "floating ribs."

The first ribs on both sides are short and make a rigid upper boundary for the thoracic inlet; the ring of the thoracic inlet is tough and is reinforced from above by the scalene muscles; the function of the thoracic inlet is to draw the lower ribs upwards during the phase of inspiration.

Indications

- Pain due to fracture of the rib.
- Postthoracotomy pain relief.
- For pain due to cancer in the intercostal region.
- Herpes zoster or postherpetic neuralgia in the thoracic region.

Contraindications

It is important to consider the following contraindications:
- local infection;
- coagulopathy;
- vital function instability;
- psychopathologies.

Technique of intercostal nerve block

Step 1. Prepare the patient before the procedure
The type of analgesia or sedation needs to be ascertained before performing the procedure. The type of sedation varies based on the status of the patient. If a diagnostic intercostal block with a local anesthetic is considered or a neurolytic agent is planned, deep sedation and analgesia may be appropriate for some patients. If RF thermocoagulation is planned, the patient needs to be awake to respond to the stimulation test. Intravenous fentanyl, midazolam, and/or propofol may be used judiciously for the patient's comfort.

Step 2. Position and monitor the patient
1. Place the patient in a prone position on the table.
2. Place a pillow under the abdomen to flex the thoracolumbar spine. The patient's head is turned to the side, and the arms are allowed to hang freely off each side of the table.
3. The intercostal nerve block may be performed at different sites of the ribs, i.e. from the front, middle, or posterior axillary line. The best method is to perform the block close to where the pain is most severe.
4. Insert an intravenous cannula for injecting medication.
5. Provide oxygen by nasal cannula.
6. Monitor vital signs (mandatory).
7. Prepare the area for needle entry in a sterile fashion.

Step 3. Drugs and equipment for intercostal nerve block
- 5 ml syringe for local infiltration;
- 1½ inch, 22 gauge needle with an extension line;
- 5 ml syringe for the intercostal block;
- 2 ml syringe for the contrast material;
- 1% lidocaine for local infiltration;
- 2 ml contrast solution (iohexol);
- 3 ml 0.05% bupivacaine and 20 mg methylprednisolone for each level if planned;
- 3 ml of 6% phenol in saline or glycerine or iohexol for the neurolytic block (only for cancer patients).

If pulsed RF is planned, use an RF machine with 2 mm electrodes.

Step 4. Mark the surface landmarks for the needle entry
1. Draw a vertical line through the posterior thoracic spinous processes. Draw another line approximately 7–8 cm from this line laterally to mark the posterior axillary line (Fig. 14.59).
2. Identify the inferior edge of each rib using a skin-marking pen.

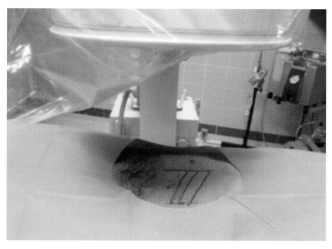
Figure 14.59 Surface landmarks for intercostal nerve block.

Step 5. Visualization

1. Place the C-arm first in a PA position; identify the ribs in this view. Then rotate the C-arm obliquely until the rib is clearly visualized with the intercostal space opened inferiorly. It is important to confirm the inferior edge of the rib under fluoroscopy (Fig. 14.60).

2. Next, pull the skin up and over the lower edge of the rib with the index finger of the left hand. Infiltrate the skin over the lower edge of the rib.

Step 6. Direction of the needle

1. A 22 gauge, 1½ inch needle with an extension line is inserted toward the rib, first perpendicular to the skin over the rib in between the index and middle fingers (Fig. 14.61).

2. Advance the needle toward the lower edge of the rib under fluoroscopy. First, a bony contact is made with the

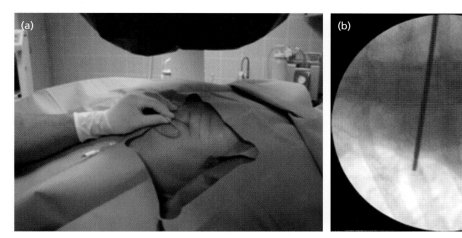
Figure 14.60 (a,b) Entry point for intercostal nerve block.

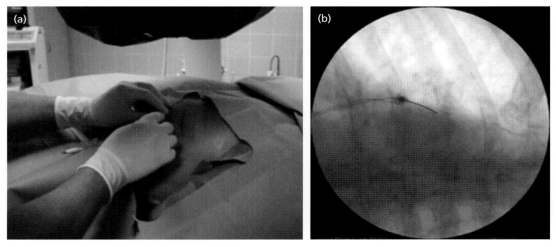
Figure 14.61 (a,b) Entry point under fluoroscopy and direction of the needle.

rib. Hold this position of the needle firm with the left hand on the patient's back. This is crucial.

3. Walk slightly off the lower edge of the rib until the resistance to the needle tip is lost. Advance slightly not deeper than 2 mm under the rib.

Step 7. Confirm the position of the needle
1. After confirmation of the needle under fluoroscopy, perform the following.
2. Aspirate first. If the aspiration test is negative, inject 2 ml of contrast solution. The contrast solution should spread along the lower edge of the rib as a smooth line. If the contrast solution is within the pleura, the patient may cough and the solution will be seen spreading in the interpleural space (Fig. 14.62).
3. It is advisable that as the physician firmly holds the needle in place, the assistant injects the various drug solutions.

Step 8. Intercostal nerve block
After the injection of the contrast solution, perform the following.
1. Inject 40 mg of methylprednisolone in 5 ml of 0.5% bupivacaine.
2. For cancer patients, one could inject 6% phenol in glycerine, saline, or iohexol for neurolysis.
There are no data on pulsed or thermocoagulation lesioning of the intercostal nerves.

Step 9. Postprocedural care
Observe the patient for at least 2 hours after the procedure. Monitoring of vital signs is mandatory. In addition, objectively document the pain relief. If pneumothorax is suspected, then a plain radiography is necessary. After a satisfactory observation, discharge the patient with appropriate and adequate instructions given to their escort. Written instructions are preferable for emergencies and they are helpful to the patient and their family.

Complications

- **Pneumothorax**

The most important complication of intercostal block is pneumothorax. In many cases it improves spontaneously. Careful performance of the block reduces the risk of development of pneumothorax.

- **Intravascular injection**

The intercostal nerve is in very close proximity with the intercostal artery and vein. An aspiration test is mandatory. To prevent local anesthetic toxicity, the maximum amount of local anesthetic should not exceed 3 ml (Fig. 14.63).

- **Hypotension**

Hypotension may develop due to intravascular injection.

- **Prolonged paresthesia**

Paresthesia of the intercostal nerve may develop due to the injection of neurolytics. Thus the first step even in cancer patients is the injection of a local anesthetic and steroid combination.

Helpful hints

Large volumes of local anesthetics should not be used for intercostal blocks in a short period, because they are more readily absorbed at this site than at any other sites. The risks associated with this block are intravascular injection and pneumothorax. Pneumothorax can be prevented if the operator is careful, slow, and confirms the anatomy of the areas before injecting the local anesthetic solution.

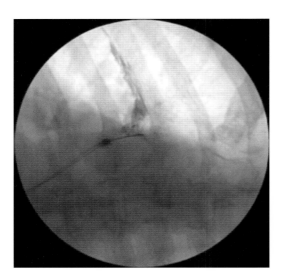

Figure 14.62 Spread of the contrast material around the intercostal nerve.

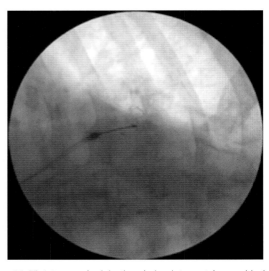

Figure 14.63 Intravascular injection during intercostal nerve block.

Resuscitative equipment and skilled personnel should always be available for cardiorespiratory collapse during the technique.

Further reading

Abram, S.E. & Boas, R.A. (1993) Sympathetic and viscera nerve blocks. In *Clinical Procedures in Anesthesia and Intensive Care* (ed. Benumof, J.L.), pp. 787–805. Philadelphia, PA: J.B. Lippincott.

Aprill, C. & Bogduk, N. (1992) High intensity zone. *British Journal of Radiology* **65**, 361–369.

Bogduk, N. (1997) Low back pain. In *Clinical Anatomy of the Lumbar Spine and Sacrum*, 3rd edition (ed. Bogduk, N.), pp. 187–214. New York: Churchill Livingstone.

Braun, H. (1914) *Local Anesthesia: Its Scientific Basis and Practical Use*. Philadelphia, PA: Lea & Febiger.

Cathelin, M.F. (1901) Mode d'action de la cocaine injecte daus l'escape epidural par le procede du canal sacre. *Comptes Rendues des Seances de la Societe de Biologie et de ses Filliales* **43**, 487.

Chua, W.H. (1994) Clinical anatomy of the thoracic dorsal rami. Presented at the 2nd Annual Scientific Meeting of the International Spinal Injection Society (ISIS), Minneapolis, MN, October 19, 1994.

Crock, H.V. (1970) A reappraisal of intervertebral disc lesions. *The Medical Journal of Australia* **1**, 983–989.

Curbelo, M.M. (1949) Continuous peridural segmental anesthesia by means of a ureteral catheter. *Current Researches in Anesthesia and Analgesia* **28**, 12–23.

Elias, M. (2000) The anterior approach for thoracic sympathetic ganglion block using a curved needle. *Pain Clinic* **12**(1), 17–24.

Erdine, S. & Talu, G.K. (2008) Sympathetic blocks of the thorax. In *Interventional Pain Management, Image-Guided Procedures* (ed. Raj, P., et al.), pp. 255–266. Philadelphia, PA: Saunders-Elsevier.

Ghormley, R.K. (1933) Low back pain: with special reference to the articular facets, with presentation of an operative procedure. *Journal of the American Medical Association* **101**, 1773–1777.

Harmon, D. & Hearty, C. (2007) Ultrasound guided suprascapular nerve block technique. *Pain Practice* **10**(6), 743–746.

Hingson, R.A. & Edwards, W.B. (1942) Continuous caudal anesthesia during labor and delivery. *Anesthesia and Analgesia* **21**(6), 301–310.

Hirsch, C. (1948) An attempt to diagnose level of disc lesion clinically by disc puncture. *Acta Orthop Scandinavica* **18**, 131–140.

Kux, E. (1954) *Thorakoskopische Eingriffe an Merran System*. Stuttgart: Georg Thieme Verlag.

Leriche, R. & Fontaine, R. (1934) L'aniskesie isolee du ganglion etile; sa technique, ses indications, ses resultats. *La Presse Médicale* **42**, 849–850.

Lindblom, K. (1948) Diagnostic puncture of the intervertebral discs in sciatica. *Acta Orthopaedica Scandinavica* **17**, 231–239.

Linton, S.J., Hellsing, A.L. & Hallden, K. (1998) Population based study of spinal pain among 35–45-year-old individuals. *Spine* **23**, 1457–1463.

Manchikanti, L., Staats, P.S., Singh, V., et al. (2003) Evidence-based practice guidelines for interventional techniques in the management of chronic spinal pain. *Pain Physician* **6**, 3–80.

Mandl, F. (1926) *Die Paravertebral Injection*. Vienna: J. Springer.

Plancarte-Sanchez, R., Guajardo-Rosas, J. & Guillen-Nunez, R. (2005) Sympathetic block: thoracic and lumbar. *Techniques in Regional Anesthesia and Pain Management* **9**, 91–96.

Raj, P.P. (2002) *Textbook of Regional Anesthesia*. New York: Churchill Livingstone.

Roofe, P.G. (1940) Innervation of the anulus fibrosus and posterior longitudinal ligament. *Archives of Neurology and Psychiatry* **44**, 100–103.

Sachs, B.L., Vanharanta, H., Spivey, M.A., et al. (1987) Dallas discogram description. A new classification of CT/discography in low-back disorders. *Spine* **12**, 287–294.

Sicard, M.A. (1901) Les injections medicamenteuse extradurales par voie saracoccygiene. *Comptes Renues des Seances de la Societe de Biologie et de ses Filliales* **53**, 396.

Skabelund, C. & Racz, G.B. (1999) Indications and techniques of thoracic 2 and thoracic 3 neurolysis. *Current Review of Pain* **3**, 400–405.

Stanton-Hicks, M. (1990) Blocks of the sympathetic nervous system. In *Pain and the Sympathetic Nervous System* (ed. Stanton-Hicks, M.), pp. 125–164. Boston: Kluwer Academic.

Stanton-Hicks, M. (2001) Thoracic sympathetic block: a new approach. *Techniques in Regional Anesthesia and Pain Management* **5**(3), 94–98.

Stanton-Hicks, M. (2007) Complications of sympathetic blocks for extremity pain. *Techniques in Regional Anesthesia and Pain Management* **11**, 148–151.

Stevens, R.A. & Ruesch, S. (1998) Sympathetic blocks of the upper extremity and their complications. *Techniques in Regional Anesthesia and Pain Management* **2**(3), 130–136.

Stolker, R.J., Vervest, A.C.M. & Groen, G.J. (1999) Percutaneous facet denervation in chronic thoracic spinal pain. *Acta Neurochirurgica* **122**, 82–90.

Stolker, R.J., Vervest, A.C.M., Ramos, L.M.P. & Groen, G.J. (1994) Electrode positioning in thoracic percutaneous partial rhizotomy: an anatomical study. *Pain* **57**, 241–251.

Swetlow, G. (1926) Paravertebral alcohol block in cardiac pain. *American Heart Journal* **1**, 393–412.

Tuohy, E.B. (1944) Continuous spinal anesthesia: its usefulness and technique involved. *Anesthesiology* **5**, 142–148.

Waldman, S.D. (2001) Thoracic sympathetic ganglion block. In *Interventional Pain Management* (ed. Waldman, S.D.), pp. 400–401. Philadelphia, PA: Saunders.

Wilkinson, H. (1984) Percutaneous radiofrequency upper thoracic sympathectomy: a new technique. *Neurosurgery* **15**, 811–814.

Wilkinson, H.A. (1996) Percutaneous RF of upper thoracic sympathectomy. *Neurosurgery* **38**, 715–725.

15

Interventional Procedures for Visceral Pain in the Thoraco-Abdominal Region

Percutaneous block and lesioning of the splanchnic nerve

History

Splanchnic nerve neurolysis or neurolytic celiac plexus block for the treatment of chronic abdominal pain was first reported by Kappis in 1914. In 1918, Wendling was the first to report an anterior transabdominal technique. This technique was considered dangerous and was soon abandoned. However, when new imaging techniques became available, this anterior technique was brought back into clinical use. Computed tomography (CT) and ultrasound-guided methods have already proved to be an effective imaging technique for citing needles in celiac plexus block. Traditionally a CT-guided posterolateral splanchnic block requires the bilateral oblique placement of needles transcrurally into the retrocrural space, which can be difficult and may be complicated by inaccurate needle placement.

Anatomy

Origin of the splanchnic nerve and its location

The splanchnic nerves are formed by the greater, lesser, and least splanchnic nerves. The greater splanchnic nerve is derived from the T5–T10 spinal roots. The lesser splanchnic nerve arises from the T10–T11 roots whereas the least splanchnic nerve arises from the T11–T12 spinal roots. All these three nerves coalesce in the celiac plexus. They are preganglionic fibers entering the celiac plexus.

These nerves lie in a narrow tubular space bounded by the vertebral body medially, pleura laterally, the posterior mediastinum ventrally, and crura of the diaphragm caudally (Figs 15.1 and 15.2).

Indications

- Pain syndromes involving upper abdominal viscera.
- Acute and chronic pancreatitis.
- Cancer pain from the upper abdominal viscera.

Contraindications

It is important to consider the following contraindications.
- Local infection.
- Coagulopathy.
- Vital function instability.
- Psychopathologies.
- Distorted anatomy due to tumor invasion.
- Abdominal aorta aneurysm.
- Pleural adhesions.

Techniques of splanchnic block and lesioning

There are two common approaches for the splanchnic block. Posterior approaches are as follows: (1) retrocrural approach (of Hartel); (2) paravertebral lateral approach.

Technique of retrocrural approach of Hartel

Step 1. Prepare the patient before the procedure
A recent CT scan is necessary to see the anatomical structures at the entry site or near the splanchnic nerve.

All patients should have an intravenous catheter inserted in a large vein and securely anchored. A 500 ml solution of dextrose-Ringer's lactate should be started, with at least 200 ml of solution infused before the procedure.

The type of analgesia or sedation needs to be ascertained before performance of the procedure. The type of sedation varies based on the technique being used. If a diagnostic epidural block with a local anesthetic is considered, some form of sedation and analgesia may be appropriate for some patients. Intravenous fentanyl, midazolam, and/or propofol may be used judiciously for the patient's comfort.

Pain-Relieving Procedures: The Illustrated Guide, First Edition. P. Prithvi Raj and Serdar Erdine.
© 2012 John Wiley & Sons, Ltd. Published 2012 by John Wiley & Sons, Ltd.

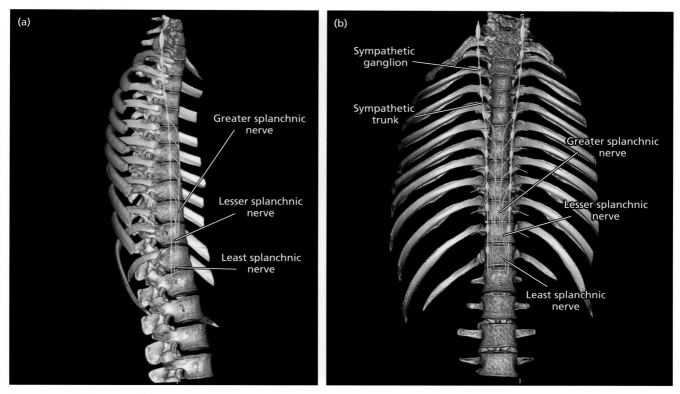

Figure 15.1 (a,b) Anatomy of the splanchnic nerves.

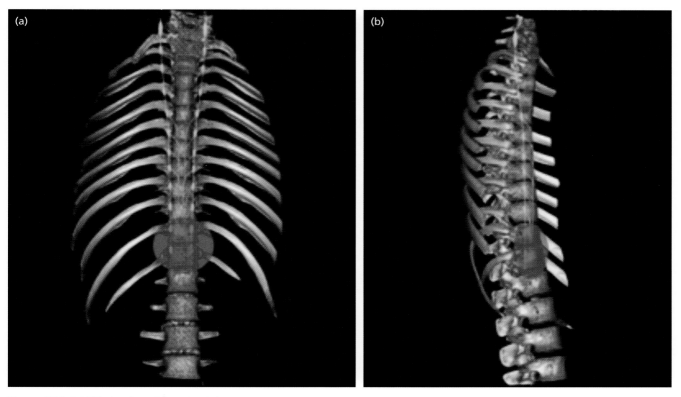

Figure 15.2 (a,b) The location of the splanchnic nerves.

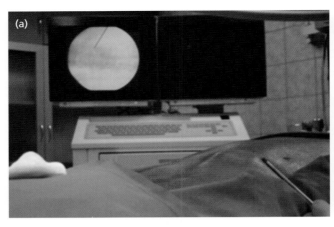
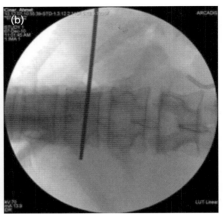

Figure 15.3 (a,b) Identify the ribs and T12 vertebral body.

Step 2. Position and monitor the patient
1. Place the patient prone on the table. Place a pillow under the abdomen to flex the thoracolumbar spine. The patient's head is turned to the side, and the arms are permitted to hang freely off each side of the table.
2. An intravenous cannula is inserted for medication injections.
3. Oxygen is provided by nasal cannula.
4. Monitoring of vital signs is mandatory.
5. The area for needle entry is prepared in a sterile fashion.

Step 3. Equipment and drugs for the technique
• 5 ml syringe for local anesthetic.
• 1½ inch needle for local infiltration.
• 10 ml syringe for the splanchnic block.
• Two 10 cm, 22 gauge needles for the splanchnic block.
• 5 ml syringe for the contrast material.
• 1% lidocaine for skin infiltration or for diagnostic injections.
• Nonionic contrast solution.
• 5 ml 0.5% bupivacaine and 40 mg methylprednisolone for each side.

For neurolysis
6% phenol in glycerine or saline or with iohexol.

Special equipment for radiofrequency
• Radiofrequency (RF) machine with cables and electrodes.
• Two 10 cm needles with 5 mm active tip electrode for the RF.

Step 4. Visualization
1. Place the C-arm for posteroanterior view of the T10–L2 region first. The anatomical landmarks to be determined are the twelfth ribs, and vertebral body of T12 and T11. To identify the T12 vertebral body easily one may first identify

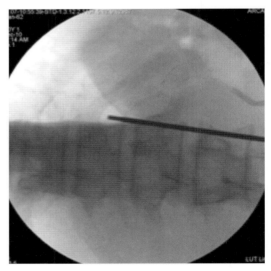

Figure 15.4 The entry point in oblique view.

the L4–L5 interspace and the posterior superior iliac crests under fluoroscopy and course upwards (Fig. 15.3).
2. Then rotate the C-arm approximately 45° to view the edge of the vertebral body and the diaphragm. The lateral side of the T12 vertebral body should be in view. Note the movement of the diaphragm during inspiration and expiration and note the image of the lateral side of the vertebral body during the expiration phase.

Step 5. Direction of the needle
1. The point of entry is at the junction of the rib and vertebral body (T10–T11) (Fig. 15.4).
2. Infiltrate the skin with 1% lidocaine. Insert a 10 cm, 22 gauge needle through the skin and advance under fluoroscopy using tunneled vision. After advancing 1–1.5 cm anteriorly, turn the C-arm laterally (Figs 15.5 and 15.6).

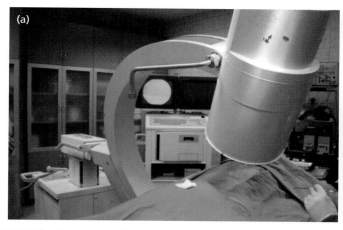
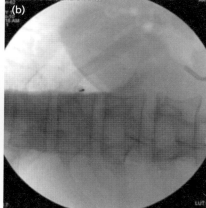

Figure 15.5 (a,b) Direction of the needle in "tunneled vision."

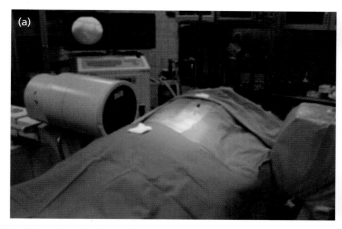
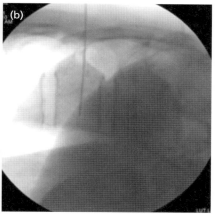

Figure 15.6 (a,b) Needle under lateral view.

3. Advance the needle until it reaches the junction of the anterior one-third and posterior two-thirds of the vertebral body. One should always have a bony contact with the vertebral body while advancing the needle.
4. Now position the C-arm for the posteroanterior view again to verify the bony contact of the needle with the vertebral body (Fig. 15.7).
5. Aspirate for blood or cerebrospinal fluid. If the aspiration test is positive, withdraw and redirect the needle. Repeat the procedure on the contralateral side (Fig. 15.8).

Step 6. Confirm the position of the needle
1. Inject 5 ml of contrast material. On the posteroanterior view the contrast material will spread adhering to the T10, T11, or T12 vertebral body. A smooth contoured image will appear in the lateral view. The tip on the lateral view should stay retrocrural to the aorta (Fig. 15.9).

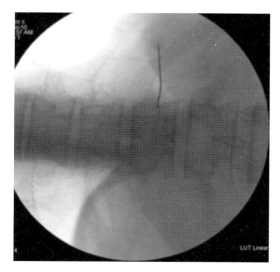

Figure 15.7 Needle position under posteroanterior view.

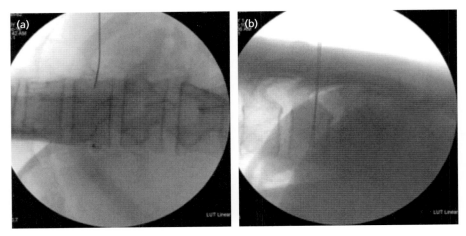

Figure 15.8 (a,b) Repeat the procedure for the contralateral side.

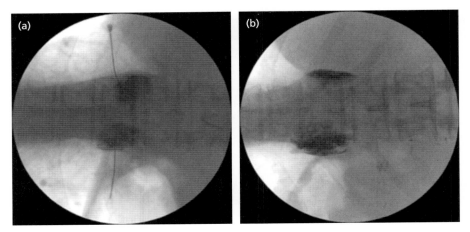

Figure 15.9 (a,b) Spread of the contrast material under posteroanterior and lateral views.

Step 7. Splanchnic block
1. For diagnostic and prognostic purposes inject 5 ml of 1% lidocaine bilaterally.
2. For neurolysis inject 5 ml of 6% phenol in glycerine or saline or with iohexol bilaterally. The risk of neuritis is higher with alcohol if that is preferred for neurolysis.
3. Repeat the same procedure on the contralateral side if bilateral block is required.

Technique of paravertebral transthoracic approach
Steps 1, 2, and 3 are as described above.

Step 4. Visualization
1. Identify the twelfth ribs under the posteroanterior view with the C-arm (Fig. 15.10).
2. Mark the entry point approximately 6 cm from the midline. Infiltrate the skin with 1% lidocaine.

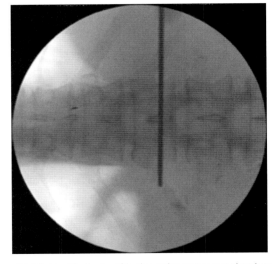

Figure 15.10 Identify the twelfth ribs under posteroanterior view.

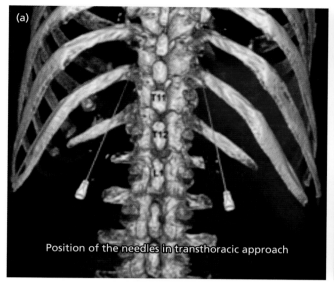

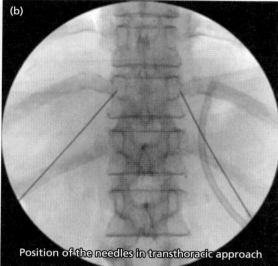

Figure 15.11 (a,b) Direction of the needles in transthoracic approach.

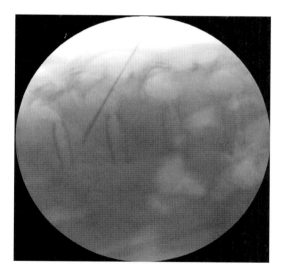

Figure 15.12 Position of the needles under lateral view.

Step 5. Direction of the needle
1. Advance the needle 45° toward the midline and about 35° cephalad towards the anterolateral aspect of the T11 vertebral body, passing beneath the eleventh rib (Fig. 15.11).
2. Then position the C-arm laterally.
3. Advance the needle until it reaches the junction of the anterior one-third and posterior two-thirds of the vertebral body. One should always have a bony contact with the vertebral body while advancing the needle (Fig. 15.12).

Step 6. Confirm the position of the needle
1. When confirmed to be in the right position, inject 2–3 ml of contrast solution. The contrast material should be con-

fined just lateral to the vertebral body on the posteroanterior view (Fig. 15.13).
2. Confirm the spread also in the lateral view.
3. Repeat the procedure for the contralateral side or bilateral block.
4. If the needle is too superficial the contrast solution may spread to the epidural space and if too deep it will contact the diaphragm (Fig. 15.14).

Step 7. Neurolytic block
After verifying the correct position of the needle, inject 3–6 ml of 6% phenol in glycerine or saline or iohexol for neurolysis.

Technique of RF lesioning of the splanchnic nerve
Because splanchnic nerves are contained in a narrow compartment they are accessible for RF lesioning. This approach has been described by P. Raj in 2002.

Steps 1 and 2 are as described above.

Step 3. Equipment for RF lesioning of the splanchnic nerves
- RF machine.
- 15 cm curved RF needle with 15 mm electrode tip.
- 14 gauge, 5 cm extracath (for skin entry before RF needle insertion).
- 2–10 ml plastic syringe with local anesthetic and steroids (for injections before lesion).
- 1–10 ml syringe with Omnipaque (contrast solution) (to confirm the correct placement the needle tip).
- 1–2 ml syringe with local anesthetic for skin infiltration.
- One extension set to help manipulate the needle and for easy injection of solutions.

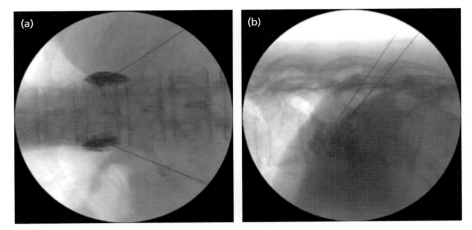

Figure 15.13 (a,b) Spread of the contrast material under posteroanterior and lateral view.

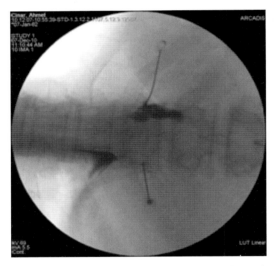

Figure 15.14 Needle in correct position on the right and near the pleura on the left side.

Step 4. Visualization
1. In the prone position, the T12 vertebral body is identified in the posteroanterior view of the fluoroscope. Keeping a mark on the T12 or T11 vertebra, the C-arm is moved to an oblique position (about 45 °C).
2. The edge of the diaphragm lateral to the vertebral body is viewed. Its movement during inspiration and expiration is noted. If the diaphragm shadows the T12 vertebra and its rib, then the T11 rib is identified.

Step 5. Mark the surface landmarks for the needle entry
The point of entry for both levels is at the junction of the rib and vertebra. Skin infiltration is made at this point. With the oblique fluoroscopic view still in place, a 14 gauge, 5 cm extracath is inserted so that the catheter transverses towards the target as a pinhead.

Step 6. Direction of the needle
1. After the extracath is inserted two-thirds of the way, the stylet is removed and the RF needle is inserted. The oblique view of the fluoroscope is maintained. Extension tubing is attached to the needle.
2. With short thrusts of 0.5 cm at a time, the tip of the needle is advanced anteriorly, keeping in mind that the needle stays hugging the lateral aspect of the T11 or T12 vertebral body, close to the costovertebral angle.

Step 7. Confirm the position of the needle
1. After advancing 1–1.5 cm anteriorly, the lateral fluoroscopic view is taken. In the lateral view, the needle is advanced until it reaches the junction of the anterior one-third and posterior two-thirds of the lateral surface of the vertebral body.
2. The needle is then aspirated for fluid, which could be blood, cerebrospinal fluid, or chyle. If negative for any fluid aspiration, then oblique views are taken to confirm the final position of the curved needle on the vertebral body. Omnipaque (5 ml) is injected to note that the solution in anteroposterior and lateral views hugs the spine. It should flow medial to the interpleural space, above the crus of the diaphragm, and anterior to the foramen.

Step 8. Stimulation test
1. Once the needle is in place, a 15 cm electrode is introduced through the RF needle. The electrical circuit is tested. The impedance should be below 250 ohms.
2. At 50 Hz, the sensory stimulation is conducted up to 1 V. The patient may report that he or she feels stimulation in the epigastric region. This is typical and satisfactory. If the stimulation is in a girdle like fashion around the intercostal spaces, then the needle needs to be pushed anteriorly.
3. At 2 Hz motor stimulation is done up to 3 V. One tries to palpate or see the intercostal muscle contraction. If this is negative then test stimulation is satisfactory.

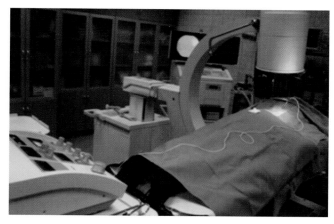

Figure 15.15 RF lesioning of the splanchnic nerve.

Step 9. RF lesioning

1. Lesion: after satisfactory test stimulation, 2–5 ml of local anesthetic (ropivacaine 0.5% with steroid, 40 mg of triamcinolone) is injected through the RF needle. After waiting for 1–2 minutes, the RF lesion is created with a setting 90 seconds at 80 °C. The second lesion at the same setting is done turning the RF needle 180°. If the procedure is for bilateral neurolysis, then the same procedure of testing and lesioning is done on the opposite site (Fig. 15.15).

2. After RF lesioning, 40 mg of triamcinolone is injected to prevent inflammation due to lesioning. The electrodes are then withdrawn.

Step 10. Postprocedure care

After the procedure is completed, the patient needs to be observed for at least 2 hours. Monitoring of vital signs is mandatory. In addition to monitoring the pain relief one should document it. After a satisfactory observation in the recovery room, the patient should be discharged to the in-patient floor to continue with the protocol for the procedure or to home with appropriate and adequate instructions given to their escort. Written instructions are preferable for emergencies and are helpful to the patient and their family.

Complications

In this section, only complications related to splanchnic nerve block are presented. Complications seen both in celiac plexus block and splanchnic nerve block are presented in the section on celiac plexus block.

- **Pneumothorax**

Pneumothorax may occur by mistakenly identifying the eleventh rib for the twelfth when outlining surface anatomy relationships. The pleural reflection can extend as low as the neck of the twelfth rib posteriorly. Use of smaller gauge needles is recommended to prevent pneumothorax.

- **Sensory and motor loss**

Injection or contact of neurolytic solutions to neural structures other than the celiac plexus may cause sensory motor loss in the lower extremities.

- **Spinal cord ischemia, paraparesis, and paraplegia**

Paraplegia generally is regarded as an idiosyncratic event that is unrelated to technique, expertise, or negligence. Although still a remote complication, paraplegia now has been reported with essentially every major posterior approach to celiac and splanchnic nerve blocks except blockade by the anterior percutaneous route.

The pyramidal and spinothalamic tracts typically are affected, with relative sparing of proprioception. Given the wide acceptance of the use of radiologic guidance and the distance between the celiac axis and the spinal canal, the most important mechanism of neurologic injury is postulated to relate to spinal cord ischemia or infarct as a consequence of disruption of small nutrient vessels by spasm, direct injury, or accidental intravascular injection. Mechanical or chemical disruption of the nutrient vessels to the spinal cord with the development of spinal cord infarction has been invoked to explain most occurrences of major neurologic morbidity after celiac and splanchnic block. Adamkiewicz's arteries (arteria radicularis magna), the largest of the cord's ventral radicular arteries, provide nutrient blood flow to the lower two-thirds of the spinal cord. After leaving the aorta, they run laterally, about 80% of the time on the left, and typically reach the cord between T8 through L4, making them vulnerable to injury during the splanchnic block.

- **Neuritis**

Neuritis may develop due to the neurolytic agents. The incidence seems to be higher with alcohol, thus phenol in saline is preferred.

- **Inadvertent epidural or intrathecal puncture**

If the entry point is more than 7.5 cm from the midline and the angle of insertion is less than 45°, there is a risk of inadvertent epidural or intrathecal puncture. However, this complication is nearly impossible if the splanchnic block is performed under fluoroscopy.

- **Chylothorax**

Inadvertent puncture of the thoracic ducts may cause chylothorax. However, it is a very rare complication.

- **Inadvertent vascular injection**

As with all techniques, there is a risk of intravascular injection. The contrast material should be administered under live imaging and an aspiration test is mandatory.

- **Hemi-diaphragmatic paralysis**

The spread of the neurolytic solution on the diaphragm may cause paralysis of the diaphragm.

Helpful hints

The fluoroscopic oblique view ensures the medial direction of the needle and the lateral view ensures that the needle stays posterior to the aorta and anterior to the foramen.

Before lesioning, the injection of the local anesthetic helps in reducing the discomfort due to the RF lesioning and decreases pain postoperatively. Steroids help in treating the occasional occurrence of neuritis by reducing edema and inflammation of the lesioned structures.

The incidence of pneumothorax related to splanchnic nerve block is higher than the celiac plexus block. The incidence of pneumothorax can be decreased if the needles are kept close to the vertebral bodies during needle placement.

Percutaneous block and lesioning of the celiac plexus

History
In 1914, Kappis introduced the percutaneous splanchnic and celiac plexus block with local anesthetic through a posterior approach and proposed it for surgical anesthesia. He rapidly gained experience with this technique and reported a series of 200 patients in 1918. At the same time, Wendling described the anterior percutaneous approach, a method of blocking the celiac plexus using a single needle placed anteriorly through the liver. Judged to be riskier than Kappis's posterior approach, it rapidly fell into disfavor. Seven decades later, an anterior approach was "rediscovered" using CT or ultrasound guidance. In 1996, a transgastric endoscopic technique was also developed.

Over the ensuing 30 years since Kappis invented his technique, Labat, Farr, and others introduced various modifications. It is important to note that the celiac plexus and splanchnic nerve block were initially used as a surgical anesthetic technique. However, because of the complexity and variable outcome of this technique, in due course it needed to be supplemented by neuroaxial anesthesia and segmental blockade of the somatic paravertebral nerves.

As celiac plexus and splanchnic nerve blocks were falling into disuse for surgical anesthesia, the clinical use of these techniques was becoming apparent in the new specialty of pain management. Jones first described alcohol neurolysis of the splanchnic nerves and celiac plexus for long-lasting relief of abdominal pain in 1957 through the classic retrocrural approach. Bridenbaugh and colleagues reported on the role of neurolytic celiac plexus block to treat the pain of upper abdominal malignancy. In 1978, Boas set apart the retrocrural technique from the transcrural. Five years later, Ischia described a transaortic one-needle injection. There is renewed interest in the anterior approach to the celiac plexus block, using CT or ultrasonography to allow more accurate needle placement.

Despite various modifications, Kappis's classic posterior approach to the celiac plexus and splanchnic nerves continues to serve as the basis for contemporary techniques. It is important to mention that none of the techniques developed show superiority in relation to safety and success. In general, the celiac plexus and splanchnic neurolytic lesions yield 70–90% long-lasting pain relief in abdominal, and mainly in pancreatic, malignancy.

Anatomy of the celiac plexus
The celiac plexus is a complex network of nerves located in the abdomen, near the celiac trunk and superior mesenteric artery of the aorta. It is located behind the stomach and the omental bursa, and lies in front of the crura of the diaphragm, at the level of the L1 vertebra.

Formation of the celiac plexus
The plexus is formed (in part) by the greater and lesser splanchnic nerves of both sides, and parts of the right vagus nerve. The celiac plexus proper consists of the celiac ganglia and a network of interconnecting fibers. The aorticorenal ganglia are often considered to be part of the celiac ganglia and, thus, part of the plexus.

The celiac plexus includes several smaller plexuses: hepatic plexus, splenic plexus, gastric plexuses, pancreatic plexus, and suprarenal plexus.

Other plexuses that are derived from the celiac plexus are the renal plexus, testicular plexus/ovarian plexus, superior mesenteric plexus, and inferior mesenteric plexus.

The celiac plexus provides innervation to the following abdominal viscera: pancreas, stomach, liver, biliary tract, spleen, kidneys, adrenals, omentum, small bowel, and large bowel (to the level of the splenic flexure).

The origin of the celiac plexus from splanchnic nerves
The greater (T5–T10), lesser (T10–11), and the least splanchnic nerves (T12) are composed of the preganglionic nerve fibers, which synapse at the celiac plexus. These splanchnic nerves traverse the posterior mediastinum and enter the abdomen through the crura of the diaphragm, a variable distance above the first lumbar vertebral body. Once the splanchnic nerves pierce the diaphragmatic crura, they form the right and left celiac ganglia. These ganglia with their dense interconnecting nerve fibers make up the celiac plexus. Ward et al. have documented that the size and position of the celiac ganglia are variable. The ganglia vary in diameter from 0.5 to 4.5 cm, and the cephalocaudad ganglia position varies from the T12–L1 disc space to the middle of the L2 vertebral body. Closely situated to the celiac plexus, on the right the vena cava is typically anterolateral, the kidneys are lateral, and the pancreas lies anterior.

Diaphragmatic crura
The anatomy of the crura of the diaphragm is important in understanding the two principal techniques of celiac plexus block. The musculotendinous crura arise from the anterior surfaces of the lumbar vertebral bodies, from the anterior

longitudinal ligament, and from the intervertebral discs. The right crus is larger and longer than the left crus. The right crus originates from the upper three lumbar vertebrae. The left crus arises from only the upper two. The right crus usually splits to enclose the esophagus as it pierces the diaphragm. The fibers of the right crus decussate beyond the elliptical opening, and make an esophageal hiatus a complete muscular sphincter. The left crus is smaller and lies farther from the median plane than the right crus, and participates in the formation of the esophageal hiatus. The medial tendinous margins of the crura meet to form an arch across the front of the aorta and distinctly create an aortic hiatus. The muscular fibers of the lateral margins of the crura are continuous with those arising from the medial lumbocostal arches. At this location, the crura are pierced by the splanchnic nerves on both the right and left sides.

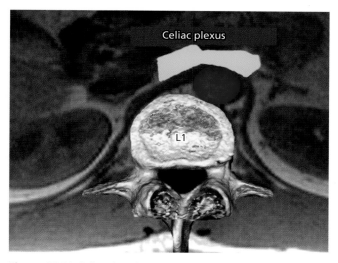

Figure 15.16 Celiac plexus in transverse section.

Composition of the celiac plexus nerve fibers

Fibers within the plexus arise from preganglionic splanchnic nerves, parasympathetic preganglionic nerves from the vagus, some sensory nerves from the phrenic and vagus nerves, and sympathetic postganglionic fibers. Afferent fibers concerned with nociception pass diffusely through the celiac plexus (Figs 15.16 and 15.17).

Nomenclature of the celiac plexus block

Anatomically, the crus of the diaphragm determines whether the block that is performed represents a true celiac plexus block or a splanchnic nerve block. If the tip of the needle lies posterior to the crus, the nerves that are blocked belong to the splanchnic nerves. When the needles are advanced anteriorly, they pass transcrurally, and the solution that is injected blocks nerve fibers of the celiac plexus. Needles placed at the T11 vertebral body are always located posterior to the crus. Below this level, the crus migrates posteriorly to attach to the T12 through L1 vertebral bodies. At the T12 or L1 level, the needles can be placed either anterior or posterior to the crus. The classical technique of needle placement at the anterior border of the vertebral body usually results in placement posterior to the crus. For reliable placement anterior to the crus, the needle must be placed transcrurally, often anterior to the abdominal aorta.

Significant structures close to the celiac plexus at T12–L1

The aorta lies anterior and slightly to the left of the anterior margin of the vertebral body. The inferior vena cava lies to the right, with the kidneys posterolateral to the aortic branches. The pancreas lies anterior to the celiac plexus. All these structures lie within the retroperitoneal space.

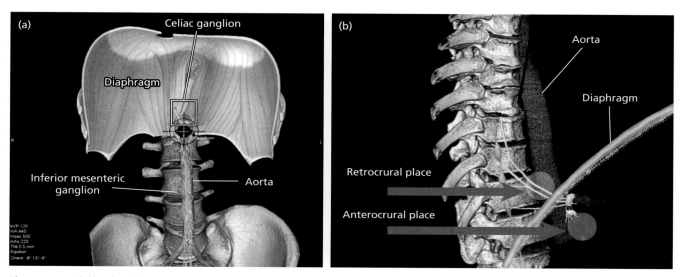

Figure 15.17 (a,b) Celiac plexus, anteroposterior and lateral views (anterocrural, retrocrural).

Indications
- For pain due to upper abdominal viscera.
- Cancer of the upper abdominal viscera (stomach and duodenum).
- Pancreatic cancer.
- Cancer of the adrenal glands.
- Chronic pancreatitis.

Contraindications
- Local or systemic infection.
- Coagulopathy and patients using anticoagulants.
- Congenital abnormalities.
- Bowel obstruction.
- Intraabdominal infection.

Techniques for celiac plexus block
There are three approaches: (1) posterior retrocrural approach; (2) posterior anterocrural approach; (3) transaortic approach.

1. Posterior retrocrural approach

Step 1. Prepare the patient before the procedure
Ascertain the type of analgesia or sedation before performance of the invasive procedure. The type of sedation varies, based on the technique being used. If a local anesthetic is considered or neurolytic block is planned, mild sedation is all that is necessary. If pulsed RF is planned, the patient needs to be awake to respond to the stimulation test. Intravenous fentanyl or midazolam may be used judiciously for the patient's comfort.

Step 2. Position and monitor the patient
1. Place the patient in a prone position on the table.
2. Place a pillow beneath the iliac crest to flatten the lumbar lordosis.

3. Insert an intravenous cannula for injecting medication.
4. Provide oxygen by nasal cannula.
5. Monitor vital signs (mandatory).
6. Prepare the area for needle entry in a sterile fashion.

Step 3. Drugs and equipment for celiac plexus block
Prepare and confirm that the following equipment, needles, and drugs are ready to be used for the procedure:
- 25 gauge, 1½ inch needle for skin infiltration;
- 5 ml syringe for local anesthetic solution;
- 10 ml syringe for contrast material (iohexol);
- two 20 ml syringes for the celiac plexus block;
- two 15 cm, 22 gauge needles for the celiac plexus block;
- 1% lidocaine for skin infiltration;
- contrast solution (iohexol);
- for the celiac plexus block (in 20 ml syringe):
  (1) 5 ml of 0.5% bupivacaine;
  (2) 5 ml of saline;
  (3) absolute alcohol.

Step 4. Visualization
Place the C-arm in the posteroanterior view first. The anatomical landmarks to be identified are the twelfth ribs and the vertebral body of L1. To identify the L1 vertebral body easily, one may first identify the L4–L5 interspace and the posterior superior iliac crests under fluoroscopy (Fig. 15.18).

Step 5. Mark the surface landmarks for the needle entry
1. Mark the spinous process of the T12 and L1 vertebral body. Draw a line from the inferior edge of the L1 vertebral body to intersect the twelfth ribs bilaterally. The intersection is approximately 7.5 cm on each side. Draw a triangle joining this line with the cephalic portion of the L1 vertebral body to form an isosceles triangle to guide needle positioning. If

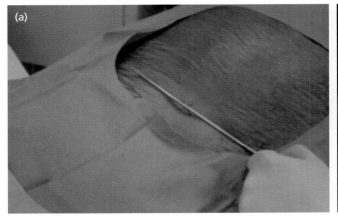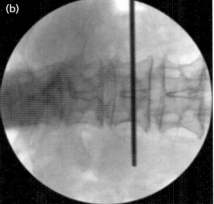

Figure 15.18 (a,b) Identify the spinous processes of the L1, T12 vertebral bodies.

the height of the triangle is more than 2.5 cm, the landmarks are incorrectly marked (Fig. 15.19).

2. These landmarks are of great importance. If lower levels are marked, there is a risk of penetrating the kidney or ureteropelvic junction. If higher levels are marked, there is a risk of pneumothorax.

Step 6. Direction of the needle

1. Infiltrate the entry points with 1% lidocaine. Insert a 20 or 22 gauge 15 cm needle, just beneath the twelfth rib, 45° with the skin toward the midline and 15° cephalad until a bony contact is made. Measure the depth of the needle during the bony contact (Fig. 15.20).

2. Withdraw the needle slightly, redirect increasing the angle to 60°, until the bony contact with the vertebral body is lost.

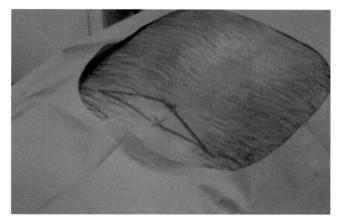

Figure 15.19 Mark the entry points.

Step 7. Confirm the position of the needle

1. Position the C-arm laterally, advance the needle 1.5–2 cm anterior to the vertebral body under lateral view (Figs 15.21 and 15.22).

2. An aspiration test should be done at this stage and should be negative for any fluids (blood, cerebrospinal fluid, or chyle) on both sides. Inject 2 ml of contrast solution and check again that the tip of the needle is not in a vessel. The contrast solution should spread as a smooth line in front of the vertebral body (Fig. 15.23).

3. Position the C-arm in the posteroanterior view again. The contrast solution should be confined to the midline beneath the T12–L1 level (Fig. 15.24).

Step 8. Celiac plexus block

1. First administer 2 ml of local anesthetic as a test dose to verify that the needle is not in the intrathecal or epidural space. One should wait for a few minutes. After repeating the aspiration test again inject 20 ml of local anesthetic, saline, and absolute alcohol solution if neurolysis is performed on each side. The alcohol concentration varies from 50 to 90% (Fig. 15.25).

2. The patient may feel severe pain for a few minutes after the alcohol injection. The patient should be informed in advance. It may be better to inject 5 ml of 2% lidocaine before injecting the alcohol solution.

3. Repeat the procedure on the contralateral side.

There is no report of RF lesioning of the celiac plexus.

2. Posterior anterocrural approach on the right side

• In this approach, the goal is to place the needle anterior to the crus of the diaphragm on the right side.

• The approach is similar to the retrocrural technique; however, the entry points are 5–6 cm away from the midline instead of 7–8 cm.

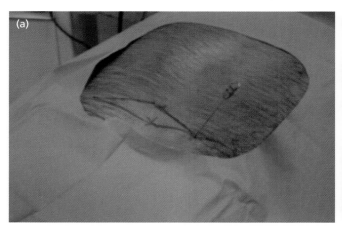
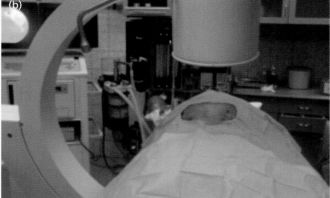

Figure 15.20 (a,b) Direction of the needle under posteroanterior view.

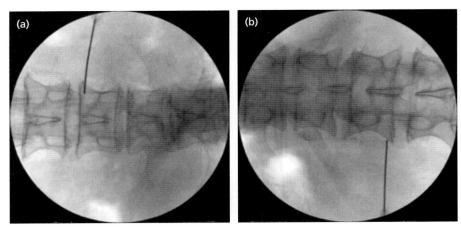

Figure 15.21 (a,b) Position of the needles under posteroanterior view.

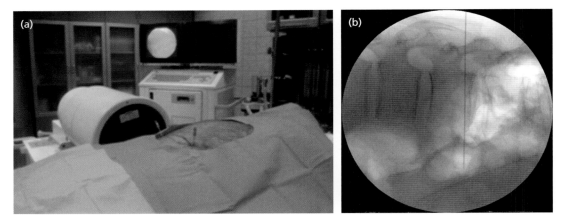

Figure 15.22 (a,b) Position of the needles under lateral view.

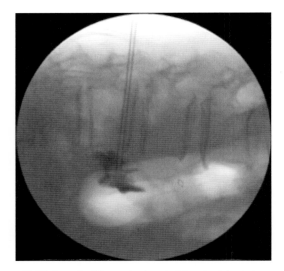

Figure 15.23 Spread of the contrast material under lateral view.

- A 22 gauge 15 cm needle is introduced with an angle of 45° in the horizontal plane until a bony contact is made with the vertebral body of L1.
- After the bony contact, the needle is withdrawn slightly, then redirected until it passes the anterolateral edge of the vertebral body.
- The needle is advanced more than for the retrocrural approach. It is not always easy to understand that the needle tip is placed anterior to the crus.
- The best anterocrural approach is transaortic, described by Ischia in 1983.

3. Transaortic approach

Steps 1, 2, and 3 are similar. On the left side the celiac plexus is in close proximity with the abdominal aorta, just anterior to the aorta. This is a one-needle approach from the left side.

Step 4. Direction of the needle

1. The entry point is as described above. A 22 gauge, 15 cm needle is introduced with an angle of 45° with the horizontal plane until a bony contact is made with the vertebral body of L1 (Figs 15.26 and 15.27).

2. After the bony contact, the needle is withdrawn slightly, then redirected until it passes the anterolateral edge of the vertebral body.

3. The C-arm is placed in the lateral position. The needle is gradually advanced until its tip rests in the posterior periaortic space. There may be a slight resistance at the wall of the aorta which can be seen pulsating the needle (Fig. 15.28).

Step 5. Confirm the position of the tip of the needle

1. Remove the stylet and advance the needle gradually until it enters the aorta. A pop may be felt as it enters the aorta. There will be a free flow of arterial blood with palpation. Continue to advance the needle within the aortic lumen until it passes the anterior wall of the aorta. At this point, free blood flow will cease.

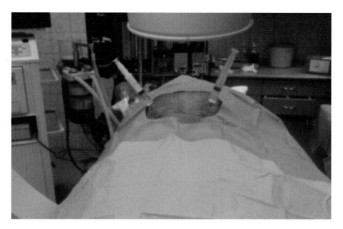

Figure 15.25 20 ml of solution injected from both needles.

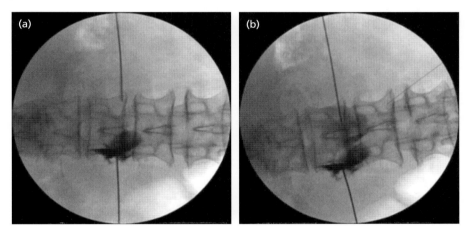

Figure 15.24 (a,b) Spread of the contrast material under posteroanterior view.

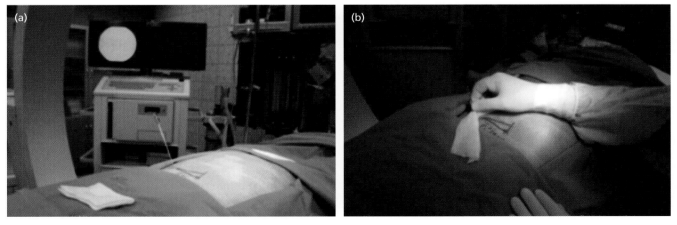

Figure 15.26 (a,b) Transaortic approach, direct the needle with 45° angle, advance the needle towards the aorta.

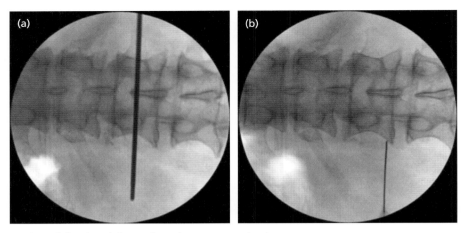

Figure 15.27 (a,b) Entry point and direction of the needle under posteroanterior view.

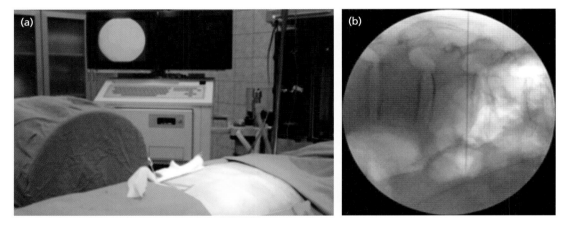

Figure 15.28 (a,b) Direction of the needle under lateral view during transaortic approach.

2. First aspirate. The aspiration test should be negative. If the aspiration test is positive, it shows that the needle is still within the aortic lumen. Advance slightly until the aspiration test is negative.

3. Inject 2–3 ml of contrast material. The contrast material should spread in a smooth line anterior to the anterior wall of the aorta. One should view the pulsation of the aorta under live and continuous imaging (Fig. 15.29). Position the arm in the posteroanterior view. The contrast material should be confined to the midline around the anterolateral borders of the aorta. If the contrast material is totally on the lateral border of the aorta the position is not correct and one should redo the procedure.

Step 6. Transaortic celiac plexus block
Inject local anesthetic solution up to 20 ml of 50% alcohol for the neurolytic block as described earlier.

Step 7. Postprocedure care
Observe the patient for at least 2 hours after the procedure. Monitoring of vital signs is mandatory. In addition, objec-tively document the pain relief. After a satisfactory observation, discharge the patient with appropriate and adequate instructions given to their escort. Written instructions are preferable for emergencies and are helpful to the patient and their family.

Complications

Complications of celiac plexus block may be classified as follows: (1) cardiovascular complications; (2) gastrointestinal complications; (3) genitourinary complications; (4) pulmonary complications; (5) systemic complications; (6) neurological complications.

1. Cardiovascular complications
• Hypotension

Hypotension, the most common complication of celiac block, is usually transient. It is a consequence of unopposed parasympathetic innervation, regional vasodilatation, and pooling within the splanchnic bed. It can usually be prevented by the intravenous administration of 500–1000 ml of balanced electrolyte solutions. Particular vigilance should be

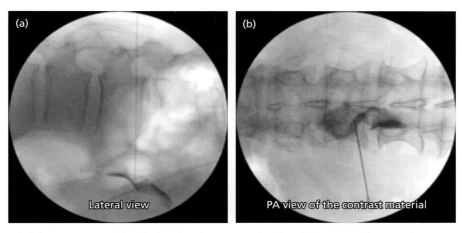

Figure 15.29 (a,b) Spread of the contrast material under lateral and posteroanterior view during transaortic approach.

maintained in elderly, debilitated, and chronically or acutely dehydrated patients to avoid hypotension and iatrogenic congestive heart failure. Monitoring of blood pressure during the procedure and recovery is mandatory.

• Hematoma

The plexus extends in front of and around the aorta. Although very rare, during the transaortic approach there may be a risk of trauma to the aorta or aorta dissection. If very severe and sudden hypotension develops after the celiac block, one should suspect hematoma in the region where the celiac plexus lies. This may be confirmed by CT scan.

There is also a risk of injury to the inferior caval vein, which lies on the anterolateral space of the vertebral body just at the right of the aorta.

2. Gastrointestinal complications

• Gastrointestinal hypermotility and intractable diarrhea

Gastrointestinal hypermotility is another consequence of unopposed parasympathetic activity. It lasts generally for 36–48 hours. However, in a very few cases, intractable diarrhea may be severe, persistent, and, if unrecognized, even life threatening.

3. Genitourinary complications

• Kidney puncture

The kidneys are sited at the T12–L3 level. The left kidney is slightly cephalad than the right one. Hematuria and hypotension may develop in case of kidney puncture.

• Loss of bladder control and impotence

Inadvertent administration of neurolytic solution to the nerves around the kidney, loss of bladder control, and urinary incontinence and impotence may develop. Renal puncture is more likely when needles are inserted more than 7.5 cm lateral to the midline and are positioned with their tips excessively lateral to the vertebral body.

4. Pulmonary complications

• Pneumothorax

Pneumothorax may occur by mistakenly identifying the eleventh rib for the twelfth rib when outlining surface anatomy relationships. The pleural reflection can extend as low as the neck of the twelfth rib posteriorly. It occurs more frequently during the splanchnic block.

5. Systemic complications

Although systemic effects of alcohol ordinarily should not be anticipated, an accidental intravascular injection of a large volume may induce intoxication, seizures, and unconsciousness. Intravascular injection or absorption of phenol may produce transient tinnitus and flushing. Higher doses may produce stimulation of the central nervous system, myoclonus, seizures, unconsciousness, hypotension, cardiac arrhythmias, and hepatic or renal insufficiency.

6. Neurological complications

• Spinal cord ischemia, paraparesis, and paraplegia

(a) Paraplegia generally is regarded as an idiosyncratic event that is unrelated to technique, expertise, or negligence. Although still a remote complication, paraplegia now has been reported with essentially every major posterior approach to celiac and splanchnic nerve blocks except blockade by the anterior percutaneous route.

The pyramidal and spinothalamic tracts typically are affected, with relative sparing of proprioception. Given the wide acceptance of the use of radiologic guidance and the distance between the celiac axis and the spinal canal, the most important mechanism of neurologic injury is postulated to relate to spinal cord ischemia or infarct because of disruption of small nutrient vessels by spasm, direct injury, or accidental intravascular injection. Mechanical or chemical disruption of the nutrient vessels to the spinal cord with the development of spinal cord infarction has been invoked to explain most occurrences of major neurologic morbidity after celiac and splanchnic block. Adamkiewicz's arteries (arteria radicularis magna), the largest of the cord's ventral radicular arteries, provide nutrient blood flow to the lower two-thirds of the spinal cord. After leaving the aorta, they run laterally, about 80% of the time on the left, and typically reach the cord between T8 through L4, making them vulnerable to injury during celiac block.

(b) Paraparesis after alcohol celiac plexus block may be reversible over an extended period. This may be possible because acute ischemic medullary damage might be related to the spasm of Adamkiewicz arteries. The ischemia may be caused either by direct mechanical damage to the arteries by a needle or by arterial vasospasm in response to localized exposure to alcohol.

• **Sensory and motor loss**

Injection or contact of neurolytic solutions to neural structures other than the celiac plexus may cause sensory motor loss in the lower extremities.

• **Genitofemoral neuralgia**

In the retrocrural approach, the neurolytic solution may spread to the T12–L1 spinal nerves as well as to the branches of the lumbar plexus. However, this is a very rare complication.

• **Inadvertent epidural or intrathecal puncture**

If the entry point is more than 7.5 cm from the midline and the angle of insertion is less than 45°, there is a risk of inadvertent epidural or intrathecal puncture. However, this complication is nearly impossible if the celiac plexus block is performed under fluoroscopy.

• **Pain**

It is not uncommon for patients to experience new, generally self-limited pain, presumably from soft tissue trauma, paresthesias, or chemical irritation. This usually manifests as dull backache or pleuritic pain after celiac or splanchnic block, respectively.

Complications of celiac plexus block are presented in Table 15.1.

Helpful hints

The celiac plexus block should only be performed by very experienced physicians. Preparation of the patient is of utmost importance prior to the procedure. A CT scan is necessary to view the recent anatomical changes in the region especially for the transaortic approach where compression of the aorta is possible.

We do not advise the blind techniques any more. The celiac plexus block should always be performed under fluoroscopy. The patient should be monitored for at least 6 hours after the procedure for possible cardiovascular changes.

The written consent of the patient and their family should be taken. The side effects and complications of the celiac plexus block should be explained in detail. The patient

Table 15.1 Complications of celiac plexus block

Hypotension
Paresthesia of the lumbar somatic nerve
Intravascular injection
Inadvertent epidural or intrathecal puncture
Diarrhea
Perforation of the kidney
Paraplegia
Pneumothorax
Chylothorax
Vascular thrombosis or emboli
Vascular injury
Injection to the psoas muscle
Abscess formation
Peritonitis
Retroperitoneal hematoma
Perforation of the ureter
Impotence
Hiccups
Pain during injection

should be aware that there may not be total pain relief but reduction of opioids and other analgesics is also a success.

Celiac plexus block is one of the few procedures that should be performed in the earlier stages of the disease.

Further reading

Abram, S.E. & Boas, R.A. (1993) Sympathetic and visceral nerve blocks. In *Clinical Procedures in Anesthesia and Intensive Care* (ed. Benumof, J.L.), pp. 787–805. Philadelphia, PA: J.B. Lippincott.

Boas, R.A. (1978) Sympathetic blocks in clinical practice. *International Anesthesiology Clinics* **16**, 159–182.

Brown, D.L. & Wright, R.M. (1990) Precautions against injection in the spinal artery during celiac plexus block. *Anesthesia* **45**, 247–248.

Chan, V.W. (1996) Chronic diarrhea: an uncommon side effect of celiac plexus block. *Anesthesia & Analgesia* **82**, 205–207.

Cousins, M.J. & Bridenbaugh, P.O. (1998) *Neural Blockade in Clinical Anesthesia and Management of Pain*, 3rd edition. New York: Lippincott-Raven.

Davies, D.D. (1993) Incidence of major complications of neurolytic celiac plexus block. *Journal of the Royal Society of Medicine* **86**, 264–266.

De Cicco, M., Matovic, M., Bortolussi, R., et al. (2001) Celiac plexus block: injectate spread and pain relief in patients with regional anatomic distortions. *Anesthesiology* **94**, 561–565.

Erdine, S. (2005) Interventional treatment of cancer pain. *European Journal of Cancer* **3**(3), 97–106.

Erdine, S. (2009) Neurolytic blocks, when, how, why. *Ağrı* **21**(4), 133–140.

Erdine, S. & Talu, G.K. (2008) Sympathetic blocks of the thorax. In *Interventional Pain Management, Image Guided Procedures* (ed. Prithvi Raj, P.P., et al.), pp. 255–266. Philadelphia, PA: Saunders-Elsevier.

Garcea, G., Thomasset, S. & Berry, D.P. (2005) Percutaneous splanchnic nerve RF ablation for chronic abdominal pain. *ANZ Journal of Surgery* **75**, 640–644.

Hilgier, M. & Rykowski, J.J. (1994) One needle transcrural celiac plexus block. Single shot or continuous technique, or both. *Regional Anesthesia* **19**, 277–283.

Ina, H., Kitoh, T. & Kobayashi, M. (1996) New technique for the neurolytic celiac plexus block: The transintervertebral disc approach. *Anesthesiology* **85**, 212–217.

Ischia, S., Ischia, A., Polati E. & Finco, G. (1996) Three posterior percutaneous celiac plexus block techniques. A prospective randomized study in 61 patients with pancreatic cancer pain. *Anesthesiology* **76**, 534–540.

Ischia, S., Luzzani, A., Ischia, A., et al. (1983) A new approach to the neurolytic block of the coeliac plexus: the transaortic technique. *Pain* **16**, 333–341.

Jackson, T.P. & Gaeta, R. (2008) Neurolytic blocks revisited. *Current Pain and Headache Reports* **12**, 7–13.

Kappis, M. (1914) Erfahrungen mit Lokalanästhesie bei Bauchoperationen. *Verhandlungen der Deutschen Gesellschaft fuer Chirurgie* **43**, 87.

Mauck, W.D. & Rho, R.H. (2010) The role of neurolytic sympathetic blocks in treating cancer pain. *Techniques in Regional Anesthesia and Pain Management* **14**, 32–39.

Mercadante, S., Catala, E., Arcuri, E. & Casuccio, A. (2003) Celiac plexus block for pancreatic cancer pain: factors influencing pain, symptoms and quality of life. *Journal of Pain and Symptom Management* **26**, 1140–1147.

Mercadante, S., La Rosa, S. & Villari, P. (2002) CT-guided neurolytic splanchnic nerve block by an anterior approach. *Journal of Pain and Symptom Management* **23**(4), 268–270.

Moore, D.C. (1979) Celiac (splanchnic) plexus block with alcohol for cancer pain of the upper intra-abdominal viscera. In *Advances in Pain Research and Therapy*, volume 2 (ed. Bonica, J.J. & Ventafridda, V.), pp. 593–596. New York: Raven Press.

Moore, D.C., Bush, W.H. & Burnett, L.L. (1980) Celiac plexus block: a roentgeno-graphic, anatomic study of technique and spread of solution in patients and corpses. *Anesthesia and Analgesia* **60**, 369–379.

Moore, D.C., Bush, W.H. & Burnett, L.L. (1982) An improved technique for celiac plexus block may be more theoretical than real. *Anesthesiology* **57**, 347–348.

Owitz, S. & Koppolu, S. (1983) Celiac plexus block: an overview. *Mount Sinai Journal of Medicine* **50**, 486–490.

Özyalçın, N.S., Talu, G.K., Camlica, H. & Erdine, S. (2004) Efficacy of coeliac plexus and splanchnic nerve blockades in body and tail located pancreatic cancer pain. *European Journal of Pain* **8**(6), 539–545.

Patt, R.B., Reddy, S.K. & Black, R.G. (1998) Neural blockade for abdominopelvic pain of oncologic origin. *International Anesthesiology Clinics* **36**, 87–104.

Plancarte-Sánchez, R., Máyer-Rivera, F., del Rocío Guillén Núñez, M., Guajardo-Rosas, J. & Acosta-Quiroz, C.O. (2003) Transdiscal percutaneous approach of splanchnic nerves. *Cirugia y Cirujanos* **71**(3), 192–203.

Prasanna, A. (1996) Unilateral celiac plexus block. *Journal of Pain and Symptom Management* **11**, 154–157.

Raj, P.P. (2001) Celiac plexus/splanchnic nerve blocks. *Techniques in Regional Anesthesia and Pain Management* **5**(3), 102–115.

Raj, P.P. (2002) *Textbook of Regional Anesthesia*. Philadelphia, PA: Churchill Livingstone.

Raj, P.P., Sahinler, B. & Lowe, M. (2002) Radiofrequency lesioning of splanchnic nerves. *Pain Practice* **2**(3), 241–247.

Rauck, R.L. & DeLeon, O.A. (2003) Sympathetic nerve block interventional techniques. In *Pain Medicine. A Comprehensive Review*, 2nd edition (ed. Raj, P.P.) pp. 250–271. St. Louis, MO: Mosby.

Rosenthal, J.A. (1998) Diaphragmatic paralysis complicating alcohol splanchnic nerve block. *Anesthesia and Analgesia* **86**, 845–846.

Singler, R.C. (1982) An improved technique for alcohol neurolysis of the celiac plexus. *Anesthesiology* **56**, 137–141.

Visentin, M., Trentin, L. & Biscuola, G. (1990) Diffusion of contrast media in relation to different techniques of celiac plexus block. *Minerva Anestesiologica* **56**, 1409–1412.

Ward, E.M., Rorie, D.K., Nauss, L.A. & Bahn, R.C. (1979) The celiac ganglia in man: normal anatomic variations. *Anesthesia and Analgesia* **58**, 461–465.

Wendling, H. (1918) Ausschaltung der Nervi splanchnici durch Leitungsanesthesie bei Magenoperationen und anderen Eingriffen in der oberen Bauchule. *Beitrag zur Klinische Chirurgie* **110**, 517.

Wong, G.Y. & Brown, D.L. (1997) Celiac plexus block for cancer pain. *Techniques in Regional Anesthesia and Pain Management* **1**(1), 18–26.

16

Interventional Pain Procedures in the Lumbar Region

Percutaneous interlaminar block of the lumbar epidural space

History

Corning was the first author to describe a technique now commonly known as epidural block. In 1885 he published his studies of administering cocaine into the spinal canal both in a dog and in man. The first publication of epidural anesthesia has been credited to Cathelin and Sicard. However, in 1942 Edwards and Hingston described continuous caudal anesthesia.

Anatomy (Figs 16.1–16.6)

The upper limit of the epidural space is the foramen magnum, which is the point where the vertebral spine meets the base of the skull. The lower limit is at the tip of the sacrum, at the sacrococcygeal ligament. The epidural space is bounded by the pedicles of the vertebral bodies and the ligamentum flavum posteriorly and the intervertebral foramina laterally, the posterior longitudinal ligament, intervertebral discs, and segmental spinal nerves anteriorly. The epidural space is 5–6 mm at the L2–L3 interspace with the lumbar spine flexed.

The epidural space at all levels contains fatty tissue, arteries, epidural venous plexuses, spinal nerve roots, and lymphatics. The epidural fat is relatively vascular and serves as a shock absorber for other contents in the spinal canal.

The venous plexus surrounds the dura in a segmental fashion. The epidural veins are concentrated principally in the anterolateral portion of the epidural space. However, in the presence of obstruction to venous run-off such as epidural scarring, there may be large distended high-pressure veins in the midposterior epidural space. These veins are valveless and so reflect both intrathoracic and intraabdominal pressures. As pressure in any of these body cavities increases, owing to Valsalva's maneuver or compression of the inferior vena cava by a gravid uterus or a tumor mass, the epidural veins distend and reduce the volume of the epidural space.

Epidural arteries

The arteries that supply the bony and ligamentous confines of the cervical epidural space, as well as the cervical spinal cord, enter the cervical epidural space by two routes: through the intervertebral foramina and through direct anastomoses from the intracranial portions of the vertebral arteries.

Arteries enter the epidural space through the neural foramina anteriorly and posteriorly at multiple levels. The anterior segmental arteries are found most commonly at lower cervical, lower thoracic, and upper lumbar levels. These anterior segmental arteries supply the anterior spinal artery. Posterior segmental arteries are more numerous and evenly distributed than anterior segmental arteries and supply the posterior spinal arteries.

There are significant anastomoses between the epidural arteries, most of which lie in the lateral portions of the epidural space. Trauma to the epidural arteries can result in epidural hematoma formation and compromise the blood supply to the spinal cord itself.

Lymphatics

The lymphatics in the epidural space are concentrated in the region of the dural nerve roots, where they scavenge foreign material from the subarachnoid and epidural spaces.

Ligaments

Posterior to the lumbar epidural space, there are subcutaneous tissue, the supraspinous ligament, interspinous ligament, and the ligamentum flavum.

The supraspinous ligament is a strong fibrous structure, attached to the apices of the spinous processes from the seventh cervical vertebra to the sacrum. It is thicker and broader in the lumbar than in the thoracic region, and intimately blended in both situations with the adjacent fascia.

Pain-Relieving Procedures: The Illustrated Guide, First Edition. P. Prithvi Raj and Serdar Erdine.
© 2012 John Wiley & Sons, Ltd. Published 2012 by John Wiley & Sons, Ltd.

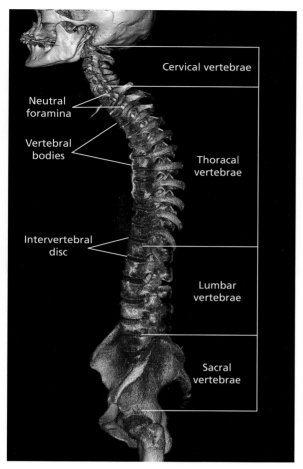

Figure 16.1 Vertebral column, cervical, thoracic, lumbar, and sacral vertebrae.

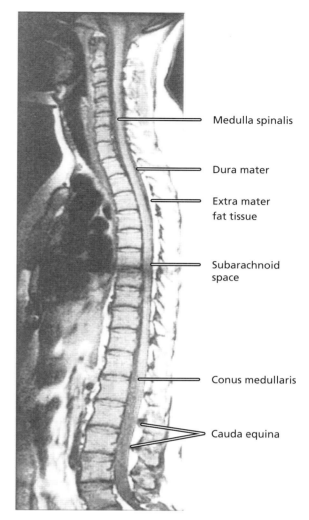

Figure 16.2 MRI showing the structures within the vertebral canal, medulla spinalis, dura mater, subarachnoid space, and cauda equina.

The interspinous ligaments are thin and membranous, connecting with adjoining spinous processes, and extending the whole length of the spinous process. The ligamenta flava lies posterior to these structures and the supraspinal ligament behind. The ligaments are narrow and elongated in the thoracic region, broader, thicker, and quadrilateral in the lumbar region, and only slightly developed in the neck.

The ligamenta flava connect the laminae of adjacent vertebrae, all the way from the occiput to the first segment of the sacrum (C2–S1). They are best seen from the interior of the vertebral canal; when viewed from the outer surface they appear short, being overlapped by the laminae.

Each ligament consists of two lateral portions, which originate on either side of the roots of the articular processes, and extend backward to the point where the laminae meet the spinous process; the posterior margins of the two portions are in contact and united.

Their marked elasticity serves to preserve the upright posture, and to assist the vertebral column in resuming it after flexion. The elastin prevents buckling of the ligament into the spinal canal during extension, which would cause canal compression. Hypertrophy of this ligament may cause spinal stenosis because it lies in the posterior portion of the vertebral canal.

Indications
- For diagnosis of lumbar spinal pain.
- Localized neural irritation and inflammation.
- Disc hernia, bulging, protrusion.
- Discogenic pain.
- Failed back surgery syndrome.

Contraindications
- Local or systemic infection.
- Coagulopathy.
- Advanced spinal stenosis, spinal instability.
- Myelomalacia.

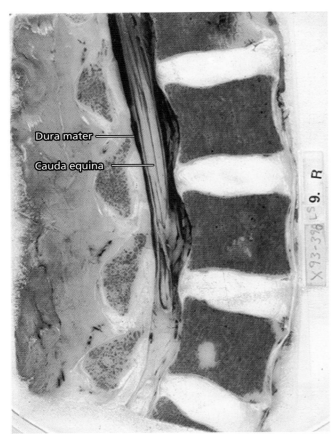

Figure 16.3 Parasagittal section of lumbar spine. The cauda equina descend in the lumbar spinal canal within the dural sac (which terminates at the S2 level); the epidural space contains a venous plexus. (Courtesy of J. Taylor.)

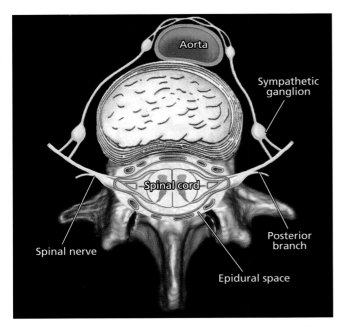

Figure 16.4 Lumbar epidural space and structures in close proximity.

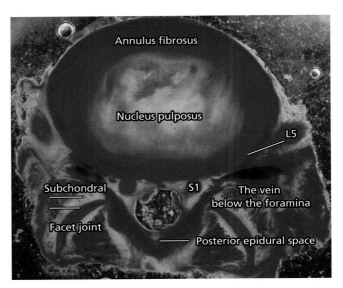

Figure 16.5 Three-dimensional CT showing the transverse section of a lumbar vertebra.

- Coexisting disease producing significant respiratory or cardiovascular compromise.
- Immunosuppression.

Technique of interlaminar approach to lumbar epidural space

Step 1. Prepare the patient before the procedure
Ascertain the type of analgesia or sedation before performing the invasive procedure. If a local anesthetic is considered or neurolytic block is planned, mild sedation is all that is necessary. If pulsed radiofrequency (RF) is planned, the patient needs to be awake to respond to the stimulation test. Intravenous fentanyl or midazolam may be used judiciously for the patient's comfort.

Step 2. Position and monitor the patient
- Lumbar epidural nerve block may be performed with the patient in a lateral or prone position.
- Lumbar epidural interlaminar block may be performed either by a median or paramedian approach using a "loss of resistance" or "hanging drop" technique.
For a lateral approach, do the following.
1. Place the patient in the lateral decubitus position on the table with their head in a hyperflexed position and the legs pulled and flexed towards their abdomen. Support the abdomen and thorax with pillows, so the patient feels comfortable.
2. Obtain an intravenous access if drugs need to be administered.
3. Monitor vital signs (mandatory in unstable patients).
4. Prepare the area for needle entry in a sterile fashion.

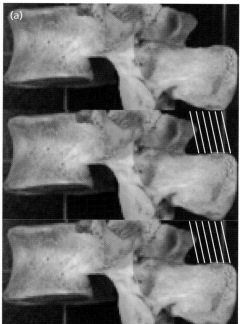

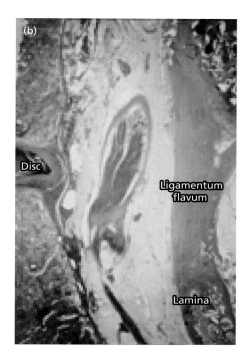

Figure 16.6 (a,b) Ligaments of posterior elements. (Courtesy of J. Taylor.)

5. The patient should not be over-sedated. The patient should remain sufficiently conscious to provide responses to any questions.

Step 3. Drugs and equipment for the lumbar interlaminar epidural block
Prepare and confirm that the following equipment, needles, and drugs are ready to be used for the procedure.
• 1½ inch, 25 gauge needle for skin infiltration.
• 5 ml syringe for local anesthetic solution.
• 2 ml syringe for the contrast material.
• 5 ml syringe for the epidural block.
• 18 gauge Tuohy type epidural needle.
• 1% lidocaine for skin infiltration.
• Contrast material, e.g. iohexol.
• Saline.
• Nonparticulate steroid solution.

Step 4. Mark the surface landmarks for needle entry
1. The initial target is the intervertebral space. This may be identified by palpating the spinous processes above and below the level one needs to enter. To ensure that the needle entry site is exactly in the midline, the physician's middle and index fingers are placed on each side of the spinous processes. In obese patients it may be difficult to identify the midline, so place the C-arm in a lateral position where the anteroposterior view of the vertebral column will appear.
2. To identify the level of approach, the anatomical landmarks are as follows.

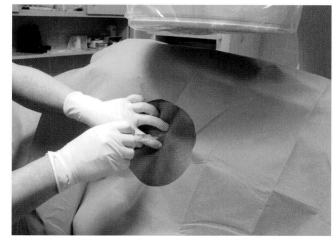

Figure 16.7 Palpate the spinous processes above and below the level one needs to enter.

3. Vertebral body of L1 just below the vertebral body of T12 where the ribs appear bilaterally.
4. The line drawn on the posterior iliac crest is between the L4–L5 intervertebral space.

Step 5. The procedure
1. Infiltrate the skin subcutaneous tissues, and supraspinous and interspinous ligament in the midline, with local anesthetic. Then insert a 10 cm, 18 or 20 gauge Tuohy needle at the midline between the above and below spinous processes (Figs 16.7 and 16.8).

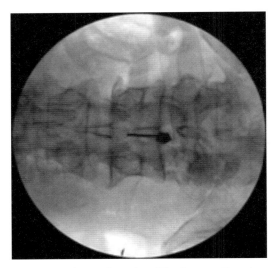

Figure 16.8 Direct the needle at the midline between the spinous processes above and below.

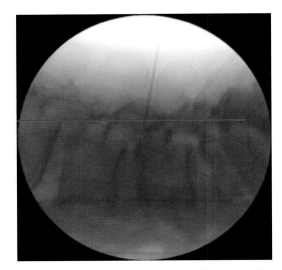

Figure 16.10 Anterior to this virtual line lies the ligamentum flavum (red arrow).

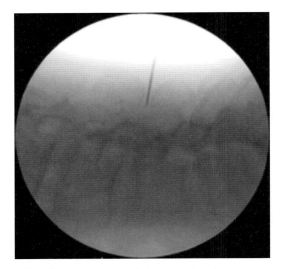

Figure 16.9 Direction of the needle between the spinous processes under lateral view.

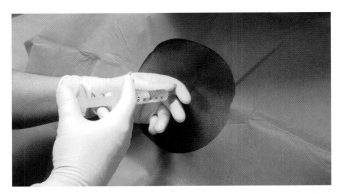

Figure 16.11 Hold the hub of the epidural needle firmly with the left thumb and index finger. Place the wrist of the left hand against the back of the patient to prevent the advance of the needle by unexpected movement of the patient.

2. Move the C-arm to the lateral view. Identify the vertebral body, intervertebral space, and spinous process in this view (Fig. 16.9). The base of the spinal process appears as a virtual line in the lateral view. Anterior to this virtual line lies the ligamentum flavum. The target of the needle is the virtual line. Advance the needle through the supraspinous and interspinous ligament under fluoroscopy. Stop at the level of the "virtual line," the line drawn at the base of the spinous process (Fig. 16.10).

3. Entry to the lumbar epidural space is possible either by a "loss of resistance" or "hanging drop" technique. We prefer the loss of resistance technique.

Loss of resistance technique

1. Remove the stylet of the needle. Attach a well-lubricated 5 ml syringe filled with saline.

2. Hold the hub of the epidural needle firmly with the left thumb and index finger.

3. Place the wrist of the left hand against the back of the patient to prevent the advance of the needle owing to unexpected movement of the patient.

4. Hold the syringe with the right hand, advance the needle under fluoroscopy with the thumb applying pressure on the plunger (Fig. 16.11).

5. As soon as the needle bevel passes through the ligamentum flavum, there will be a "loss of resistance" and the plunger slides easily.

6. Gentle aspiration is required. If blood is aspirated, withdraw the needle outside the epidural space, redirect, and enter the epidural space again. If blood is again aspirated terminate the procedure.

7. If cerebrospinal fluid is aspirated, terminate the procedure for another day.

Step 6. Confirm the position of the needle

1. Inject 2–5 ml of contrast material. A "straight line image" view will be visualized in lateral vision. With negative aspiration of blood or cerebrospinal fluid, one should wait about 30 seconds to see if the contrast solution stays in the epidural space. Rapid clearance of the contrast solution can signify that the needle is in the subarachnoid space (Figs 16.12–16.15).

2. If the needle is within the subdural space, injection of a very small amount of contrast material will appear like a

thin direct line at multiple levels. Unlike the injection of the contrast solution in the subarachnoid space, the contrast solution does not disappear (Fig. 16.16).

Step 7. Interlaminar epidural block

For therapeutic epidural block, inject 10 ml of 0.25% preservative-free bupivacaine in combination with 80 mg of depo methylprednisolone slowly.

Technique of interlaminar epidural block for prone paramedian approach

After all the steps have been taken as described in the lateral interlaminar approach (vide supra), position the patient in the prone position.

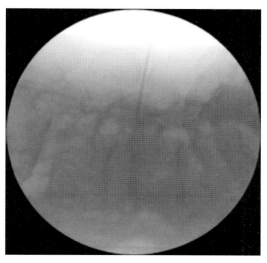

Figure 16.12 The needle is within the epidural space in lateral view.

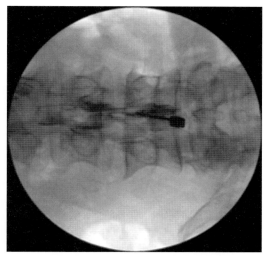

Figure 16.14 Spread of the contrast material in posteroanterior view.

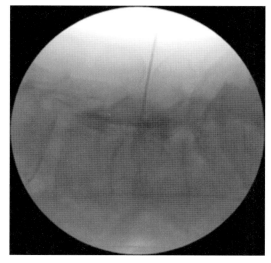

Figure 16.13 Spread of the contrast material in lateral view.

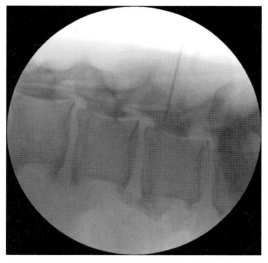

Figure 16.15 Subarachnoid spread of the contrast material.

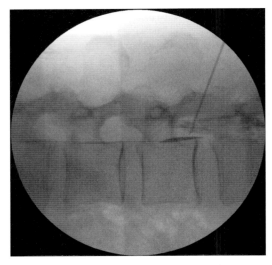

Figure 16.16 Subdural spread of the contrast material.

• Prepare and drape the area in a sterile fashion.
• The patient should not be over-sedated. The patient should remain sufficiently conscious to provide responses to any questions.

Step 4. Visualization
Steps 1–3 are as described previously.
1. Place the C-arm in a posteroanterior position. Identify the midpoint of the intervertebral space at the target level.
2. Infiltrate the skin with local anesthetic solution using a short 25 gauge needle down to the lamina.

Step 5. Direction of the needle
1. Introduce the needle about 1 cm paramedian at the level of the tip of the spinous process. The needle is then angled slightly medial and advanced to make contact with the lamina. Once the bony contact is made, redirect the needle with an angle of 45° with the parasagittal and 15° axial plane medial and cephalad.
2. Then position the C-arm laterally and advance the needle with the loss of resistance technique as explained above (Figs 16.17–16.20).

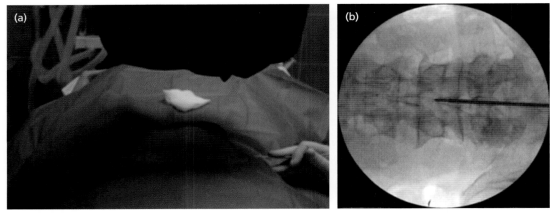

Figure 16.17 (a,b) Identify the midpoint of the intervertebral space.

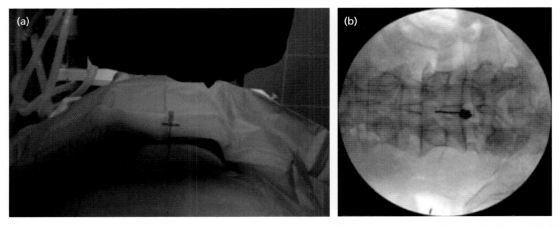

Figure 16.18 (a,b) Introduce the needle about 1 cm paramedian at the level of the tip of the spinous process with an angle of 45° with the parasagittal and 15° axial plane medial and cephalad.

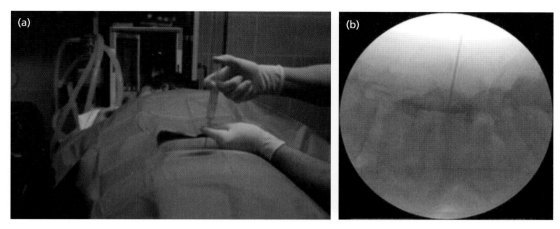

Figure 16.19 (a,b) Place the C-arm laterally and advance the needle with the loss of resistance technique.

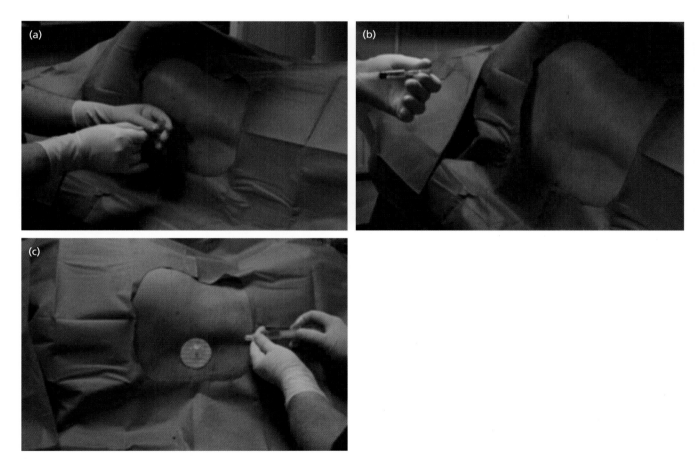

Figure 16.20 (a–c) Insertion of epidural catheter.

Technique of epidural catheter placement in the lumbar epidural space

• Enter the lumbar epidural space (vide supra).
• Verify that the bevel of the needle is in the lumbar epidural space by injecting contrast solution both in posteroanterior and lateral views.

• Inject the epidural catheter with 5–10 ml of saline before inserting the catheter through the needle.
• Insert and advance the catheter through the needle under fluoroscopy in the lateral view. The catheters have marks showing centimeters, which measure the length of the catheter inserted through the needle. Introduce the catheter up to the level that is predetermined.

• Aspirate. If blood comes, advance the catheter several millimeters, and aspirate again. If the aspiration test is positive, withdraw the catheter with the needle and interrupt the procedure.

• If the aspiration test is negative, inject contrast material through the catheter to verify the tip of the catheter in the epidural space both in posteroanterior and lateral views.

• Anchor the catheter on the skin firmly with adhesive tape or suture.

Step 8. Postprocedure observation

After the procedure is completed, the patient needs to be observed for up to 2 hours. Monitoring of vital signs is mandatory. In addition, the pain relief should be objectively documented. After a satisfactory observation, the patient should be discharged with appropriate and adequate instructions given to their escort. Written instructions are preferable for emergencies and are helpful to the patient and their family.

Helpful hints for epidural catheter insertion

Because the catheter is marked at every 5 cm from the tip, when advancing the catheter one should be aware of the length of the catheter introduced within the epidural space. For a single block or therapeutic purposes, introduce the catheter up to 5 cm ideally.

For long-term use, the tip of the catheter should be at least 10 cm within the epidural space. In some cases advancing the catheter within the epidural space may be difficult: the ligamentum flavum may be attached to the anteroinferior surface of the lower lamina; epidural fibrosis may prevent the advance of the catheter; loss of resistance may be felt while the needle enters the epidural space, but only a part of the needle tip may be within the epidural space; the needle may be in close contact with the dura, which will not allow the catheter to be advanced. One should not insist on advancing the catheter, as inadvertent dural puncture may occur.

The tip of the catheter may enter a vein. If blood is aspirated, try to advance the catheter for a few centimeters, aspirate again; if blood is aspirated again, terminate the procedure. The final position of the catheter should be verified under fluoroscopy by injecting contrast solution. In some cases the tip of the catheter may go out of the epidural space through an intervertebral foramen. Long-term catheter placement needs to be monitored closely for sterility and early appearance of infection.

Complications related to the technique
• **Inadvertent dural puncture**

There is a risk of inadvertent dural puncture, even in the most experienced hands. During the dural puncture, cerebrospinal fluid may not be aspirated. Rapid clearance of the contrast material can signify that the needle is in the subarachnoid space.

• **Inadvertent subdural puncture**

The subdural space is a potential space between the subarachnoid and epidural spaces. Injection of a very small amount of contrast material will appear like a thin direct line at multiple levels. Unlike injection of the contrast material in the subarachnoid space, contrast solution does not disappear. Administration of local anesthetic solution to the subdural space will appear with total spinal block after 20 minutes.

• **Spinal nerve injury**

The needle may contact the spinal segmental nerve or its ventral ramus while advanced through the intervertebral foramen. Immediate severe pain and paresthesia will develop at that instant. The patient should remain sufficiently conscious to provide a response to such an event. The needle is then to be replaced. If the same symptoms recur, the procedure should be interrupted.

• **Inadvertent intravascular injection**

During the aspiration test, blood may not be aspirated. The contrast solution should slowly be injected under live imaging. If the needle is within the vertebral artery, the contrast material spreads vertically and disappears immediately. If the needle is within the segmental artery it will spread medially towards the spinal cord. The spread of the contrast solution within the epidural or paraspinous veins is slower. During the puncture of anterior or posterior segmental arteries, if nonparticulate steroid solutions are injected, serious complications may not occur. Particulate solutions injection has the risk of emboli or infarct.

• **Epidural hematoma**

Bleeding within the epidural space is a significant complication if hematoma develops. The most important cause of epidural hematoma is the bleeding of venous plexuses within the lumbar epidural space. Bleeding due to mechanical damage of the arteries within the epidural space gives rise to early signs and symptoms. Bleeding in the venous plexus may give rise to such findings at a later stage. If severe pain, paresthesia, and loss of strength in the extremities develop within hours or days, one should suspect epidural hematoma.

• **Spinal cord injury**

The disadvantage of the interlaminar lumbar epidural block is that there is a risk of causing immediate injury to the spinal cord by advancing the epidural needle too far and a greater risk of delayed injury by causing an epidural hematoma or abscess.

In some patients there may be gaps in the ligamentum flavum in the midline at the lumbar levels. To prevent this complication, an intermittent lateral fluoroscopic view should be used while advancing the needle. The patient may not feel pain or paresthesia when the needle contacts the spinal cord. They may feel pain only if the needle contacts the sensory fibers. If local anesthetics are injected around the meninges they may not feel this sensation. Permanent damage within the spinal cord may also develop owing to the injection of local anesthetics.

• **Inadvertent intradiscal puncture**

This is a very rare complication for interlaminar epidural block.

Side effects related to drugs

- **Infection**

Although uncommon, infection in the epidural space remains an ever-present possibility, especially in the immunocompromised AIDS or cancer patient. Especially in patients with an epidural catheter for a prolonged period, one should be very careful about infection. A possible cause of infection is seeding the infectious agents from the entry site at the skin. *Staphylocccus aureus*, *Streptococcus*, and *Staphylococcus epidermidis* are the common agents.

- **Epidural abscess**

If epidural abscess occurs, surgical drainage of the abscess to avoid spinal cord compression and irreversible neurologic deficit is required. Early detection and treatment of infection is crucial to avoid potentially significant deleterious sequelae. Epidural abscesses may not be diagnosed in the early stages until neurological signs develop.

- **Meningitis**

Meningitis is a rare complication. However, it should be kept in mind.

Helpful hints

Interlaminar epidural steroid injection is one of the most commonly used procedures in interventional pain management. At many pain centers, the blind technique is still used. We do not advise the blind technique for pain management.

The use of fluoroscopy is mandatory if an epidural catheter is to be inserted; this helps to verify the final position of the catheter tip. The final position of the catheter should be verified under fluoroscopy by injecting contrast material. In some cases the tip of the catheter may go out of the epidural space through an intervertebral foramen.

The physician may feel the "loss of resistance" while passing the interspinous ligament that runs obliquely between the spinous processes.

The patient should not be over-sedated. The patient should remain sufficiently conscious to provide responses to the physician's questions.

Inadvertent dural and subdural puncture are the most significant complications to be avoided. The use of fluoroscopy is crucial while performing the interlaminar epidural block.

Percutaneous transforaminal block of the lumbar epidural space

History

The first description of transforaminal epidural block was through the S1 posterior sacral foramen, in 1952, by Robecchi and Capra. The use of fluoroscopy for interventional procedures facilitated the use of the transforaminal route. Derby and Bogduk reviewed the technique in 1993, and Kikuchi described the anatomic variants of the dorsal root ganglia in 1994.

Anatomy

There are anterior, neuroaxial, and posterior compartments within the spinal column. The anterior compartment consists of the vertebral body and intervertebral disc, whereas the neuroaxial compartment consists of structures within the epidural space and neural pathways. The posterior compartment is formed by facet joints and associated bony vertebral arch structures. The neuroaxial compartment includes all structures within the osseous and ligamentous boundaries of the spinal canal, including the posterior longitudinal ligament, ligamentum flavum, epidural, and epiradicular membranes (Figs 16.21 and 16.22).

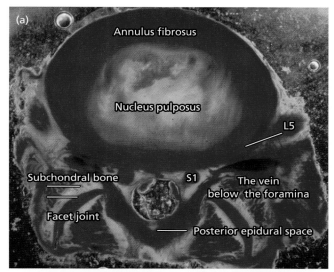

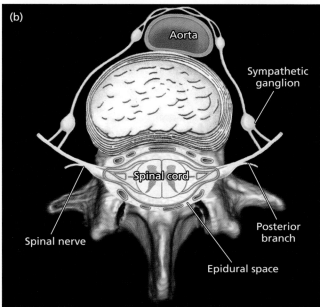

Figure 16.21 (a,b) L5–S1 transverse section, nerves exiting through the foramen. (Courtesy of J. Taylor.)

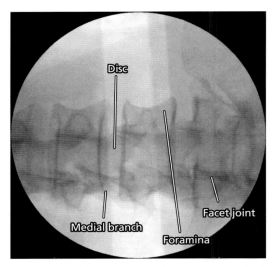

Figure 16.22 X-ray of the lumbar spine showing structures in close proximity with the neural foramen.

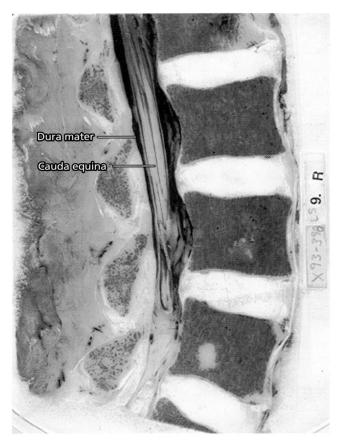

Figure 16.23 Parasagittal section of lumbar spine. The cauda equina descend in the lumbar spinal canal within the dural sac (which terminates at S2 level); the epidural space contains a venous plexus. (Courtesy of J. Taylor.)

The anterior wall of the vertebral column is formed by the posterior surfaces of the lumbar vertebrae, the discs, and the posterior longitudinal ligament; the posterior wall is formed by the laminae of the vertebrae and ligamentum flavum; the lateral walls of the vertebral canal are formed by the pedicles of the lumbar vertebrae.

Each intervertebral foramen is bounded anteriorly by an intervertebral disc, the adjacent lower third of the vertebral body above, and uppermost portion of the vertebral body below; posteriorly by vertebral lamina and a facet joint; and above and below by a pedicle.

The intervertebral foramen looks like an oval, round, or inverted teardrop-shaped window. The anterior aspect of the intervertebral foramen is bounded by the posterior aspect of the adjacent vertebral bodies, the intervertebral disc, the posterior longitudinal ligament, and anterior longitudinal venous sinus.

The posterior aspect of the foramen is bounded by the superior and inferior articular process of the facet joint at the same level, and the lateral prolongation of the ligamentum flavum. The medial canal border contains the dural sleeve. The lateral boundary is a fascial sheet and overlying psoas muscle. A distal and proximal oval perforation is seen in the fascia. The distal perforation houses the nerve root, and the smaller proximal perforation regularly has blood vessels traversing through it.

The height of the foramen is dependent upon the vertical height of the corresponding intervertebral disc. With aging and disc degeneration there will be a loss of disc height, which will decrease the availability of space for neurovascular structures to pass.

Resting on the floor of the vertebral canal is the dural sac, which is posterior to the backs of the vertebral bodies and the intervertebral discs covered by the posterior longitudinal ligament; and, posteriorly, the dural sac is related to the roof of the vertebral canal, the laminae, and ligamentum flavum.

In adults, the spinal cord generally extends inferiorly to the L1 or L2 level. However, the surrounding dural sac extends inferiorly in the sacrum to approximately the S2 level within the bony sacral canal and then terminates at the sacral hiatus at the S4 or S5 level (Figs 16.23 and Fig. 16.24).

When spinal nerve roots leave the dural sac, they do so just above the level of each intervertebral foramen by penetrating the dural sac in an inferolateral direction, taking with them an extension of dura mater and arachnoid mater referred to as the dural sleeve.

This sleeve encloses the nerve roots as far as the intervertebral foramen and spinal nerve, where the dura mater merges with, or becomes, the epineurium of the spinal nerve. The nerve roots are sheathed with pia mater embedded in spinal fluid. Further, immediately proximal to its junction with the spinal nerve, the dorsal root forms an

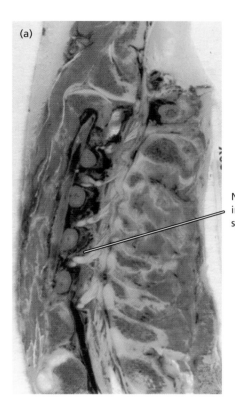

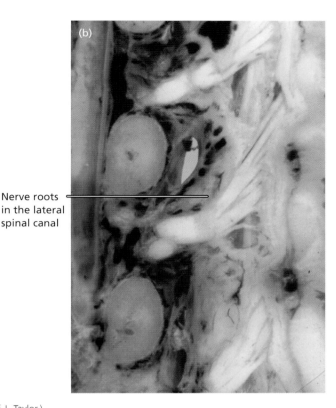

Nerve roots in the lateral spinal canal

Figure 16.24 (a,b) Sagittal section of nerve roots. (Courtesy of J. Taylor.)

enlargement, the dorsal root ganglion, which contains the cell bodies of sensory fibers in the dorsal root. Thus, the ganglion lies within the dural sleeve of the nerve root and occupies the upper, medial part of the intervertebral foramen but may lie further distally in the foramen if the spinal nerve is short.

The spinal nerve that exits through the neural foramen follows a variable course as the nerve root leaves the spinal canal, depending on the level of the spine. In the lumbar spine, the nerve roots travel inferiorly and exit in a lateral plane. Thus, the lumbar roots exit under the pedicle with a downward course of 40–50° from horizontal and occupy the superior portion of each foramen. It is common consensus that the upper portion of the foramina just beneath the adjacent pedicle is a safe zone to place the injectate close to the lumbar nerve root.

In addition, the angle at which each pair of nerve roots leaves the dural sac varies, as the L1 and L2 root sleeve of the dural sac leave at an obtuse angle, but the dural sleeves of the lower nerve roots form increasingly acute angles with the lateral margins of the dural sac. Thus, the angles formed by the L1 and L2 roots are about 80° and 70°, whereas the angles of the L3 and L4 roots are each about 60°, with the angle of the L5 root around 45°. Similarly, the level of origin of the nerve root sleeves also varies from L1 downwards, with the L1 sleeve arising behind the L1 body, and

the L2 sleeve arising behind the L2 body; but successive origins of the nerve root sleeves arise increasingly higher behind the vertebral bodies, until the sleeve of the L5 nerve root, which arises behind the L4/5 intervertebral disc (Figs 16.25–16.27).

Each spinal nerve root is connected to the spinal cord by a dorsal and ventral root centrally. However, each spinal nerve divides into a larger ventral ramus and a smaller dorsal ramus. The spinal nerve roots join the spinal nerve in the intervertebral foramen, and the ventral and dorsal rami are formed just outside the foramen. Consequently, the spinal nerves are quite short, as each one is no longer than the width of the intervertebral foramen in which it lies. The dorsal root of each spinal nerve transmits sensory fibers from the spinal nerve to the spinal cord, whereas the ventral root largely transmits motor fibers from the cord to the spinal nerve; however, it also transmits some sensory fibers. In addition, the ventral roots of L1 and L2 spinal nerves transmit preganglionic, sympathetic, efferent fibers.

Indications
- For diagnostic purposes to verify the pain source.
- Localized neural irritation and inflammation.
- Disc hernia, bulging, protrusion.
- Discogenic pain.
- Failed back surgery syndrome.

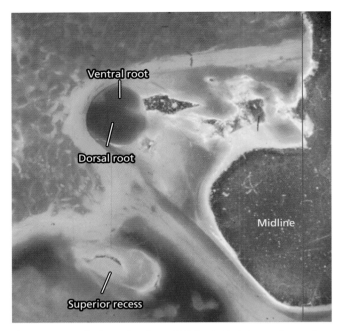

Figure 16.25 The large dorsal root (DR) lies behind the small ventral root in the fat of the lateral recess of the spinal canal (thick unstained transverse section). The fat of the facet joint superior recess (SR) is seen behind the lamina.

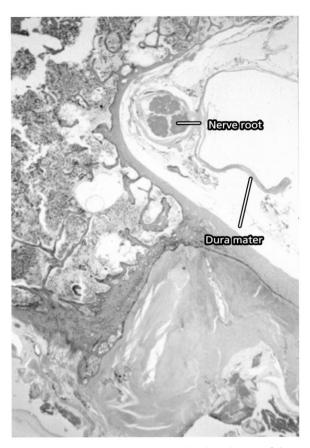

Figure 16.26 Transverse section at L3–L4. The lateral recess of the spinal canal contains the nerve root budding off the dura in its root sleeve of dura and arachnoid. (Courtesy of J. Taylor.)

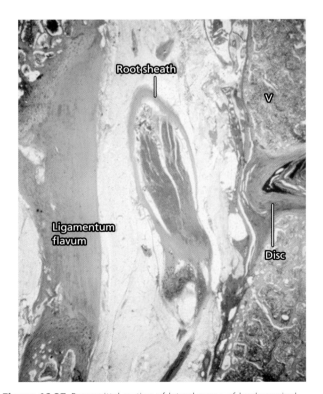

Figure 16.27 Parasagittal section of lateral recess of lumbar spinal canal. The anterior and posterior nerve roots descend obliquely in their root sleeve towards the intervertebral foramen. (Courtesy of J. Taylor.)

Contraindications

- Local or systemic infection.
- Coagulopathy.
- Advanced spinal stenosis, spinal instability.
- Myelomalacia.
- Coexisting disease producing significant respiratory or cardiovascular compromise.
- Immunosuppression.

Technique of transforaminal epidural space approach: prone technique

Step 1. Prepare the patient before the procedure
Ascertain the type of analgesia or sedation before performing the invasive procedure. If a local anesthetic is considered or neurolytic block is planned, mild sedation is all that is necessary. If pulsed RF is planned, the patient needs to be awake to respond to the stimulation test. Intravenous fentanyl or midazolam may be used judiciously for the patient's comfort.

Step 2. Position and monitor the patient

1. Place the patient prone on the table. Place a pillow under the abdomen to flatten the lumbar lordosis.

2. Obtain an intravenous access if drugs need to be administered.

3. Monitor vital signs (mandatory in unstable patients).

4. Prepare the area for needle entry in a sterile fashion.

5. The patient should not be over-sedated. The patient should remain sufficiently conscious to provide responses to any questions.

Step 3. Drugs and equipment for the lumbar transforaminal block

- 1½ inch, 25 gauge needle for skin infiltration.
- 5 ml syringe for local anesthetic solution.
- 2 ml syringe for the contrast material.
- 5 ml syringe for the epidural block.
- 10 cm, 22 gauge needle with extension line for the epidural block.
- 10 cm, 2-5 mm active-tip electrode (for RF).

- 1% lidocaine for skin infiltration.
- Contrast solution (iohexol).
- Preservative-free saline.
- Deposteroid.

Step 4. Visualization

1. Place the C-arm in a posteroanterior position first. Identify the midpoint of the intervertebral space at the target level. Adjust the lower endplate of the target vertebral body to be aligned by moving the C-arm in a cephalocaudal direction (Fig. 16.28).

2. Oblique the C-arm in the coronal plane approximately 20°, until the facet joint is delineated. Then oblique the C-arm 15° in the caudocephalad direction ipsilaterally to align the superior articular process of the vertebra below with the 6 o'clock position of the pedicle above (Fig. 16.29).

Step 5. Mark the surface landmarks for the needle entry

1. Infiltrate the skin with local anesthetic solution using a short 25 gauge needle down to the lamina.

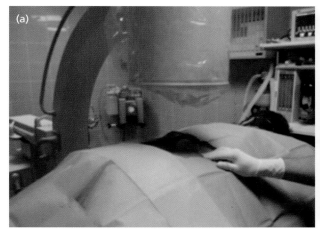
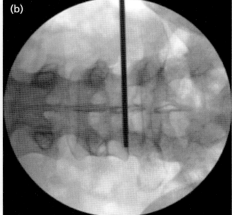

Figure 16.28 (a,b) Mark the level of entry for lumbar transforaminal block.

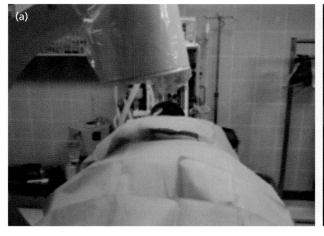
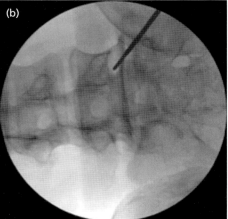

Figure 16.29 (a,b) C-arm in the oblique position, point of entry for the L5–S1 level.

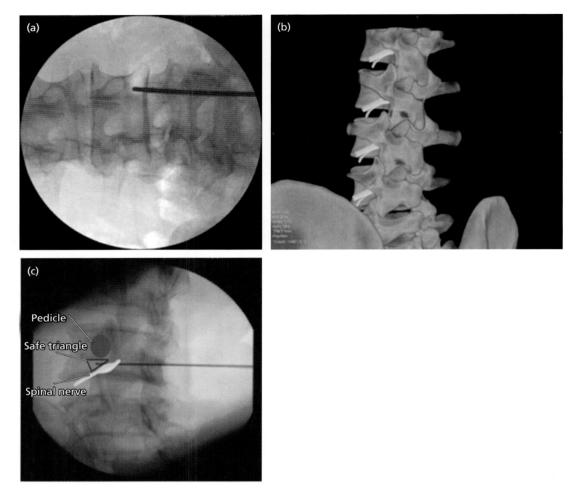

Figure 16.30 (a–c) Entry point for the L4 level and the safe zone to introduce the needle.

2. The entry point should be the "safe triangle" at this location, with three sides corresponding to the horizontal base of the pedicle, the outer vertical border of the intervertebral foramen, and the connecting diagonal nerve root and dorsal ganglion. Thus, a needle placed into the safe triangle will lie above and lateral to the nerve root (Fig. 16.30).

Step 6. Direction of the needle
1. Advance a 10 cm, 22 gauge needle under tunneled vision just lateral to the tip of the superior articular process of the level below the indicated neural foramen until the tip impinges on bone over the pedicle lateral to the 6 o'clock position (Figs 16.31–16.33).
2. Move the C-arm to a lateral position. In the lateral view, ideal placement of the needle is with the tip in the cephalo-dorsal corner, at the level of the ventral border of the foramen. Do not go further ventrally; if the needle is misdirected, inadvertent puncture of the intervertebral disc is possible.

3. Move the C-arm to a posteroanterior position to verify that the needle is not medial to the 6 o'clock position on the pedicle to avoid the needle being deeper in the spinal canal.
4. If the patient feels paresthesia or sudden pain, withdraw the needle and redirect.
5. An aspiration test is mandatory. If blood is aspirated, withdraw the needle and redirect. Note that blood may not be aspirated sometimes, even though the needle tip may be in a blood vessel. Injection of contrast material under continuous live imaging will reveal an inadvertent vascular injection.

Step 7. Confirm the position of the needle
1. The spread of the contrast material should delineate the nerve root only, with no spread in the epidural space or onto the peripheral plexus (Figs 16.34 and 16.35).
2. Inject 0.5 ml of contrast material; the contrast material should flow proximally around the pedicle into the epidural space.

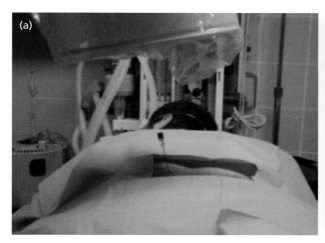

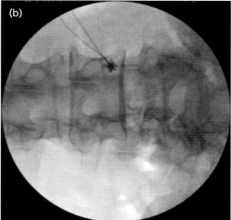

Figure 16.31 (a,b) Direction of the needle under oblique view.

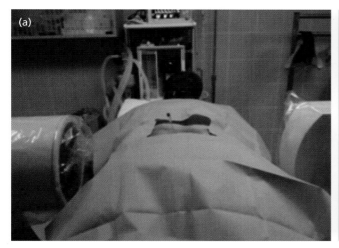

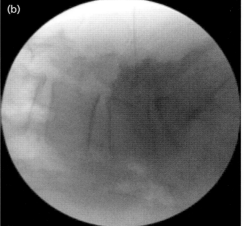

Figure 16.32 (a,b) Position of the needle under lateral view.

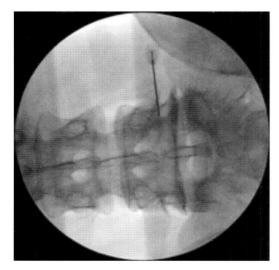

Figure 16.33 Position of the needle under posteroanterior view.

3. If the needle is deeper, the contrast material will spread in the epidural space. In patients with spinal stenosis, the contrast material spreads in multiple levels. In patients with epidural fibrosis due to a previous operation, the contrast material spreads caudally.

4. There should be no evidence of subarachnoid, subdural, or intravascular spread of the contrast.

Step 8. Lumbar transforaminal epidural block
1. Inject 20–40 mg of deposteroid in saline solution or with 0.5% bupivacaine 2–3 ml for each level.
2. Even if the pain is unilateral, bilateral transforaminal injection may be preferred because of a possible inflammation on the contralateral side (Fig. 16.36).

Adjusting the C-arm according to levels

To align the lower endplates of the vertebral bodies for L1, L2, and L3, slight movement of the C-arm in cephalad or

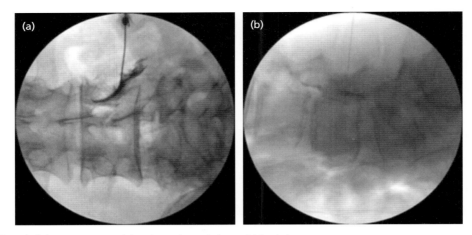

Figure 16.34 (a,b) Spread of the contrast material under posteroanterior and lateral views.

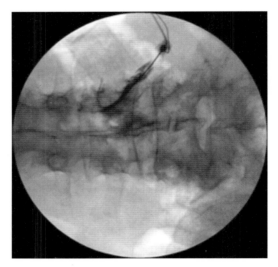

Figure 16.35 Spread of the contrast material into the epidural space.

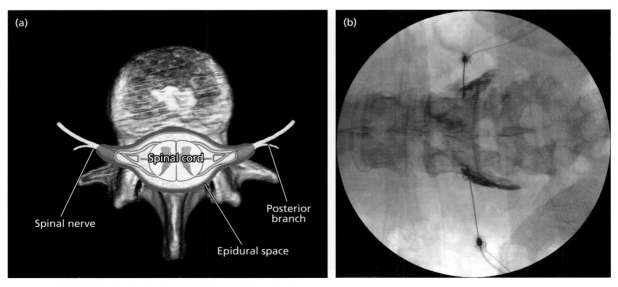

Figure 16.36 (a,b) Bilateral transforaminal injection due to bilateral inflammation.

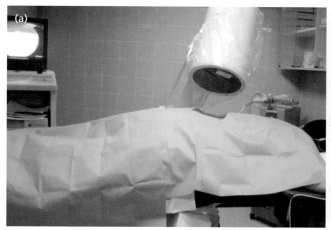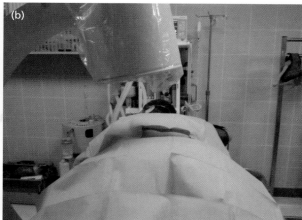

Figure 16.37 (a,b) Adjusting the C-arm according to levels.

caudal directions will be enough. For the L4 level, the C-arm should be placed more caudally, whereas for the L5 level it should be more cephalad (Fig. 16.37).

Step 9. Postprocedure observation

After the procedure is completed, the patient needs to be observed for up to 2 hours. Monitoring of vital signs is mandatory. In addition the pain relief should be objectively documented. After a satisfactory observation, the patient should be discharged with appropriate and adequate instructions given to their escort. Written instructions are preferable for emergencies and are helpful to the patient and their family.

Complications related to the technique
• Inadvertent dural puncture

The risk of inadvertent dural puncture is possible even in the most experienced hands. During the dural puncture, cerebrospinal fluid may not be aspirated. Rapid clearance of the contrast material can signify that the needle is in the subarachnoid space (Fig. 16.38).

• Inadvertent subdural puncture

The subdural space is a potential space between the subarachnoid and epidural space. Injection of a very small amount of contrast material will appear like a thin direct line in multiple levels. Unlike injection of the contrast material to the subarachnoid space, contrast material does not disappear. Administration of local anesthetic solution to the subdural space will end with total spinal block.

• Spinal nerve injury

The needle may contact the spinal segmental nerve or its ventral ramus while advanced through the intervertebral foramen. Immediate severe pain and paresthesia develop at that instant. The patient should remain sufficiently conscious to provide a response to such a complication. The needle is then to be replaced. If the same symptoms recur, the procedure should be interrupted.

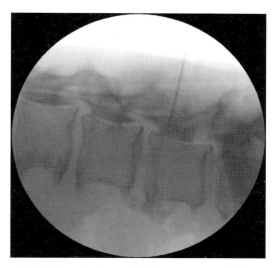

Figure 16.38 Subarachnoid spread of the contrast material.

• Inadvertent intravascular injection

During the aspiration test, blood may not be aspirated. The contrast material should slowly be given under uninterrupted live imaging. If the needle is within the vertebral artery, the contrast material spreads vertically. If the needle is within the segmental artery, it will spread medially towards the spinal cord. The spread of the contrast material within the epidural or paraspinous veins is slower. During the puncture of anterior or posterior segmental arteries if nonparticulate steroid solutions are injected, serious complications will not occur. Only if particulate solutions are used is there the risk of emboli or infarct (Fig. 16.39).

• Epidural hematoma

Bleeding within the epidural space is a major complication if hematoma develops. The most important cause of epidural hematoma is the bleeding of the venous plexus within the lumbar epidural space. Bleeding due to mechanical damage of the arteries within the epidural space gives rise to early findings while bleeding in the venous plexus may give rise to findings in later stages, even some days after. Hematoma in the lumbar epidural space can have a mass effect on arterial or venous blood flow, which results in spinal cord ischemia.

If severe pain, paresthesia, and loss of strength in the upper extremities develop within hours or days, one should suspect epidural hematoma.

- **Spinal cord injury**

The risk of spinal cord injury during transforaminal injection is low. If the site of entry is too lateral, the needle may be directed towards the spinal cord.

Permanent damage within the spinal cord may also develop owing to the injection of local anesthetics or other solutions.

- **Inadvertent intradiscal puncture**

If the needle is directed toward the disc, there is a risk of inadvertent intradiscal puncture. Thus one should be very

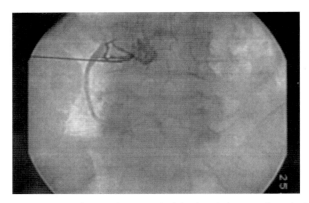

Figure 16.39 Inadvertent intravascular injection during transforaminal epidural block.

careful with the site of entry. It should be below the pedicle and should not be directed toward the disc. The needle should be advanced under a lateral view (Fig. 16.40).

Side effects related to drugs

- **Infection**

Although uncommon, infection in the epidural space remains an ever-present possibility, especially in the immunocompromised AIDS or cancer patient. Especially in patients with an epidural catheter for a longer period, one should be very careful about infection. A possible cause of infection is seeding of the infectious agents from the entry site at the skin and their subsequent hematogenous spread. *Staphylocccus aureus*, *Streptococcus*, and *Staphylococcus epidermidis* are the common agents.

- **Epidural abscess**

If epidural abscess occurs, emergent surgical drainage to avoid spinal cord compression and irreversible neurologic deficit is usually required. Early detection and treatment of infection is crucial to avoid potentially life-threatening sequelae. Epidural abscesses may not be diagnosed in the early stages until neurological signs develop.

- **Meningitis**

Meningitis is a rare complication. However, it should be kept in mind.

Helpful hints

The objective of an epidural steroid injection is to deliver corticosteroid close to the site of pathology, presumably onto an inflamed nerve root.

The epidural space may be divided as anterior and posterior. During the interlaminar epidural block, the target is the posterior epidural space. The injectate within the epidural

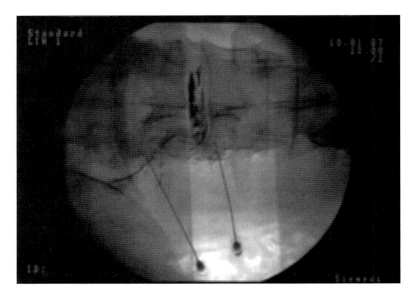

Figure 16.40 Inadvertent intradiscal puncture during transforaminal epidural block.

space spreads in an uncontrollable manner during the interlaminar approach.

Although not preferable, it may be performed by blind technique.

Ligaments or fibrosis within the epidural space may prevent the solution from spreading to the inflamed part of the nerve or the disc.

The disadvantages of interlaminar epidural block are that higher volumes of solutions are injected, extradural injection, inadverdent intravascular, subarachnoid and subdural injection, spinal cord injury.

The disadvantages of transforaminal lumbar epidural block are inadvertent intravascular injection, subdural puncture, intraneural injection, and segmental spinal nerve injury.

Transforaminal epidural block can only be performed under fluoroscopy.

The contrast material should be injected under live fluoroscopic imaging to identify any intravascular injection.

Although subarachnoid injection is less likely compared to intralaminar injection, it is still a possibility. The contrast material in the subarachnoid space will reveal initially a smooth contoured anterior spread slightly posterior to the posterior border of the vertebral body.

Performing transforaminal lumbar epidural block is one of the first steps for a trainee. Although it may be seen to be an easy technique, taking into consideration the complications one should be very careful while performing the block.

The trainee should be competent in the procedure, including neurological and fluoroscopic anatomy and imaging. Detailed knowledge of pharmacology, adverse effects of agents injected, knowledge of risks, complications, benefits, and alternatives to the procedure are required.

The risks and complications of the procedure should be thoroughly explained to the patient before a written consent is taken.

The risks include infection, bleeding, and nerve injury.

The patient should be given instructions about activity limitations. The patient should be followed up weekly for the first month and then on a monthly basis.

Percutaneous block and lesioning of the lumbar facet joint and medial branch

History

In 1941, Badgley was the first clinician to associate facet arthritis with nerve root irritation as a cause of low back pain and sciatica. Hirsch in 1963 demonstrated that low back pain along the sacroiliac and gluteal regions with radiation to the greater trochanter could be induced by injecting hypertonic saline in the region of the lumbar facet

joints. In 1971, Rees proposed a surgical approach to severing the posterior primary rami. In 1975 Shealy first described the RF denervation of the medial branch of lumbar facet joints.

Anatomy of the lumbar zygapophyseal (facet) joint

The zygapophyseal joints or facet joints are formed by the inferior articular process of the vertebra above and the superior articular process of the vertebra below. The concavity of the superior articular process accommodates in the convexity of the inferior articular process. The facet joints in the region are a part of the intervertebral foramen.

The facet joints are synovial joints; the inferior and superior articular processes are lined with articular cartilage. Every lumbar zygapophyseal joint is enclosed by a fibrous capsule. This capsule is made up of collagen fibers passing from one articular surface to the other along the posterior, inferior, and superior joint margins. The anterior margin of the joint effaces the ligamentum flavum, which replaces the fibrous joint capsule anteriorly. Posteriorly, the capsule attaches about 2 mm from the edge of the articular cartilage. At the superior and inferior poles, this attachment is even further from bone, creating subscapular pockets that contain fat and communicate with extracapsular fat through capsular foramina superiorly and inferiorly.

The facet joint capsule is approximately 1 mm thick, attached 2 mm below the articular margin, and contains a space with a maximal volume capacity of 1–2 ml of synovial fluid. The synovium of the lumbar zygapophyseal joints attaches along the margin of the cartilage of one articular process and crosses the joint to the opposite articular process, lining the surface of the fibrous capsule posteriorly, superiorly, and inferiorly, and lining the ligamentum flavum anteriorly (Figs 16.41–16.43).

A capsule that is lined by a synovial membrane surrounds each joint. In the superior and inferior recesses of the facet joints, the capsule appears to be redundant, forming two meniscoid structures: one superior and one inferior.

Innervation of the facet joint

The nerve supply to the lumbar facet joints is via the medial branches of the posterior primary rami of L1–L5 (Fig. 16.44).

At the origin, the posterior and anterior primary rami of a nerve root diverge at the intervertebral foramen. The posterior ramus passes dorsally and caudally through a foramen in the intertransverse ligament. At a point 5 mm from its origin, it divides into medial, lateral, and intermediate branches. The medial branch supplies the lower pole of the facet joint at its own level and the upper pole of the facet joint below.

Each medial branch supplies the joints above and below its course, except for L5, which sends an ascending articular

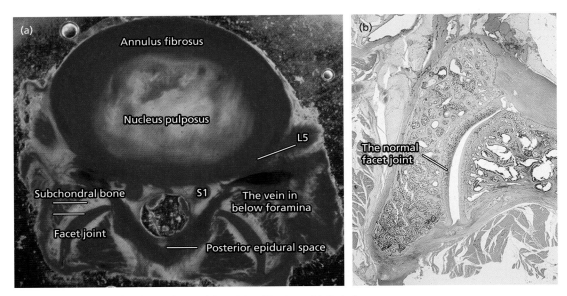

Figure 16.41 (a,b) Facet joint in axial section and normal facet joint. (Courtesy of J. Taylor.)

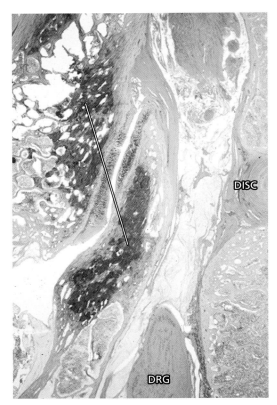

Figure 16.42 Sagittal section of the lumbar facet joint. DRG, dorsal root ganglion. (Courtesy of J. Taylor.)

branch only to the L5–S1 joint. Conversely, each zygapophyseal joint is supplied by the two medial branches that drape over the transverse processes at the levels comprising the joint. Thus, the L3–L4 joint is supplied by the medial branches that cross the L3 and L4 transverse processes, which are the medial branches of the posterior primary rami of L2 and L3. Similarly, the L5–S1 joint is innervated by the L4 and L5 medial branches, which cross the transverse process of L5 and the ala of the sacrum, respectively. Each medial branch of the posterior primary ramus also supplies the multifidus, interspinales, and intertransversarii medialis muscles and the ligaments and periosteum of the neural arch.

The L5 medial branch arises from the longer L5 posterior primary ramus and runs in the groove formed by the junction of the superior articular process and sacral ala. The L5 medial branch then travels medially around the base of the L5–S1 joint, sending an articular branch to this joint and then supplying the multifidus muscle. The medial branches of the lumbar posterior primary rami innervate the facet joints, multifidus muscle, and interspinous ligament and muscle. The lateral branches innervate the iliocostalis quadratus lumborum muscle and often become cutaneous at L1, L2, and L3, innervating the skin over the buttock. The intermediate branches innervate the longissimus muscle.

Indications

- Facet joint syndrome.
- Facet joint arthropathy.
- Spinal lumbar stenosis.
- Chronic low back pain without radiculopathy.
- Postlaminectomy syndrome.

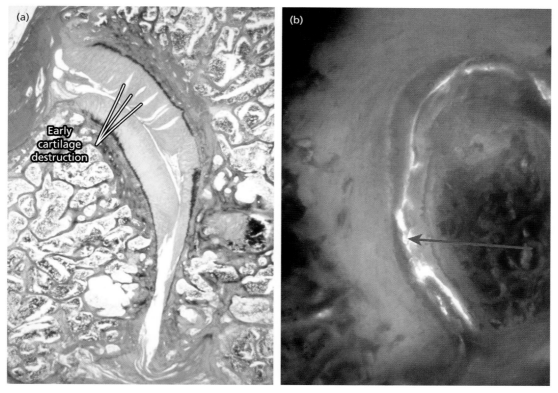

Figure 16.43 (a,b) Destruction in the facet joints. (Courtesy of J. Taylor.)

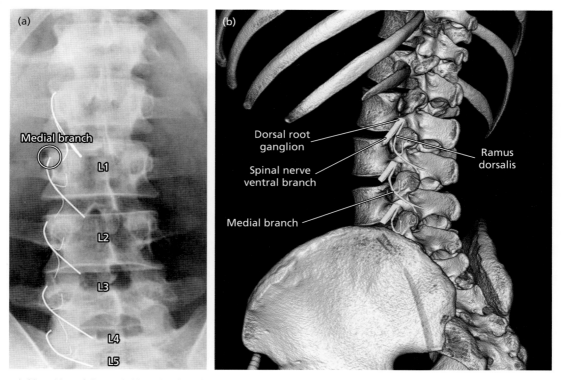

Figure 16.44 (a,b) Position of the medial branch of the facet joint under fluoroscopic view and three-dimensional CT scan.

Contraindications
- Local infection or sepsis.
- Coagulopathy.
- Vital functions instability.
- Psychopathologies.

Technique of facet joint block

Step 1. Prepare the patient before the procedure
The type of analgesia or sedation needs to be ascertained before performance of the invasive procedure. If a local anesthetic is considered or neurolytic block is planned, mild sedation is all that is necessary. If pulsed RF is planned, the patient needs to be awake to respond to the stimulation test. Intravenous fentanyl or midazolam may be used judiciously for the patient's comfort.

Step 2. Position and monitor the patient
1. Place the patient prone on the table. Place a pillow under the abdomen to flatten the lumbar lordosis.
2. An intravenous cannula is inserted for medication injections.
3. Monitoring of vital signs is mandatory.
4. Oxygen is provided by nasal cannula.
5. The area for needle entry is prepared in a sterile fashion.

Step 3. Drugs and equipment for lumbar facet joint block
- 5 ml syringe for skin infiltration.
- 1½ inch, 25 gauge needle for skin infiltration.
- 5 ml syringe for contrast material.
- 10 cm, 22 gauge needle for facet joint block.
- 1% lidocaine for skin infiltration.
- Contrast material, e.g. iohexol.
- Deposteroid.
- 0.5% bupivacaine.
- Saline.

Step 4. Visualization
1. Place the C-arm in a posteroanterior position first. Identify the midpoint of the intervertebral space at the target level. Adjust the lower endplate of the target vertebral body to be aligned by moving the C-arm in cephalocaudal direction.
2. Turn the C-arm in the oblique direction approximately 45° for L4–L5 and L5–S1 levels, and 30° for upper levels, until the facet joint comes into view. One should be able to view the "Scottie dog" in this position (Figs 16.45–16.48).

Step 5. Direction of the needle
Infiltrate the skin with 1% lidocaine. Advance the needle under fluoroscopic guidance in a tunneled vision fashion toward the inferior aspect of the facet joint to pass the inferior subscapular recess.

Step 6. Confirm the position of the needle
1. Inject 0.2 ml contrast solution. If the needle tip is within the joint space, a straight line will appear.
2. Move the C-arm laterally to reconfirm the depth of the needle (Fig. 16.49).

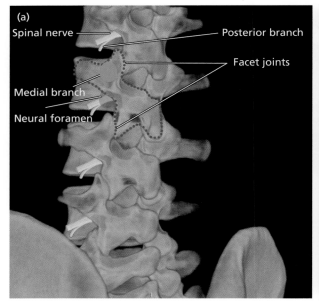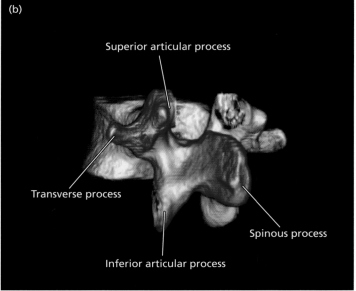

Figure 16.45 (a,b) "Scotty dog" and structures in close proximity .

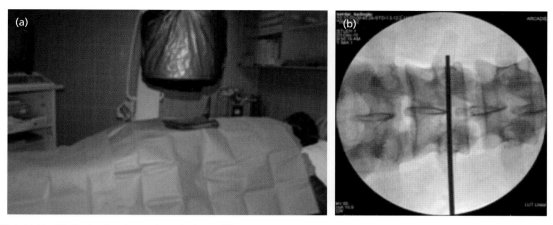

Figure 16.46 (a,b) Identify the level under posteroanterior position.

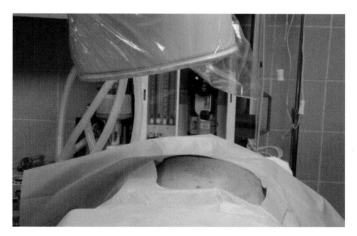

Figure 16.47 Position of the C-arm for the oblique view of the lumbar facet.

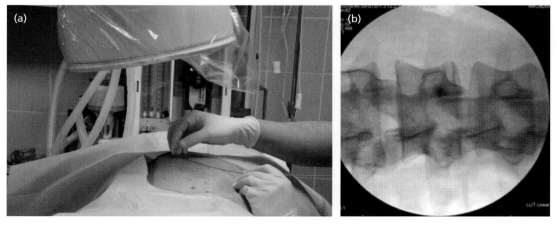

Figure 16.48 (a,b) The needle in position within the facet joint under "tunneled vision."

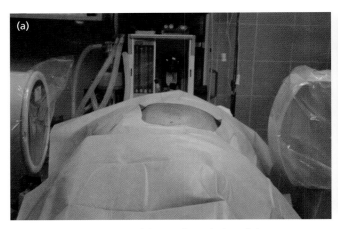
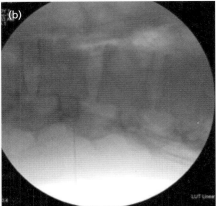

Figure 16.49 (a,b) Confirm the position of the needle under lateral view.

Step 7. Lumbar facet joint block

1. After confirming the correct position of the needle, inject 1 ml of deposteroid local anesthetic combination for each facet joint.

Note: do not force during injection, which may cause rupture of the joint capsule and exacerbate the pain.

2. If the facet joint block is performed for diagnostic purposes, periarticular injection of local anesthetic may be sufficient.

Technique of lumbar facet medial branch block and RF lesioning

Steps 1 and 2. These are similar to those described with the facet joint block (vide supra).

Step 3. Drugs and equipment for medial branch block and RF denervation
- 5 ml syringe for skin infiltration.
- 1½ inch, 25 gauge needle for skin infiltration.
- 5 ml syringe for contrast solution.
- 10 cm, 22 gauge needle for facet joint block.
- 10 cm, 2–5 mm active-tip electrode for RF.
- RF machine.
- 1% lidocaine for skin infiltration.
- Contrast solution, e.g. iohexol.
- Deposteroid.
- 0.5% bupivacaine.
- Saline.

Step 4. Visualization

1. The level chosen to be blocked is identified under fluoroscopic view in the posteroanterior projection. The lower endplate of the target vertebral body needs to be aligned by moving the C-arm in a cephalocaudal direction (Fig. 16.50).

2. Then rotate the C-arm in an oblique fashion toward the lateral projection slowly until a view of the "Scottie dog"

is obtained. The "Scottie dog" is formed by the superior as well as the inferior pars of the same vertebra. The "ear" of the dog is the superior articular process (pars) and the "front legs" of the dog are the inferior articular process (pars) (Figs 16.51–16.53).

Step 5. Direction of the needle or electrode

1. Once this view has been obtained, the optimal point of contact with the bone by the needle should be the "eye of the dog," which is the junction of the superior articular process and the transverse process.

2. After infiltrating the skin, a 22 gauge, 10 cm needle is introduced and advanced toward the target until a bony contact is made. The needle tip should rest on the bone.

Step 6. Confirm the position of the needle

1. Then rotate the C-arm laterally to confirm the position of the needle. The needle tip should be in line with the facet column, not beyond this point, posterior to the intervertebral foramen (Fig. 16.54).

2. On the posteroanterior view, the needle should be at the junction of the superior articular process and the medial most aspect of the transverse process (Fig. 16.55).

3. The needle may slide about 1 mm at the junction of the superior articular process and transverse process.

Step 7. Test stimulation

1. A sensory stimulation test at 50 Hz is conducted. The patient should feel paresthesia or a tingling sensation in the back at approximately 0.5 V. If the patient feels sensations in the lower extremity, the needle tip is too close to the segmental nerve root and it should be slightly withdrawn, and the stimulation test needs to be repeated.

2. Then a motor stimulation test is conducted at 2 Hz. The patient should feel local contractions of the multifidus muscles. If any contraction of the leg or leg muscles occurs, the needle tip should be repositioned.

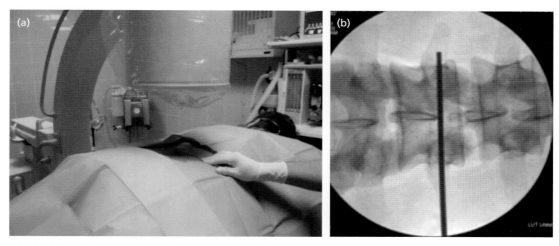

Figure 16.50 (a,b) Adjust the lower endplate of the target vertebral body.

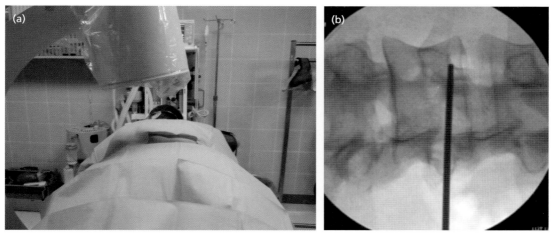

Figure 16.51 (a,b) C-arm in oblique position, the target for the medial branch block.

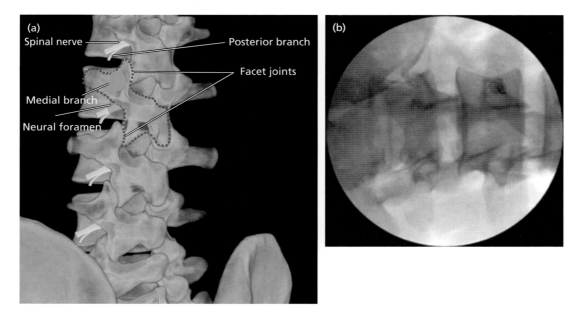

Figure 16.52 (a,b) Target point for medial branch block and the needle in position.

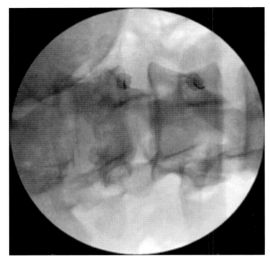

Figure 16.53 Needles in position on two levels.

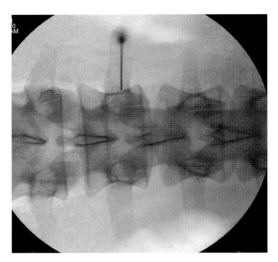

Figure 16.55 Position of the needle under posteroanterior view.

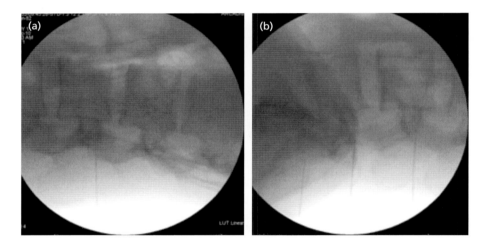

Figure 16.54 (a,b) Confirm the position of the needles under lateral view.

3. At this point, an aspiration test is done. If blood is aspirated, reposition the needle and aspirate again. In the case where cerebrospinal fluid is aspirated, check if the needle is too deep, withdraw and terminate the procedure.

Step 8. Medial branch block and/or RF denervation

1. At this point, after careful negative aspiration, the local anesthetic is injected. This should be repeated at each level corresponding to the medial branch innervating the facet joint targeted.

Note: the lumbar zygapophyseal joints are innervated by the medial branches found at the same levels comprising the joint but named for the source of the segmental nerve from which it came. Thus, the L4–L5 zygapophyseal joint is innervated by the L3 and L4 medial branches.

2. RF lesioning at 67°C for 60 seconds is performed at each level.

3. If pulsed RF is to be performed, do this at 45 V for two cycles of 120 seconds.

Block and RF lesioning of the median branch of L5

The medial branch at the L5 level lies in the groove formed by the superior articular process of the sacrum and the ala of this bone. It then gives the medial and intermediate branches. There is no pedicle at this level.

1. Place the C-arm in a posteroanterior position. To view the junction as a curve, the C-arm may be rotated in a cephalocaudal fashion (Fig. 16.56).

2. Advance the needle or the electrode in a tunneled vision fashion toward the junction.

3. Move the C-arm to the lateral position. In the lateral view, the tip should stay over the posterior border of the facet column outside and posterior to the neural foramen.

4. The rest of the procedure is the same as described above (Fig. 16.57).

Parallel placement of electrodes

In many centers, the electrodes are placed on the medial nerve by a tunneled vision approach perpendicularly. However, there are centers that place the electrode accurately on the target nerves parallel to the nerves rather than perpendicular. It has been speculated that when placed in this manner, the electrodes coagulate a substantial length of the target nerves (Fig. 16.58).

Step 9. Postprocedural care

After the procedure is completed, the patient needs to be observed for up to 2 hours. Monitoring of vital signs is mandatory. In addition, the pain relief should be objectively documented. After a satisfactory observation, the patient should be discharged with appropriate and adequate instructions given to their escort. Written instructions are prefer-

able for emergencies and are helpful to the patient and their family.

Complications

• **Transient backache and muscle spasm**

This complication may occur especially after RF lesioning. Injecting deposteroid solution after lesioning is recommended.

• **Neuritis**

Neuritis may develop after RF lesioning.

• **Segmental spinal nerve injury**

If the needle or electrode is placed toward the neural foramen, segmental spinal injury and numbness in the related dermatome may develop. Thus the final position of the needle or electrode tip should be confirmed by lateral view as well as by sensorial and motor stimulation tests.

• **Infection**

The incidence of infection is the same as with the other procedures.

Helpful hints

In the upper lumbar spine, approximately 80% of the facet joints are curved and 20% are flat. In the lower lumbar spine, the situation is reversed and approximately 80% of the facet joints are flat. The upper lumbar facets are more oriented in the sagittal plane, and by the L5–S1 level they have rotated to a more oblique angle. The facet joints are oriented lateral to the sagittal plane from the midline posteriorly as follows: the L1–L2 joint 30° or less, the L2–L3 joint 15–45°, and the L3–L4 joints 30–75°. The lumbar facets are all almost vertically oriented, being tipped approximately 10° with the cephalad end of the joint farther anterior than the caudal end of the joint. Because of the curvature of the upper lumbar facet joints, the posterior opening is usually more in the sagittal plan than the overall angle of the joint. This usually means that the accessible posterior joint space opening is usually 5–10° less oblique than the best fluoroscopic image, which shows the angle of the joint overall.

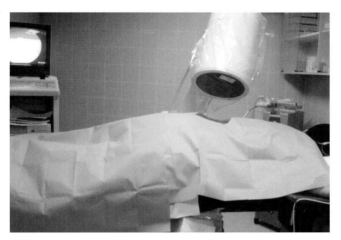
Figure 16.56 Position of the C-arm for the L5–S1 level.

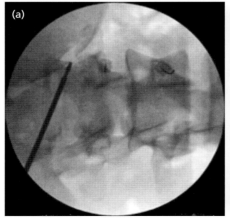
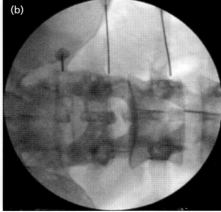
Figure 16.57 (a,b) L5 medial branch block or RF.

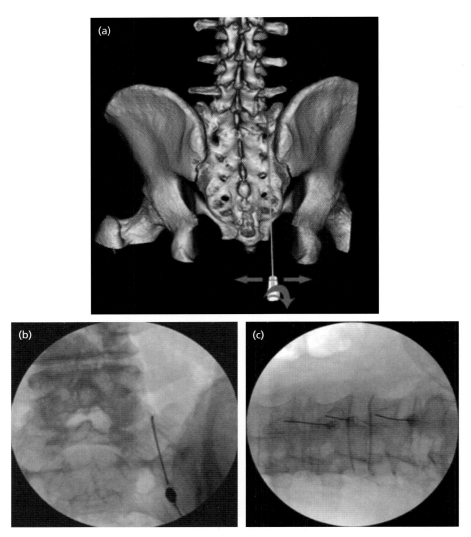

Figure 16.58 (a–c) Parallel positioning the electrodes for medial branch block.

The medial branch approach is preferred to the lumbar facet joint block. One should not insist on entering the joint, because the volume of the joint is very small and it may be destroyed. It is better first to perform a medial branch block and if it is effective then perform RF lesioning.

Percutaneous block and lesioning of the lumbar sympathetic ganglia

History
Historically the first report of lumbar sympathetic block seems to be attributed to Brunn and Mandl. In 1924 they described Sellheim's technique of injecting the lumbar sympathetic nerves as a component of his paravertebral approach to blocking the mixed spinal outflow in the lumbar region. Kappis also described the technique of lumbar sympathetic

block and surgical resection of the lumbar sympathetic nerves about this time. Others associated with expansion of the technique are von Gaza; Mandl and Lawen in Germany; Jonnesco and Fountain in France; and White in the United States. During the 1950s, Bonica, and Moore and Arnulf, described in detail the importance of lumbar sympathetic blockade, particularly its relationship to the treatment of causalgia and posttraumatic reflex dystrophies in servicemen after World War II. Although the technique described by Mandl in 1926 remains one of the most popular approaches to the lumbar sympathetic trunk, Reid and colleagues, in a large series published in 1970, described a more lateral approach that avoids contact with the transverse process. Two techniques are described in this chapter: the "classic" technique first described by Kappis and Mandl, and the lateral technique first described by Mandl and redefined by Reid and colleagues.

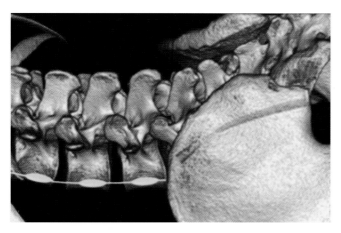

Figure 16.59 Three-dimensional CT scan showing the position of the lumbar sympathetic chain.

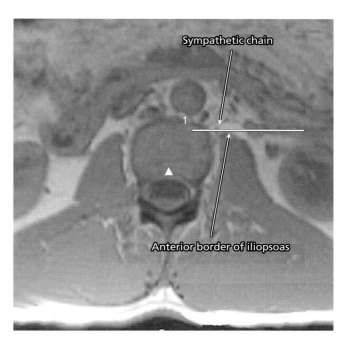

Figure 16.60 MRI showing the lumbar sympathetic chain, transverse section.

Anatomy

Location of the lumbar sympathetic ganglion

The sympathetic ganglia of the lumbar sympathetic chain are variable in both number and position. Rarely are five ganglia found on each side in the same individual. In most cases, only four are found. There tends to be fusion of the L1 and L2 ganglia in most patients, and ganglia are aggregated at the L2–L3 and L4–L5 discs. Considerable variability is noted in the size of the ganglia, some being fusiform and as long as 10–15 mm, others being round and approximately 5 mm long.

The L2 ganglion is situated at the caudal one-quarter segment of the vertebral body close to the anterior border of the L2, the L3 ganglion is situated as a mirror image, the L2 ganglion at the cephalad one-fourth of the L3 vertebral body, L4 and L5 are variable and lie in between (Figs 16.59 and 16.60).

Composition and course of the sympathetic chain

The sympathetic nervous system consists of preganglionic and postganglionic fibers that innervate deep somatic structures, skin, and viscera.

The preganglionic fibers traverse with their corresponding nerves as white rami communicantes, which communicates with considerable convergence in the paravertebral ganglia with postganglionic efferents and in the prevertebral ganglia with postganglionic efferents to the pelvic viscera. A small percentage of postganglionic fibers pass directly to ganglia in the aortic plexus and the superior and inferior hypogastric plexuses.

The postganglionic fibers leave the sympathetic trunk as gray rami communicantes, some passing to the L1 nerve to contribute to the iliohypogastric and genitofemoral nerve territories, some to the L2–L5 nerves, and some to the upper three sacral nerves, where they pass on to their respective destinations in the lumbosacral plexus.

Each lumbar sympathetic chain enters the retroperitoneal space under the right and left crura, continuing inferiorly in the interval between the anterolateral aspect of the vertebral bodies and the origin of the psoas muscle to enter the pelvis and the L5–S1 disc. Posteriorly, the periosteum overlies the vertebral bodies and the fibroaponeurotic origin of the psoas muscles and their fascial coverings. Anterior is the parietal reflection of the peritoneum, the aorta lying anteromedial to the left trunk and the vena cava anterior to the right trunk. The white and gray rami communicantes pass to their respective ganglia beneath the fibrous arcades of the psoas attachments to each vertebral body. They also tend to pass alongside the middle of the vertebral body.

Indications

Peripheral vascular disorders.
- Arteriosclerotic vascular disease.
- Raynaud's phenomenon and disease.
- Burger's disease.
- Diabetic neuropathy.
- For perioperative vascular surgery.
  Complex regional pain syndrome type I and II of the lower extremities.
- Posttraumatic syndrome.
- Perioperative orthopedic surgery.
  Miscellaneous
- Hyperhidrosis.

- Post amputation early stump pain.
- Phantom pain.
- Frostbite.
- Sympathetically mediated pain of any origin.

Contraindications
- Local infection or sepsis.
- Coagulopathy.
- Vital function instability.
- Psychopathologies.

Technique of lumbar sympathetic block and lesioning: prone approach

The procedure of lumbar sympathetic block is commonly done in either prone or lateral positions. The blind technique is not recommended. We prefer the fluoroscopic technique.

Step 1. Prepare the patient before the procedure
Ascertain the type of analgesia or sedation before performing the invasive procedure. It is important to start an intravenous infusion with normal saline as hypotension may occur with this procedure. If a local anesthetic is considered or neurolytic block is planned, mild sedation is all that is necessary. If pulsed RF is planned, the patient needs to be awake to respond to the stimulation test. Intravenous fentanyl or midazolam may be used judiciously for the patient's comfort.

Step 2. Position and monitor the patient
1. Place the patient in a prone position on the table.
2. Place a pillow under the abdomen to flatten the lumbar lordosis.
3. Obtain an intravenous access if drugs need to be administered.
4. Monitor vital signs (mandatory in unstable patients).
5. Prepare the area for needle entry in a sterile fashion.

Step 3. Drugs and equipment for the lumbar sympathetic block
Prepare and confirm that the following equipment, needles, and drugs are ready to be used for the procedure.
- 5 ml syringe for skin infiltration.
- 1½ inch, 25 gauge needle for skin infiltration.
- 5 ml syringe for contrast solution.
- 15 cm, 22 gauge needle for sympathetic block.
- 1% lidocaine for skin infiltration.
- Nonionic contrast solution.
- 5 ml of 0.5% bupivacaine and 40 mg methylprednisolone. If RF is desired:
- 2–5 mm active-tip electrode for RF lesioning.
- RF machine.

Step 4. Visualization
1. Place the C-arm in a posteroanterior position first. Identify the midpoint of the intervertebral space at the target level, at any chosen level from L3 to L4. Adjust the lower endplate of the target vertebral body to be aligned by moving the C-arm in a cephalocaudal direction (Fig. 16.61).
2. Next, rotate the C-arm obliquely to the ipsilateral side until the tip of the transverse process almost disappears behind the lateral side of the vertebral body. While rotating the C-arm, identify the width of the transverse process. The entry point is just at the inferior border of the transverse process (Fig. 16.62).

Step 5. Mark the surface landmarks for the needle entry
Infiltrate the point of entry with lidocaine. Next, introduce a 15 cm, 22 gauge needle and advance the needle in tunneled vision until the bony contact is made at the paravertebral edge of the vertebral body (Fig. 16.63).

Step 6. Confirm the position of the needle
1. Next, rotate the C-arm laterally. The needle tip should be located at the anterior border of the vertebral body; the

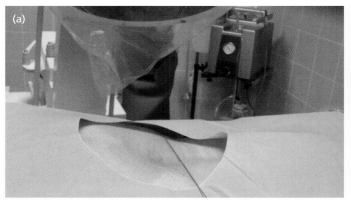
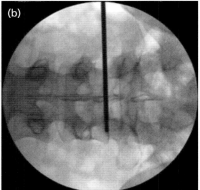

Figure 16.61 (a,b) Identify the intervertebral space.

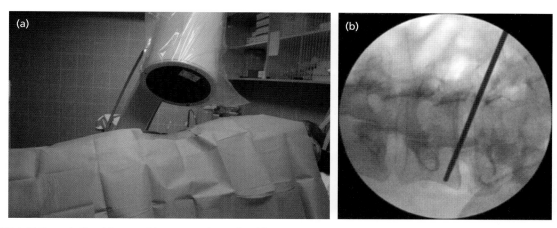

Figure 16.62 (a,b) C-arm in the oblique position, entry point under oblique view.

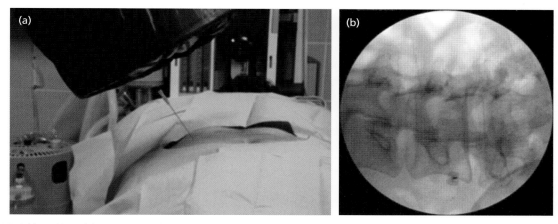

Figure 16.63 (a,b) Position of the C-arm and direction of the needle in "tunneled vision."

needle should be placed at the bottom one-fourth of the L2 and the upper one-fourth of the L3 and L4 vertebral bodies, and the lower one-third for the L5 vertebral body (Fig. 16.64).
2. Then rotate the C-arm back to the posteroanterior position. The needle tip should be confirmed at the level of the facet joint, approximately 1 cm deep and hugging the vertebral body.

Step 7. Injection of local anesthetic or steroid
1. After negative aspiration inject up to 5 ml of contrast solution. The contrast solution should spread as a straight line at the anterior border of the vertebral body in the lateral view and close to the vertebral body in the posteroanterior view (Figs 16.65 and 16.66).
2. After confirming the correct positioning of the needle, one should administer 5 ml of a combination of 40 mg methylprednisolone in 0.5% bupivacaine at a single site and smaller amounts if injected at multiple levels.
3. If a neurolytic block is planned (only for cancer patients), 5 ml of 6% phenol in glycerine (iohexol) may be administered.

Lateral approach
The lateral approach by Reid is described. The position of the patient is lateral in this approach.
Step 1 is as described above.

Step 2. Position and monitor the patient
Place the patient in the lateral decubitus position on the table with the head in the hyperflexed position and the legs pulled and flexed towards the abdomen. Support the abdomen and thorax with pillows, so the patient feels comfortable.

Step 3. Mark the surface landmark for entry point
With the patient in a lateral position, a skin wheal is made 10–14 cm lateral to the superior border of the spinous processes of L1 and L4. Usually, L3 is chosen aiming to have a spread of a contrast over L2–L4 sympathetic ganglia. The point of entry is infiltrated with a local anesthetic.

Step 4. Visualization and direction of the needle
A 6–8 inch sympathectomy needle is inserted at an angle of 60° to the sagittal plane, toward the body of the L3 vertebra. The needle is then advanced until it contacts the vertebral body. Fluoroscopy in two planes will confirm its position and the angle to assume for redirection of the needle to its final position at the anterolateral aspect of the vertebral body

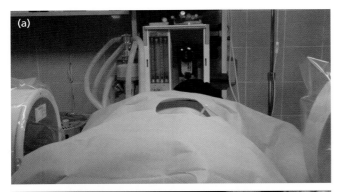

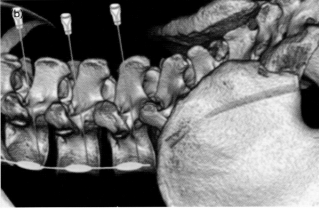

Figure 16.64 (a,b) Position of the needle under lateral view and a three-dimensional CT scan showing the position of the needles in each level, L3, L4, and L5.

with the fluoroscopy positioned laterally. Any final adjustments can be made to ensure that the needle tip lies exactly at the anterolateral edge of the vertebral body.

Step 5. Confirm the position of the needle
A small amount of contrast material will identify the correct tissue plane. The dye should spread to form a line conforming to the anterolateral margin of the vertebral bodies (L2–L4). If the spread of contrast dye is restricted to one ganglion, the procedure is then repeated with the second needle at an adjacent level, i.e., the L2 or L4 vertebral body.

Step 6. Injection of local anesthetic
A long-acting agent such as bupivacaine or ropivacaine is advantageous for both therapy and prognosis, because it enables enough time to evaluate the effects of sympatholysis and any effect this might have on the pain. A concentration of 0.5% bupivacaine or 0.5% ropivacaine gives optimal duration without the need for an added vasoconstrictor. However, a short-acting local anesthetic is commonly used first to obtain a quick skin response (temperature elevation, plethysmography curve heightening, galvanic skin response), then a long-acting agent is injected.

RF lesioning of the lumbar sympathetic chain
After the steps are taken to position the patient as described earlier, the RF needle electrode is inserted as described in the prone position with or without cannulae. A 10 or 15 cm, 5 mm active-tip electrode is positioned and confirmed as described above.

Step 5. Stimulation test
Stimulation is performed at 50 Hz for sensory and 2 Hz for motor stimulation. There should be an absence of fasciculation at the ventral root, dorsal plexus, or genitofemoral nerve during motor stimulation at 2 Hz up to 2 V. The patient may feel slight paresthesia at the back during sensory stimulation at 50 Hz at 0.2–0.5 V.

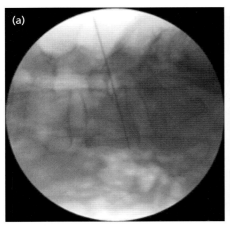

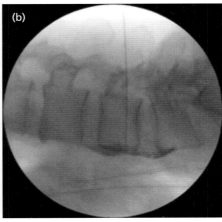

Figure 16.65 (a,b) Spread of the contrast material under lateral view.

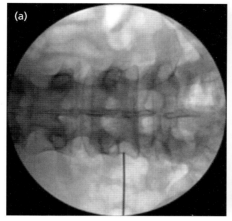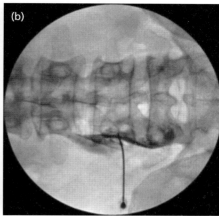

Figure 16.66 (a,b) Spread of the contrast material under posteroanterior view.

Step 6. Thermocoagulation of the sympathetic ganglia
1. Before RF lesioning inject 1 ml of 1% lidocaine. A lesion is made at each level at 60° for 60–90 seconds. The lesion diameter should be approximately 10 mm for L2 and 15 mm for L3 and L4. Thus multiple lesioning may be necessary by moving the tip of the electrode. Before each lesioning procedure, a motor and sensory stimulation test should be repeated.
2. If pulsed RF is planned, it may be applied at 20 ms/s at 45 V for two cycles for 120 seconds.

Step 7. Postprocedure observation
After the procedure is completed, observe the patient for up to 2 hours. In case of hypotension, intravenous electrolyte solutions should be administered. Monitoring of vital signs is mandatory. In addition, objectively document pain relief. After a satisfactory observation, discharge the patient with appropriate and adequate instructions given to their escort. Written instructions are preferable for emergencies and are helpful to the patient and their family.

Complications

Complications of lumbar sympathetic block may be classified as (a) neurological complications, (b) renal and ureteric complications, or (c) vascular complications.

Neurological complications
• **Neuritis**
Neuritis may develop owing to the spread of the neurolytic agent to a somatic nerve or lumbar plexus. The incidence of neuritis is higher with alcohol. Alcohol should not be preferred as the neurolitic agent.
• **Neuralgia**
Neuralgia, especially genitofemoral neuralgia, is one of the most important complications of lumbar sympathetic block with neurolytic agents. The patient complains of hyperesthesia in the groin. Normally it lasts 2–6 weeks.

Genitofemoral neuralgia develops especially if the lumbar sympathetic block is performed at the L4–L5 level. The genitofemoral nerve is in close proximity with the lumbar sympathetic chain along the fascia of the psoas muscle. Owing to the effect of the local anesthetic or neurolytic agent, minor sensory loss or motor weakness at the quadriceps muscle may develop. Another cause of neuralgia may be spread of the neurolytic agent to the rami communicantes, which has connections with the lateral cutaneous nerve of the thigh.
• **Inadvertent dural puncture**
Dural puncture particularly may occur if the lumbar sympathetic block is performed by a blind technique. It is almost impossible when using fluoroscopy and confirming the final position of the needle by contrast material. Paraplegia may occur if neurolytic agents are used.
• **Paraplegia**
This is a very rare complication, which may develop to the ischemia of the anterior spinal artery.
• **Inadvertent epidural or subdural puncture**
This complication may occur again only with the blind technique.
• **Inadvertent intradiscal puncture**
If the needle is directed more medially at the L4–L5 level, intradiscal puncture is possible. There will be an increase of resistance at the tip of the needle. If the needle tip is within the disc, 1 ml of 50 mg cephalosporin should be administered.
• **Low back pain and muscle spasm**
Low back pain or muscle spasm in the area may occur lasting 4–5 days after the procedure.

Renal or ureteric complications
• **Penetration of the kidney or ureter**
Penetration of the kidney, its capsule, or the ureter may occur owing to the wide lateral approach. The entry point should not exceed 6 or 7 cm from the midline.

• **Transient hematuria, renal colic, or dysuria**
These complications may be due to renal puncture.
• **Impotence**
Impotence may develop owing to the spread of the neurolytic solution to the genitofemoral nerve. One should avoid using neurolytic agents in males.
• **Retrograde ejaculation**
This is a very rare complication.

Vascular complications
• **Inadvertent inferior vena cava puncture**
This is one of the most important complications that may occur. The needle tip should stay just at the anterior border of the vertebral body. The inferior vena cava lies at a distance of 0.5–1 cm dorsal to the anterior border of the vertebral body. An aspiration test is mandatory. In the case of a positive aspiration test, one should change the position of the needle; if bleeding continues the procedure has to be terminated.
• **Retroperitoneal hematoma**
In patients with bleeding diathesis, retroperitoneal hematoma may develop. It is an absolute contraindication to perform lumbar sympathetic block in such patients.
• **Hypotension**
Owing to the sympathetic blockade, hypotension may develop. Administration of approximately 500 ml of lactate solution before the procedure is recommended.
• **Systemic and toxic reactions**
Intravascular injection of local anesthetics or neurolytics may cause systemic and toxic reactions.

Helpful hints
To perform a lumbar sympathetic block is one of the first steps in training a pain physician. However, one should consider the complications. It should not be performed by blind technique, and even if performed under fluoroscopy, every step should be confirmed meticulously.

The advantages of percutaneous RF lumbar sympathectomy are as follows.
• The lesion is controllable, it can be repeated, and there is no potential risk of neurolytic agents spreading to other neural structures.
• The risk of hypotension is less than with other sympatholytic procedures.
• The incidence of genitofemoral neuralgia is less with appropriate motor and sensory stimulation.

Percutaneous block and lesioning of the rami communicantes

History
The history is as described in the section on percutaneous block and lesioning of the lumbar sympathetic ganglia.

Anatomy
The communicating rami of the sympathetic chain originate off the segmental nerve immediately after it exits the intervertebral foramen. While the segmental nerve continues its path in a caudal, lateral, and anterior direction, the communicating rami run anteriorly, in close contact with the vertebral body en route to the regional sympathetic chain.

Although there are anatomic variations, the typical communicating ramus runs deep to the psoas muscle; however, it also may run between the psoas fibers or may be embedded in the connective tissue of the intervertebral disc. Two communicating rami may even branch off from one segmental nerve. Therefore, the relationship with the vertebral body is variable, but the proximal part of the communicating rami usually runs adjacent to the middle or caudal part of the vertebral body (Fig. 16.67).

Indications
• Discogenic pain at a single or multiple levels.
• Complex pain of vertebral structures.

Contraindications
• Local or systemic infection.
• Coagulopathy.

Technique of lesioning of the rami communicantes

Step 1. Prepare the patient before the procedure
Ascertain the type of analgesia or sedation before performing the invasive procedure. It is important to start an intravenous infusion with normal saline as hypotension may

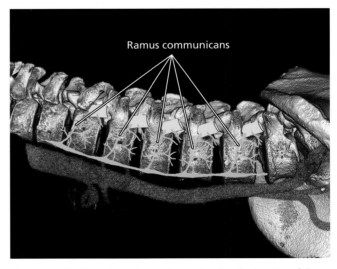

Figure 16.67 Three-dimensional CT scan showing the location of the ramus communicantes.

occur with this procedure. If a local anesthetic is considered or neurolytic block is planned, mild sedation is all that is necessary. If pulsed RF is planned, the patient needs to be awake to respond to the stimulation test. Intravenous fentanyl or midazolam may be used judiciously for the patient's comfort.

Step 2. Position and monitor the patient
1. Place the patient in a prone position on the table.
2. Place a pillow under the abdomen to flatten the lumbar lordosis.
3. Obtain an intravenous access if drugs need to be administered.
4. Monitor vital signs (mandatory in unstable patients).
5. Prepare the area for needle entry in a sterile fashion.

Step 3. Drugs and equipment for L2 communicating ramus
Prepare and confirm that the following equipment, needles, and drugs are ready to be used for the procedure:
- 1½ inch, 25 gauge needle for skin infiltration.
- 5 ml syringe for local anesthesia.
- 2 ml syringe for aspiration test.
- 1% lidocaine for skin infiltration.

- Contrast solution.
- 0.5% bupivacaine.
- Deposteroid.
  If RF is desired:
- RF machine.
- 10 cm, 5 mm active-tip electrode.

Step 4. Visualization
1. Place the C-arm in a posteroanterior position first. Identify the midpoint of the intervertebral space at the target level. Adjust the lower endplate of the target vertebral body to be aligned by moving the C-arm in a cephalocaudal direction (Fig. 16.68).
2. Then turn the C-arm obliquely towards the ipsilateral side, approximately 30°. Locate the anatomical landmarks, the transverse process and the neural foramen, at the targeted site (Fig. 16.69).

Step 5. Mark the surface landmarks for the needle entry
The entry point is just below the transverse process, in line with the lateral edge of the vertebral body, approximately 6–7 cm from the midline.

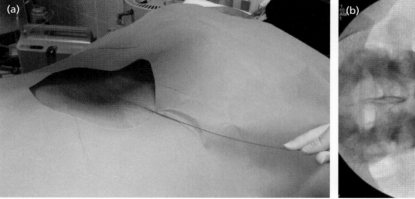
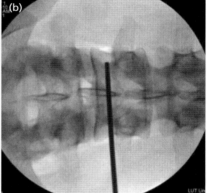

Figure 16.68 (a,b) Adjust the lower endplate of the target vertebral body to be aligned by moving the C-arm in a cephalocaudal direction.

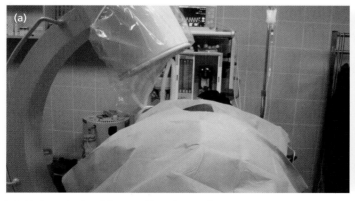
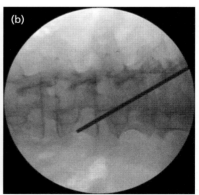

Figure 16.69 (a,b) C-arm in the oblique position, the needle entry point.

Step 6. Direction of the needle
Infiltrate the entry point with 1% lidocaine and advance the needle in a tunneled vision toward the lateral edge of the vertebral body until a bony contact is made. If the needle contacts the segmental nerve, the patient will complain of a sudden pain; correct the needle position in a more cranial direction (Fig. 16.70).

Step 7. Confirm the position of the needle
1. Position the C-arm laterally; the tip of the needle or electrode should be in the middle portion of the vertebral body, with a bony contact. Inject 1 ml of contrast material. The contrast should spread behind the facet line, parallel to the needle, unlike the view during the lumbar sympathetic block where the spread is like a straight line at the anterior border of the vertebral body (Figs 16.71 and 16.72).
2. Place the C-arm back to the posteroanterior position. The contrast material should be closely lateral to the vertebral body just caudal to the transverse process.
3. An aspiration test should be negative.

Step 8. Stimulation test
1. Sensory stimulation is made between 0 and 1 V, at 50 Hz. The patient will feel discomfort from 0.2 to 0.5 V. If pain radiating to the groin occurs at the L2 level, close proximity to the genitofemoral nerve is indicated and the needle should be repositioned for retesting.
2. During motor stimulation at 2 Hz up to 1 V, no response should be elicited.

Step 9. RF lesioning
1. After confirming the position of the electrode, inject 0.5 ml of 1% lidocaine, followed by RF lesioning at 60 °C for 60 seconds.
2. Pulsed RF at 45 V for two cycles of 120 seconds not exceeding 42 °C may also be performed.

Step 10. Postprocedure observation
After the procedure is completed, observe the patient for up to 2 hours. In case of hypotension, intravenous electrolyte solutions should be administered. Monitoring of vital signs is mandatory. In addition, objectively document pain relief. After a satisfactory observation, discharge the patient with appropriate and adequate instructions given to their escort. Written instructions are preferable for emergencies and are helpful to the patient and their family.

Complications
Segmental nerve injury.
Inadvertent puncture of the paravertebral artery.
Genitofemoral nerve injury.

Helpful hints
L2 communicating ramus lesion or block may be used in pain of discal origin. The communicating ramus RF lesioning should be performed after a progrostic block with 0.5 ml of 1% lidocaine. If the pain disappears, one should continue with RF lesioning.

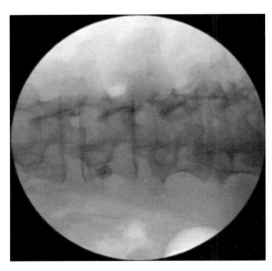

Figure 16.70 Direction of the needle in "tunneled vision."

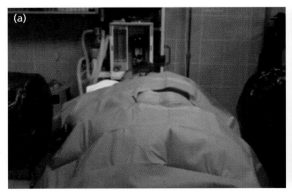
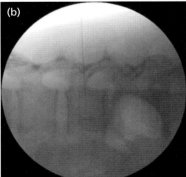
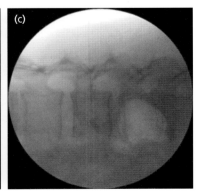

Figure 16.71 (a–c) C-arm in the lateral position, final location of the needle and the spread of the contrast material.

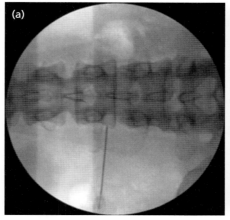

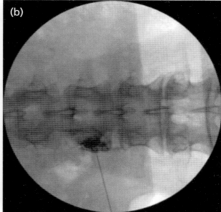

Figure 16.72 (a,b) Position of the needle under posteroanterior view, spread of the contrast material under posteroanterior view.

Percutaneous discography and lesioning of the lumbar disc

History

In 1948, Hirsch injected procaine into a herniated disc and reported relief of sciatica.

In 1940 Roofe described the annulus fibrosus innervation, which led to the conceptualization that the disc is a pain source independent of a neurocompressive neurological phenomenon. In 1944, Lindblom demonstrated the presence of radial annular fissures upon injecting a dye in a disc of a cadaver.

Hirsch followed this with a clinical study to determine how the ruptures or tears in the annulus would lead to pathologic processes producing pain. He hypothesized that putting pressure on a ruptured or degenerated disc would reproduce pain. His technique used saline to pressurize the disc and procaine solution to modulate the pain response generated.

In 1970, Crock advanced the theory of internal disc disruption. He showed that these patients have abnormal discograms and that pain is reproduced by a small volume (0.3 ml) of solution injected, owing to hypersensitivity of pain fibers in the disc. Discographic patterns on radiographs were shown to be abnormal. In 1987 Sachs described the Dallas Discogram Scale.

Bogduk in 2004 followed it up with a description of the cardinal component of discography. The characteristic grade I lesion is a radial fissure extending to the inner third, a grade II to the middle third, and grade III to the outer third. Seventy-five percent of grade III disruptions are associated with exact or similar pain reproduction, and 77% of discs with exact pain reproduction were found to have a grade III tear. Bogduk stated that discography is a diagnostic tool designed only to obtain information about the source of a patient's pain.

Anatomy

The intervertebral discs are complex structures that consist of a thick outer ring of fibrous cartilage termed the annulus fibrosus, which surrounds a more gelatinous core known as the nucleus pulposus; the nucleus pulposus is sandwiched inferiorly and superiorly by cartilage endplates.

Structure of the nucleus pulposus

The central nucleus pulposus contains collagen fibers, which are organized randomly, and elastin fibers (sometimes up to 150 μm in length), which are arranged radially; these fibers are embedded in a highly hydrated aggrecan-containing gel. Interspersed at a low density (approximately 5000/mm) are chondrocyte-like cells, sometimes sitting in a capsule within the matrix. Outside the nucleus is the annulus fibrosus, with the boundary between the two regions being very distinct in the young individual (<10 years).

Structure of the annulus

This is made up of a series of 15–25 concentric rings, or lamellae, with the collagen fibers lying parallel within each lamella. The fibers are oriented at approximately 60° to the vertical axis, alternating to the left and right of it in adjacent lamellae. Elastin fibers lie between the lamellae, possibly helping the disc to return to its original arrangement following bending, whether it is flexion or extension. They may also bind the lamellae together as elastin fibers pass radially from one lamella to the next. The cells of the annulus, particularly in the outer region, tend to be fibroblast-like, elongated, thin, and aligned parallel to the collagen fibers. Toward the inner annulus the cells can be more oval. Cells of the disc, both in the annulus and nucleus, can have several long, thin cytoplasmic projections, which may be more than 30 μm long. Such features are not seen in cells of articular cartilage. Their function in disc is unknown but it has been suggested that they may act as sensors and communicators of mechanical strain within the tissue.

Structure of the endplate

The third morphologically distinct region is the cartilage endplate, a thin horizontal layer, usually less than 1 mm thick, of hyaline cartilage. This interfaces the disc and the vertebral body. The collagen fibers within it run horizontal and parallel to the vertebral bodies, with the fibers continuing into the blood vessels and nerve supply of the disc.

The healthy adult disc has few (if any) blood vessels, but it has some nerves, mainly restricted to the outer lamellae, some of which terminate in proprioceptor. The cartilaginous endplate, like other hyaline cartilages, is normally totally avascular and aneural in the healthy adult. Blood vessels present in the longitudinal ligaments adjacent to the disc and in young cartilage endplates (less than about 12 months old) are branches of the spinal artery (Figs 16.73–16.83).

Nerves in the disc have been demonstrated, often accompanying these vessels, but they can also occur independ-

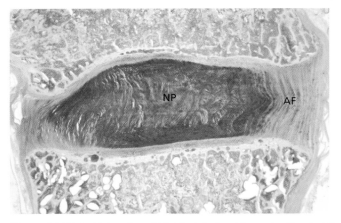

Figure 16.73 Sagittal section of L3–L4 adult disc. AF, annulus fibrosis; NP, nucleus pulposus. (Courtesy of J. Taylor.)

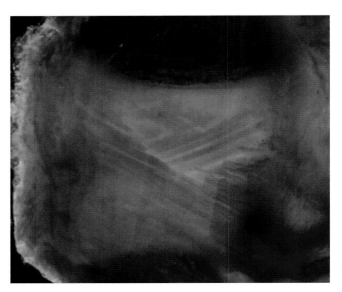

Figure 16.75 Alternating fiber direction in adjacent layers of outer annulus, 2.5 mm thick section. (Courtesy of J. Taylor.).

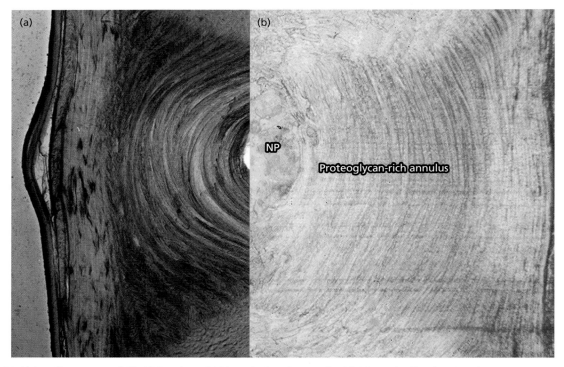

Figure 16.74 (a) Lamellar structure of AF; (b) 2 regions of AF in sagittal section anterior AF. AF, annulus fibrosis; NP, nucleus pulposus. (Courtesy of J. Taylor.)

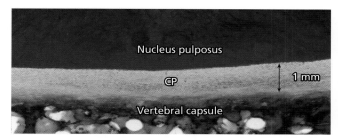

Figure 16.76 Cartilage plate (CP), hyaline cartilage, 1 mm thick, caps end surface of vertebra attached to vertebral body by thin calcified layer, which is penetrated by small vascular buds. Pathway for diffusion of nutrients to disc, barrier between avascular proteoglycan-rich nucleus and vascular spongiosa of vertebra. (Courtesy of J. Taylor.)

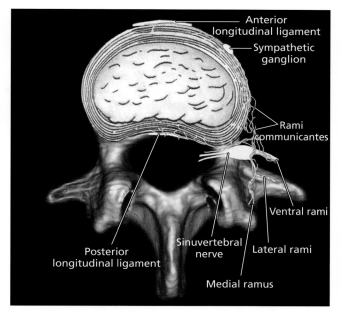

Figure 16.77 Three-dimensional CT scan showing the lumbar disc and structures in close proximity.

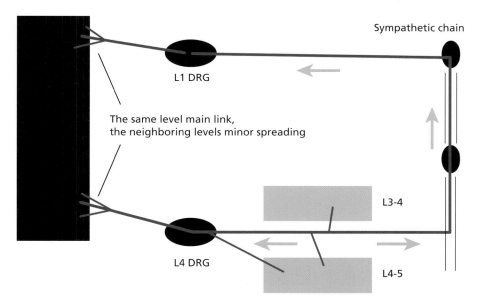

Figure 16.78 The innervation of the lumbar disc.

ently, being branches of the sinuvertebral nerve or derived from the ventral rami or gray rami communicantes. A meningeal branch of the spinal nerve, known as the recurrent sinuvertebral nerve, originates near the disc space. This nerve exits from the dorsal root ganglion and enters the foramen, when it then divides into a major ascending and a lesser descending branch. It has been shown in animal studies that further afferent contributions to the sinovertebral nerve arise through the rami communicantes from multiple superior and inferior dorsal root ganglia. In addition, the anterior longitudinal ligament receives afferent innerva-

tion from branches that originate in the dorsal root ganglion. The posterior longitudinal ligament is richly innervated by nociceptive fibers from the ascending branch of the sinovertebral nerve. These nerves also innervate the adjacent outer layers of the annulus fibrosus. Some of the nerves in discs also have glial support cells, or Schwann cells, alongside them.

In a painful disc, substance P and phospholipase A2 enzyme activity increase. These inflammatory chemical substances cause a chronic chemical sensitization within the disc and cause pain.

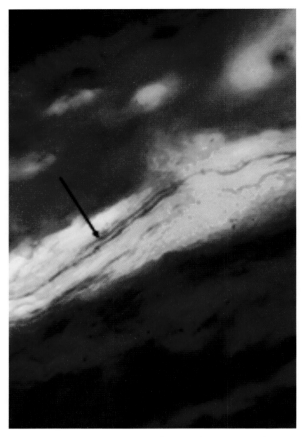

Figure 16.79 Silver stain of annulus fibrosus showing nerve fibers which penetrate to six lamellae deep from the surface. (Courtesy of J. Taylor.)

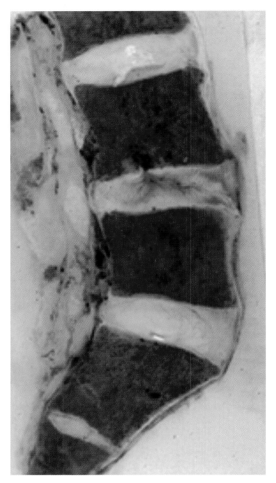

Figure 16.81 The cauda equina, descending in the lumbar spinal canal within the dural sac (which terminates at the S2 level); the epidural space contains a venous plexus (parasagittal section of lumbar spine). (Courtesy of J. Taylor.)

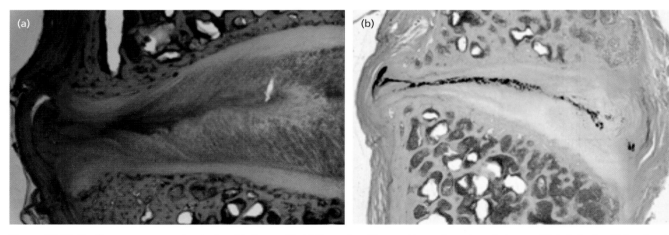

Figure 16.80 The fissures are more extensive in subjects over 35. (a) Fissure in a 22-year-old man through posterior one-third of disc (sagittal sections). (b) Extensive fissure in a 36-year-old man (demonstrated by injection of carbon particles into center of disc before fixation and sectioning).

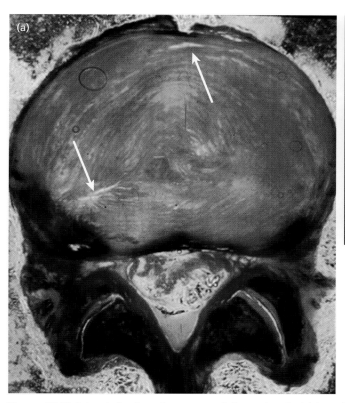

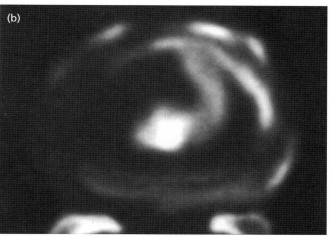

Figure 16.82 Internal disc disruption, a cause of discogenic pain. (a) Spread of contrast from NP circumferential fissures. (b) Radial fissure into cadaver disc. (Courtesy of J. Taylor.)

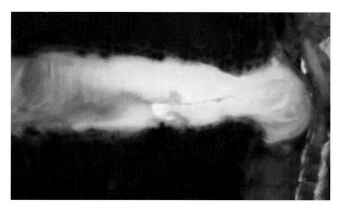

Figure 16.83 Protrusion of the disc at the lumbar level. (Courtesy of J. Taylor.)

During growth and skeletal maturation, the boundary between annulus and nucleus becomes less obvious, and with increasing age the nucleus generally becomes more fibrotic and less gel-like. With age and degeneration, the disc changes in morphology, becoming increasingly disorganized. Often the annular lamellae become irregular, bifurcating, and interdigitating, and the collagen and elastin networks appear to become more disorganized. There is frequently cleft formation with fissures forming within the disc, par-

ticularly in the nucleus. Nerves and blood vessels are increasingly found with degeneration. Cell proliferation occurs, leading to cluster formation, particularly in the nucleus. Cell death also occurs, with the presence of cells with necrotic and apoptotic appearance. It has been reported that more than 50% of cells in adult discs are necrotic. Discs from individuals as young as 2 years of age have some very mild cleft formation and granular changes to the nucleus. With increasing age comes an increased incidence of degenerative changes, including cell death, cell proliferation, mucous degeneration, granular change, and concentric tears. It is difficult to differentiate changes that occur solely because of aging from those that might be "pathological."

Classification of disc degeneration
Disc lesions can be classified as contained or herniated. The progression of disc degeneration can further be classified as follows (Fig. 16.84).

Grade 0. Normal nonleaking nucleus.

Grade 1. Annular tearing confined to the inner region of the annulus fibrosus. In grade 1, a tear or fissure becomes visible. It extends from the nucleus radially into the inner one-third of the annulus fibrosus. This is described as a grade 1 radial annular tear, or grade 1 internal disc disruption (IDD).

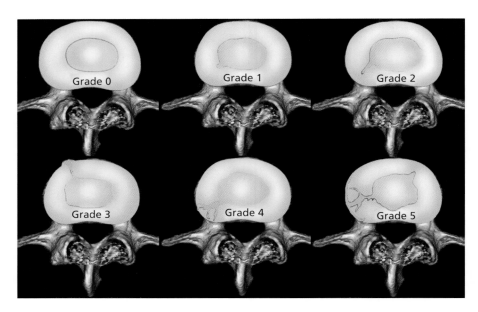

Figure 16.84 Classification of disc degeneration.

Grade 2. In this condition, annular tears have completely disrupted the disc architecture but do not affect the outer contour of the annulus. The entire annulus is disrupted. There is no leakage of injected dye on discography from the disc, nor bulging or protrusion of the disc. This state of the disc is classified as grade 2 IDD or a grade 2 radial annular tear. There is no compressive effect on the corresponding nerve root. Many of these patients (with grade 2 IDD) complain of lower back pain, which may travel into the lower limb and even past the knee into the lower leg and foot.

Grade 3. In this situation, tears have completely disrupted the annulus and the posterior longitudinal ligament and deformed the contour of the posterior portion of the disc. There is a full thickness annular tear in which the outer annulus (Sharpey's fibers) and posterior longitudinal ligament have been completely ruptured. During discography, contrast material leaks out of the back of the disc into the epidural space. The presence of a disc bulge and/or disc herniation is also included in this category. This condition is classified as grade 3 IDD, or grade 3 radial annular tear. This disc pathology produces the same incidence of patients having sciatica as the grade 2 IDD patients. This indicates the nerve fibers in the posterior annulus are a strong trigger of annular tears. This classification has been modified by perception of sciatic pain in the lower limbs.

Computed tomography classification of annular tears

The following classification was finalized in the 1990s and is the "gold standard" for the computed tomography (CT) classification of annular tears. This classification was modified by Bogduk et al. in 1992, then further modified by Schellhas et al. in 1996. There are five possible severities of the radial annular tear as seen on an axial CT image.

Grade 0 is a normal disc, where no contrast material injected in the center of the disc has leaked from the confines of the nucleus pulposus. The grade 1 tear has leaked contrast material but only into the inner one-third of the annulus. In the grade 2 tear, the contrast has leaked from the nucleus into the outer two-thirds of the annulus. The grade 3 tear has leaked contrast completely through all three zones of the annulus. This tear is believed to be painful because the outer one-third of the disc has many tiny nerve fibers that are irritated. The grade 4 tear is a more serious form of the grade 3 tear, in that now the contrast has spread circumferentially around the disc, often resembling a ship's anchor. To qualify as a grade 4 tear, the spread must encompass greater than 30° of the disc circumference. Pathologically, this represents the merging of a full thickness radial tear with a concentric annular tear. The grade 5 tear includes either a grade 3 or grade 4 radial tear that has completely ruptured the outer layers of disc and is leaking contrast material from the disc into the epidural space. This type of tear is thought to have the ability to induce a severe inflammatory reaction in the adjacent neural structures. In some patients, this inflammatory process is so severe that it causes a painful chemical radiculopathy and sciatica without the presence of nerve root compression.

Mechanism of discogenic pain

In 1979, Brodsky and Binder characterized the mechanism for the provocation of pain with discography. Their findings included (1) stretching of the fibers of an abnormal annulus, (2) extravasation of extradurally irritating substances such as glycosaminoglycans, lactic acid, and acidic media, (3) pressure on nerves posteriorly caused by bulging of the annulus, (4) hyperflexion of posterior joints on disc injection, and (5) the presence of vascular granulation tissue, with pain caused by scar distension. Another mechanism speculated was pain generators in the endplates that may be provoked by endplate deflection.

Provocation discography

The "gold standard" in making the diagnosis of IDD is a very painful and invasive test called provocation discography with follow-up CT discogram. There are two components to provocation discography. The first is an attempt by the physician to provoke the patient to feel their usual pain (concordant pain) by pressurizing the disc with a contrast material. The second is a painless discogram in the adjacent discs.

The International Society for the Study of Pain, in its taxonomy, has adapted the following set of criteria for diagnosing IDD: (1) no visible disc herniations seen on magnetic resonance imaging (MRI) or CT; (2) during provocation discography injection of the suspected disc, recreation of the patient's exact back and/or leg pain must occur; (3) injection of the disc above or below the suspect disc must be nonpainful, which acts as a control disc or normal disc; and (4) a grade 3 or 4 radial annular fissure must be demonstrated on CT discography.

Gadolinium-DTPA-enhanced MRI

Although provocation discography with CT discography is the "gold standard" to make the diagnosis of symptomatic IDD, the procedure itself can damage the disc and spread degenerative disc disease. As an alternative, the use of gadolinium (contrast) enhancement may be considered. Gadolinium-dimethoxypropane (Gd-diethylene triamine pentaacetic acid), when injected into the vein during the MRI, will "light up" the granulation tissue that forms within a healing/healed full-thickness annular disc tear.

Hyperintensity zone

A hyperintensity zone is a focal high intensity signal in the posterior annulus fibrosus distinct from the nucleus without disc protrusion. This phenomenon also gives another clue that IDD might be involved in the patient's pain syndrome, although this T2-weighted MRI finding is highly controversial (Fig. 16.85).

Indications

- Chronic, intrusive low back pain for greater than 3 months.
- Failure to achieve adequate improvement with comprehensive nonoperative treatment.
- No neurologic deficit.
- Normal straight-leg raise with radicular pain.
- Nondiagnostic MRI scan for diagnosis of spinal pain.
- No evidence for segmental instability, spondylolisthesis at target level.
- No greater than 25% loss of disc height.

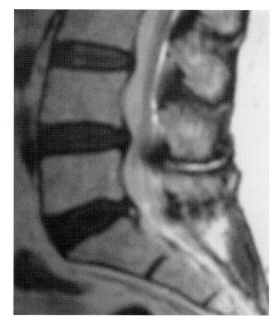

Figure 16.85 High-intensity zone.

- Surgical planning of lumbar fusion.
- To identify a painful disc among multiple degenerative discs.
- To evaluate an intervertebral disc adjacent to a structural abnormality such as spondylolisthesis or fusion.
- Evaluating suspected lateral or recurrent disc herniation.
- To access failed surgeries to determine whether there is a painful pseudoarthrosis or symptomatic disc in a posteriorly fused segment.
- To help select an appropriate surgical technique, like annula denervation and/or percutaneous procedures.

Contraindications

Absolute
- If contrast solution cannot be used because of known anaphylactic reaction.
- The patient has evidence of an untreated localized infection in the procedural field.
- Known bleeding diathesis.
- Anticoagulants.

Relative
- Allergy to injectates.
- Anatomical derangements, congenital or surgical, which compromise the safe and successful conduct of the procedure.
- The patient has known systemic infection.
- Coexisting disease producing significant respiratory or cardiovascular compromise.
- Immunosuppression.

Technique of provocation discography

Lumbar discography (disc stimulation or provocative discography) is a technique that is used to properly identify a painful intervertebral disc in a patient in whom a diagnosis of discogenic pain is suspected. It is defined as a procedure in which contrast media is instilled into the nucleus of the disc to delineate its morphology and identify if there is an exact and/or similar reproduction of a patient's clinical pain syndrome.

Step 1. Prepare the patient before the procedure
The patient should be aware of why they are having this procedure done, what to expect from the procedure and from the team. All complications and side effects should be explained in detail, before the procedure. Valid written consent should be obtained.

The type of analgesia or sedation needs to be ascertained before performance of the invasive procedure. Intravenous fentanyl, midazolam, and/or propofol may be used judiciously for the patient's comfort. Patient response should be monitored and the dosage titrated to establish a level of sedation allowing the patient to be conversant and responsive after needle placements. Because the disc is avascular, there is an increased risk of disc space infection, and most discographers use prophylactic antibiotics. Prophylactic intravenous antibiotics 20 minutes before the procedure are recommended. Usual prophylaxis consists of intravenous administration of cefazolin 900–950 mg given intravenously 15–60 minutes before beginning the procedure. For patients allergic to cefazolin, clindamycin 600 mg, ciprofloxacin 400 mg, or vancomycin 900 mg may be preferred.

Step 2. Position and monitor the patient
1. Place the patient in a prone position on the table. Place a pillow under the abdomen to flatten the lumbar lordosis.
2. Fix the head on the table with a strip of adhesive tape.
3. Insert an intravenous cannula for injecting medication.
4. Provide oxygen by nasal cannula.

5. Monitoring of vital signs is mandatory.
6. Prepare the area for needle entry in a sterile fashion.

Step 3. Drugs and equipment for discography
Prepare and confirm that the following equipment, needles, and drugs are ready to be used for the procedure.
• 5 ml syringe for skin infiltration.
• 22 gauge, 1½ inch needle for local anesthesia.
• 18 gauge, 10 cm needle for discography.
• 10 ml syringe for discography.
• Manometry.
• 1% lidocaine for skin infiltration.
• Nonionic contrast material for discography.
• Antibiotic, for administration at both intradiscal and intravenous access.

Step 4. Visualization
1. Place the C-arm in a posteroanterior position first. Identify the midpoint of the intervertebral space at the target level. Adjust the lower endplate of the target vertebral body to be aligned by moving the C-arm in a cephalocaudal direction (Fig. 16.86).
2. Rotate the C-arm in the oblique projection so that the superior articular process is positioned at the junction of the posterior and middle thirds of the cephalad vertebral body (Fig. 16.87).

Step 5. Direction of the needle
1. Infiltrate the skin with local anesthetic solution using a short 25 gauge needle down to the lamina.
2. The needle is introduced on the opposite side of the patient's symptoms, to prevent the confusion of pain, i.e. whether it is from the procedure or the pathology (Figs 16.88 and 16.89).

Step 6. Confirm the position of the needle
1. A 10 cm, 22 gauge spinal needle is advanced in tunneled view to the anterior of the superior articular process. As

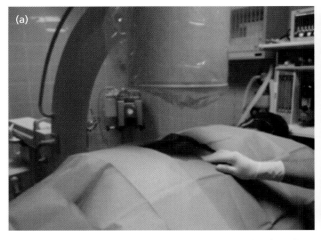
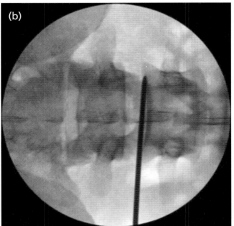

Figure 16.86 (a,b) Patient in supine position, the lower endplate to be aligned.

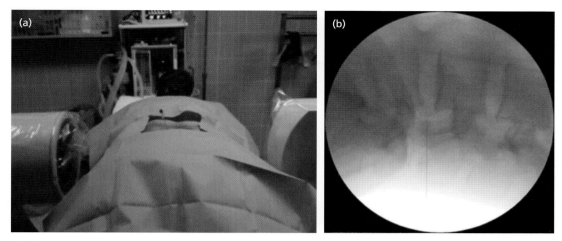

Figure 16.87 (a,b) C-arm in the oblique position, the superior articular process is positioned at the junction of the posterior and middle thirds of the cephalad vertebral body.

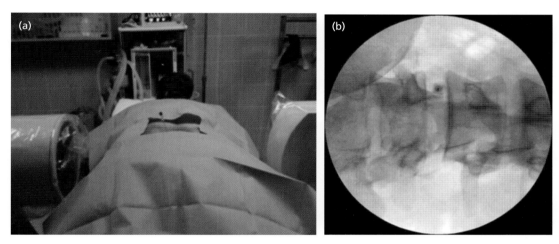

Figure 16.88 (a,b) Direction of the needle in "tunneled vision."

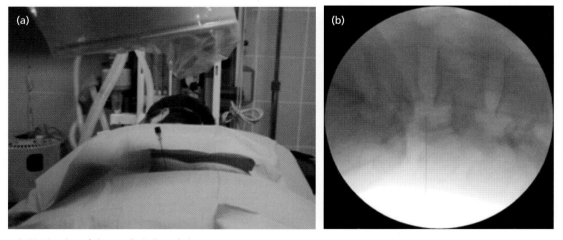

Figure 16.89 (a,b) Direction of the needle in lateral view.

soon as the needle is seen to be close to the annulus, place the C-arm laterally and advance the needle toward the center of the intervertebral disc (Fig. 16.90).

2. Move the C-arm to the posteroanterior position and confirm that the needle is within the disc. The needle tip should be in the middle of the disc on an anteroposterior view (Fig. 16.91).

3. Approach to the L5–S1 disc is difficult. The C-arm should be rotated obliquely in the cephalad direction until the iliac crest does not prevent the opening of the intervertebral discs (Fig. 16.92).

Note: if the needle tip is in the middle of the disc on an anteroposterior view, but anterior on the lateral view, the needle entered the disc too laterally. If the needle tip is centered on the anteroposterior view but posterior on the lateral image, the needle entered the disc too medially.

Step 7. Discography

1. Once the needle position is confirmed in the center of the disc, contrast should be injected in 0.5–1 ml increments, while the pressure of the injection and the patient's response are recorded (Fig. 16.93).

2. Injection into the disc can be performed using a pressure-controlled injection (discomanometry). This is performed using a specially designed injection device and a pressure monitoring system. The opening pressure of the disc and the pressure at which the concordant pain is elicited can be accurately monitored using this method. A concordant pain is defined as a pain which matches the patient's spontaneous pain in terms of the location, quantity, and intensity (Figs 16.94–16.96).

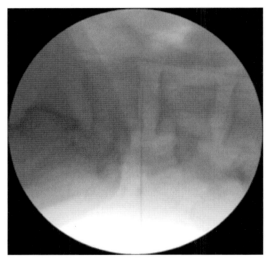

Figure 16.90 The needle within the disc.

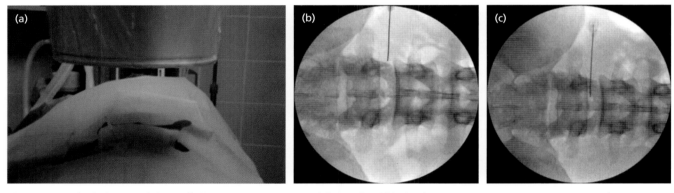

Figure 16.91 (a–c) Direction of the needle in posteroanterior view and the needle within the disc.

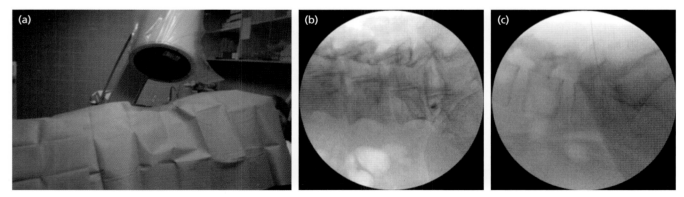

Figure 16.92 (a–c) Position of the C-arm for the L5–S1 level, direction of the needle in oblique and lateral views.

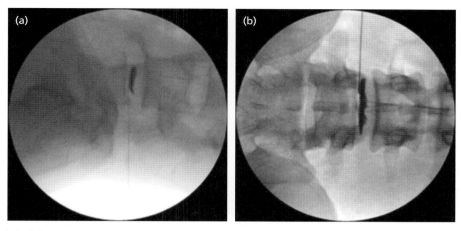

Figure 16.93 (a,b) Spread of the contrast material in lateral and posteroanterior views.

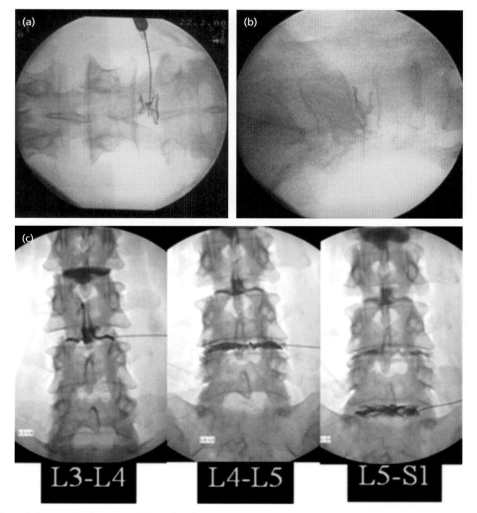

L3-L4   L4-L5   L5-S1

Figure 16.94 (a–c) Several discography pictures at different levels.

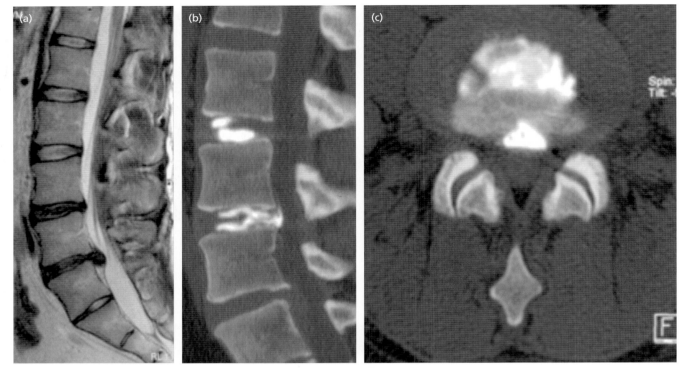

Figure 16.95 (a–c) Discography under CT scan, sagittal and transverse sections.

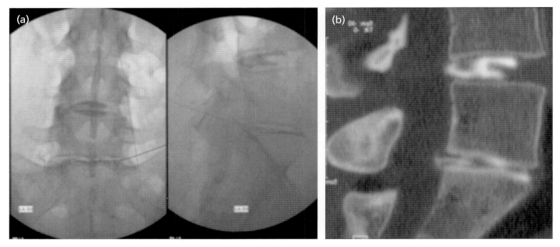

Figure 16.96 (a,b) Discography at L4–L5 and L5-S1evels and CT scan.

3. After discography, 50–100 mg of cefazoline is injected in the disc.

Step 8. Postprocedure care
After completing the procedure, observe the patient for at least 2 hours. Monitoring of vital signs is mandatory. The patient should be followed up for any evidence of subcutaneous bleeding or hematoma immediately after the discogram, and again 30 minutes later. In addition, objectively document the pain relief. The patient should be warned about postprocedure discomfort

and back pain after lumbar discography. After a satisfactory observation, discharge the patient with appropriate and adequate instructions given to their escort. Written instructions are preferable for emergencies and are helpful to the patient and their family. Complications of discography are shown in Table 16.1.

Complications of discography (Table 16.1)
- During the procedure and in the first 24 hours:
  - Cauda equina syndrome.
  - Acute disc hernia.

- ○ Anaphylaxis due to contrast solution.
- ○ Bleeding.
- ○ Muscle spasm.
- 1 day, 7–14 days:
  - ○ Discitis.
  - ○ Vertebral osteomyelitis.
  - ○ Epidural abscess formation.
  - ○ Causalgia.
- 2 weeks and later:
  - ○ Causalgia.
  - ○ Discitis.

Table 16.1 Complications associated with discography. Reproduced from Pino et al. (2009) with permission from author and Elsevier

Hematoma
Superficial infection/abscess
Paraspinous/retroperitoneal hematoma
Paraspinous/retroperitoneal infection/abscess
Intradural injection
Meningitis
Epidural abscess
Direct needle trauma to nerve root
Other complications
Allergic/anaphylactic reaction to radiographic contrast

Complications

- **Discitis**

The incidence of discitis is around 0.1–1.3%. It may be due to the contamination from skin flora. The most frequent microorganisms are *Staphylococcus aureus* and *Staphylococcus epidermidis*. It may also develop owing to Gram-negative bacteria. The patient complains of increasing pain. To prevent discitis, intradiscal antibiotics are recommended.

- **Epidural abscess**

Epidural abscess formation is very rare, but it should still be considered.

- **Urticaria**

Urticaria may develop owing to the drugs used during the procedure.

- **Retroperitoneal hemorrhage**

If the needle passes the disc and enters the retroperitoneal space, retroperitoneal hemorrhage may develop. The final position of the needle should be confirmed by lateral view.

- **Nausea and vomiting**

This may be due to the irritation of the disc or inadvertent dura puncture.

- **Headache**

This may be due to dural puncture or an irritation of the disc. Especially during cervical discography, headache may develop.

- **Disc hernia due to discography**

Repeated puncture of the disc may cause disc hernia. Thus the physician should try to enter the disc in one attempt.

Helpful hints: discographic metrics that allow for correct discogenic pain

Derby has divided discs into four different categories based on their pressure. These comprise the following.

Chemically sensitive. Discs that are painful at less than 15 p.s.i. (pounds per square inch) above opening pressure.

Mechanically sensitive. Discs that are painful between 15 and 50 p.s.i. above opening pressure.

Indeterminate. Discs that are painful at greater than 50 p.s.i. above opening pressure.

Normal. Discs that are not painful despite pressure above 50 p.s.i. that can reasonably be generated.

The normal lumbar disc in the lateral decubitus position has an average opening pressure of 27 p.s.i. and in the sitting position 85 p.s.i. Using discomanometry, Derby reported that patients with chemically sensitive or low-pressure discs (15 p.s.i.) are better served by interbody fusion techniques than posterolateral techniques.

Nucleography

A nucleogram is obtained on fluoroscopy after contrast is instilled into the disc both using anteroposterior and lateral fluoroscopic views; then in the axial plane using CT imaging. These two-dimensional views can be interpreted to reveal normal or degenerative patterns. Adams and coworkers classified the degree of degeneration by appearance as follows (Sachs et al. 1987).

1. Cottonball. No signs of degeneration. Correlates with grade 0 Dallas Discogram criteria.

2. Lobular. Mature disc with nucleus starting to degenerate into fibrous lumps. Correlates with grade 0 Dallas Discogram criteria.

3. Irregular. Degenerated disc with fissures and clefts in the nucleus and inner annulus. Correlates with grade 1 or 2 Dallas Discogram criteria.

4. Fissured. Degenerated disc with radial fissure leading to the outer edge of the annulus. Correlates with grade 3 or 4 Dallas Discogram criteria.

5. Ruptured. Disc has a complete radial tear that allows injected fluid to escape. Correlates with grade 5 Dallas Discogram criteria.

Percutaneous intradiscal procedures

History

The origin of intradiscal procedures goes back to the end of World War II. In 1941 Jansen and Balls produced the chymopapain enzyme from the papaya fruit. In 1956 Thomas discovered the chemical structure of this material. In 1964 Smith first injected chymopapain inside the disc. Intradiscal electrothermal therapy was initially popularized by the Saal brothers in 1998 (Fig. 16.98). However, one should credit Menno Sluijter when, in 1994, he described intradiscal RF thermocoagulation (Fig. 16.97). Ozone chemonucleolysis

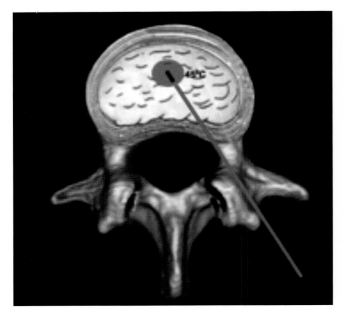

Figure 16.97 Intradiscal RF (Sluijter 1994).

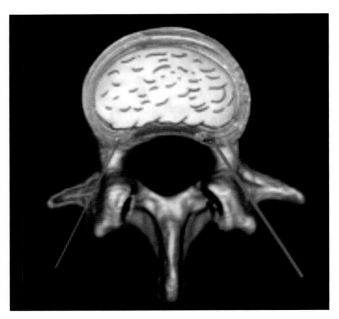

Figure 16.99 DiscTRODE (Finch 2000).

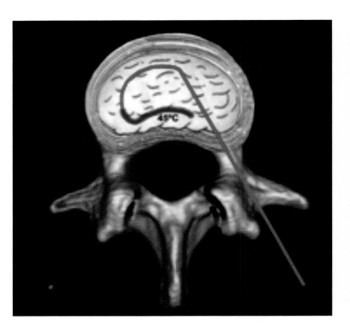

Figure 16.98 IDET (Saal and Saal 1998).

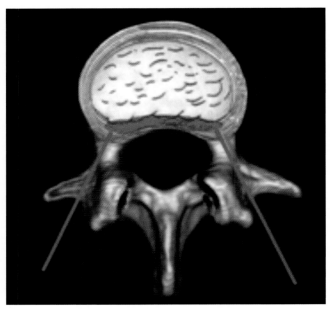

Figure 16.100 Biacuplasty. (Sagittal sections).

has been described by Verga in 1983 (Raj, 2008). In 2004 Finch described a discTRODE procedure and recently biacuplasty has been popularized (Figs 16.99 and 16.100).

Anatomy

The anatomy of the lumbar intervertebral disc is described in the previous section. Only some special points will be described here.

Changes in the disc due to aging

During growth and skeletal maturation, the boundary between annulus and nucleus becomes less obvious, and with increasing age the nucleus generally becomes more fibrotic and less gel-like. With age and degeneration, the disc changes in morphology, becoming increasingly disorganized. Often the annular lamellae become irregular, bifurcating, and interdigitating, and the collagen and elastin networks appear to become more disorganized. There is frequently cleft formation with fissures forming within the disc, particularly in the nucleus. Nerves and blood vessels are increasingly found with degeneration. Cell proliferation occurs, leading to cluster formation, particularly in the nucleus. Cell death also occurs, with the presence of cells with necrotic and apoptotic appearance. It has been reported that more than 50% of cells in adult discs are necrotic. Discs from individuals as young as 2 years of age have some very mild cleft formation and granular changes to the nucleus. With increasing age comes an increased incidence of degenerative changes, including cell death, cell proliferation, mucous degeneration, granular change, and concentric tears. It is difficult to differentiate changes that occur solely because of aging from those that might be "pathological."

Biochemistry of the normal disc

The mechanical functions of the disc are served by the extracellular matrix; its composition and organization govern the disc's mechanical responses. The main mechanical role is provided by two major macromolecular components.

Collagen fibers

The collagen network, formed mostly of type I and type II collagen fibrils and making up approximately 70 and 20% of the dry weight of the annulus and nucleus, respectively, provides tensile strength to the disc and anchors the tissue to the bone.

Aggrecan

Aggrecan, the major proteoglycan of the disc, is responsible for maintaining tissue hydration through the osmotic pressure provided by its constituent chondroitin and keratin sulfate chains. The proteoglycan and water content of the nucleus (around 15 and 80% of the wet weight, respectively) are greater than in the annulus (approximately 5 and 70% of the wet weight, respectively).

Matrix

The matrix is a dynamic structure. Its molecules are continually being broken down by proteinases, such as the matrix metalloproteinases (MMPs) and aggrecanases, which are also synthesized by disc cells. The balance between synthesis, breakdown, and accumulation of matrix macromolecules determines the quality and integrity of the matrix, and thus the mechanical behavior of the disc itself. The integrity of the matrix is also important for maintaining the relatively avascular and aneural nature of the healthy disc.

The intervertebral disc is often likened to articular cartilage. However, there are significant differences between the two tissues, one of these being the composition and structure of aggrecan. Disc aggrecan is more highly substituted with keratin sulfate than that found in the deep zone of articular cartilage. In addition, the aggrecan molecules are less aggregated (30%) and more heterogeneous, with smaller, more degraded fragments in the disc than in articular cartilage (80% aggregated) from the same individual. Disc proteoglycans become increasingly difficult to extract from the matrix with increasing age.

Pathophysiology

Loss of proteoglycan

The most significant biochemical change to occur in disc degeneration is loss of proteoglycan.

The aggrecan molecules become degraded, with smaller fragments being able to leach from the tissue more readily than larger portions. This results in loss of glycosaminoglycan; this loss is responsible for a fall in the osmotic pressure of the disc matrix and therefore a loss of hydration.

Even in degenerate discs, however, the disc cells can retain the ability to synthesize large aggrecan molecules with intact hyaluronan-binding regions, which have the potential to form aggregates. Less is known about how the small proteoglycan population changes with disc degeneration, although there is some evidence that the amount of decorin, and more particularly biglycan, is elevated in degenerate human discs compared with normal ones.

Loss of collagen fibers

Although the collagen population of the disc also changes with degeneration of the matrix, the changes are not as obvious as those of the proteoglycans. The absolute quantity of collagen changes little but the types and distribution of collagens can be altered. For example, there may be a shift in proportions of types of collagen found and in their apparent distribution within the matrix. In addition, the fibrillar collagens, such as type II collagen, become more denatured, apparently because of enzymic activity; the amount of denatured type II collagen increases with degeneration. However, collagen cross-link studies indicate that, as with proteoglycans, new collagen molecules may be synthesized, at least early in disc degeneration, possibly in an attempt at repair.

Increase in fibronectin

Other components can change in disc degeneration and disease in either quantity or distribution. For example, fibronectin content increases with increasing degeneration and it becomes more fragmented. These elevated levels of fibronectin could reflect the response of the cell to an altered environment. Whatever the cause, the formation of fibronectin fragments can then feed into the degenerative cascade because they have been shown to downregulate aggrecan synthesis but to upregulate the production of some MMPs in in-vitro systems.

Enzymatic activity

The biochemistry of disc degeneration indicates that enzymatic activity contributes to this disorder, with increased fragmentation of the collagen, proteoglycan, and fibronectin populations. Several families of enzymes are capable of breaking down the various matrix molecules of disc, including cathepsins, MMPs, and aggrecanases. Cathepsins have maximal activity in acid conditions. In contrast, MMPs and aggrecanases have an optimal pH that is approximately neutral. All of these enzymes have been identified in the disc.

Functional changes of the disc owing to degeneration

The loss of proteoglycan in degenerate discs has a major effect on the disc's load-bearing behavior. With loss of proteoglycan, the osmotic pressure of the disc falls and the disc is less able to maintain hydration under load; degenerate discs have a lower water content than do normal age-matched discs, and when loaded they lose height and fluid more rapidly: the discs tend to bulge. Loss of proteoglycan and matrix disorganization has other important mechanical effects; because of the subsequent loss of hydration, degenerated discs no longer behave hydrostatically under load. Loading may thus lead to inappropriate stress concentrations along the endplate or in the annulus; the stress concentrations seen in degenerate discs have also been associated with discogenic pain produced during discography.

Such major changes in disc behavior have a strong influence on other spinal structures, and may affect their function and predispose them to injury. For instance, as a result of the rapid loss of disc height under load in degenerate discs, apophyseal joints adjacent to such a disc may be subject to abnormal loads and eventually develop osteoarthritic changes. Loss of disc height can also affect other structures. It reduces the tensional forces on the ligamentum flavum and hence may cause remodeling and thickening. With consequent loss of elasticity, the ligament will tend to bulge into the spinal canal, leading to spinal stenosis – an increasing problem as the population ages.

Loss of proteoglycans also influences the movement of molecules into and out of the disc. Aggrecan, because of its high concentration and charge in the normal disc, prevents movement of large uncharged molecules such as serum proteins and cytokines into and through the matrix. The fall in concentration of aggrecan in degeneration could thus facilitate loss of small, but osmotically active, aggrecan fragments from the disc, possibly accelerating a degenerative cascade. In addition, loss of aggrecan would allow increased penetration of large molecules such as growth factor complexes and cytokines into the disc, affecting cellular behavior and possibly the progression of degeneration. The increased vascular and neural ingrowth seen in degenerate discs and associated with chronic back pain is also probably associated with proteoglycan loss because disc aggrecan has been shown to inhibit neural ingrowth.

It is now clear that herniation-induced pressure on the nerve root cannot alone be the cause of pain because more than 70% of "normal," asymptomatic people have disc prolapses pressurizing the nerve roots but no pain. A past and current hypothesis is that, in symptomatic individuals, the nerves are somehow sensitized to the pressure, possibly by molecules arising from an inflammatory cascade from arachidonic acid through to prostaglandin E2, thromboxane, phospholipase A2, tumor necrosis factor-α, the interleukins, and MMPs. These molecules can be produced by cells of herniated discs and because of the close physical contact between the nerve root and disc following herniation they may be able to sensitize the nerve root. The exact sequences of events and specific molecules that are involved have not been identified.

Nutritional pathways of disc degeneration

One of the primary causes of disc degeneration is thought to be failure of the nutrient supply to the disc cells. Like all cell types, the cells of the disc require nutrients such as glucose and oxygen to remain alive and active. In vitro, the activity of disc cells is very sensitive to extracellular oxygen and pH, with matrix synthesis rates falling steeply at acidic pH and at low oxygen concentrations, and the cells do not survive prolonged exposure to low pH or glucose concentrations. A fall in nutrient supply that leads to a lowering of oxygen tension or of pH (arising from raised lactic acid concentrations) could thus affect the ability of disc cells to synthesize and maintain the disc's extracellular matrix and could ultimately lead to disc degeneration. The disc is large and avascular and the cells depend on blood vessels at their margins to supply nutrients and remove metabolic waste. The pathway from the blood supply to the nucleus cells is precarious because these cells are supplied virtually entirely by capillaries that originate in the vertebral bodies, penetrating the subchondral plate and terminating just above the cartilaginous endplate. Nutrients must then diffuse from the capillaries through the cartilaginous endplate and the dense extracellular matrix of the nucleus to the cells, which may be as far as 8 mm from the capillary bed

The nutrient supply to the nucleus cells can be disturbed at several points. Factors that affect the blood supply to the vertebral body such as atherosclerosis, sickle cell anemia, Caisson disease, and Gaucher's disease all appear to lead to a significant increase in disc degeneration. Long-term exercise or lack of it appears to have an effect on movement of nutrients into the disc, and thus on their concentration in the tissue.

The mechanism is not known but it has been suggested that exercise affects the architecture of the capillary bed at the disc–bone interface. Finally, even if the blood supply remains undisturbed, nutrients may not reach the disc cells if the cartilaginous endplate calcifies; intense calcification of the endplate is seen in scoliotic discs.

Effect of mechanical load and injury to the disc

Abnormal mechanical loads are also thought to provide a pathway to disc degeneration. For many decades, it was suggested that a major cause of back problems is injury, often work-related, that causes structural damage. It is believed that such an injury initiates a pathway that leads to disc degeneration and finally to clinical symptoms and back pain. Although intense exercise does not appear to affect discs adversely and discs are reported to respond to some long-term loading regimens by increasing proteoglycan content, experimental overloading or injury to the disc can induce degenerative changes.

Genetic factors in disc degeneration

More recent work suggests that the factors that lead to disc degeneration may have important genetic components. Several studies have reported a strong familial predisposition for disc degeneration and herniation. Findings from two different twin studies conducted in 1989 (Heikkila et al. 1989) showed heritability exceeding 60%. MRI in identical twins was very similar with respect to the spinal columns and the patterns of disc degeneration.

Genes associated with disc generation have been identified. Individuals with a polymorphism in the aggrecan gene were found to be at risk for early disc degeneration. Studies of transgenic mice have demonstrated that mutations in structural matrix molecules such as aggrecan, collagen II, and collagen IX can lead to disc degeneration. Mutations in genes other than those of structural matrix macromolecules have also been associated with disc degeneration.

Options for treatment of discogenic pain

- Intradiscal injections.
  - Chemonucleolysis.
  - Ozone injection.
- Annuloplasty.
  - Intradiscal electrothermal therapy (IDET).
  - RF posterior annuloplasty (RFA).
  - Biacuplasty.
- Percutaneous disc decompression.
  - Laser discectomy.
  - RF coblation (plasma discectomy).
  - Mechanical disc decompression (Dekompressor®).
  - Manual percutaneous lumbar discectomy (PLD).
- Endoscopic percutaneous discectomy.

Indications

- Radicular pain.
- Discal hernia.
- Positive straight leg test.
- Provocative tests positive.
- Paresthesia and pain at the segmental innervation.

The approach towards the disc is similar for all procedures. Thus, first the intradiscal approach will be described in detail and differences among the techniques will then be compared.

Step 1. Prepare the patient before the procedure
1. A recent MRI, CT, and plain radiography necessary are before the procedure. Plain radiography will clarify the disc height and scolisosis and calcifications in the region; MRI will clarify the disc height, soft tissues, and compression on the spinal nerves; CT will clarify the surrounding tissues around the disc and bony structure.
2. Ascertain the type of analgesia or sedation before performing the invasive procedure. If a local anesthetic or neurolytic block is planned, mild sedation is all that is necessary. If pulsed RF is planned, the patient needs to be awake to respond to the stimulation test. Intravenous fentanyl or midazolam may be used judiciously for the patient's comfort.
3. Detailed information related to the procedure, side effects, and complications should be thoroughly explained to the patient and their family. The patient should be aware of why they are having this procedure done, and what to expect from it. All complications and side effects should be explained in detail, before the procedure. Valid written consent should be obtained.

Step 2. Position and monitor the patient
1. Place the patient in a prone position on the table. Place a pillow under the abdomen to flatten the lumbar lordosis.
2. Insert an intravenous cannula for injecting medication.
3. Provide oxygen by nasal cannula.
4. Monitor vital signs (mandatory).
5. Prepare the area for needle entry in a sterile fashion.

Step 3. Drugs and equipment for the technique
Prepare and confirm that the following equipment, needles, and drugs are ready for the procedure.
- 5 ml syringe for skin infiltration.
- 1½ inch, 25 gauge needle.
- 10 ml syringe for discography.
- For intradiscal injection or procedure.
  - 18 gauge, 10 cm needle.
  - 18 gauge, 15 mm active-tip electrode.
  - IDET kit.
  - Disctrode kit.
  - Nucleoplasty kit.
  - Biaculoplasty kit.
  - Decompressor kit.
  - Laser discectomy kit.
- 1% lidocaine for skin infiltration.
- Nonionic contrast solution for discography.
- 50 mg cephalosporine for intradiscal injection.
- IV antibiotic.

Step 4. Visualization

1. Place the C-arm in a posteroanterior position first. Identify the midpoint of the intervertebral space at the target level. Adjust the lower endplate of the target vertebral body to be aligned by moving the C-arm in a cephalocaudal direction (Fig. 16.101).

2. Oblique the C-arm in the coronal plane approximately 25–30°, until the spinous processes are lateral; the facet line should appear midline. Infiltrate the skin with local anesthetic solution using a short 25 gauge needle down to the lamina (Fig. 16.102).

3. The entry point is at the midpoint of the superior articular process, at the lateral edge.

4. Infiltrate the skin with 1% lidocaine with a 25 gauge, 1½ inch needle.

Step 5. Direction of the needle

1. Advance a 10 cm, 22 gauge needle under tunneled vision just lateral to the midpoint of the superior articular process (Fig. 16.103).

2. Rotate the C-arm laterally and advance the needle until it touches the posterior wall of the disc, the annulus fibrosus. The tip of the needle should be at the midpoint of the disc and the direction of the needle should be parallel to the upper and lower endplates of the vertebral bodies (Fig. 16.104).

3. Rotate the C-arm to a posteroanterior position again to view the direction of the needle (Fig. 16.105).

4. Advance the needle into the disc. As the needle passes the annulus fibrosus, there will be a slight resistance and then loss of resistance as the needle is within the disc.

5. For the L5–S1 level, the angle of the C-arm should be cephalocaudal (Fig. 16.106).

Step 6. Confirm the position of the needle

Inject 2 ml of contrast material into the disc: the contrast material should spread within the disc which should be confirmed by posteroanterior and lateral views (Fig. 16.107).

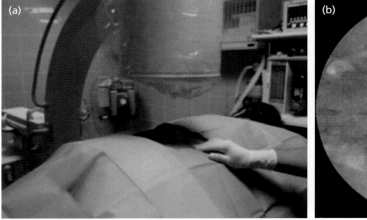
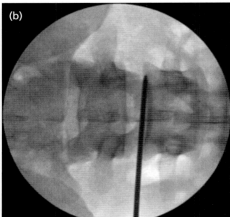

Figure 16.101 (a,b) Patient in supine position, the lower endplate to be aligned.

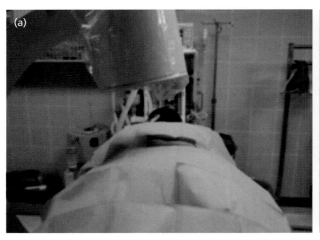
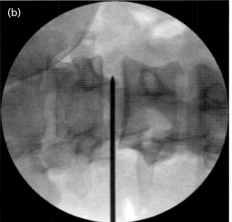

Figure 16.102 (a,b) C-arm in the oblique position, the superior articular process positioned at the junction of the posterior and middle thirds of the cephalad vertebral body.

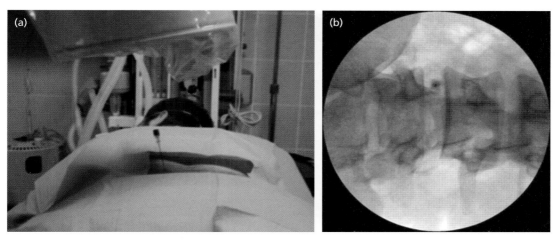

Figure 16.103 (a,b).Direction of the needle in "tunneled vision."

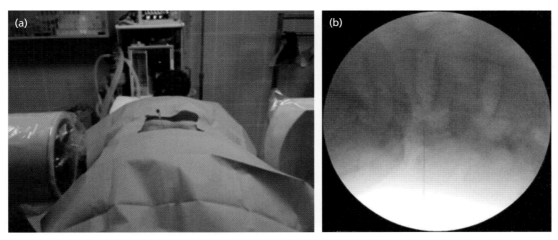

Figure 16.104 (a,b) Direction of the needle in lateral view.

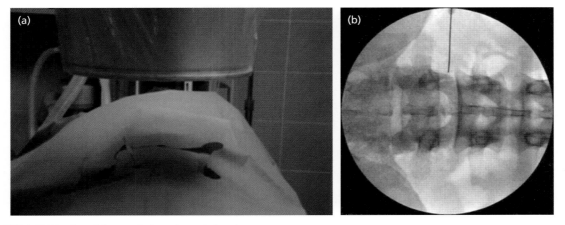

Figure 16.105 (a,b) Direction of the needle in posteroanterior view.

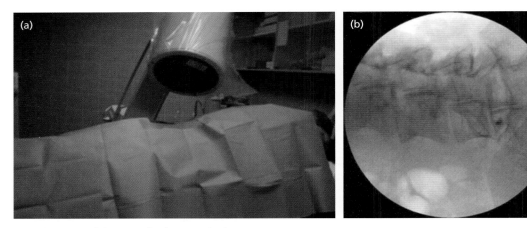

Figure 16.106 (a,b) Position of the C-arm for the L5–S1 level.

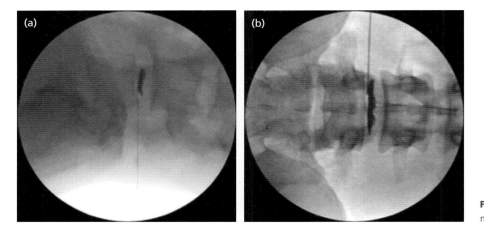

Figure 16.107 (a,b) Spread of the contrast material in lateral and posteroanterior view.

Step 7. Stimulation test

1. Impedance monitoring is crucial to verify that the tip of the electrode is within the disc. The impedance should be around 200–250 ohms, otherwise one should check the position of the needle.

2. Motor stimulation at 2 Hz up to 1–2 V. If there are strong motor contractions at the lower extremities, change the site of the electrode.

Step 8. RF lesioning

1. Intradiscal injections

(a) Chemonucleolysis

Chymopapain works by depolymerizing the proteoglycan and glycoprotein molecules in the nucleus pulposus. These large molecules are responsible for water retention and turgidity. When exposed to chymopapain, the water content within the disc plummets; shrinkage follows and causes a reduction in disc height and girth. The bulging disc, therefore, shrinks (Fig. 16.108).

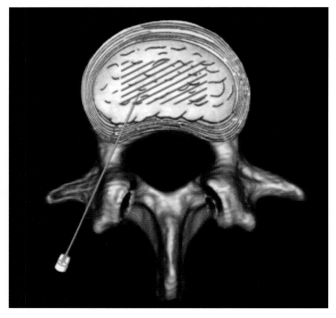

Figure 16.108 Chymopapain.

Use of chymopapain has been approved by FDA; however, it has not been manufactured within the United States since 1999.

To prevent anaphylaxis, reported in 1% of cases, a chymopapain test should be performed one day before the procedure, and H1 and H2 receptor blockers should be administered.

One should avoid general anesthesia as it may mask the signs of anaphylaxis and it should be performed under light sedation.

At first 200 units of chymopapain is injected to test the hypersensitivity. Some authors prefer to inject 1000 units. Chymopapain is then injected into the nucleus pulposus in amounts ranging from 1000 to 4000 units very slowly over a period of 5 minutes. The number of units injected decreases if more than one disc is to be treated.

To prevent muscle spasms and low back pain after chymopapain injection, some authors recommend injection of local anesthetics to the paradiscal region.

Anaphylactic reactions generally develop within the first 15 minutes after injection. The patient should be kept in the theater for one hour and followed up for at least 6 hours in recovery.

Low back pain may occur for several days. Bed rest for one week may be recommended.

Anaphylaxis, reported in 1% of cases, proved to be the most severe complication. It became clear that good patient selection, proper surgical training and technique, preoperative hypersensitivity testing, and antihistamine administration could greatly reduce the complication rate when using chymopapain.

(b) Ozone chemonucleolysis

The method involves the administration of 40/60 ml of ozone gas (O_2–O_3 mixture) at a concentration of 20/30 μg/ml, repeated 8–14 times. The injection is generally made into the paravertebral musculature, and in the hernia zone. The injection itself, except for a slight sense of localized pain of short duration, is generally painless and well tolerated.

There are insufficient published data to conclude that this technique is a promising alternative method.

2. Intradiscal procedures

(a) Intradiscal electrothermal therapy: IDET annuloplasty

• Keep the introducer needle facing the posterior wall of the discs as it enters the annulus. The annulus will provide resistance and feel "gritty" to the physician as the needle passes. This will be followed by a sudden loss of resistance.
• The needle should be placed in this transitional zone between the annulus and the nucleus; this should be confirmed in both the posteroanterior and lateral views.
• Once the introducer needle is properly placed, the navigable catheter is threaded through the needle hub. When using the spine-CATH system, the curve at the tip of the catheter and the white line on the catheter handle should be aligned with the bevel marker on the needle hub and facing the posterior aspect of the disc.
• As the catheter is advanced into the needle, note when the first bold depth marker on the catheter enters the needle hub. This indicates the tip of the catheter has reached the tip of the introducer needle.
• Using continuous fluoroscopic guidance, in the lateral view the catheter will pass in the transitional zone between the annulus and the nucleus and curl inside the disc at the interface of the nucleus and the interior annular wall (Fig. 16.109).
• Ideal placement is the posterior third of the disc, across the midline of the posterior wall, and centered between the plates. Note that the catheter must not be outside of the disc wall. Also, note that when the second bold marker of the proximal shaft enters the needle, the heater end has completely exited the tip of the needle into the disc.
• The fluoroscope is then rotated cephalocaudal to view the catheter from the top of the disc. This should be observed as radiopaque markers of the resistive coil being outside of the introducer needle.

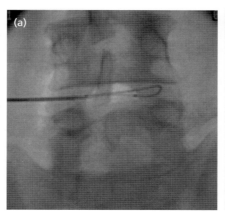 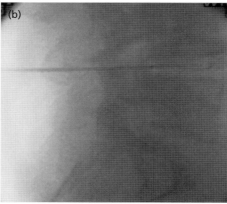

Figure 16.109 (a,b) IDET.

- Care must be taken not to force the catheter, or kinking will result.
- If the physician observes significant resistance to movement, especially during withdrawal of the catheter through the introducer needle, both the needle and the catheter should be immediately removed together.
- After proper catheter placement, the catheter is heated to 65 °C. The temperature is then raised 1 °C every 30 seconds until the desired therapy level is reached. Ideally, this is between 80 and 90 °C, for 4–6 minutes, to distribute the heat thoroughly.
- The total time for a heating lasts between 14 and 17 minutes. As the temperature increases, the patient is continuously evaluated for back pain and any other signs of nerve root irritation such as extremity pain. It is expected that there may be reproduction of back or extremity pain concordant with the patient's normal symptoms.
- It is important to monitor the impedance. Before placement of the catheter, this should be checked and verified that it is within the acceptable range of 120–200 ohms. This range should be maintained throughout the thermocoagulation and is an indicator of a functioning power circuit.
- After the thermocoagulation is complete, gently remove the catheter. This may require some rotation. Intradiscal antibiotics (1 ml of 5 mg/ml cefazolin) should be administered through the needle.
- After removal of the introducer needle, the site is covered with antibiotic ointment and a Band-Aid dressing.

(b) DiscTRODE

- The discTRODE™ procedure is quite similar to IDET, except that the wire or electrode is introduced into the outer part of the disc, whereas the IDET goes to the inner part. The Radionics discTRODE™ RF Catheter Electrode is a navigable, semi-rigid RF electrode that is introduced percutaneously into an intervertebral disc through a cannula introducer.
- A cannula introducer with a curved tip is posterolaterally introduced percutaneously into an intervertebral disc. Impedance monitoring may be used as an aid, in addition to fluoroscopy, to place the cannula to the desired depth.
- After disc space visualization and local anesthetic infiltration of the skin and the subcutaneous tissues with 2% lidocaine, the introducer of the discTRODE is introduced just lateral to the facet joint (superior pars) in the middle of the disc using a tunneled vision.
- The entry point is approximately 5–7 cm from the midline. The introducer is advanced through the disc. After entering the disc, the placement of the introducer is confirmed with posteroanterior and lateral fluoroscopic views (Fig. 16.110).
- The tissue impedance is measured as an aid, in addition to fluoroscopy, to evaluate the desired depth and has to be less than 250 ohms (Fig. 16.111).

- A lateral view is used to provide the accurate depth of the introducer facing the posterior wall of the disc as it enters the annulus (Fig. 16.112).
- The introducer stayed at the annulus and not at the nucleus. After inserting the introducer; the navigable, semi-rigid discTRODE catheter is passed through the introducer and directed medially and contralaterally along the posterior nuclear–annular interface (Fig. 16.113).
- Before initiating the treatment, the SMK Thermocouple Electrode is placed in the outer annulus on the contralateral side to monitor local tissue temperatures. The tissue impedance is measured to aid in the placement, similar to the introducer placement. These local temperatures register on the external temperature monitor attached to the RFG-3C Plus Lesion Generator.
- Before the RF application, motor stimulation at 2 Hz is applied to see whether the tip of the catheter is very close

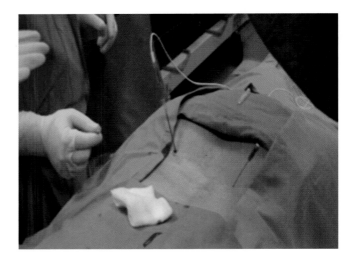

Figure 16.110 Direction of the electrodes for discTRODE.

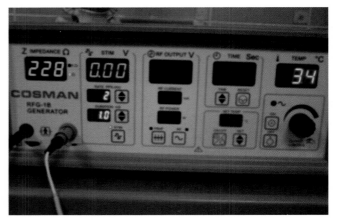

Figure 16.111 Impedance monitoring during intradiscal procedures.

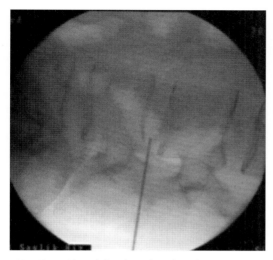

Figure 16.112 Position of the electrode in lateral view.

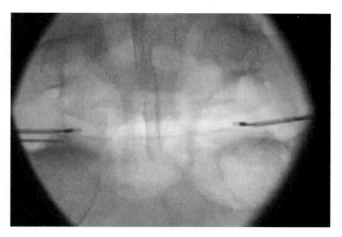

Figure 16.114 Biacuplasty.

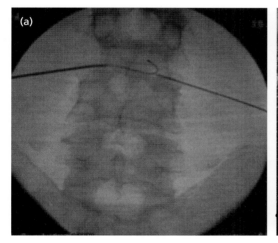

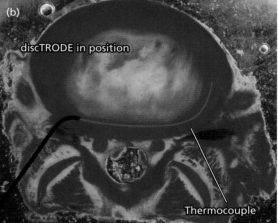

Figure 16.113 (a,b) Electrodes in position for discTRODE.

to the nerve root or not. Before procedure initiation, the RFG-3C Plus Lesion Generator treatment time is set at 10 minutes. The treatment temperature is manually increased in a stepwise progression from 50 to 65 °C every 2 minutes.
• Intraoperative and postoperative prophylactic cefazolin 50 mg intradiscally and 1000 mg intravenously should be administered.

Biacuplasty
The new annuloplasty procedure termed intradiscal biacuplasty (Baylis Medical, Montreal, Canada) uses a bipolar system that includes two cooled, RF electrodes placed on the posterolateral sides of the intervertebral annulus fibrosus. The electrodes are placed fluoroscopically. Two 17 gauge transdiscal introducers are placed in the posterior annulus using a posterolateral, oblique approach. Then, RF probes are positioned through each of the introducers bilaterally to

create a bipolar configuration. There is a gradual increase of the temperature of the electrodes to 55 °C over 11 minutes (Fig. 16.114).

Disc decompression techniques

Nucleoplasty
• The first nucleoplasty was performed in 2000. RF coblation combines disc removal and thermal coagulation to decompress a contained herniated disc.
• Indications for this procedure include low back pain with or without radiculopathy, MRI confirmation of contained herniated disc, and failed conservative therapy. Patients who should be excluded from receiving this procedure include those with spinal stenosis, a loss of disc height of 50%, severe disc degeneration, spinal fracture, or tumor.

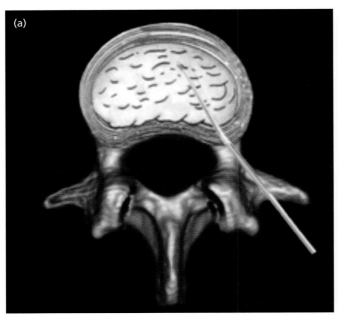

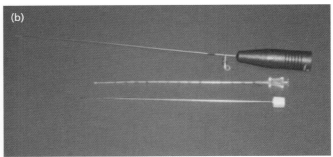

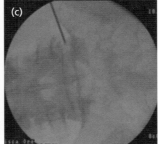

Figure 16.115 (a–c) Nucleoplasty.

• A 17 gauge obturator stylet is introduced inside the disc. A discogram may take place at this time to confirm location and for a positive provocation test.

• Taking care not to contact the anterior annulus, the nucleus pulposus is first ablated with RF waves as the wand is advanced, causing a molecular dissociation process converting tissue into gas, which is removed through the needle.

• As the wand is withdrawn, coagulation takes place thermally treating the channel, which leads to a denaturing of nerve fibers adjacent to the channel within the nucleus pulposus.

• This process is repeated up to six times within an individual disc turning the tip of the catheter at 2–4–6–8–10–12 o'clock positions (Fig. 16.115).

Mechanical disc decompression (Dekompressor®)

• The Dekompressor® is a disposable, self-contained, battery-operated handpiece connected to a helical probe. The outer cannula measures 1.5mm, with an inner rotating probe.

• When activated, the probe rotates, creating suction to pull the milled nucleus pulposus from the disc up the cannula to a suction chamber at the base of the handheld unit.

• Approximately 0.5–2 ml of nucleus pulposus is removed.

• This efficient removal of disc material decreases surgical procedure times to approximately 30 minutes, with the actual time of use for the probe not exceeding 10 minutes. This procedure is performed under fluoroscopic guidance.

• The Dekompressor® technique specifically has yet to be studied in a controlled clinical trial and results with this new automated technique are limited.

Laser discectomy

• Medical lasers have been used since the early 1960s. Ascher et al. published their experiences with the use of a neodymium:yttrium–aluminum–garnet (Nd:YAG) laser on the lumbar spine for nucleolysis (Chay 1995).

• There are several types of laser in use for the lumbar spine, the most common being the holmium:yttrium–aluminum–garnet (Ho:YAG) laser; the others are potassium–titanyl–phosphate, and the neodymium (Nd):YAG lasers. The Ho:YAG laser is most commonly paired with an endoscope for disc ablation and removal capabilities. This laser-assisted technique combines two effective but limited approaches.

• Indications for laser discectomy include those with back and leg pain with a confirmed disc herniation. A ruptured annulus and lateral recess stenosis are not contraindications.

• As the affected tissues absorb the laser, light is converted to heat. At 100 °C, tissue vaporizes and ablation takes place. As a small amount of nucleus pulposus is vaporized, intradiscal pressure decreases, allowing the disc to return to its normal state. If any disc material needs to be removed, endoscopic tools can be used to do so.

• An 18 gauge, 7 inch needle is introduced just anterior to the superior articular process and superior to the transverse process through a so-called "triangular safe zone." Using fluoroscopy, the needle is placed 1 cm beyond the annulus into the nucleus pulposus just parallel to the disc axis, preferably halfway between the superior and inferior endplates.

• If the procedure is endoscopically assisted, dilators are placed over the guide needle for visualization and the introduction of the endoscope. Irrigation with saline allows for better visualization of the spaces.

- Depending on the type, the laser is either fired as a pulse or continuously. The Ho:YAG laser is pulse-fired. Newer laser models offer side-firing capabilities. This advance helps to provide more control of laser placement, better observation, and can help reduce the risk of injury to several areas, especially those anterior to the spinal column.
- Larger fragments, which are more difficult to remove through the endoscope, can be laser ablated. After firing the laser and adequate nucleus pulposus has been removed/ablated, the laser and dilators are removed. The incision can be closed with sutures or surgical adhesives. The patient is moved to recovery and sent home later in the day.
- After the procedure is completed, observe the patient for up to 2 hours. Monitoring of vital signs is mandatory. In addition, objectively document the pain relief. After a satisfactory observation, discharge the patient, with appropriate and adequate instructions given to their escort. Written instructions are preferable for emergencies and are helpful to the patient and their family.

Step 9. Postprocedural care

In the first month, all patients are encouraged to walk and perform low-intensity leg stretches, exercising the hamstrings and gastrosoleus muscles. In the second month, most patients are told to resume low-intensity stabilization floor exercises gradually. In the third month, the intensity of exercise is slightly increased. Athletic activities such as skiing, running, and tennis are delayed until the fifth or sixth month.

Complications

- Early complications
  - Spinal nerve injury due to the misplacement of the electrode or catheter.
  - Injury to retroperitoneal viscera due to the placement of the catheter outside the disc.
  - Kinking or breaking of the catheter.
  - Thermal injury.
  - Cauda equina syndrome.
  - Spinal cord injury.
- Late complications
  - Infection.
  - Discitis.
  - Epidural abscess formation.
  - Meningitis.
  - Severe low back pain.
  - Disc hernia after IDET.

Further reading

Abdi, S., Datta, S., Trescot, A.M., et al. (2007) Epidural steroids in the management of chronic spinal pain: a systematic review. *Pain Physician* **10**(1), 185–212.

Alo, K.M., Wright, R.E., Sutcliffe, J. & Brandt, S.A. (2004) Percutaneous lumbar discectomy: clinical response in an initial cohort of fifty consecutive patients with chronic radicular pain. *Pain Practice* **4**, 19–29.

Aprill, C. & Bogduk, N. (1992) High intensity zone. *British Journal of Radiology* **65**, 361–369.

Arnulf, G. (1954) *Practique des Infiltrations Sympathetiques*. Lyon: Camgli.

Badgley, C.E. (1941) The articular facets in relation to low back pain and sciatic radiation. *Journal of Bone and Joint Surgery America* **23**, 481–496.

Benedetti, E.M., Siriwetchadarak, R., Stanec, J. & Rosenquist, R.W. (2009) Epidural steroid injections: complications and management. *Techniques in Regional Anesthesia and Pain Management* **13**(4), 236–250.

Benzon, H.T., Chew, T.L., McCarthy, R.J., Benzon, H.A. & Walega, D.R. (2007) Comparison of the particle sizes of different steroids and the effect of dilution. A review of the relative neurotoxicities of the steroids. *Anesthesiology* **106**(2), 331–338.

Bogduk, N. (ed.) (2004) *Practice Guidelines for Spinal Diagnostic and Treatment Procedures*. San Francisco, CA: International Spinal Intervention Society.

Bonica, J.J. (1953) *The Management of Pain*. Philadelphia, PA: Lea & Febiger.

Boswell, M., Trescot, A. & Datta, S. (2007) Interventional techniques: evidence based practice guidelines in the management of chronic spinal pain. *Pain Physician* **10**(1), 7–111.

Brodsky, A.E. & Binder, W.F. (1979) Lumbar discography. *Spine* **4**, 110–120.

Brown, D. (1996) Update on chemonucleolysis. *Spine* **21**, 62S–68S.

Brunn, F. & Mandl, F. (1924) Die paravertebrale Injektion zur Bekaempfung viszeraler Schmerzen. *Wiener Klinische Wochenschrift* **37**, 511.

Buenaventura, R.M., Shah, R.V., Patel, V., Benyamin, R. & Singh, V. (2007) Systematic review of discography as a diagnostic test for spinal pain: an update. *Pain Physician* **10**, 147–164.

Calodney, A. (2004) Radiofrequency denervation of the lumbar zygapophysial joints. *Techniques in Regional Anesthesia and Pain Management* **8**(1), 35–40.

Cathelin, M.F. (1901) Mode d'action de la cocaine injecte daus l'escape epidural par le procede du canal sacre. *Comptes Rendues des Seances de la Societe de Biologie et de ses Filliales* **43**, 487.

Chay, D.S. (1995) Clinical experience and results with 389 PLDD procedures with the Nd:YAG laser, 1986–1995. *Journal of Clinical Laser Medicine and Surgery* **13**(3), 209–213.

Conn, A., Buenventura, R.M., Datta, S., Abdi, S. & Diwan, S. (2009) Systematic review of caudal epidural injections in the management of chronic low back pain. *Pain Physician* **12**(1), 109–136.

Corning, J.L. (1885) Spinal anaesthesia and local medication of the cord. *New York Medical Journal* **42**, 483–485.

Crock, H.V. (1970) A reappraisal of intervertebral disc lesions. *Medical Journal of Australia* **1**, 983–989.

Deer, T., Ranson, M., Kapural, L. & Diavan, S.A. (2009) Guidelines for the proper use of epidural steroid injections for the chronic pain patient. *Techniques in Regional Anesthesia and Pain Management* **13**(4), 288–295.

Derby, R., Bogduk, N. & Kine, G. (1993) Precision percutaneous blocking procedures for localizing spinal pain. Part 2. The lumbar neuraxial compartment. *Pain Digest* **3**, 175–188.

Derby, R., Lee, SH. & Chen, Y. (2005) Discograms: cervical, thoracic, and lumbar. *Techniques in Regional Anesthesia and Pain Management* **9**(2), 97–105.

Erdine, S. & Talu, G.K. (2002) Precautions during epidural neuroplasty. *Pain Practice* **2**(4), 308–314.

Finch, P.M. (2004) Radiofrequency denervation of the annulus fibrosus: A rationale. *Techniques in Regional Anesthesia and Pain Management* **8**(1), 41–45.

Gajraj, N.M. (2004) Selective nerve root blocks for low back pain and radiculopathy. *Regional Anesthesia and Pain Medicine* **29**(3), 243–256.

Gharibo, C., Koo, C., Chung, J. & Moroz, A. (2009) Epidural steroid injections: an update on mechanisms of injury and safety. *Techniques in Regional Anesthesia and Pain Management* **13**, 266–271.

Hadjipavlou, A.G., Tzermiadianos, M.N., Bogduk, N. & Zindrick, M.R. (2008) The pathophysiology of disc degeneration: a critical review. *Journal of Bone and Joint Surgery, British Volume* **90**(10), 1261–1270.

Heikkila, J.K., Koskenvuo, M., Heliovaara, M., et al. (1989) Genetic and environmental factors in sciatica. Evidence from a nationwide panel of 9365 adult twin pairs. *Annals of Medicine* **21**, 393–398.

Hingston, R.A. & Edwards, W.B. (1942) Continuous caudal anesthesia during labor and delivery. *Anesthesia and Analgesia* **21**, 301–310.

Hirsch, C. (1948) An attempt to diagnose level of disc lesion clinically by disc puncture. *Acta Orthopaedica Scandinavica* **18**, 131–140.

Hirsch, C., Inglemark, B. & Miller, M. (1963) The anatomical basis for low back pain. *Acta Orthopaedica Scandinavica* **33**, 1.

Jansen, E.F. & Balls, A.K. (1941) Chymopapain: a new crystalline proteinase from papaya latex. *Journal of Biological Chemistry* **137**, 459–460.

Jonnesco, R. (1920) Angine de poitrien guerie par le resection du sympathique cervico-thoradique. *Bulletin of the Academy of Medicine* **84**, 93.

Kappis, M. (1923) Weitere Erfahrungen mit der Sympathektomie. *Klinische Wochenschrift* **2**, 1441.

Kapural, L. & Cata, J.P. (2007) Complications of percutaneous techniques used in the diagnosis and treatment of discogenic lower back pain. *Techniques in Regional Anesthesia and Pain Management* **11**(3), 157–163.

Kapural, L., Nageeb, F., Kapural, M., Cata, J.P., Narouze, S. & Mekhail, N. (2008) Cooled radiofrequency system for the treatment of chronic pain from sacroilitis: the first case-series. *Pain Practice* **8**(5), 348–354.

Kikuchi, S., Sato, K., Konno, S. & Hasue, M. (1994) Anatomic and radiographic study of dorsal root ganglia. *Spine* **19**, 6–11.

Kloth, D.S., Fenton, D.S., Andersson, G.B. & Block J.E. (2008) Intradiscal electrothermal therapy (IDET) for the treatment of discogenic low back pain: patient selection and indications for use. *Pain Physician* **11**(5), 659–668.

Kushnerik, V., Altman, G. & Gozenput, P. (2009) Pharmacology of steroids used during epidural steroid injections. *Techniques in Regional Anesthesia and Pain Management* **13**(4), 212–216.

Lawen, A. (1922) Ueber segmentare Schmerzaufhebungen durch paravertebrale Novokaininjektion zur differentialen Diagnose intraabdominaler Erkranbungen. *Munchen Medizinische Wochenschrift* **69**, 1423.

Lindblom, K. (1944) Protrusion of the discs and nerve compression in the lumbar region. *Acta Radiologica* **25**, 195–212.

Mandl, F. (1926) *Die Paravertebrale Injektion*. Vienna: J. Springer.

Moore, D.C. (1954) *Stellate Ganglion Block*. Springfield, IL: Charles C. Thomas.

Nelson, J.W. (2004) Percutaneous radiofrequency lumbar sympathectomy. *Techniques in Regional Anesthesia and Pain Management* **8**(1), 53–56.

Patel, V.B. (2009) Techniques for epidural injections. *Techniques in Regional Anesthesia and Pain Management* **13**(4), 217–228.

Pino, C.A., Ivie, C.S. & Rathmell, J.P. (2009) Lumbar discography: diagnostic role in discogenic pain. *Techniques in Regional Anesthesia and Pain Management* **13**(2), 85–92.

Raj, P.P. (2008) Intervertebral disc: anatomy–physiology–pathophysiology–treatment. *Pain Practice* **8**(1), 18–44.

Rees, W.E.S. (1971) Multiple bilateral subcutaneous rhizolysis of segmental nerves in the treatment of the intervertebral disk syndrome. *Annals of General Practice* **16**, 126.

Reid, W., Watt, J.K. & Gray, R.G. (1970) Phenol injection of the sympathetic chain. *British Journal of Surgery* **57**, 45.

Robecchi, A. & Capra, R. (1952) L'idrocortisone (composto F). Prime esperienze cliniche in campo reumatologico. *Minerva Medica* **98**, 1259–1263.

Roofe, P.G. (1940) Innervation of the anulus fibrosus and posterior longitudinal ligament. *Archives of Neurology and Psychiatry* **44**, 100–103.

Saal, J.S. & Saal, J.A. (2000) Management of chronic discogenic low back pain with a thermal intradiscal catheter: a preliminary report. *Spine* **25**(3), 382–388.

Sachs, B.L., Vanharanta, H., Spivey, M.A., et al. (1987) Dallas discogram description. A new classification of CT/discography in low-back disorders. *Spine* **12**, 287–294.

Sharps, L.S. & Issac, Z. (2002) Percutaneous disc decompression using nucleoplasty. *Pain Physician* **5**(2), 121–126.

Shealy, C.N. (1975) Percutaneous radiofrequency denervation of spinal facets: treatment for chronic back pain and sciatica. *Journal of Neurosurgery* **43**, 448–451.

Sicard, M.A. (1901) Les injections medicamenteuse extradurales par voie saracoccygiene. *Comptes Rendues des Seances de la Societe de Biologie et de ses Filliales* **53**, 396.

Singh, V. & Derby, R. (2006) Percutaneous lumbar disc decompression. *Pain Physician* **9**(2), 139–146.

Sluijter, M.E. (1994) Intradiscal RF procedures for discogenic pain. *Pain Clinic* **7**, 193–198.

Smith, L., Garvin, P.J., Gesler, R.M. & Jennings, R.B. (1963) Enzyme dissolution of the nucleus pulposa. *Nature* (London) **198**, 1311.

Soin, A., Kapural, L. & Mekhail, N. (2007) Imaging for percutaneous vertebral augmentation. *Techniques in Regional Anesthesia and Pain Management* **11**(2), 90–94.

Thomas, L. (1956) Reversible collapse of rabbit ears after intravenous papain and prevention of recovery by cortisone. *Journal of Experimental Medicine* **104**, 245–252.

von Gaza, W. (1924) Die Resektion der paravertebralen Nerven und die isolierte Durchschneidung des Ramus communicans. *Archiv fuer Klinische Chirurgie* **133**, 479.

17 Interventional Pain Procedures in the Pelvic and Sacral Regions

Percutaneous interlaminar block of the caudal epidural space

History

The caudal approach to the epidural space is the earliest known technique for epidural steroid injection. It was first reported in 1901 by Cathelin, Pasquier, and Sicard. The caudal block was introduced again in 1925 by Viner with its use for treating sciatica. It was popularized only after 1952 when a corticosteroid was added to the local anesthetic for acute and chronic pain by Robecchi and Capra in 1952 and Lievre in 1957.

Anatomy

The caudal epidural technique is very difficult to perform because of the many variations in anatomic structure from patient to patient, and because it is often hard to palpate the sacral coccygeal hiatus.

Sacrum

The sacrum is a large, triangular bone at the base of the spine and at the upper and back part of the pelvic cavity, where it is inserted like a wedge between the two hip bones. Its upper part connects with the last lumbar vertebra, and bottom part with the coccyx.

The base of the sacrum, which is broad and expanded, is directed upward and forward.

The ala of sacrum is a large triangular surface, which supports the psoas major and the lumbosacral trunk. In the articulated pelvis it is continuous with the iliac fossa.

The pelvic surface of the sacrum is concave from above downward, and slightly so from side to side.

It is curved upon itself and placed obliquely (that is, tilted forward). It is kyphotic – that is, concave facing forward. The base projects forward as the sacral promontory internally and articulates with the last lumbar vertebra to form the prominent sacrovertebral angle. The central part is curved outward toward the posterior, allowing greater room for the pelvic cavity. The pelvic surface of the sacrum is concave from above downward, and slightly so from side to side. The dorsal surface of the sacrum is convex and narrower than the pelvic surface. The lateral surface of the sacrum is broad above, but narrows into a thin edge below. The base of the sacrum, which is broad and expanded, is directed upward and forward. The apex of the sacral bone is directed downward, and presents an oval facet for articulation with the coccyx. The sacrum articulates with four bones: the last lumbar vertebra above, the coccyx (tailbone) below, and the ilium portion of the hip bone on either side. It is called the sacrum when referring to all of the parts combined, but sacral vertebrae when they are referred to individually. The sacrum is noticeably sexually dimorphic. In the female it is shorter and wider than in the male; the lower half forms a greater angle with the upper; the upper half is nearly straight, the lower half presenting the greatest amount of curvature. The bone is also directed more obliquely backward; this increases the size of the pelvic cavity and renders the sacrovertebral angle more prominent. In the male the curvature is more evenly distributed over the whole length of the bone, and is altogether greater than in the female.

The vertebral canal (canalis sacralis; sacral canal) runs throughout the greater part of the bone; above, it is triangular in form; below, its posterior wall is incomplete, from the non-development of the laminae and spinous processes. It lodges the sacral nerves, and its walls are perforated by the anterior and posterior sacral foramina through which these nerves pass out. There are four anterior sacral foramina through which the sacral nerves exit and the lateral sacral arteries enter. The posterior surface of the sacrum is convex. Laterally, one can identify four dorsal sacral foramina. They transmit the posterior divisions of the sacral nerves (Figs 17.1–17.3).

There are rudimentary spinous processes from the first three or four sacral segments in the midline. The laminae unite to form a sacral groove. The laminae of the fifth sacral

Pain-Relieving Procedures: The Illustrated Guide, First Edition. P. Prithvi Raj and Serdar Erdine.
© 2012 John Wiley & Sons, Ltd. Published 2012 by John Wiley & Sons, Ltd.

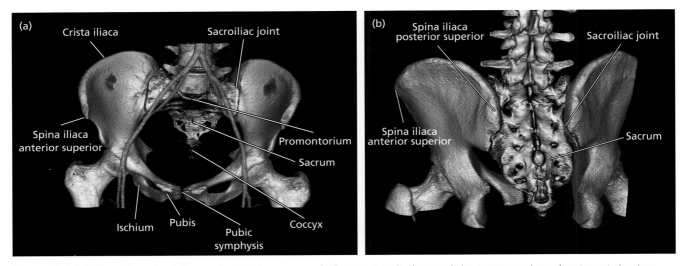

Figure 17.1 (a,b) Three-dimensional CT scan showing the sacrum and other structures in close proximity, anteroposterior and posteroanterior views.

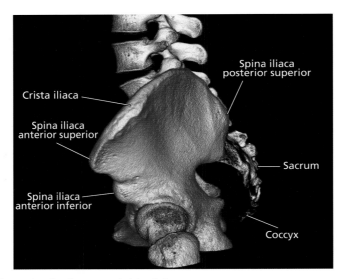

Figure 17.2 Three-dimensional CT scan showing the sacrum in lateral view.

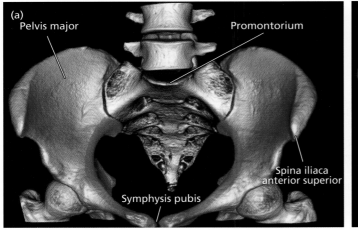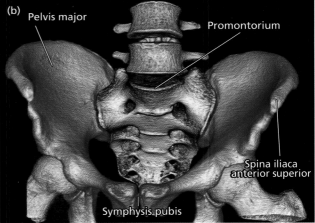

Figure 17.3 (a) Pelvis in the female. (b) Pelvis in the male.

vertebra fail to unite posteriorly to form a sacral hiatus, which is U- or V-shaped. The tubercles that represent the inferior articular processes make up the sacral corona and are connected inferiorly to the coccygeal cornua.

The sacral hiatus is covered by the sacrococcygeal membrane. Just beneath the sacrococcygeal membrane lies the caudal border of the epidural space. Anatomically the sacral hiatus varies greatly. The apex of the sacral hiatus is at the level one-third above the lower border of S4. The sacral canal contains the epidural venous plexus down to the level of S4. It also contains some epidural fat. The termination of the thecal sac varies depending on age, and varies between the lower border of the S1 foramen in adults and the S3 foramen in children. This is of significance when judging the optimum placement of the epidural needle tip and avoiding dural puncture and postdural puncture headache. The coccyx is the final segment of the apex vertebral column. Comprising three to five separate or fused vertebrae (the coccygeal vertebrae) below the sacrum, it is attached to the sacrum by a fibrocartilaginous joint, the sacrococcygeal symphysis.

In each of the first three segments may be traced a rudimentary body and articular and transverse processes; the last piece (sometimes the third) is a mere nodule of bone. The transverse processes are most prominent and noticeable on the first coccygeal segment. All the segments are destitute of pedicles, laminae, and spinous processes. The first is the largest; it resembles the lowest sacral vertebra, and often exists as a separate piece; the last three diminish in size from above downward.

The anterior surface is slightly concave and marked with three transverse grooves that indicate the junctions of the different segments. It gives attachment to the anterior sacrococcygeal ligament and the levatores ani and supports part of the rectum. The posterior surface is convex, marked by transverse grooves similar to those on the anterior surface, and presents on either side a linear row of tubercles, the rudimentary articular processes of the coccygeal vertebrae. Of these, the superior pair is large, and is called the coccygeal cornua; they project upward, and articulate with the cornua of the sacrum, and on either side complete the foramen for the transmission of the posterior division of the fifth sacral nerve.

The lateral borders are thin and exhibit a series of small eminences, which represent the transverse processes of the coccygeal vertebrae (Fig. 17.4).

Of these, the first is the largest; it is flattened from front to back, and often ascends to join the lower part of the thin lateral edge of the sacrum, thus completing the foramen for the transmission of the anterior division of the fifth sacral nerve; the others diminish in size from above downward, and are often wanting. The borders of the coccyx are narrow, and give attachment on either side to the sacrotuberous and sacrospinous ligaments, to the coccyges in front of the ligaments, and to the gluteus maximus behind them.

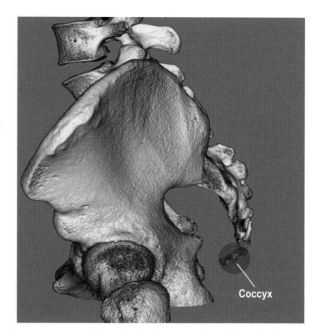

Figure 17.4 Three-dimensional CT scan showing the lateral view of the coccyx.

The apex is rounded, and has attached to it the tendon of the sphincter ani externus. It may be bifid.

Sacrococcygeal and intercoccygeal joints are variable and may be (1) synovial joints, (2) thin discs of fibrocartilage, (3) intermediate between these two, or (4) ossified sacral canal.

The vertebral canal (sacral canal) runs throughout the greater part of the sacral bone; above, it is triangular in form; below, its posterior wall is incomplete, from the non-development of the laminae and spinous processes.

It lodges the sacral nerves, and its walls are perforated by the anterior and posterior sacral foramina through which these nerves pass out.

The average capacity of the sacral canal is 12–65 ml, with a range of 30–34.5 ml.

Filum terminale exit the dura and continue through the sacral canal to exit at the sacral hiatus. Sacral venous plexus, a part of the internal epidural plexus, generally ends at the S4 level; however, in some cases it may continue all along the canal. The sacral canal also contains epidural fat.

Sacral and coccygeal nerves

The five sacral nerves emerge from the sacrum. Although the vertebral components of the sacrum are fused into a single bone, the sacral vertebrae are still used to number the sacral nerves (Fig. 17.5).

Posteriorly, they emerge from the posterior sacral foramina, and form the posterior branches of sacral nerves (including the medial clunial nerves).

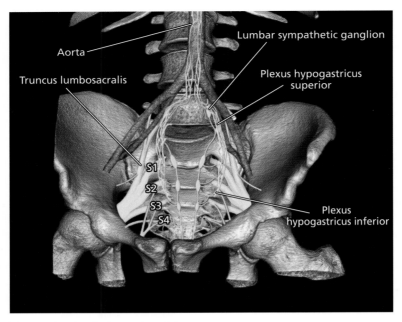

Figure 17.5 Three-dimensional CT scan showing the innervation of the sacrum.

Anteriorly, they emerge from the anterior sacral foramina, and contribute to the sacral plexus (S1–S4) and coccygeal plexus.

Indications
- Coccydinia.
- Lumbar sprain.
- Spondylolisthesis.
- Herniated disc with nerve root irritation.
- Herniated disc without nerve root compression.
- Chemical neuritis.
- Scoliosis with nerve root entrapment.
- Spinal stenosis.

Contraindications
- Local or systemic infection.
- Coagulopathy.
- Previous operations in the region.

Technique of interlaminar block of the caudal epidural space

Step 1. Prepare the patient before the procedure
1. The history, physical examination, and radiological studies are important before the procedure. All complications should be explained to the patient in detail, including the risks of numbness in the region, infection, and bowel and bladder dysfunction. Laboratory studies including prothrombin time, partial thromboplastin time, bleeding time, C-reactive protein (CRP), and urine analysis should be made. A recent magnetic resonance imaging (MRI) is mandatory, especially in patients with failed back-surgery syndrome.
2. The patient should be aware of why this procedure is being done, and what to expect from it and the team. All complications and side effects should be explained in detail, before the procedure. Valid written consent should be obtained.
3. The type of analgesia or sedation needs to be ascertained before performance of the invasive procedure. Intravenous fentanyl, midazolam, and/or propofol may be used judiciously for the patient's comfort.

Step 2. Position and monitor the patient
1. Place the patient prone on the table.
2. Place a pillow beneath the iliac crest to flatten the lumbar lordoses.
3. Obtain an intravenous access.
4. Administer oxygen by nasal cannula.
5. Monitor the vital signs noninvasively.
Prepare and drape the intergluteal crease, anus, and surrounding area in a sterile fashion. One should be especially careful in preparing this region, due to the risk of infection.

Step 3. Equipment and drugs for caudal epidural block
- 5 ml syringe for local anesthetic solution.
- 1½ inch 25 gauge needle for skin infiltration.
- 22 gauge 3½ inch needle for caudal epidural block.
- 5 ml syringe for contrast material, iohexol.
- 10 ml syringe for caudal epidural block.

• 5 ml of 1% lidocaine for skin infiltration.
• 5 ml contrast material, iohexol.
• 10 ml of 0.5% bupivacaine combined with depomedrol.

Step 4. Mark the surface landmarks for the needle entry
1. The gluteal fold does not prolapse over the lower middle portion of the sacrum, where palpation of the sacral coccygeal hiatus is performed.
2. The thumb and second finger are placed on the prominent sacral tuberosity just below the articular processes of the fifth lumbar vertebrae, and the middle finger is swept downward and medial to palpate the sacral cornua.
3. With the finger in place over the sacral cornua, the skin is moved slightly cephalad a few millimeters and a 25 gauge needle is inserted for skin analgesia. An amount less than 0.125–0.25 ml is needed for a 1 cm wheal. Leave the needle used for skin infiltration in that position (Fig. 17.6).

Step 5. Visualization
1. Place the C-arm in the posteroanterior position. Mark the sacral hiatus after palpation, the needle should be near to the midline.
2. Rotate the C-arm in the lateral position, view the coccyx and the sacral–caudal canal (Figs 17.7 and 17.8).

Step 6. Direction of the needle
1. Insert a 22 gauge, 3½ inch needle toward the inferior lateral angle of the sacral cornua, approximately at a 45° angle to the skin, through the sacrococcygeal membrane into the caudal epidural space. A loss of resistance will occur while the needle enters the caudal space (Fig. 17.9).
2. Advance the needle 2 cm more cephalad into the caudal epidural space with the needle between the dorsal and ventral plates of the sacrum.

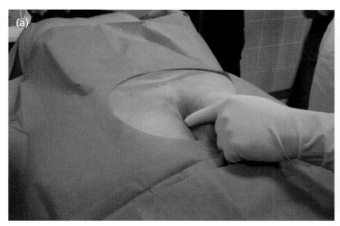
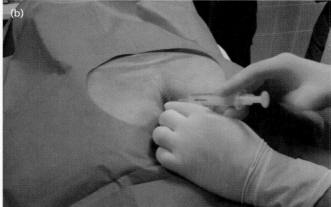

Figure 17.6 (a,b) Palpate the sacral cornu, infiltrate the skin.

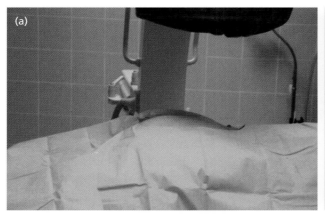
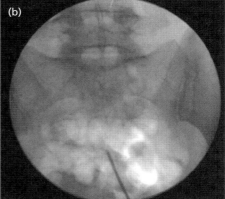

Figure 17.7 (a,b) C-arm in posteroanterior position, mark the entry point.

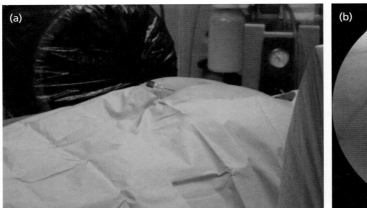

Figure 17.8 (a,b) C-arm in lateral position.

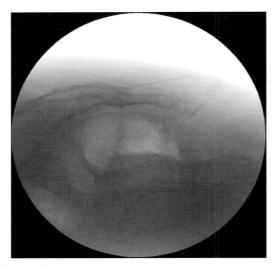

Figure 17.9 Position of the needle in lateral view.

3. One should aspirate, and be careful about damaging a large connection of venous plexus lying within the caudal epidural space. If blood is aspirated, advance the needle one more centimeter, aspirate again, and if blood is aspirated, terminate the procedure.

Step 7. Confirm the position of the needle

If the aspiration test is negative, inject 3–5 ml of contrast material. The contrast material should spread cephalad; if not, one should suspect fibrosis or stenosis in the caudal canal. If contrast material spreads properly a Christmas-tree-like view will appear (Fig. 17.10).

Step 8. Caudal epidural block

1. After verifying the tip of the needle is in the caudal epidural space under fluoroscopy, inject contrast solution and 5–10 ml of 0.5% bupivacaine with 40 mg methylprednisolone.

2. Some physicians prefer to inject an excessive amount of local anesthetic up to 25 ml; normally injection of 10 ml solution will spread up to the L5 level. Intraocular hemorrhage has been reported owing to an increase in intraocular pressure if an excessive amount of solution is injected.

Step 9. Postprocedure care

After the procedure the patient should be observed for a reasonable time for the risk of hypotension. In case of hypotension, intravenous electrolyte solutions should be administered. The recovery and observation time depends on the sedation and analgesia used, and facilitates the assessment of any impairment of intellectual function, tolerance of oral intake, assessment of the immediate results of the neural blockade, and pain response to the procedure.

The patient should be provided with all instructions, including whom to call or where to go for any postprocedure urgent/emergency care. The patient should be discharged accompanied by a responsible adult.

Complications

- **Infection**

Infection is a real risk for this procedure owing to the site of injection in close proximity with the anus. Strict care for aseptic preparations is essential.

- **Postinjection pain at the sacral hiatus**

Postinjection pain at the sacral hiatus, which is the site of needle entry, may be prolonged but usually lasts no more than 2–6 months.

- **Inadvertent intrathecal injection**

Inadvertent intrathecal injection may occur if the needle is advanced too far or due to dural puncture if a catheter is advanced through the needle. The patient will complain of numbness in the lower extremities soon after the injection, which will not occur after epidural injection. If the injectate spreads to upper levels, there is risk of respiratory distress

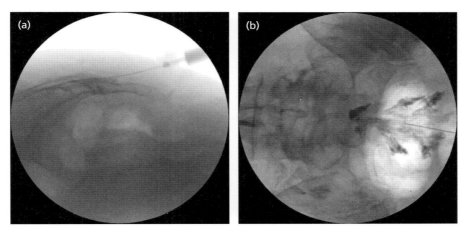

Figure 17.10 (a,b) Spread of the contrast material in lateral and posteroanterior view.

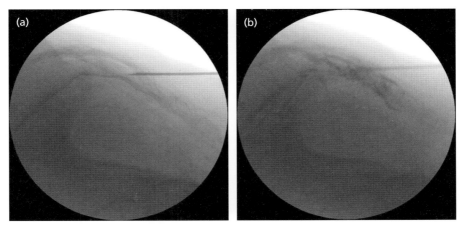

Figure 17.11 (a,b) Intraosseous injection and vascularization.

or even arrest due to total spinal anesthesia. Postpuncture headache may also occur.

- **Intravascular injection**

The caudal canal is rich with many venous plexuses. An aspiration test is mandatory. The aspiration test may be negative in the case of intravascular injection. A small amount of test dose of the local anesthetic before injecting the total amount will prevent severe complications such as local anesthetic toxicity.

- **Intraosseous injection**

If a resistance is encountered while advancing the needle within the caudal space, one should not insist; slightly withdraw the needle, and redirect again. Intraosseous injection of local anesthetic may cause toxic reactions (Fig. 17.11).

Helpful hints

In patients who have no significant anatomic variation, needle entry into the epidural space is quick and reliable. However, in some cases the caudal epidural technique is very difficult to perform because of the many variations in anatomic structure from patient to patient, and because it is often hard to palpate the sacral coccygeal hiatus.

There are other potential causes of difficulty in entering the caudal epidural space. In patients with short stature of less than 5 feet (approximately 1.52 meters), some of these difficulties may be due to the following: short sagittal descension of the sacrum; tip of the needle above the level of the anterior foramen of S1 in the anteroposterior view; atypical anatomy within the sacral canal, including presence of a tethered cord; acute angle of sacral dorsal convexity; inability to identify anatomic landmarks; severe to morbid obesity blocking radiologic (fluoroscopic) visualization; deformity of sacral coccygeal area secondary to previous trauma or birth defect; sealed sacra; hiatus, relatively long coccyx with "superior" location of sacral hiatus; and developmental fusion of sacral canal.

The procedure should not be performed by the blind technique. The needle may not enter the sacral canal or may enter the canal but leave through the foramen dorsally, resulting in the injection of the solution out of the epidural space.

Preexisting arachnoiditis, whether clinical or subclinical, can lead to prolonged block in caudal epidural steroid injection.

Complications have been reported with injections of high volumes into the epidural space, with increases in intraocular pressure with retinal hemorrhage.

Percutaneous technique of caudal epidural neuroplasty

History
Caudal epidural neuroplasty may be defined as inserting an epidural catheter through the caudal space and injecting a combination of local anesthetic steroid, hypertonic saline, and hyaluronidase.

In 1901 Cathelin performed the first caudal block. The initial epidurography was performed serendipitously in 1921 by Sicard and Forestier. Payne and Rupp in 1950 combined hyaluronidase with local anesthetic. Lievre reported the first use of corticosteroid injected into the epidural space for the treatment of sciatica in 1957. Hypertonic saline was first administered by Hitchcock in 1967 for the treatment of chronic back pain when he injected cold saline intrathecally. Hypertonic saline was subsequently used by Ventafridda and Spreafico in 1974 for intractable cancer pain by intrathecal administration.

In the late 1970s Claude Duval described the use of epidural hypertonic saline without fluoroscopy for chronic pain. Racz and Holubec in 1989 reported the first use of epidural hypertonic saline to facilitate lysis of adhesions, and hyaluronidase was introduced as an alternative agent by Stolker and associates in 1994. Then Racz introduced the Racz catheter, with less risk of shearing, obstructing, and migration.

Anatomy
The sacrum is a large, triangular bone, situated below L5. Distally the apex of the sacrum articulates with the coccyx. Its anterior surface is concave. Anteriorly, four transverse ridges cross its median part. The portions of the bone between the ridges are the bodies of the sacrum. There are four anterior sacral foramina through which the sacral nerves exit and lateral sacral arteries enter. The posterior surface of the sacrum is convex. There are rudimentary spinous processes from the first three or four sacral segments in the midline. The laminae unite to form the sacral groove. The sacral hiatus is formed by the failure of the laminae of S5 to unite posteriorly. The tubercles that represent remnants of the inferior articular processes are known as the sacral cornua; they are connected inferiorly to the coccygeal cornua. Laterally one can identify four dorsal sacral foramina.

They transmit the posterior divisions of the sacral nerves. The sacrum may have many variations. The bodies of S1 and S2 may fail to unite or the sacral canal may remain open throughout its length.

The caudal canal has a variable orientation in the anterior–posterior plane, necessitating an epidural needle skin entry point inferior to the sacral hiatus. The sacrum may curve in, resembling a kyphotic shape, placing the inferior sacral canal posterior to the sacral hiatus.

In a lateral view, the caudal canal appears as a slight step off on the most posterior part of the sacrum. The median sacral crest is seen as an opaque line posterior to the caudal canal. While still in the lateral view, the sacral hiatus is usually visible as a translucent opening at the base of the caudal canal. To aid identification of the sacral hiatus, the coccyx can be seen articulating with the inferior surface of the sacrum.

On the anteroposterior view, the intermediate sacral crests are seen as opaque vertical lines on either side of the midline. The sacral foramina are seen as translucent near-circular areas lateral to the intermediate sacral crests. Note that the presence of bowel gas can make recognition of these structures difficult (Fig. 17.12).

Indications
- Failed back surgery syndrome.
- Epidural fibrosis.
- Lumbar radiculopathy.
- Spinal stenosis.
- Lateral recess stenosis.
- Back pain and radiculopathy.
- Herniated discs.
- Radicular neuropathic pain.
- Postradiation neuropathy.
- Postmeningitis epidural scarring.

Contraindications
- Infection.
- Coagulopathies.
- Unstable lumbar spine.
- Inability to lie in prone position.
- Arachnoiditis.

Technique of caudal neuroplasty

Step 1. Prepare the patient before the procedure
The history, physical examination, and radiological studies are important before the procedure. All complications should be explained to the patient in detail, including the risks of numbness in the region, infection, bowel and bladder dysfunction. Laboratory studies including prothrombin time, partial thromboplastin time, bleeding time, CRP, and urine analysis should be made. A recent MRI is mandatory, especially in patients with failed back surgery syndrome.

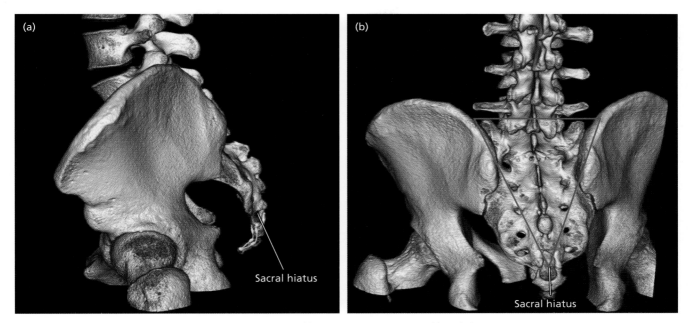

Figure 17.12 (a,b) Three-dimensional CT scan showing the sacral hiatus in posteroanterior and lateral view.

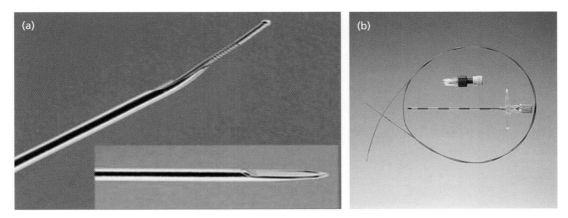

Figure 17.13 (a,b) Racz needle and the tip of the Racz catheter.

Step 2. Position and monitor the patient
1. Place the patient prone on the table. Place a pillow under the abdomen to flatten the lumbar lordosis. Abduction of the legs and internal rotation of the feet facilitates entry into the sacral hiatus.
2. Obtain an intravenous access.
3. Administer oxygen by nasal cannula; monitor the vital signs noninvasively.
4. Prepare and drape the area in a sterile fashion. Prepare and drape the intergluteal crease, anus, and surrounding area in a sterile fashion. One should be especially careful when preparing this region because of the risk of infection. Insert a pad between the sacral hiatus and anus.
5. The patient should not be over-sedated. They should remain sufficiently conscious to provide responses to any

questions. It may be necessary to sedate the patient with 1–2 mg midazolam and 25–50 μg of fentanyl. Intravenous injection of 1 g of ceftriaxone (Rocephin) is recommended.

Step 3. Equipment and drugs for the technique
• 25 gauge, ¾ inch infiltration needle.
• 18 gauge, 1½ inch needle.
• 15–16 gauge Epimed RX Coude epidural needle (Fig. 17.13).
• Epimed Tun-L or Epimed Brevi-stiff catheter for dense scarring.
• 5 ml syringe for skin infiltration.
• Two 10 ml syringes.
• 1% lidocaine for skin infiltration.
• 2% preservative-free lidocaine.
• 0.25% levobupivacaine or bupivacaine.

- 0.9% preservative-free normal saline.
- 10% preservative-free hypertonic saline.
- 1500 units of hyaluronidase.

Step 4. Visualization
Place the C-arm in the posteroanterior position. The sacrum and coccyx have to be visualized (Fig. 17.14**)**.

Step 5. Mark the surface landmarks for the needle entry
1. Note the gluteal fold does not cover over the lower middle portion of the sacrum, where palpation of the sacral coccygeal hiatus is performed.
2. The thumb and second finger are placed on the prominent sacral tuberosities just below the articular processes of the fifth lumbar vertebrae, and the middle finger is swept downward and medially to palpate the sacral cornua (Fig. 17.15).
3. Contralateral from the symptomatic side, 1 inch from the midline and 2 inches from the sacral hiatus on the gluteal

mound, the skin is infiltrated with a 25 gauge, 1½ inch needle with local anesthetic. With the finger in place over the sacral cornua, the skin is moved slightly cephalad a few millimeters, and a 25 gauge needle is inserted for skin analgesia. An amount less than 0.125–0.25 ml is needed for a 1 cm wheal. Leave the needle used for skin infiltration in that position.

Step 6. Direction of the needle
1. Insert a 15 gauge RX needle toward the inferior lateral angle of the sacral cornua, approximately at a 45° angle to the skin, through the sacrococcygeal membrane into the caudal epidural space. A loss of resistance will occur while the needle enters the caudal space (Fig. 17.16).
2. Verify the position of the needle within the caudal space with fluoroscopy under posteroanterior and lateral views (Fig. 17.17).
3. Advance the needle 2 cm more cephalad into the caudal epidural space with the needle between the dorsal and

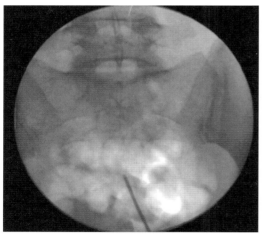

Figure 17.14 The entry point for the Racz needle.

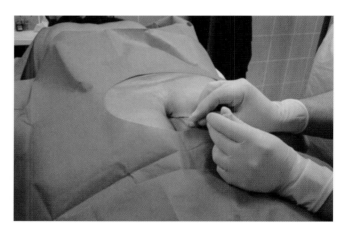

Figure 17.16 Advance the needle through the sacral hiatus.

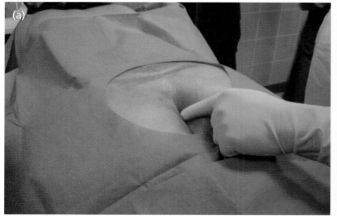

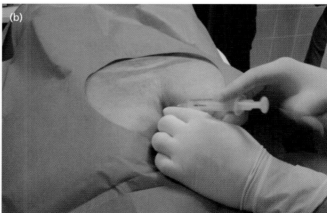

Figure 17.15 (a,b) Palpate the sacral hiatus and infiltrate the skin.

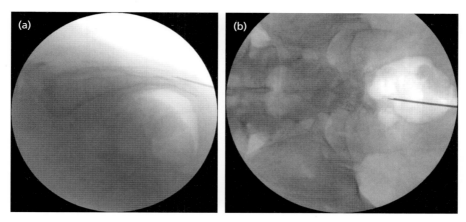

Figure 17.17 (a,b) Direction of the Racz needle in lateral and posteroanterior view.

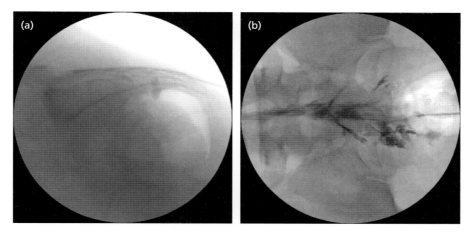

Figure 17.18 (a,b) Spread of the contrast material in lateral and posteroanterior view. The spread of the contrast material in posteroanterior view. Christmas-tree-like view.

ventral plates of the sacrum to a level not more than S3 foramen to avoid damaging the sacral nerve roots.

4. One should aspirate, and be careful about damaging a large connection of venous plexus lying within the caudal epidural space. If blood is aspirated, advance the needle one more centimeter; aspirate again. If blood is aspirated, terminate the procedure.

5. If the aspiration test is negative, inject 3–5 ml of contrast material.

Step 7. Confirm the position of the needle

Inject 3–5 ml of contrast material. The contrast solution should spread cephalad; if not, one should suspect fibrosis or stenosis in the caudal canal. If contrast solution spreads properly, a Christmas-tree-like view is seen. In the case of epidural adhesions, the dye will not spread over the involved nerve roots, forming a "filling defect" image (Fig. 17.18).

Step 8. Inserting and placing the catheter in the epidural space

1. After confirming that the tip of the needle is within the caudal space, insert a stainless-steel, fluoropolymer-coated spiral tipped Racz catheter through the needle (Fig. 17.19).

2. The bevel of the needle should be facing the ventrolateral aspect of the caudal canal of the affected side. This turning of the needle facilitates passage of the catheter to the desired side, and decreases the chance of shearing the catheter.

3. Because scar formation is usually uneven, multiple passes may be necessary to place the catheter into the scarred area. For this reason, it is best to use a 15 gauge RX epidural needle, which has been specially designed to allow multiple passes of the catheter.

4. The catheter should be placed in the anterior epidural space and it should be confirmed under lateral vision. If the catheter is placed in the posterior epidural space, it should be reinserted because epidural fibrosis is significant in the

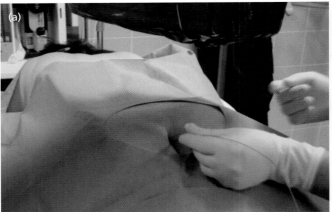 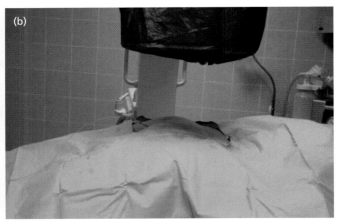

Figure 17.19 (a,b) Introduce the Racz catheter through the Racz needle.

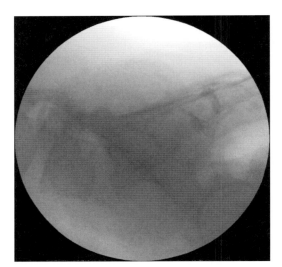

Figure 17.20 Position of the catheter within the anterior epidural space.

anterior epidural space (Figs 17.20 and 17.21). It may be difficult to advance the catheter in the scarred area. If resistance develops against the catheter, one should not persist to push it; withdraw the catheter, inject 5 ml of preservative-free saline, and try to reinsert the catheter again.

5. After negative aspiration, inject 5–10 ml of contrast material through the catheter. If the tip of the catheter is within a vein or venous plexus, one should reposition the tip of the catheter.

6. Caution: the tip of the catheter may puncture the dura, when resistance is felt while advancing the catheter. If one suspects dura puncture, administer contrast solution again to view if the tip of the catheter is within the subarachnoid space. The contrast material will suddenly fade if the catheter is within the subarachnoid space. In the case of inad-

vertent dural puncture, the procedure has to be aborted to be repeated another day.

7. The tip of the catheter should be on the side of the scarred area. After confirming the correct position of the catheter, the needle is withdrawn carefully. Caution must be taken to not puncture the catheter with the needle, and not to cut the catheter. Triple-antibiotic ointment, such as polymyxin, and two 2 inch × 2 inch split gauze pads are used to cover the catheter exit site. The surrounding skin is sprayed or covered with tincture of benzoin and, with a single loop of the catheter toward midline, all of the above area is covered with a 4–6 inch sterile transparent surgical dressing to prevent postprocedure infection from the buttock area.

8. Inject a test dose of 2 ml of 1% lidocaine to confirm that the catheter is within the epidural space; there should be no signs of motor block including the ability to flex the hip.

Step 9. Injection of local anesthetic and other solutions

1. After negative aspiration inject a combination of 9 ml of 0.25% bupivacaine, 40 mg triamcinolone and 1500 units of hyaluronidase. Wait for 30 minutes after the first injection, then inject 10 ml of 10% hypertonic saline slowly for 30 minutes with an infusion pump.

2. On days 2 and 3, the catheter is injected once a day with 10 ml of 0.2% ropivacaine after negative aspiration from the catheter. Fifteen minutes later, 9 ml of 10% saline is infused over 20 minutes for the patient's comfort. As with all hypertonic saline infusion series, the catheter must be flushed with 1.5 ml of preservative-free normal saline. On day 3, the catheter is removed 10 minutes after the last injection. A triple-antibiotic ointment is placed on the wound and is covered by a bandage or other appropriate dressing.

Step 10. Postprocedural care of the patient

In the recovery room after the first procedure of epidural neuroplasty, for the infusion of hypertonic saline, the patient is placed in the lateral position with the painful side down,

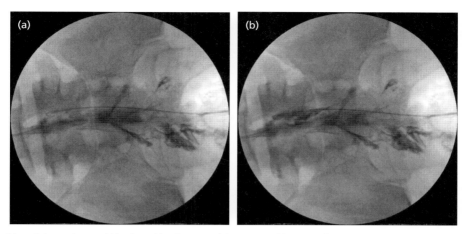

Figure 17.21 (a,b) Position of the catheter within the epidural space, Christmas-tree-like view of the contrast material, and the filling defect.

and remains in this position for 30 minutes following the completion of the infusion. Occasionally, the patient may complain of severe burning pain during the infusion. The burning is usually from the introduction of hypertonic saline to unanesthetized epidural tissue. Should this occur, the infusion must be stopped and a 3–5 ml bolus of additional local anesthetic is injected. After 5 minutes, the hypertonic saline infusion can be restarted without incident. Following completion of the hypertonic saline infusion, 1.5 ml of preservative-free normal saline is used to flush the catheter.

During the time that the catheter is indwelling, the patient should keep the insertion site dry and prevent infection.

Complications
- Related to the drugs administered.
- Related to the procedure.

Complications and side effects related to drugs administered
- Complications and side effects related to the drugs administered.
  - Allergy.
  - Related to antibiotics.
  - Related to iodine containing contrast material.
  - Related to disinfectants.
  - Related to local anesthetics.
  - Related to hyaluronidase.
- Toxicity related to overdose of the following.
  - Local anesthetics.
  - Steroids.

Complications related to the procedure
- Pain.
  - At the site of entry.
  - Due to increased inflammation.
  - Due to hypertonic saline.

- Excessive amount of solutions.
  - Barotrauma.
  - Ischemia on the spinal nerves and spinal cord.
  - Retinal hemorrhage.
- Nonsterile technique.
  - Infection at the site of entry.
  - Infection at the epidural space.
  - Epidural abscess.
  - Meningitis.
- Epidural hematoma.
- Shearing and tearing of the catheter.
- Blocking of the catheter.
- Inadvertent puncture of the catheter.
  - Intravascular.
  - Subarachnoid.
  - Subdural.
- Neurological complications.
  - Paresthesia.
  - Bowel and bladder dysfunction.
  - Sexual disfunction.

Complications and side effects related to the drug administered
- **Allergic reactions**

Agents used during epidural lysis with allergenic potential include iodine containing radiopaque contrast and surgical disinfectants, antibiotics, local anesthetics and hyaluronidase. It is important to obtain an accurate history to identify patients predisposed to allergic reactions to the substances mentioned and to avoid, if possible, using the substances. Documented anaphylactic reactions to local anesthetics and hyaluronidase are rare.

- **Hypertonic saline**

Injection of hypertonic saline into the epidural space is very painful. Five milliliters of 1% lidocaine should be injected at least 30 minutes before hypertonic saline injection. In patients with severe spinal stenosis, permanent paresthesia, bowel and bladder dysfunction, or sexual dysfunction may develop owing to hypertonic saline. The incidence of permanent paresthesia is higher if the tip of the catheter lies at the L5–S1 level. Thus, if the catheter cannot be advanced to higher levels it is better not to administer hypertonic saline in those patients. Inadvertent subarachnoid injection of hypertonic saline causes more serious complications such as muscle cramps, hypertension, cardiac arrhythmia, pulmonary edema, and cerebral infarct. Hemiplegia, permanent paresthesia, and bladder and bowel dysfunction may also develop.

- **Steroids**

Preservatives in steroid solutions may cause adhesive arachnoiditis. Particulate steroids may cause emboli. Subarachnoid administration of steroids may cause arachnoiditis and aseptic meningitis.

- **Contrast material**

In the past, contrast material containing oil caused more complications. However, with the use of nonionic contrast material, problems related to contrast material are very rare except allergy.

- **Local anesthetics**

Intravascular injection of bupivacaine may cause cardiac arrest. The tip of the catheter should be confirmed by contrast material under continuous imaging. A serious amount of local anesthetic solution is delivered to the epidural space during the procedure, which may cause hemodynamic instability, especially in hemodynamically impaired patients with cardiovascular diseases or chronic illnesses. In high-risk patients, intravenous crystalloids or colloids must be administered before the procedure. In addition, the patients should be monitored during the whole procedure, and intravenous solutions should be given to prevent hypotension from occurring.

Complications related to the procedure

Pain
- At the site of entry.
- Due to increased inflammation.
- Due to hypertonic saline.

Pain may be due to the injury at the site of entry owing to the larger gauge of needles used. It may last for several days.

Injection of hypertonic solutions into the normal epidural space is quite painful unless preceded by local anesthetic. If the hypertonic saline spread is greater than the coverage area of the local anesthetic, the patient may have severe pain. The pain caused by the hypertonic saline in the epidural space rarely persists more than 5 minutes.

Excessive amount of solutions
- Barotrauma and ischemia on the spinal nerves and spinal cord.
- Retinal hemorrhage.

Barotrauma and ischemia
Injection of fluid into a closed compartment in the epidural space or into the subdural space can have the net effect of creating a space-occupying lesion that produces direct barotrauma to underlying tissue and/or blocks blood flow to the spinal cord or cauda equina thereby producing ischemic injury. The term loculation is used for this phenomenon. The fluid fills one compartment, and as the pressure–volume effect is pushed beyond just filling the compartment, fluid finds the weakest spot in the compartment and overflows into adjoining compartments, which in turn will fill.

Injection of hypertonic saline solution into a closed, loculated compartment within the epidural space can produce direct trauma by pressing on adjacent neural structures. In addition, hypertonic saline is hyperosmolar and will cause fluid shifts that will further increase the volume and pressure within the loculated compartment as osmosis draws fluid to the space to regain iso-osmolar status. To reach equilibrium, the 10% sodium chloride must reach 0.9% and in the process the volume expands 11 times over the injected volume. In the epidural space, the lateral recesses communicate with the neuroforamen to the outside of the spinal canal. So long as there is documented outlet from the epidural space, acting as a pressure relief mechanism, infusing pressure does not compress the nerves, the spinal cord, and the nerve roots through which blood supply is carried to the spinal cord.

Somatomotor, somatosensory, visceral, and autonomic dysfunctions are consequences of injury due to barotrauma or ischemic injury. The symptoms may last for only hours or may be irreversible. The injury is minimized or prevented by assuring that closed spaces are opened to establish drainage during the lysis procedure. The spread of the dye within the epidural space should be confirmed under a lateral view, and if the dye is confined to a limited space the tip of the catheter should be repositioned.

Retinal hemorrhage
One feared complication of any volume injection into the epidural space is the development of retinal hemorrhage, which has occurred after uncontrolled injections of relatively large volumes. There is no specific volume known to produce retinal hemorrhage. If the catheter is in the midline or the subdural or the subarachnoid space, the consequences of volume injection could very well result in significant pressure increase of the cerebrospinal fluid, giving rise to retinal hemorrhage. Complete recovery of vision usually occurs over a matter of days to months.

Nonsterile technique
- Infection at the site of entry.
- Infection at the epidural space.
- Epidural abscess.
- Meningitis.

Because hygienic conditions at the entrance site of the caudal canal are not optimal, infection is an important possible complication of the procedure. Infection may either occur at the entrance site of the catheter, in the caudal canal, or in the epidural space.

Delayed overwhelming infection has been seen after epidural injection in patients with preexisting chronic infections. The usual symptoms include increased pain, neck pain, headache, photophobia, numbness, weakness; the signs are elevated temperature, meningitis, and some neural deficits. Abnormalities in the laboratory findings include elevated white blood counts, elevated erythrocyte sedimentation rate, and spinal fluid abnormalities.

Epidural infections usually respond to antibiotic treatment administered for 5–10 days.

Epidural infection or abscess formation may be due to hematogenous spread or extension of superficial skin infections. Immunocompromised patients, diabetic patients, steroid-dependent patients, and those with malignancies are at higher risk for infection. Epidural abscess formation may not be recognized at the beginning because it is localized, and fever and increased white blood count may not always accompany this serious infection. In time, however, fever will rise as the abscess develops.

Meningismus signs may be observed. MRI evaluation is necessary to verify the extent of the problem but may not always reveal any findings at the very beginning of abscess formation.

Bleeding in the epidural space
Bleeding occurs, especially in patients who had previous back surgery, in whom the hygienic conditions of the epidural space are disrupted secondary to their surgery. In those cases where blood is aspirated from the epidural space during the introduction of the needle and/or the catheter, the catheter and the epidural space must be rinsed with normal saline and a few minutes should elapse before introducing the needle again.

If blood aspiration continues after saline rinsing, the entry site of the needle should be changed. If, after moving the tip of the catheter within the epidural space, blood ceases to be aspirated, it is safe to continue with the procedure. Although it has not been reported as a risk, epidural hematoma may follow bleeding. If epidural hematoma does occur, neurologic findings such as severe lumbar pain, bilateral lower extremity weakness, diffuse diminished pinprick sensation, paresthesia, and hypesthesia may be found. If an epidural hematoma is suspected, MRI evaluation may be required.

It may not be easy to identify an epidural hematoma if the procedure was performed despite epidural bleeding during the insertion of the catheter. Local anesthetic agents administered will, like an epidural hematoma, also give rise to paresthesia for several hours, which may mask the neurologic signs while hematoma does develop. The best precaution for epidural hematoma is to cease the procedure if excessive blood is aspirated through the needle or the catheter or at least postpone drug administration until neurologic assessment is performed.

Bending of the tip of the needle
The tips of the needles used to introduce catheters may bend or be damaged during insertion through the sacral hiatus. If this occurs, catheters would not be able to be directed to the targeted area (Fig. 17.22).

If bony structures are encountered while introducing an epidural needle with the stylet in place, a different angle of approach of the needle must be tried. Otherwise, the tip of the needle might become damaged or become bent, which would make introduction of the catheter through the needle difficult. Bent needles may enter the caudal space, which may be confirmed by injecting contrast material. However, the catheter might not be introduced easily through the needle, and if introduced, its withdrawal might lead to severe problems, which will be discussed later. If this problem is encountered, it is much safer to proceed using a different needle.

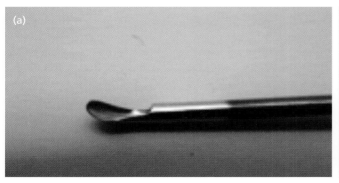
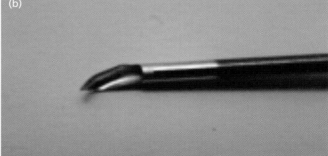

Figure 17.22 (a,b) Bending of the tip of the needle.

Pain-Relieving Procedures

Shearing of the catheter

Catheter shearing and its retention within the epidural space is one of the major complications that can occur during epidural neuroplasty. The Racz catheter is a wire-embedded catheter with a fine sheath around the embedded wires. Although the needle and the catheter have been specially designed for this procedure, while the catheter is moved forwards and backwards there is always the risk of shearing and tearing. In those cases where the catheter passes through a bent tip of the needle, the risk of tearing and shearing is much higher when moving the catheter within the needle. To prevent shearing and tearing of the catheter, one should be very cautious during the introduction of the catheter through the needle, especially when it is known that the tip of the needle was bent during its introduction (Fig. 17.23).

Using a needle that is one size smaller than it should be increases the risk of shearing catheters. The direction of the catheter and the direction of the tip of the needle must be similar. If the direction of the catheter is different from the opening of the needle, the sharp edge of the needle will cut into the outer plastic coating of the spring wire or the plastic catheter if the catheter is withdrawn through the needle.

One must be cognisant that there should be no resistance to the catheter while introducing it through the needle or moving it back through the needle. If there is any resistance to movement of the catheter within the needle, it is far safer to withdraw the needle and the catheter together and check the tip of the needle and unity of the sheath of the catheter than to just withdraw the catheter alone.

The sheath of the catheter may be torn completely off the catheter and remain in the epidural space. In such instances there are only two options: either to leave the torn segment within the epidural space or to remove it surgically. It may also be removed using arthroscopy forceps.

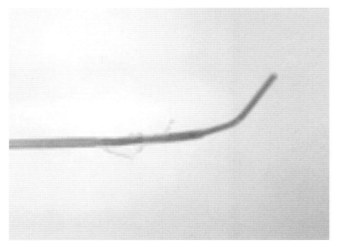

Figure 17.23 Shearing of the catheter.

Blocking of the catheter

The catheter may be blocked owing to clot formation around the tip of the catheter or to the artifacts of deposteroids administered through the catheter. Thus, before and after each use, the catheter should be rinsed with normal saline and especially after delivering deposteroids and hypertonic saline.

Misplacement of the catheter

- Intravascular.
- Subarachnoid.
- Subdural.

Although all catheters are inserted under fluoroscopic guidance during this procedure, there still remains a risk of misplacement of the catheters. Catheters should be placed very carefully as close to the targeted area as possible after epidurography.

The possibilities for catheter misplacement are the catheter entering a vein, or the catheter entering the paravertebral space, the subdural space, or the intrathecal space while advancing within the epidural space.

Because hygienic conditions within the epidural space are not favorable, especially in those patients who have had spinal surgery, there is always the risk of entering a vein near the target site or dural puncture. The catheter may enter the vein either during the initial insertion or after it is introduced into the epidural space.

There is always a risk of dural penetration while introducing the Racz catheter if the stylet is completely inside the catheter. The tip of the catheter may tear the dura and enter the intrathecal space. Because of increased adhesive tissue, dural penetration is more common in patients who have had back surgery. To prevent this complication the stylet should be withdrawn 0.3–0.5 mm back from its tip so the tip of the catheter may slightly move and bend when it comes across dural resistance. However, in some cases, this procedure of moving the stylet back may increase the difficulty of placing the catheter close to the targeted area.

After completing the initial procedure of catheter placement, even if the tip of the catheter is performed under fluoroscopy and the epidural space is verified, it is imperative that, during the second and third injections, a test dose of local anesthetic (2% lidocaine) is injected through the catheter to prevent any complications that might arise due to migration of the catheter. Otherwise, both local anesthetic and the hypertonic saline may be administered into the intrathecal space.

When hypertonic saline is injected intrathecally, like with other neurolytic agents, severe pain and muscle cramps, hypertension, cardiac arrhythmia, pulmonary edema, and cerebral infarction may occur. Localized paresis lasting hours, paresthesia lasting for weeks, transient hemiplegia, and persistent loss of sphincter control with sacral anesthesia have been reported.

Besides intrathecal misplacement, the catheter may also be placed into the subdural space despite fluoroscopic placement. During epidural insertion, if the catheter enters the subdural space, there exists the potential hazard of serious side effects, especially because of the drugs delivered. The local anesthetic in the mixture may cause total spinal block. Hypertonic saline in the mixture may cause permanent sensory damage.

The midline catheter is more likely to enter the subdural space, and if the patient suffers from non-recognized arachnoiditis with preexisting problems, very distressing complications of bowel and/or bladder dysfunction may result. Subdural contrast spread, and subdural contrast, local anesthetic, and steroid injection result in motor block, and with or without additional hypertonic saline can give rise to denervated bowel and bladder.

Placing the catheter properly and verifying its position under fluoroscopy does not always prevent later penetration of the dura. Owing to the changes in position of the patient, migration of the tip of the catheter, or the effect of the pressure of the injected volume, the catheter may penetrate the dura in the days after its initial placement.

Neurogenic complications

- Paresthesia.
- Numbness in perineal region.
- Bowel and bladder dysfunction.
- Sexual dysfunction.

Perineal numbness probably is one of the most common symptoms following the caudal transsacral hiatus lysis procedure. It is usually self-limiting and likely the consequence of neuropraxia produced by pressure from the needle and the catheter on the S5 nerve roots as they exit through the sacral hiatus. We believe it is possible for nerves to be cut during needle insertion. The numbness is usually without consequence. In rare instances, the sacral hiatus area may be painful, possibly because of a neuroma that usually responds to injection of local anesthetics into the painful neuroma site. In rare instances, one of the S5 nerves may be cut by the needle tip, and prolonged or permanent perineal numbness can occur.

Neurogenic complications include bowel, bladder, and sexual dysfunction, especially if there is preexisting pathology such as arachnoiditis. In the presence of arachnoiditis, fluids can reach the subdural space even though the injecting needle or catheter is a long way from the dura. Injected fluids take the path of least resistance and enter the subdural space though a surgical tear or congenital weakness in the dura. This fluid becomes loculated within the subdural space. Under these circumstances, compression of the blood supply is a distinct possibility, which leads to weakness, numbness, paralysis, and infarction of the cord.

Helpful hints

This procedure is usually followed by significant improvement in pain and motor function. With improvement of pain, it is important to initiate aggressive physical therapy to improve muscle strength and tone, which is usually decreased from lack of use secondary to pain. Often it is not possible to lyse existing epidural adhesions completely because of the extensive amount of scar tissue. If necessary, one can repeat the procedure. Because of the steroids used, a 3 month delay between procedures is necessary, during which time the patient should be encouraged to continue intense physical therapy. This therapy should begin immediately, when possible. Initiation of neural flossing techniques, especially while the local anesthetic is still active, provides a prime opportunity to maximize the adhesiolysis process with the least discomfort to the patient. One month of aquatic therapy followed by aggressive, graded physical therapy and work hardening is also recommended.

After negative aspiration is noted, all solutions should be injected slowly. Observation of the fluoroscopies often initially reveals massive epidural scar formation. After injection of 10 ml of Omnipaque 240, one can see the dye preferentially spreading toward one side, opening up the L4–L5 and S1–S2 nerve roots on that side, whereas there is a complete filling defect on the other side at L4 and S1 and partial filling of the L5 nerve root. Immediate monitoring is for acute effects of spinal local anesthetic and mechanical complications. The initial 4 hours should include bed rest or supervised walking, as partial motor block may be present. Bladder function and motor recovery should be present before the patient is allowed to ambulate independently.

Patients should be warned that perianal numbness may be transiently present, especially in those with spinal stenosis due to a transient neuropraxia. In the presence of persistent neuropraxia, an MRI should be considered to evaluate possible complications, especially loculation and spinal cord compression.

Delayed monitoring is aimed at hematoma formation and infection.

Epiduroscopy

History

An attempt to view spinal anatomy and pathology through an endoscope is not new! In fact, the first published attempts date back to the early 1930s. In 1931 Michael Burman examined cadaver spines using arthroscopic equipment. Because the endoscope was rigid and the light source poor, Burman was greatly limited in what he could see. Despite these obstacles, he concluded that myeloscopy is a useful procedure and was only limited only by the available technology.

In 1942 Lawrence Pool performed myeloscopy before surgery. He noted that he could often establish or confirm a diagnosis with the aid of a myeloscope. During his observations he was able to identify neuritis, herniated nucleus pulposus, hypertrophied ligamentum flavum, primary and metastatic neoplasms, varicose vessels, and arachnoid adhesions.

In the late 1960s and early 1970s Yoshio Ooi developed an endoscope for intradural and extradural examinations. He used a rigid endoscope, but of a smaller diameter than Pool or Burman. One advantage he had was improved fiberoptic light technology, which allowed enough light for photography of what he saw through the endoscope.

In the mid- to late 1980s Blomberg published a method of epiduroscopy. He was still using rigid scopes, because his studies were primarily concerned with placement of epidural needles and catheters for epidural analgesia.

In 1991, Lloyd Saberski began studies using fiber-optic systems for epiduroscopy, which led to the current modalities practiced today.

In 1991, James Heavner continued this development by advancing the flexible epiduroscope.

Anatomy

Successful application of epiduroscopy requires unique knowledge of the anatomy of the contents of the bony vertebral canal.

The spinal cord ends in the adult at about L1 or L2. It is surrounded by the pia mater, cerebrospinal fluid, arachnoid mater, and dura mater. The filum terminale and lumbar, sacral, and coccygeal anterior and posterior nerve roots continue in the caudal sac. The caudal sac is filled with cerebrospinal fluid and is bounded outwardly first by the arachnoid and then by the dura.

The upper limit of the epidural space is the foramen magnum, which is the point where the spine meets the base of the skull. The lower limit is at the tip of the sacrum, at the sacrococcygeal membrane. The epidural space is limited by the periosteum of the pedicles of the vertebral bodies and intervertebral foramina laterally, posterior longitudinal ligament, intervertebral discs, and segmental spinal nerves anteriorly, and ligamentum flavum posteriorly. The lumbar epidural space is 5–6 mm at the L2–L3 interspace with the lumbar spine flexed. The epidural space contains fatty tissue, arteries, epidural venous plexus, spinal nerve roots, and lymphatics. The epidural fat is relatively vascular and serves as a shock absorber for other contents in the epidural space.

The vascular and lymphatic network is described anatomically in Chapter 16 and will not be described here.

Structures most commonly seen through the epiduroscope

When the epiduroscope tip approaches an intervertebral foramen, nerve roots are more readily identified, as are larger blood vessels that pass through the foramen. In the posterior epidural space, the ligamentum flavum and less peridural fat are usually viewed. The plica mediana dorsalis, a connective tissue band in the dorsomedial epidural space attached at one end to the posterior dura and to the periosteum of the vertebral arch at the other, may or may not be seen. Careful examination of lateral intervertebral spaces may reveal articular surfaces and vertebral pedicles. Examination with epiduroscopy is usually limited to the posterior, posterolateral, lateral, and anterolateral epidural space.

Indications
- Observation of pathology and etiopathology of changes in the epidural space.
- Cytology and biopsy of the visual epidural contents.
- Epidural neuroplasty.
- Placing electrodes and catheters.
- Endoscopic surgery.
- Placing of epidural drug directly.

Contraindications
- Local or systemic infection.
- Coagulopathy.
- Space-occupying lesions in the central nervous system.
- Psychopathology.
- Vital function instability.

Technique of epiduroscopy
The most common approach is through the caudal space.

Step 1. Prepare the patient for the procedure
1. Physical examination (including examination of the entry site for local infection and distorted anatomy), lumbosacral magnetic resonance imaging, urology evaluation (if necessary), and laboratory studies, including complete blood count with platelets, prothrombin time, partial thromboplastin time, platelet function studies and bleeding time, and urine analysis, are required.
2. For preoperative medication, use the standard recommendations for conscious sedation given by the American Society of Anesthesiologists. Preprocedure sedatives, analgesics, and ancillary drugs are administered as needed in the surgical holding area. The patient is given 1 g of ceftriaxone (Rocephin) intravenously before the start of the procedure. (Ciprofloxin [Cipro], 400 mg, given 1 hour before epiduroscopy is started, but may be substituted if there is concern about allergy.)

Step 2. Position and monitor the patient
1. The patient is placed prone on the table. A pillow is placed under the abdomen to flatten the lumbar lordosis.
2. An intravenous cannula is inserted for medication injections.
3. Oxygen is provided by nasal cannula.

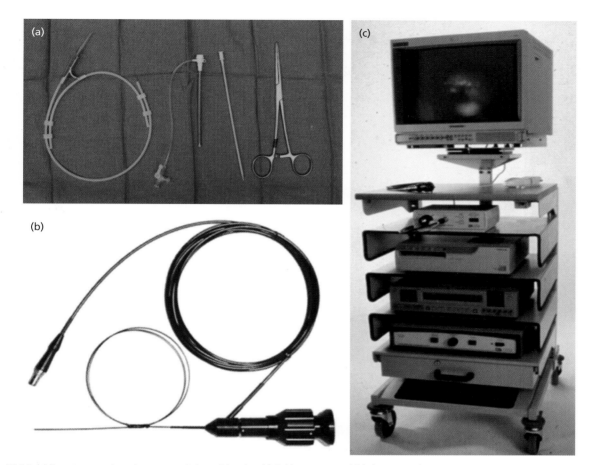

Figure 17.24 (a) Percutaneous introducer set and the guide wire. (b) Epiduroscope and (c) the TV monitor.

4. Vital signs monitoring is mandatory.

5. The area for needle entry is prepared in a sterile fashion.

Step 3. Drugs and equipment for epiduroscopy (Fig. 17.24)
- 0.8–1.0 mm fiber-optic epiduroscope.
- TV monitor.
- Percutaneous introducer set, a 9- or 10-French Super Arrow-Flex vascular access.
- Guidewire.
- No. 10 blade scalpel.
- Syringes of different sizes, 5 ml, 10 ml, 20 ml.
- Two three-way stopcocks and an intravenous set with extensions.
- 25 gauge needle.
- 18 gauge Tuohy needle or equivalent.
- 1% lidocaine for skin infiltration.
- 0.25% bupivacaine.
- Preservative-free saline.
- 1500 units of hyaluronidase.
- Deposteroid.
- Contrast solution, e.g. iohexol.

Step 4. Mark the surface landmarks for the needle entry Palpate the sacral cornu. A skin wheal is raised over the sacral hiatus using 1–2 ml of 1% lidocaine and a 25 gauge needle (Fig. 17.25).

Step 5. Visualization

1. Position the C-arm laterally.

2. An 18 gauge Tuohy epidural needle is then inserted through the puncture site and into the sacral hiatus. One should inject 5 ml of contrast material into the epidural space to perform an epidurography, to verify that the Tuohy needle is within the epidural space (Figs 17.26 and 17.27).

3. A guidewire is inserted through the needle and advanced to approximately the L5 or S1 level. The level of the guidewire should be verified by lateral and posteroanterior views (Fig. 17.28).

4. A small incision is made through the skin and the underlying tissue and sacrococcygeal ligament with a no. 10 blade scalpel.

5. The epidural needle is withdrawn and a 10-French dilator is then inserted over the guidewire into the sacral canal (Fig. 17.29).

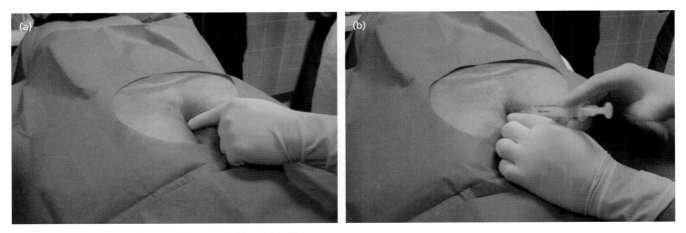

Figure 17.25 (a,b) Palpate the sacral hiatus and infiltrate the skin.

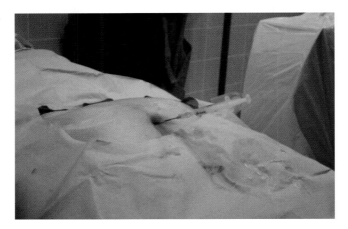

Figure 17.26 Introduce the needle through the sacral hiatus.

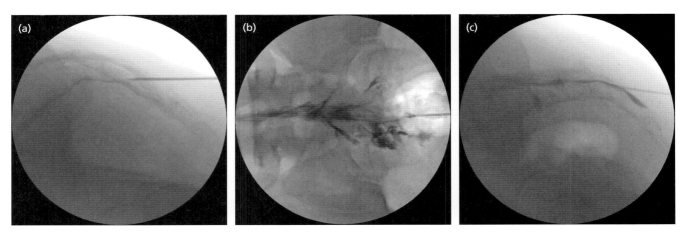

Figure 17.27 (a–c) Position of the needle within the caudal canal, spread of the contrast material in lateral and posteroanterior view.

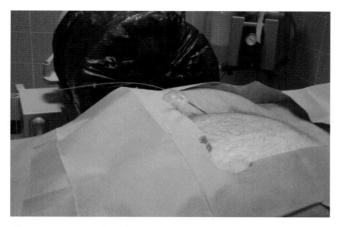

Figure 17.28 Introduce the guide wire through the epidural needle.

6. Then the dilator is removed, and the dilator with a sheath is placed over the guidewire into the space. It is important to check the guidewire for freedom of movement to avoid kinking it. It is also important to advance the dilator and sheath together until the sheath passes through the sacro-coccygeal ligament.

7. The dilator and guidewire are removed, leaving the sheath in place, then 5 ml of saline is injected through the sheath to expand the epidural space.

Step 6. Confirm the position of the epiduroscope
1. The epiduroscope is inserted through the sheath; proper placement should be verified under fluoroscopy with both posteroanterior and lateral views (Figs 17.30 and 17.31).

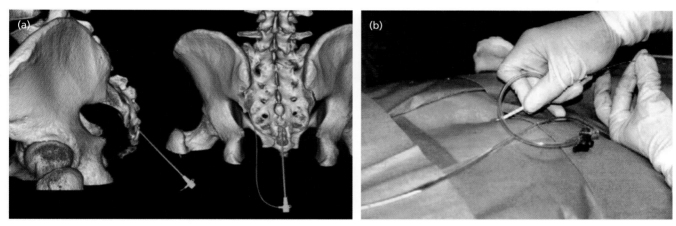

Figure 17.29 (a) Three-dimensional CT scan showing the direction of the dilator in posteroanterior and lateral view. (b) The dilator is inserted over the guidewire.

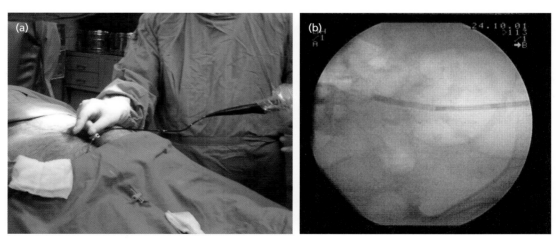

Figure 17.30 (a,b) Epiduroscope inserted through the sheath of the dilator.

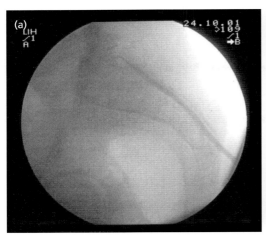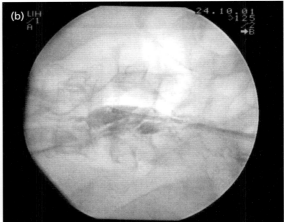

Figure 17.31 (a,b) Epiduroscope within the epidural space, lateral and anteroposterior views.

2. Preservative-free 0.9% saline is injected through the working channel of the epiduroscope to expand the epidural space and to flush away tissue debris and any extra vasalated blood to provide optimal viewing.

3. The total volume infused should generally not exceed 100 ml, because this may cause postprocedure cerebral edema. In addition to monitoring the volume infused, epiduroscopy time should be monitored. Care must be taken to use the minimal amount of saline: measure it carefully.

Step 7. Epiduroscopy

1. Examination of the epidural space may extend from the sacrum to as far cephalad as the posterior border of L2, depending on the patient's area of symptoms and the extent of abnormalities encountered.

2. The epiduroscope allows for three-dimensional direct visual observation. During epiduroscopy, equipment is used that displays both the epiduroscopic and the fluoroscopic images on a monitor.

Step 8. Postprocedure care

1. The epiduroscopy is usually done accompanying caudal neuroplasty. The postoperative care of caudal neuroplasty should be integrated with the care for that procedure.

2. After the treatment is finished, the epiduroscope and the sheath are removed. The site is covered with antibiotic ointment and occlusive dressing. The patient is observed until criteria for discharge from the hospital are met.

Complications

• **Infection**

Because hygienic conditions at the entrance site of the caudal canal are not optimal, infection is an important possible complication of the procedure. Infection may either occur at the entrance site of the catheter, in the caudal canal, or in the epidural space. Delayed overwhelming infection has been seen after epidural injection in patients with preexisting chronic infections. The usual symptoms include increased pain, neck pain, headache, photophobia, numbness, and weakness; the signs are elevated temperature, meningitis, and some neural deficits. Abnormalities in the laboratory findings include elevated white blood counts, elevated erythrocyte sedimentation rate, and spinal fluid abnormalities.

Epidural infections usually respond to antibiotic treatment administered for 5–10 days.

Epidural infection or abscess formation may be due to hematogenous spread or extension of superficial skin infections. Immunocompromised patients, diabetic patients, steroid-dependent patients, and those with malignancies are at higher risk for infection. Epidural abscess formation may not be recognized at the beginning because it is localized, and fever and increased white blood count may not always accompany this serious infection. However, in time, fever will rise as the abscess develops.

• **Bleeding**

Bleeding occurs especially in patients who had previous back surgery, in whom the hygienic conditions of the epidural space are disrupted secondary to their surgery. In those cases where blood is aspirated from the epidural space during the introduction of the needle and/or the catheter, the catheter and the epidural space must be rinsed with normal saline and a few minutes should go by before introducing the needle again. If blood aspiration continues after saline rinsing, the entry site of the needle should be changed. If, after moving the tip of the catheter within the epidural space, blood ceases to be aspirated, it is safe to continue with the procedure.

• **Epidural hematoma**

Although it has not been reported as a risk, epidural hematoma may follow bleeding. If epidural hematoma does occur, neurologic findings such as severe lumbar pain, bilateral lower extremity weakness, diffuse diminished pinprick sensation, paresthesia, and hypesthesia may be found. If an epidural hematoma is suspected, MRI evaluation may be required. It may not be easy to identify an epidural hematoma if the procedure was performed despite epidural bleeding during the insertion of the catheter. Local anesthetic agents administered will, like an epidural hematoma, also give rise to paresthesia for several hours, which may mask the neurologic signs while hematoma does develop. The best precaution for epidural hematoma is to cease the procedure if excessive blood is aspirated through the needle or the catheter, or at least postpone drug administration until neurologic assessment is performed

• **Inadvertent dural puncture**
There is always a risk of dural penetration while introducing the Racz catheter if the stylet is completely inside the catheter. The tip of the catheter may tear the dura and enter the intrathecal space. Because of increased adhesive tissue, dural penetration is more common in patients who have had back surgery. To prevent this complication, the stylet should be withdrawn 0.3–0.5 mm back from its tip so the tip of the catheter may slightly move and bend when it comes across dural resistance. However, in some cases, this procedure of moving the stylet back may increase the difficulty of placing the catheter close to the targeted area.

After completing the initial procedure of catheter placement, even if the tip of the catheter placement is performed under fluoroscopy and the epidural space is verified, it is imperative that, during the second and third injections, a test dose of local anesthetic (2% lidocaine) should be injected through the catheter to prevent any complications that might arise due to migration of the catheter. Otherwise, both local anesthetic and the hypertonic saline may be administered into the intrathecal space.

• **Postdural puncture headache**
Postdural puncture headache generally occurs within the next 48 hours. The cardinal feature is severe bilateral, frontal, and occipital headache, worsening in the upright position, improving with recumbency.

• **Retinal hemorrhage and visual disturbances**
One feared complication of any volume injection into the epidural space is the development of retinal hemorrhage that has occurred after uncontrolled injections of relatively large volumes. There is no specific volume known to produce retinal hemorrhage. On the other hand, if the catheter is in the midline or the subdural or the subarachnoid space, the consequences of volume injection could very well result in significant cerebrospinal fluid pressure increase, giving rise to retinal hemorrhage. Complete recovery of vision usually occurs over a matter of days to months.

• **Nerve root injury**
Nerve injury may occur while advancing the epiduroscope within the epidural space. Perineal numbness may also occur as a consequence of neuropraxia produced by pressure

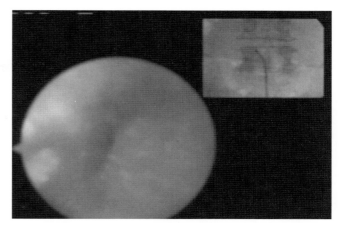
Figure 17.32 Normal epidural space and fat tissue. (Courtesy of James Heavner.)

from the needle and the catheter on the S5 nerve roots as they exit through the sacral hiatus. In rare instances, the sacral hiatus area may be painful, possibly because of a neuroma that usually responds to injection of local anesthetics into the painful neuroma site. In rare instances one of the S5 nerves may be cut by the needle tip and prolonged or permanent perineal numbness can occur.

• **Bowel, bladder, or sexual dysfunction**
Neurogenic complications include bowel, bladder, or sexual dysfunction, especially if there is preexisting pathology such as arachnoiditis. In the presence of arachnoiditis, fluids can reach the subdural space even though the injecting needle or catheter is a long way away from the dura.

Endoscopic views during epiduroscopy are shown in Figs 17.32–17.39.

Helpful hints
Before inserting the epiduroscope, be sure it is in focus and color balanced. Establish a neutral or reference position for the scope to aid orientation and to establish up/down, right/left for scope tip manipulation, as well as for image interpretation. When advancing the scope, rotate it and deflect the tip so the scope follows the spinal canal. Identification of the correct spinal level is almost impossible without simultaneous fluoroscopy.

Anteroposterior and lateral fluoroscopic viewing should be used as needed to assure that the dilator and sheath follow the guidewire and are directed as straight as possible toward the sacral hiatus.

Avoid introducing air into the injected fluid. This causes distortion of the epiduroscopic image and can be difficult to move out of the visual field.

Recognition of structures and pathology is challenging. It is absolutely essential to be familiar with the anatomy of the epidural space and other contents of the spinal canal, especially as viewed through an epiduroscope. Also essential is

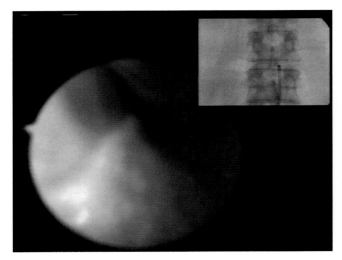

Figure 17.33 L4 nerve root. (Courtesy of James Heavner and Hemmo Bosscher.)

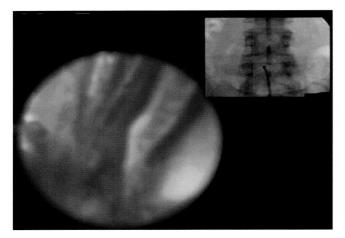

Figure 17.34 Increase of vascularity. (Courtesy of James Heavner and Hemmo Bosscher.)

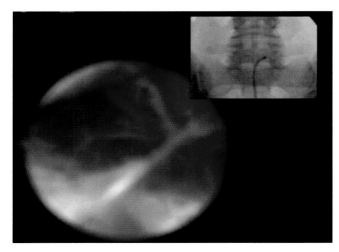

Figure 17.35 Inflamed and edematous L4 nerve root. (Courtesy of James Heavner and Hemmo Bosscher.)

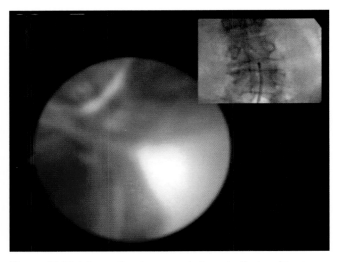

Figure 17.36 Inflammation, hypervascularity, and adhesion. (Courtesy of James Heavner and Hemmo Bosscher.)

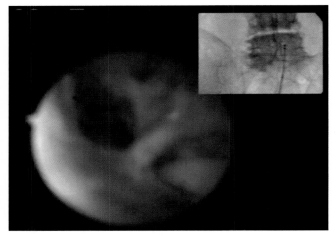

Figure 17.37 Adhesion and inflammation. (Courtesy of James Heavner and Hemmo Bosscher.)

familiarity with the type and appearance of pathology that might be encountered. Skill is required to manipulate the epiduroscope through the bony vertebral canal and to direct the scope tip to areas of interest.

If the patient has unilateral symptoms, the epidural space is examined first contralateral to the symptomatic side. This provides the general appearance of the "normal" epidural space for the patient. Next, the symptomatic side is examined with emphasis on viewing the area where the nerve or nerves that innervate the symptomatic side transverse the epidural space and pass through the intervertebral foramen. The presence or absence and the character of fat, blood vessels, and fibrous tissue, as well as the presence of abnormal tissue and of inflammation, should be noted.

Abnormalities observed include discrete or diffuse inflammation and diffuse or discrete fibrosis that ranges from mild (through which the scope easily passes) to a dense, solid

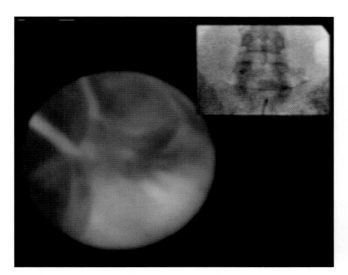

Figure 17.38 Fibrosis and adhesion. (Courtesy of James Heavner and Hemmo Bosscher.)

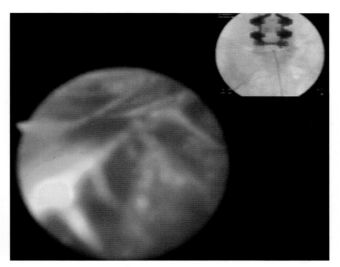

Figure 17.39 Inflammation and adhesion. (Courtesy of James Heavner and Hemmo Bosscher.)

mass through which the scope cannot be passed. Increased vascularity (small and/or larger vessels) and/or engorged, distended blood vessels may be seen. Fibrous scars may be avascular or have varying degrees of vascularity.

It is not easy to advance the epiduroscope within the epidural space. The risk of epidural hematoma is higher; one should be very careful, especially in elderly patients and in patients with spinal stenosis.

If resistances more than expected develop while advancing the epiduroscope, one should not insist continuing against a risk of dural puncture. If this resistance is immediately lost and the epiduroscope moves freely, immediately inject contrast material to verify that the tip of the fiberscope is within the epidural space.

After the diagnostic phase of the procedures, one may proceed with treatment, which is epidural lysis. This can be accomplished by using mechanical force moving the tip of the epiduroscope and injecting hyaluronidase.

There are problems with epiduroscopy such as use of an excessive amount of saline, which may generate significant epidural pressure. Identification of the spinal level is also a problem. The visuals from the epiduroscope vary for every device and are generally poor.

There are still questions to be asked such as whether epiduroscopy provides diagnostic advantages over CT scans and MRI, whether epiduroscopy-directed steroid injection is superior to low-technology, less invasive traditional injections, and whether epiduroscopy is a high-technology gadget for clinical application.

There is a need for studies to establish appropriate indications based on risk–benefit analysis.

Epiduroscopy can be safely performed but a strict protocol must be adhered to as there is potential to do serious harm to patients; specific safety guidelines are mandatory.

Percutaneous block and lesioning of the sacral nerve

History
Transsacral block was first performed by Pauchet and Laewen in 1909.

Anatomy
The sacrum is a large, triangular bone at the base of the spine and at the upper and back part of the pelvic cavity, where it is inserted like a wedge between the two hip bones. Its upper part connects with the last lumbar vertebra, and bottom part with the coccyx.

Although the vertebral components of the sacrum are fused into a single bone, the sacral vertebrae are still used to number the sacral nerves.

Location of the sacral foramina
There are four anterior sacral foramina through which the sacral nerves exit and the lateral sacral arteries enter. The posterior surface of the sacrum is convex. Laterally, one can identify four dorsal sacral foramina.

The dorsal S1 foramen is located approximately 1 cm medial to the posterior superior iliac spine, whereas the S2 foramen is 1 cm medial and 1 cm inferior to the posterior superior iliac spine. The S4 foramen is immediately lateral and just superior to the sacral cornu. The S3 foramen is located midway between the S2 and S4 foramina. The sacral foramina are somewhat rounded in form and diminish in size from above downward.

Innervation and their course
Nerves initially course through soft tissue spaces; the initial courses of the segmental sacral nerves are within the bony

sacrum. Nerve roots divide into anterior and posterior divisions that exit the sacrum through their respective sacral foramina (S1–S4). The fifth sacral nerve and the coccygeal nerve exit inferiorly through the sacral hiatus.

Posteriorly, they emerge from the posterior sacral foramina, and form the posterior branches of sacral nerves (including the medial cluneal nerves).

Anteriorly, they emerge from the anterior sacral foramina, and contribute to the sacral plexus (S1–S4) and coccygeal plexus.

Posterior divisions supply the skin and musculature of the gluteal region. Anterior divisions, with the anterior divisions of L4 and L5, form the sacral plexus, which innervates the pelvic structures, perineum, and much of the lower extremity, mostly through its large sciatic nerve (L4–S3) (Figs 17.40 and 17.41).

Indications
- Diagnostic evaluation of radicular symptoms.
- Prognostic sacral blocks (not recommended).

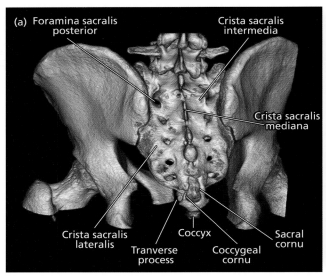 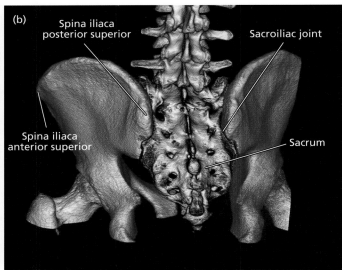

Figure 17.40 (a,b) Posterior views of the sacrum.

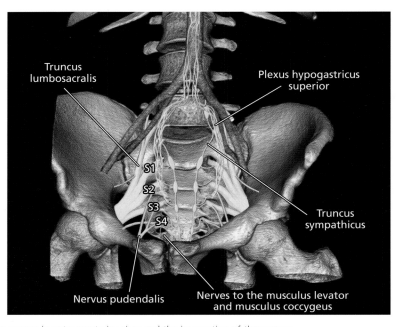

Figure 17.41 Anatomy of the sacrum in anteroposterior view and the innervation of the sacrum.

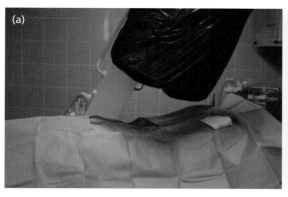
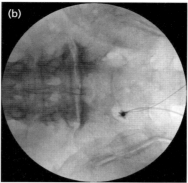
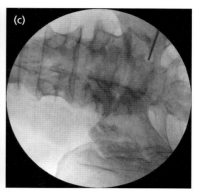

Figure 17.42 (a–c) Position of the C-arm and the view of the S1 foramen under posteroanterior view, and entrance point.

- Nerve root compression.
- Acute or postherpetic neuralgia in the region.

Contraindications
- Local or systemic infection.
- Coagulopathy.
- Anatomic derangements or previous operations.
- Vital function instability.
- Psychopathology.

Technique of sacral nerve block

Step 1. Prepare the patient before the procedure
1. The history, physical examination, and radiological studies are important before the procedure. All complications should be explained to the patient. A recent MRI is mandatory, especially in patients with failed back-surgery syndrome.
2. The patient should be aware of why they are having this procedure done, and what to expect from the procedure. All complications and side effects should be explained in detail before the procedure. Valid written consent should be obtained.
3. The type of analgesia or sedation needs to be ascertained before performance of the invasive procedure. Intravenous fentanyl, midazolam, and/or propofol may be used judiciously for the patient's comfort.

Step 2. Position and monitor the patient
1. Place the patient prone on the table.
2. Place a pillow beneath the iliac crest to flatten the lumbar lordoses.
3. Obtain an intravenous access.
4. Administer oxygen by nasal cannula.
5. Monitor the vital signs noninvasively.
6. Prepare and drape the sacral area.

Step 3. Equipment and drugs for sacral nerve block
- 5 ml syringe for local anesthetic solution.
- 1½ inch, 25 gauge needle for skin infiltration.
- 22 gauge, 3½ inch needle for sacral nerve block.

- 10 ml syringe for sacral nerve block.
- 5 ml of 1% lidocaine for skin infiltration.
- 5 ml contrast solution, e.g. iohexol.
- 10 ml of 0.5% bupivacaine combined with depomedrol.

Block of the sacral nerve roots is done with the posterior sacral foramen approach.

Step 4. Visualization
1. Place the C-arm in the posteroanterior position. Visualize the S1 foramen in this view.
2. The site of entry is visualized by adjusting the fluoroscopic beam to align the chosen posterior foramen with the anterior foramen (Fig. 17.42).
Note: the first foramen to be visualized is at the S2 level. To verify the position of the S1 foramen, one needs to measure the distance from the posterior iliac crest (approximately 1–2 cm superiorly). If the distance is longer, then it is the S2 foramen.

Step 5. Direction of the needle
1. Within the foramen, the nerve root extends from medial lateral path at the sacral pedicule. Thus the needle should be directed from the lateral side of the foramen medially and cephalad (Fig. 17.43).
2. Rotate the C-arm laterally, and advance the needle toward the anterior foramen until the tip is just anterior to the anterior sacral plate on the lateral view. One should not advance deeper than the anterior part of the foramen to prevent any damage to the viscera in close proximity.

Step 6. Confirm the position of the needle
Inject a small amount (1 ml) of nonionic, water-soluble contrast (iohexol); inject slowly to avoid trauma to the nerve root. The spread of the contrast medium should delineate the nerve root only, with no spread into the epidural space or onto the perineal plexus (Fig. 17.44).

Step 7. Sacral nerve block
If resistance is felt or vascular spread is noted, the needle must be redirected. After negative aspirate, inject 1–1.5 ml

of local anesthetic (1–2% lidocaine or 0.25–0.5% bupivacaine) under fluoroscopic guidance. The patient should not feel any pain or paresthesia during injection.

Step 8. Radiofrequency of the sacral nerve roots
Insert the electrode as described above.

Step 9. Stimulation test
1. A sensory paresthesia should be felt in the desired dermatome at less than 1.0 V at 50 Hz stimulation. Ideal stimulation should be felt between 0.4 and 0.6 V. If stimulation is felt at less than 0.4 V, the tip of the needle is too close to the dorsal root ganglion (DRG), and if stimulation is felt at greater than 0.6 V, the tip is too far away from the DRG.
2. Motor stimulation is then performed at 2 Hz. There should be a clear dissociation between motor and sensory

stimulation; that is, the voltage required to see motor fasciculations at 2 Hz should be at least twice the voltage that produces sensory stimulation at 50 Hz. Thus, if good sensory stimulation at 50 Hz is noted at 0.5 V, the motor fasciculations at 2 Hz should not be seen at voltages less than 1.0.

Step 10. Pulsed radiofrequency
Pulsed radiofrequency (RF) is done at this site two or three times for 120 seconds and at 42 °C.

Step 11. Postprocedure care
After the procedure the patient should be observed for a reasonable time for the risk of hypotension. In the case of hypotension, intravenous electrolyte solutions should be administered. The recovery and observation time depends on the sedation and analgesia used, and facilitates the assessment of any impairment of intellectual function, tolerance of oral intake, assessment of the immediate results of the neural blockade, and pain response to the procedure.

The patient should be provided with all instructions including whom to call or where to go for any postprocedure urgent/emergency care. The patient should be discharged accompanied by a responsible adult.

Complications
• **Nerve root injury**
One of the biggest concerns is damage to the nerve root while positioning the needle. Thus one should carefully and slowly advance the needle. If the patient complains of a sudden, sharp pain in the region one should stop immediately and redirect the needle.
• **Compression neuropathy**
If high amounts of contrast material or local anesthetic are injected into the sacral space, compression neuropathy may develop, especially in patients having fibrosis in the region.

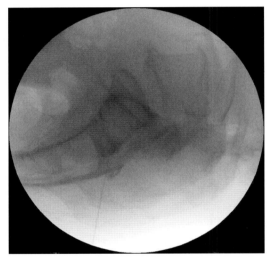

Figure 17.43 Position of the needle in lateral view.

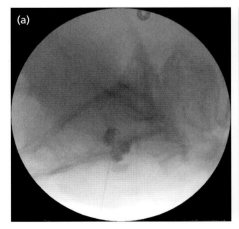
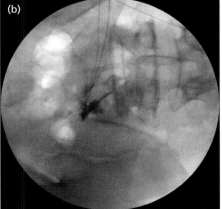

Figure 17.44 (a,b) Spread of the contrast material in lateral and posteroanterior views.

• **Neuritis**

Neuritis may develop if a neurolytic agent is used for the sacral nerve block.

• **Permanent paresthesia**

If conventional mode is used for RF, permanent paresthesia may develop. It is preferable to use pulsed RF.

• **Intravascular injection**

Sacral space has a high vascularity. An aspiration test is mandatory.

• **Bowel and bladder incontinence**

Bowel and bladder incontinence may develop due to the injury of sacral nerves.

• **Infection**

Infection risk is the same as with other procedures.

Helpful hints

One of the biggest concerns is damage to the nerve root while positioning the needle. Using a blunt-tip needle, one can reduce this complication.

Hypesthesia or anesthesia in the pelvic region is unacceptable in these patients. This will alter their sexual function, reproductive capacity, sphincter control, and in some even postural balance. Thus one should be very careful while performing RF lesioning. Pulsed RF is preferable to conventional RF.

Percutaneous block and lesioning of the superior hypogastric plexus

History

The superior hypogastric plexus block was first described by Plancarte and colleagues in 1990.

Anatomy

Location

The superior hypogastric plexus is located anterior to the L5 vertebra between the promontory of the sacrum and the bifurcation of the aorta in the reproperitoneal space. The ureter is just lateral to the superior hypogastric plexus.

It is a continuation of the celiac plexus and lumbar sympathetic chain. The hypogastric nerves are formed by the separation of fibers in the superior hypogastric plexus into right and left branches. The hypogastric nerve joins with the preganglionic parasympathetic fibers from S2 to S4; together they form the inferior hypogastric plexus.

The inferior hypogastric plexus descends on each side to the pelvic wall innervating the pelvic viscera.

Innervation

The superior hypogastric plexus innervates the pelvic viscera, the bladder, the uterus, the vagina, the prostate, and the rectum.

The superior hypogastric plexus receives fibers from the pelvic afferent and efferent sympathetic branches of the aortic plexus, fibers from the splanchnic nerves and parasympathetic fibers from S2 to S4 (Fig. 17.45).

Indications

• Pain originating from the pelvic viscera.
• Gynecologic disorders.
• Endometriosis.
• Adhesions.
• Interstitial cystitis, irritable bowel syndrome.
• Cancer pain originating from pelvic viscera.

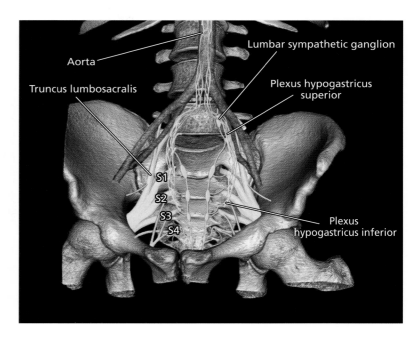

Figure 17.45 The anatomy of the superior hypogastric plexus and the nerves in close vicinity.

Contraindications
- Local or systemic infection.
- Coagulopathy.
- Anatomical variations in the pelvic region.
- Vital function instability.
- Psychopathology.

Technique of superior hypogastric plexus block
Commonly this procedure is performed in a prone position, either paramedially or laterally. Rarely, some physicians perform an anterior approach. The anterior approach will not be discussed here.

Step 1. Prepare the patient before the procedure
1. The history, physical examination, and radiological studies are important before the procedure. All complications should be explained to the patient in detail including the risks of numbness in the region, infection, and bowel and bladder dysfunction. Laboratory studies including prothrombin time, partial thromboplastin time, bleeding time, CRP, and urine analysis should be made. A recent MRI is mandatory especially in patients with failed back-surgery syndrome.
2. The patient should be aware of why this procedure is being done, and what to expect from the procedure. All complications and side effects related to the procedure should be explained in detail, before the procedure. A valid written consent should be obtained.
3. The type of analgesia or sedation needs to be ascertained before performance of the invasive procedure. Intravenous fentanyl, midazolam, and/or propofol may be used judiciously for the patient's comfort.

Step 2. Position and monitor the patient
1. Place the patient prone on the table.
2. Obtain an intravenous access.
3. Administer oxygen by nasal cannula.
4. Monitor the vital signs noninvasively.

5. Place a pillow beneath the iliac crest to flatten the lumbar lordoses.
6. Prepare and drape the area in a sterile fashion.

Step 3. Equipment and drugs for the superior hypogastric plexus block
- 25 gauge, 1½ inch needle for skin infiltration.
- 5 ml syringe for local anesthetic solution.
- 5 ml syringe for contrast material, e.g. iohexol.
- 10 ml syringe for the superior hypogastric plexus block.
- Two 15 cm, 22 gauge needles for the superior hypogastric plexus block.
- 1% lidocaine for skin infiltration.
- Contrast solution (iohexol).
- 10 ml of 0.25% bupivacaine and 40 mg methylprednisolone.
- 6% phenol in saline or glycerine or iohexol (mainly for cancer patients).

Step 4. Mark the surface landmarks for the needle entry
The superior hypogastric plexus block can be performed by (a) lateral approach or (b) transdiscal approach.

Lateral approach
1. Place the C-arm on the posteroanterior view first to identify the L4–L5 interspace under the fluoroscopy. Mark the spinous process of the L5 vertebra (Fig. 17.46).
2. Draw a line at the L4–L5 interspace bilaterally, and mark the entry points 7 cm to the midline. Inject local anesthetic solution to these points (Fig. 17.47). Introduce a 15 cm 18 gauge needle first 45° off the coronal plane and 30° caudally toward the anterolateral aspect of the bottom of the L5 vertebral body (Fig. 17.48).

Step 5. Visualization
If the iliac crest and the transverse process of the L5 vertebra prevents the needle passage, withdraw the needle up to the subcutaneous tissue, redirect slightly cephalad and caudally

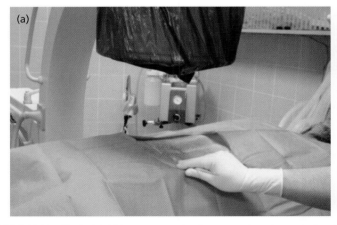 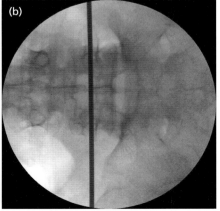

Figure 17.46 (a,b) Identify the L4–L5 interspace under fluoroscopy in anteroposterior views.

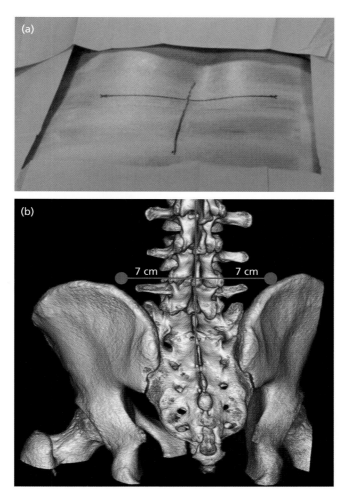

Figure 17.47 (a,b) Draw a line at the L4–L5 interspace, mark the entry points bilaterally 7 cm to the midline.

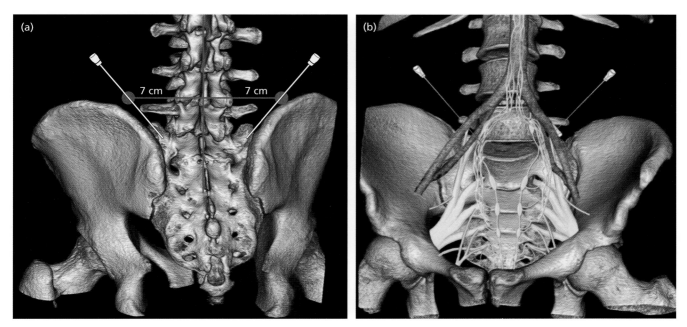

Figure 17.48 (a,b) Three-dimensional CT scans showing the direction of the needles in anteroposterior and posteroanterior views.

to slip the vertebral body. Then advance the needle 1 cm past the anterior border of the L5 vertebral body. Introduce the second needle on the contralateral side in a similar manner.

Step 6. Direction of the needle
1. In the anterolateral view, the needle tips should be located at the junction of the L5 and S1 vertebral bodies (Fig. 17.49).
2. At this time, turn the C-arm to the lateral position. Confirm the site of the needle tips just beyond the anterolateral margin of the vertebral body (Fig. 17.50).

Step 7. Confirm the position of the needle
1. Aspirate; if blood is aspirated, change the site of the needle slightly, and aspirate again. Inject 3 ml of contrast solution (iohexol) through each needle. In the lateral view a smooth posterior line, at the anterolateral margin of the vertebral body, confirms that the needle is properly located (Fig. 17.51).
2. Turn the C-arm to the posteroanterior view again. The contrast solution should be confined to the paramedian region (Fig. 17.52).

Step 8. Superior hypogastric block
1. After a negative aspiration test, inject 5 ml of 0.25% bupivacaine or 1% lidocaine together with 25 mg of triamcinolone or 40 mg of methylprednisolone through both needles.
2. In cancer patients, 5 ml of 6% phenol in saline or glycerine or with iohexol may be injected.

Transdiscal approach
In the lateral approach, the iliac crest and the transverse process of the L5 vertebral body may not allow the needle to penetrate to the target site. In such cases, a transdiscal approach is preferred. There is also another similar paramedian approach used by some physicians. This will not be described here.

Step 1. Prepare and position the patient
1. Place the patient prone on the table.
2. Obtain an intravenous access.
3. Administer oxygen by nasal cannula.
4. Monitor the vital signs noninvasively.
5. Place a pillow beneath the iliac crest to flatten the lumbar lordoses and facilitate the opening of the intradiscal space.

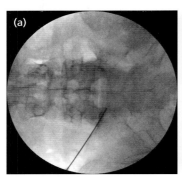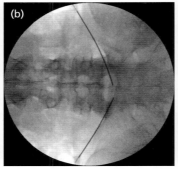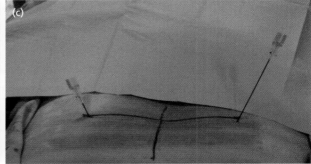

Figure 17.49 (a–c) Direction of the needles in posteroanterior view.

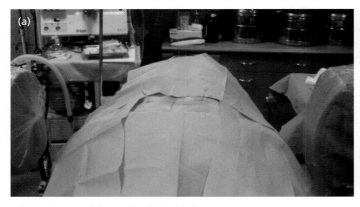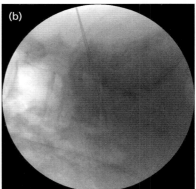

Figure 17.50 (a,b) Direction of the needles in lateral view.

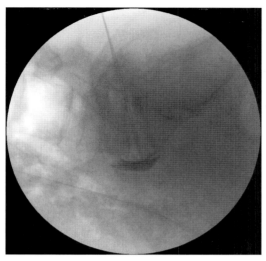

Figure 17.51 Spread of the contrast material in lateral view.

6. Prepare and drape the area in a sterile fashion.
7. Place the C-arm in the posteroanterior view, first identify the L5–S1 intradiscal space.

Step 2. Visualization
Rotate the C-arm 15–20° cephalad to align the inferior endplates of the vertebral body (Figs 17.53 and 17.54).

Step 3. Mark the surface landmarks for the needle entry
Then rotate the C-arm obliquely 25–30° until the spinous processes are seen to pass laterally and the facet line is visualized. The entry point at the skin is 5–7 cm from the midline (Fig. 17.55).

Step 4. Direction of the needle
Infiltrate the skin with local anesthetic solution. Introduce a 22 gauge, 15 cm needle lateral to the inferior aspect of the

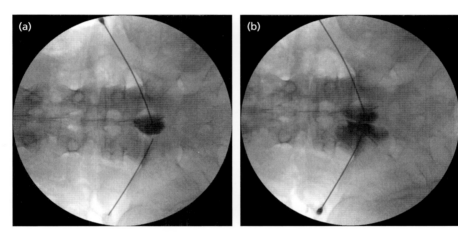

Figure 17.52 (a,b) Spread of the contrast material in posteroanterior view.

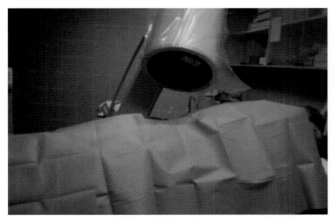

Figure 17.53 Position of the C-arm for intradiscal hypogastric plexus block.

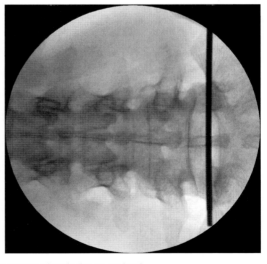

Figure 17.54 Identify the L5–S1 level.

facet joint by tunneled vision until the needle contacts the edge of the disc (Fig. 17.56).

Step 5. Confirm the position of the needle
1. Rotate the C-arm laterally, introduce the needle through the disc. Bring the C-arm to a posteroanterior position and verify that the needle is within the disc (Fig. 17.57).
2. Rotate the C-arm laterally again. Inject 1 ml contrast solution and verify that the needle tip is within the disc by lateral vision. Advance the needle more through the disc under lateral view with a 5 ml syringe until the resistance within the disc is lost. Administer 2 ml of contrast solution. A smooth posterior line at the anterolateral margin of the vertebral body confirms that the needle is properly located (Figs 17.58 and 17.59).

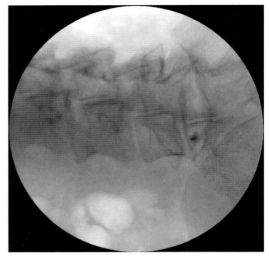

Figure 17.56 Direction of the needle under "tunneled vision."

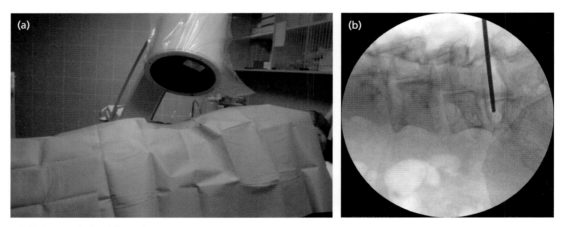

Figure 17.55 (a,b) Entry point in oblique view.

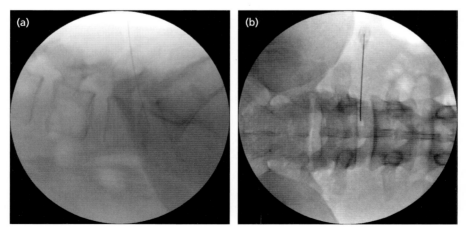

Figure 17.57 (a,b) The needle within the disc, lateral and posteroanterior view.

Step 6. Transdiscal superior hypogastric block

1. Rotate the C-arm to a posteroanterior position. The contrast solution should be confined to the paramedian region at the L5–S1 level.

2. Administer 5 ml 0.5% bupivacaine together with 40 mg methylprednisolone. 5 ml of 6% phenol in saline may be used in cancer patients.

3. Inject 1 ml air before you withdraw the needle back inside the disc. Administer antibiotic inside the disc (1 ml of 50 mg cefazolin) before withdrawing the needle.

Step 7. Postprocedure care

After the procedure the patient should be observed for a reasonable time for the risk of hypotension. In case of hypotension, intravenous electrolyte solutions should be admin-

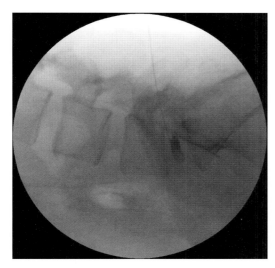

Figure 17.58 Spread of the contrast material within the disc.

istered. The recovery and observation time depends on the sedation and analgesia used, and facilitates the assessment of any impairment of intellectual function, tolerance of oral intake, immediate results of the neural blockade, and pain response to the procedure.

The patient should be provided with all instructions including whom to call or where to go for any postprocedure urgent/emergency care. The patient should be discharged accompanied by a responsible adult.

Complications

• **Injury to the L5 nerve root**

The risk of injury to the L5 nerve root is higher with the lateral approach. If the C-arm is not rotated properly during the transdiscal approach, contact with the L5 nerve root is possible. If the patient complains of sudden severe pain, withdraw and redirect the needle immediately.

• **Inadvertent puncture of vessels**

The superior hypogastric plexus is in close proximity with the bifurcation of the common iliac vessels. There is a risk of hematoma. The risk of intravascular injection is higher with the lateral approach. During the transdiscal approach, do not advance more than 1 cm once the needle passes the anterolateral margin of the vertebral body. Aspirate every time before injecting any solution.

• **Placement of the needle too laterally**

The iliac crest can be a potential barrier to needle passage and the needle may be placed more laterally. Advancing the needle in this position may injure the pelvic viscera in close proximity.

• **Discitis after transdiscal approach**

There is a potential risk of discitis with the transdiscal approach; however, it is very rare. Fifty milligrams of cefazolin in 1 ml of saline is injected into the disc before withdrawing the needle.

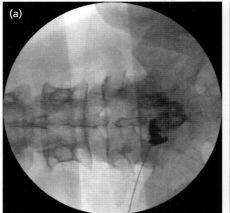
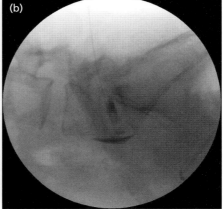

Figure 17.59 (a,b) Transdiscal hypogastric plexus block, posteroanterior and lateral view.

Percutaneous block of the impar ganglion

History
The first report on impar ganglion block was described by Plancarte in 1990.

Anatomy
The ganglion impar is a solitary retroperitoneal ganglion connected to a chain of sympathetic fibers, descending from the lumbar to the sacral region bilaterally. It is located at the level of the sacrococcygeal junction. It is the termination of the paired paravertebral sympathetic chains (Fig 17.60).

Indications
- Burning pain of unknown etiology, localized in the perineal region.
- Neuropathic pain together with tenesmus.
- Cancer pain originating from rectum, perineum, and vagina.

Contraindications
- Local or systemic infection.
- Coagulopathy.
- Distorted anatomy.

Technique of ganglion impar block
Ganglion impar block may be performed by (a) lateral approach or (b) intradiscal approach.

Lateral approach

Step 1. Prepare the patient before the procedure
1. The history, physical examination, and radiological studies are important before the procedure. All complications should be explained to the patient in detail including the risks of numbness in the region, infection, and bowel and bladder dysfunction. Laboratory studies including prothrombin time, partial thromboplastin time, bleeding time, CRP, and urine analysis should be made. A recent MRI is mandatory, especially in patients with failed back-surgery syndrome.
2. The patient should be aware of why this procedure is being done and what to expect from it. All complications and side effects should be explained in detail before the procedure. Valid written consent should be obtained.
3. The type of analgesia or sedation needs to be ascertained before performance of the invasive procedure. Intravenous fentanyl, midazolam, and/or propofol may be used judiciously for the patient's comfort. If RF thermocoagulation or pulsed RF is planned, the patient needs to be awake to respond to the stimulation test.

Step 2. Position and monitor the patient
1. Place the patient in the lateral decubitus position.
2. Obtain an intravenous access.
3. Administer oxygen by nasal cannula.
4. Monitor the vital signs noninvasively.
5. Prepare and drape the intergluteal crease, anus, and surrounding area in a sterile fashion.

Step 3. Equipment and drugs for ganglion impar block
- 5 ml syringe for local anesthetic solution.
- 1½ inch, 25 gauge needle for skin infiltration.
- 22 gauge, 3½ inch needle for ganglion impar block.
- 5 ml syringe for contrast material, iohexol.
- 5 ml syringe for the ganglion impar block.
- 5 ml of 1% lidocaine for skin infiltration.
- 5 ml contrast solution, e.g. iohexol.
- 5 ml of 0.5% bupivacaine combined with depomedrol.
- 6% phenol in saline for neurolytic block (only for cancer patients).

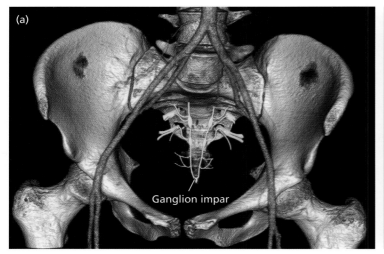 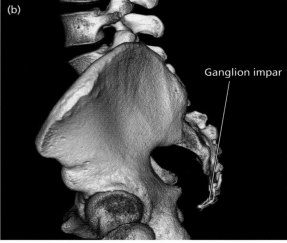

Figure 17.60 (a,b) Three-dimensional CT scans showing ganglion impar, anteroposterior and lateral views.

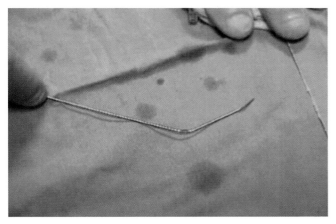

Figure 17.61 Preparation of the needle for ganglion impar block.

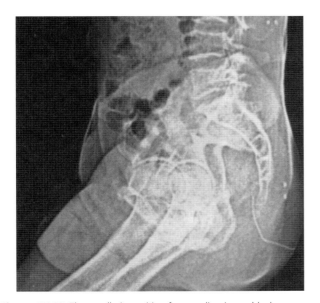

Figure 17.62 The needle in position for ganglion impar block in lateral view.

Step 4. Mark the surface landmarks for the needle entry
1. Remove the stylet from a 22 gauge 3½ inch needle which should be bent about 1 inch from the hub at a 25–30° angle (Fig. 17.61).
2. Infiltrate the skin over the coccyx with 1% lidocaine solution.
3. Place the C-arm in a posteroanterior position with the table.

Step 5. Direction of the needle
Insert the needle with its concavity posteriorly under fluoroscopy, anterior to the coccyx until the needle tip reaches the sacrococcygeal junction retroperitoneally (Fig. 17.62).

Step 6. Confirm the position of the needle
1. Inject 2 ml contrast solution, for example iohexol. A smooth line image should be viewed in this position.
2. Rotate the C-arm in a lateral position with the table. The contrast solution will be seen at the sacrococcygeal junction in the posteroanterior view (Fig. 17.63).

Step 7. Ganglion impar block
1. Inject 5 ml of 1% lidocaine or 0.5% bupivacaine together with deposteroid solution.
2. In cancer patients, inject 4–5 ml of 6% phenol in saline.

Transdiscal approach
Steps 1–3 are as described above.

Step 4. Mark the surface landmarks for the needle entry
1. Place the patient in the prone position on the table.
2. Palpate the sacrococcygeal junction.
3. Place the C-arm in a posteroanterior position. Mark the sacrococcygeal junction after palpation (Figs. 17.64 and 17.65).

Step 5. Visualization
1. Rotate the C-arm in a lateral position
2. Infiltrate the skin with 1% lidocaine solution on the sacrococcygeal junction (Fig. 17.66).

Step 6. Direction of the needle
Insert a 3½ inch needle perpendicular to the skin. Direct the needle through the sacrococcygeal junction, stopping as soon as the tip of the needle passes the anterior border of the junction (Figs 17.67 and 17.68).

Step 7. Confirm the position of the needle
1. Inject 2 ml of contrast material, e.g. iohexol; it should spread as a smooth line on the anterior border of the junction (Fig. 17.69).
2. Rotate the C-arm to a posteroanterior position. The contrast material should be viewed at the sacrococcygeal junction.
3. Inject 5 ml of 1% lidocaine or 0.5% bupivacaine together with deposteroid solution.
4. In cancer patients, inject 4–5 ml of 6% phenol in saline.

Step 8. Postprocedure care
After the procedure, the patient should be observed for a reasonable time for the risk of hypotension. In the case of hypotension, intravenous electrolyte solutions should be administered. The recovery and observation time depends on the sedation and analgesia used, and facilitates the assessment of any impairment of intellectual function, tolerance of oral intake, immediate results of the neural blockade, and pain response to the procedure.

The patient should be provided with all instructions including whom to call or where to go for any postprocedure

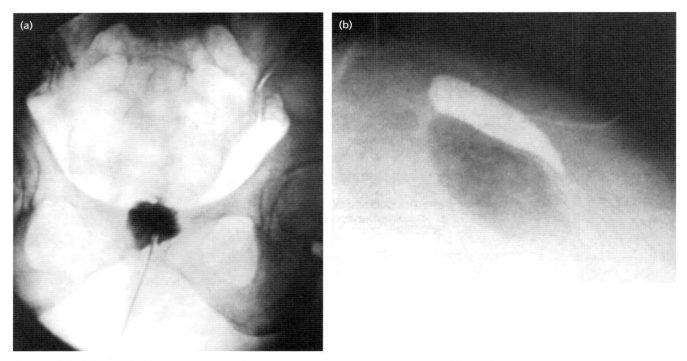

Figure 17.63 (a,b) Spread of the contrast material during ganglion impar block, posteroanterior and lateral view.

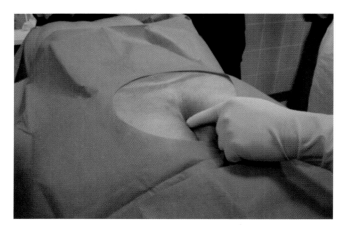

Figure 17.64 Palpate the sacrococcygeal junction.

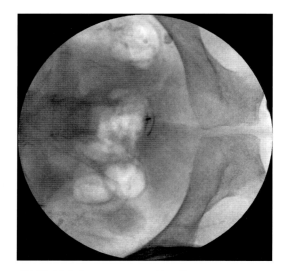

Figure 17.65 Mark the sacrococcygeal junction.

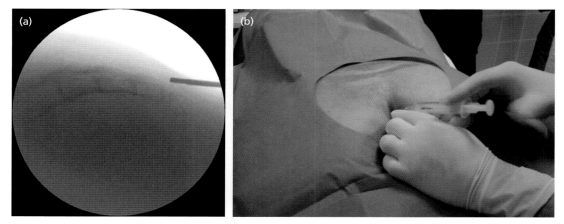

Figure 17.66 (a,b) Lateral view of the coccyx, infiltrate the skin.

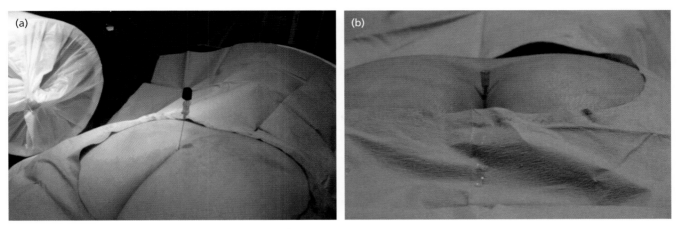

Figure 17.67 (a,b) Introduce the needle perpendicular to the skin.

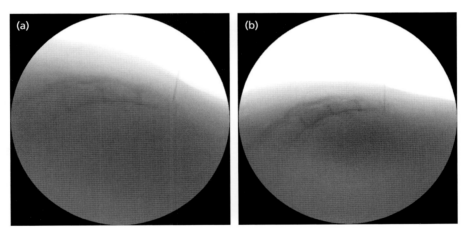

Figure 17.68 (a,b) Direction of the needle for transdiscal approach.

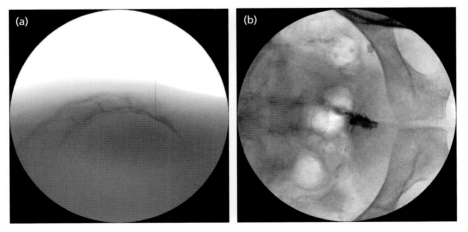

Figure 17.69 (a,b) Spread of the contrast material in lateral and posteroanterior view.

urgent/emergency care. The patient should be discharged accompanied by a responsible adult.

Complications
• Inadvertent puncture of the rectum
There is a potential risk of rectum puncture, especially if the lateral approach is preferred.
• Injection of neurolytic agent into the rectum or to a nerve in close proximity
The risk is again higher in the lateral approach.
• Neuritis
There is always a risk of neuritis if a neurolytic agent is used.

Helpful hints
Impar ganglion block should be performed by transdiscal approach. It is easier to approach the ganglion with less risk of complications.

Percutaneous block and lesioning of the sacroiliac joint

History
The history of the sacroiliac joint (SIJ) and its painful syndromes have been controversial for hundreds of years. Although Meckel first described motion in the joint in 1816, the quantity and quality of motion within the articular mechanism is still debated. There is also controversy about the etiology of the gradual anatomical changes observed in the articular surfaces throughout life. Some believe these changes represent pathological degradation, others believe the changes are a physiological adaptation. These controversies plague the physician who wishes to determine the role of the SIJ in a patient's pain with a history of low back pain.

Anatomy
The SIJs are the largest axial joints in the body that are formed between the articular surfaces of the sacrum and the ilium bones. The two SIJs move together as a single unit and are considered bicondylar joints (where the two joint surfaces move together). The S1 is a synovial (diarthrodial) joint that is more mobile in youth than later in life. The upper two-thirds of the joint become more fibrotic in adulthood (Fig. 17.70).

Composition of the SIJ
The joints are covered by two different kinds of cartilage: the sacral surface has hyaline cartilage and the ilial surface has fibrocartilage. The stability of the SIJ is maintained mainly through some bony structure and very strong intrinsic and extrinsic ligaments. The characteristics of the SIJ change as the patient's age increases.

Ligaments and muscles of SIJ
The ligaments of SIJ are the anterior sacroiliac ligament, interosseous sacroiliac ligament, posterior sacroiliac ligament, sacrotuberous ligament, and sacrospinous ligament. The main function of this ligamentous system is to limit motion in all planes of movement.

Age-related changes in the SIJ begin in puberty and continue throughout life. Degenerative changes on the sacral side generally lag 10–20 years behind those affecting the iliac surface. In the sixth decade, motion at the joint may become markedly restricted as the capsule becomes increasingly collagenous and fibrous ankylosis occurs. By the eighth decade

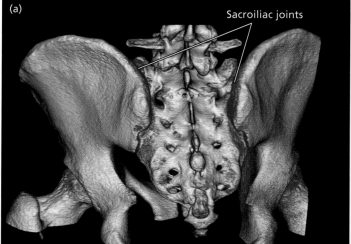
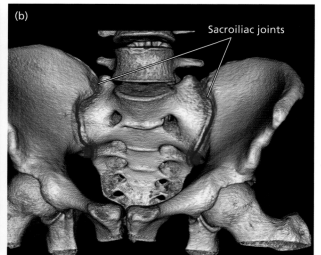

Figure 17.70 (a,b) Anatomy of the SIJ.

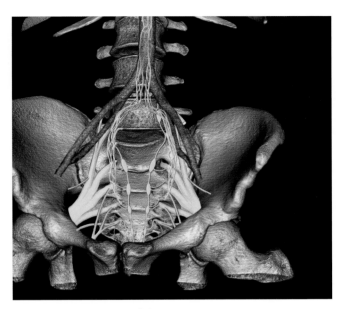

Figure 17.71 Innervation of the SIJ.

of life, erosions and plaque formation are inevitable and ubiquitous.

Major muscles attached to the S1 include the gluteus maximus, gluteus medius, latissimus dorsi, multifidus, biceps femoris, psoas, piriformis, obliquus, and transversus abdominis.

Innervation

The SIJ line is densely innervated by several levels of spinal nerves. The lateral branches of the L4–S3 posterior primary rami are the major contributors to the innervations to the posterior SIJ, whereas the anterior joint is innervated by L2–S2, L4–S2, and the L5–S2 rami (Fig. 17.71).

Pain of SIJ is typically on one side or the other (unilateral posterior superior iliac spine pain) but the pain can occasionally be bilateral.

Indications

Intraarticular pain due to
- osteoarthritis;
- spondyloarthropathy;
- metabolic diseases;
- idiopathic (capsular) strain.
  Extraarticular pain from ligaments and muscles.

Contraindications

- Local or systemic infection.
- Coagulopathy.
- Anatomic derangements or previous operations at the region.
- Psychopathology.

Procedures performed on or around the SIJ

- Intraarticular injections
  - Injection of local anesthetic steroid combination.
  - Injection of 6% phenol in saline or glycerine (recommended only in cancer patients).
- RF techniques
  - RF denervation surrounding the joint.
  - Sacroiliac joint pulsed RF.
  - Sacroiliac joint lateral branch neurotomy.
  - Lateral branch (cooled RF).
  - Bipolar lateral branch neurotomy.
  - Bipolar ligamentous RF denervation.
  - Bipolar SIJ denervation.

All the above techniques are performed in a prone position. They will all be done with the following steps.

Sacroiliac joint block

Step 1. Prepare the patient before the procedure
1. The history, physical examination, and radiological studies are important before the procedure. All complications should be explained to the patient in detail, including the risks of numbness in the region, infection, bowel and bladder dysfunction. A recent MRI is mandatory especially in patients with failed back-surgery syndrome.
2. The patient should be aware of why this procedure is being done, and what to expect from the procedure. All complications, side effects related to the procedure should be explained in detail, before the procedure. Valid written consent should be obtained.
3. The type of analgesia or sedation needs to be ascertained before performance of the invasive procedure. Intravenous fentanyl, midazolam, and/or propofol may be used judiciously for patient comfort. If RF is going to be performed, the patient should be awake to respond to stimulation tests.

Step 2. Monitor and position the patient
- Place the patient prone on the table.
- Place a pillow beneath the iliac crest to flatten the lumbar lordoses.
- Obtain an intravenous access.
- Administer oxygen by nasal cannula.
- Monitor the vital signs noninvasively.
- Prepare and drape the sacral area.

Step 3. Equipment and drugs for SIJ block
- 5 ml syringe for local anesthetic solution.
- 1½ inch, 25 gauge needle for skin infiltration.
- 22 gauge, 3½ inch needle for SIJ block.
- 5 ml syringe for contrast solution, iohexol.
- 10 ml syringe for SIJ block.
- 5 ml of 1% lidocaine for skin infiltration.
- 5 ml contrast solution, e.g. iohexol.
- 10 ml of 0.5% bupivacaine combined with depomedrol.

Step 4. Visualization
1. Position the C-arm in the posterioanterior view, then rotate it toward the oblique view until a clear view of the SIJ is obtained (Fig. 17.72).
2. One should first find the L5–S1 disc space at L5–S1 then rotate cephalic 15–25°, enough to open the disc space at L5–S1. Second, start with the oblique view, then rotate toward the anteroposterior view to visualize the widest space at the most inferior aspect of the S1 joint. The lines of the posterior and the anterior aspects of the joint are seen to overlap. Tilting the C-arm longitudinally in relation to the patient (cephalocaudally) can sometimes help the clinician distinguish between the anterior and posterior articulations.

Step 5. Direction of the needle
1. Infiltrate the skin 1–2 cm cranially from the lower edge of the SIJ.

2. Introduce a 22 gauge, 10 cm needle toward the inferior edge of the joint. One should feel that the tip of the needle is within the joint (Fig. 17.73).

Step 6. Confirm the position of the needle
1. To advance toward the joint, the tip of the needle may be slightly bent.
2. Inject 0.5–1 ml of contrast solution into the joint. The contrast solution should spread from the inferior toward the posterior edge of the joint with opacification of the ventral and dorsal joint lines (Fig. 17.74).

Step 7. Sacroiliac joint block
Inject up to 5 ml of 0.5% bupivacaine with 40 mg of triamcinolone into the joint. For cancer patients, 2.5 ml of 6% phenol in saline or glycerine may be used but is not recommended.

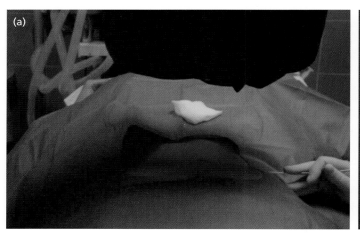
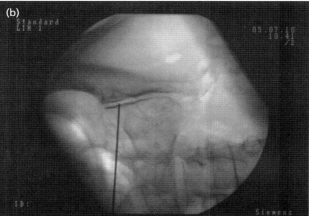

Figure 17.72 (a,b) Position the C-arm in posteroanterior view and mark the inferior edge of the sacroiliac joint.

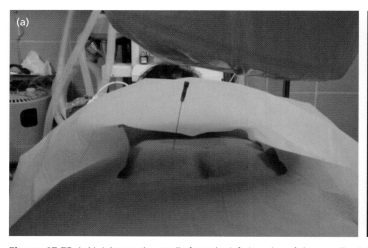
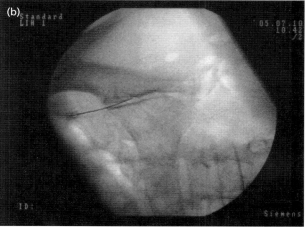

Figure 17.73 (a,b) Advance the needle from the inferior edge of the sacroiliac joint.

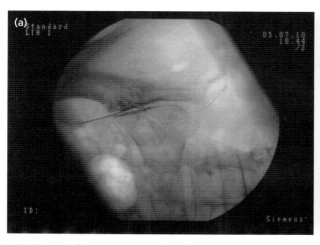
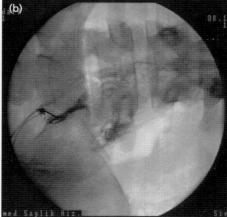

Figure 17.74 (a,b) Spread of the contrast material within the joint.

RF lesioning around the SIJ

Step 1. Placing the electrodes
Four 10 cm, 2 mm active-tip electrodes are placed from the inferior aspect of the posterior tip of the SIJ perpendicularly.

Step 2. Stimulation test
Before lesioning, a test motor stimulation should be performed at 2 Hz frequency and 1.5–2 V intensity. There should be no radicular or sphincter motor contraction. During sensory testing at 50 Hz, paresthesia of the zone must be noted above 0.5 V.

Step 3. RF lesioning
Inject 1 ml of 2% lidocaine before the lesion RF at 80 °C for 90 seconds. Multiple lesions are done along the entire posterior joint line (Fig. 17.75).

Lateral branch neurotomy of the SIJ
The L5, S1–S3 posterior primary rami are targeted with this technique.

Step 1. Visualization
Position the C-arm in the posteroanterior view first, then adjust the C-arm so that the sacral foramina can be optimally seen.

Step 2. Direction of the electrode
1. Place the first electrode at the sulcus forming the junction of the sacral ala and the root of the superior articular process of S1.
2. Inject 0.5 ml of local anesthetic before lesioning the L5 posterior ramus at this position. One RF lesion should be made at the base of the sulcus with a second 1 to 2 mm

lateral to the first lesion and a third 1 to 2 mm medial to the first lesion (Fig. 17.76).
3. Then one should distribute 1 ml of local anesthetic a few millimeters lateral to the lateral border of the foramen, approximately 0.25 ml at the 12 o'clock, 2 o'clock, 4 o'clock, and 6 o'clock positions on the right side, and the 12 o'clock, 10 o'clock, 8 o'clock, and 6 o'clock positions on the left side (Figs 17.77 and 17.78).

Step 3. Confirm the position of the electrode
An introducer with stylet is inserted onto the bone endpoint of the posterior sacrum. When inserted, the stylet extends 6 mm beyond the tip of the introducer. The RF probe, which is subsequently inserted through the same introducer, extends only 4 mm beyond the tip of the introducer.

Step 4. Stimulation test
Correct placement should be confirmed using electrostimulation at 50 Hz, with concordant pain being noted at below 0.6 V at all levels from L4–S2. Before lesioning, a test motor stimulation should be performed at 2 Hz frequency and 1.5–2 V intensity to ensure no radicular or sphincter motor contraction occurs. Position the C-arm laterally, to ensure that the tips of the electrodes are not deeper than the posterior sacral cortex.

Step 5. RF lesioning
Two or three lesions are created at each sacral level. Typically, these lesions are spaced about 1 cm apart from one another, creating a continuous strip of ablated tissue lateral to each foramen. RF energy is delivered for 2 minutes (30 seconds per lesion) with a target electrode temperature of 60 °C.

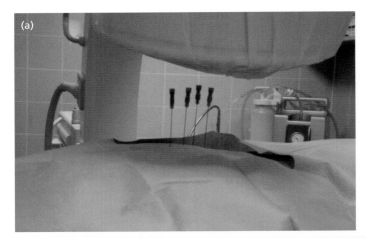

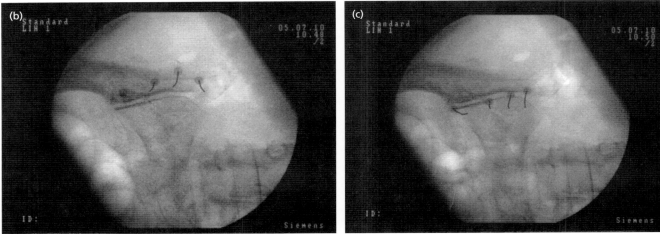

Figure 17.75 (a–c) RF lesioning of the SIJ.

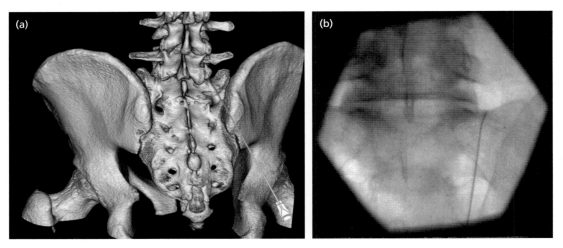

Figure 17.76 (a,b) RF lesioning of the sacral ala.

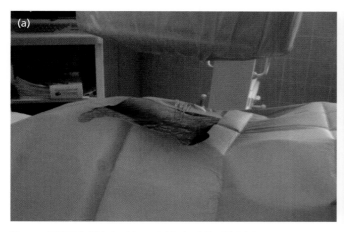
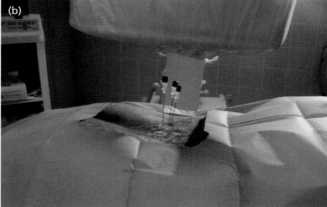

Figure 17.77 (a,b) Lateral branch block of the SA joint.

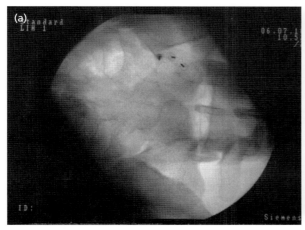
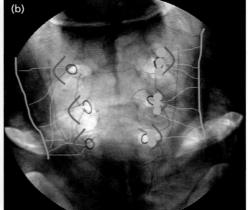

Figure 17.78 (a,b) Lateral branch block of the SA joint.

Simplicity

Simplicity is a multi-electrode RF probe which may be inserted using a single entry point for the RF lesioning of the nerves innervating the SIJ (Figs 17.79 and 17.80).

Step 1. Prepare and position the patient
The patient is prepared as described earlier.

Step 2. Visualization
Place the C-arm in the posteroanterior position, centered on the inferior border of the ipsilateral sacrum.

Step 3. Mark the surface landmark for electrode entry
The entry point is the lateral inferior border of the sacrum, 1 cm lateral to and below the S4 foramen.

Step 4. Direction of the electrode
1. Infiltrate the skin and the track of the Simplicity electrode with a 10 cm, 25 gauge spinal needle with 1% lidocaine. The track may be infiltrated in two attempts, first from the lower edge then the middle of the track.
2. Introduce the Simplicity electrode until the tip of the electrode contacts the inferolateral border of the sacrum. The electrode should be advanced meticulously and enter the periosteum.

Step 5. Confirm the position of the electrode
1. Advance the Simplicity electrode with continuous contact with the sacrum, cephalad and slightly lateral, staying lateral to the sacral foramina, medial to the SIJ, and ventral to the ilium until it contacts the sacral ala.

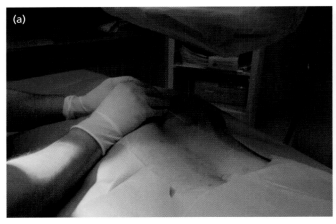

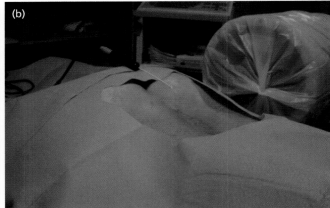

Figure 17.79 (a,b) Simplicity.

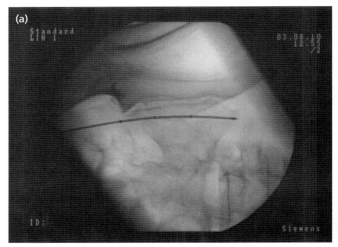

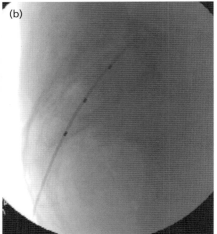

Figure 17.80 (a,b) Simplicity.

2. The electrode may be slightly moved to position the independent active electrodes adjacent to the S1, S2, S3, and S4 lateral branch innervation pathways.

3. Position the C-arm laterally to confirm that the electrode remains in contact with the posterior aspect of the sacrum over the periosteum, following the curvature of the sacrum up to the sacral ala. The three independent electrodes should be in position to lesion the lateral branches of S1, S2, S3, and S4.

Step 6. RF lesioning
RF lesioning at 85 °C for 90 minutes is made for each electrode.

Step 7. Postprocedure care (for all procedures described in this chapter)
After the procedure, the patient should be observed for a reasonable time for the risk of hypotension. In case of hypo-

tension, intravenous electrolyte solutions should be administered. The recovery and observation time depends on the sedation and analgesia used, and facilitates the assessment of any impairment of intellectual function, tolerance of oral intake, immediate results of the neural blockade, and pain response to the procedure.

The patient should be provided with all instructions, including whom to call or where to go for any postprocedure urgent/emergency care. The patient should be discharged accompanied by a responsible adult.

Complications
- **Hematoma formation**

Hematoma formation may occur especially during the RF techniques where multiple electrodes are used.
- **Neural damage**

One should be very careful to place the electrodes and handle the electrodes meticulously.

- **Trauma to the sciatic nerve**

Although very rare, there is a risk of trauma to the sciatic nerve.

- **Weakness secondary to extraarticular extravasation**
- **Temporary worsening of pain due to temporary neuritis**

Further reading

Alshab, A.K., Goldner, J.D. & Panchal, S.J. (2007) Complications of sympathetic blocks for visceral pain. *Techniques in Regional Anesthesia and Pain Management* **11**(3), 152–156.

Blomberg, R. (1985) A method for spinal canal endoscopy and spinaloscopy: presentation of preliminary results. *Acta Anaesthesiologica Scandinavica* **21**, 113–116.

Bogduk, N. (ed.) (2004) Sacroiliac joint blocks. In *Practice Guidelines for Spinal Diagnostic and Treatment Procedures*, 1st edition, pp. 66–85. San Francisco, CA: International Spine Intervention Society.

Buijs, E.J., Kamphuis, E.T. & Groen, G.J. (2004) Radiofrequency treatment of sacroiliac joint-related pain aimed at the first three sacral dorsal rami: a minimal approach. *The Pain Clinic* **16**, 139–146.

Burman, M.S. (1931) Myeloscopy or the direct visualization of the spinal cord. *Journal of Bone and Joint Surgery* **13**, 695–696.

Cathelin, M.F. (1901) Mode d'action de la cocaine injecte daus l'escape epidural par le procede du canal sacre. *Comptes Rendues des Seances de la Societe de Biologie et de ses Filliales* **43**, 487.

Cohen, S.P. (2005) Sacroiliac joint pain: a comprehensive review of anatomy, diagnosis, and treatment. *Anesthesia & Analgesia* **101**(5), 1440–1453.

Cohen, S.P. & Abdi, S. (2003) Lateral branch blocks as a treatment for sacroiliac joint pain: a pilot study. *Regional Anesthesia and Pain Medicine* **28**(2), 113–119.

Day, M. (2008) Sympathetic blocks: the evidence. *Pain Practice* **8**(2), 98–109.

De Medicis, E. & De Leon-Casasola, O.A. (2001) Ganglion impar block: critical evaluation. *Techniques in Regional Anesthesia and Pain Management* **5**(3), 120–121.

Erdine, S., Yucel, A., Celik, M. & Talu, G.K. (2003) Transdiscal approach for hypogastric plexus block. *Regional Anesthesia and Pain Medicine* **28**(4), 304–308.

Ferrante, F.M., King, L.F., Roche, E.A., et al. (2001) Radiofrequency sacroiliac joint denervation for sacroiliac syndrome. *Regional Anesthesia and Pain Medicine* **26**, 137–142.

Gundavarpu, S. & Lema, M.J. (2001) Superior hypogastric nerve block for pelvic pain. *Techniques in Regional Anesthesia and Pain Management* **5**(3), 116–119.

Hitchcock, E. (1967) Hypothermic subarachnoid irrigation for intractable pain. *Lancet* **i**, 1133–1135.

Lievre, J.A., Block-Michel, H. & Attali, P. (1957) L'injection transscree étude clinique et radiologrique. *Bulletins et Mémoires de la Société Médicale des Hôpitaux de Paris* **73**, 1110–1118.

Ooi, Y., Satoh, Y. & Morisaki, N. (1973) Myeloscopy. *Orthopaedic Surgery (Japan)* **24**, 181–186.

Payne, J.N. & Rupp, N.H. (1951) The use of hyaluronidase in caudal block anesthesia. *Anesthesiology* **12**, 164–172.

Plancarte, R., Amescua, C., Patt, R.B. & Aldrete, J.A. (1990) Superior hypogastric plexus block for pelvic cancer pain. *Anesthesiology* **73**, 236.

Plancarte, R., Amescua, C., Patt, R.B. & Allende, S. (1990) Presacral blockade of the ganglion of Walther (ganglion impar). *Anesthesiology* **73**, A751.

Plancarte, R., Guajardo, J. & Guillen, R. (2005) Superior hypogastric plexus block and ganglion impar (Walther). *Techniques in Regional Anesthesia and Pain Management* **9**(2), 86–90.

Pool, J.L. (1942) Myeloscopy: intraspinal endoscopy. *Surgery* **11**, 169–182.

Racz, G.B. & Holubec, J.T. (1989) Lysis of adhesions in the epidural space. In *Techniques of Neurolysis* (ed. Raj, P.), pp. 57–72. Boston, MA: Kluwer.

Robecchi, A. & Capra, R. (1952) L'idrocortisone (composto F). Prime esperienze cliniche in campo reumatologico. *Minerva Medica* **98**, 1259–1263.

Saberski, L.R. & Brull, S.J. (1995) Spinal and epidural endoscopy: a historical review. *Yale Journal of Biology and Medicine* **68**, 7–15.

Sicard, J.A. & Forestier, J. (1921) Methode radiographique d'exploration de la cavite epidurale par le Lipiodol. *Revue Neurologique* **28**, 1264–1266.

Sicard, M.A. (1901) Les injections medicamenteuse extradurales par voie saracoccygiene. *Comptes Rendues des Seances de la Societe de Biologie et de ses Filliales* **53**, 396.

Stolker, R.J., Vervest, A.C.M. & Gerbrand, J.G. (1994) The management of chronic spinal pain by blockades: a review. *Pain* **58**, 1–19.

Ventafridda, V. & Spreafico, R. (1974) Subarachnoid saline perfusion. *Advances in Neurology* **4**, 477–484.

Viner, N. (1925) Intractable sciatica – the sacral epidural injection. An effective method of giving pain relief. *Canadian Medical Association Journal* **15**, 630–634.

Wemm, K. Jr & Saberski, L. (1995) Modified approach to block the ganglion impar (ganglion of Walther). *Regional Anesthesia* **20**(6), 544–545.

18 Advanced Techniques

Technique of intraspinal continuous analgesia

History

The discovery of opioid receptors in 1971 and their natural location in the nerve tissue, especially their discovery in the brain and spinal cord in 1973, were the first steps for clinical use in intraspinal analgesia. In 1974 Terenius and Walström further identified endorphins as a natural chemical in humans. Based on that discovery, in 1976 Yaksh and Rudy demonstrated the mechanism of analgesia mediated by a direct spinal action of opioids. In 1979, Wang reported the intrathecal bolus use of morphine for cancer-related pain. Immediately after, Behar reported the first use of epidural analgesia. Intraspinal analgesia prolonged the duration of pain relief by the introduction of implantable, programmable, continuous drug delivery systems in the early 1980s.

In this chapter the term "intraspinal analgesia" includes both the epidural and intrathecal analgesic methods.

Anatomy

A knowledge of lumbar anatomy is required for intraspinal analgesia. Lumbar anatomy has been described elsewhere (vide supra) and will not be repeated here.

Indications

- When other systemic analgesic methods are ineffective or produce excessive, unacceptable side effects.
- When intraspinal analgesia has been shown to provide better pain relief by previous trial testing.
- When the drug delivery systems are cost effective on a prolonged basis and pain relief has been demonstrated previously.

Contraindications

- Coagulopathy and bleeding disorders.
- Local or systemic infection.
- Metabolic disorders.
- Preexisting structural abnormalities.
- Psychiatric disorders.
- Drug addiction.

Technique of intraspinal analgesia

There are two clinically viable methods: (1) intrathecal and (2) epidural drug delivery systems. Both are performed similarly except for the different location of the catheter, either epidural space or subarachnoid space, by following the usual early steps.

Technique of implanting a drug delivery system

Step 1. Prepare the patient before the procedure
1. Physical examination (including examination of the entry site) is mandatory to identify distorted anatomy. Lumbosacral magnetic resonance imaging (MRI) is also essential. Before the procedure, biochemical data need to be analyzed carefully and corrected as required for safety and prevention of postprocedure complications.
2. For preoperative medication, use the standard recommendations for conscious sedation by the American Society of Anesthesiologists. Preprocedure sedatives, analgesics, and ancillary drugs are administered as needed in the surgical holding area. The patient is given 1 g of ceftriaxone (Rocephin) intravenously before the start of the procedure. Ciprofloxin (Cipro), 400 mg, is also given 1 hour before it.
3. Before the implantation, one should decide on the site of the reservoir and port or pump device. The most appropriate location for the implantation of large devices is the right or left lower quadrant of the abdomen. The pump should not be very close to the iliac crest, the symphysis pubis, the ilioinguinal ligament, and the costal margin when seated.
4. The anatomic constraints tend to be the iliac crest, the symphysis pubis, the ilioinguinal ligament, and the costal margin.

Pain-Relieving Procedures: The Illustrated Guide, First Edition. P. Prithvi Raj and Serdar Erdine.
© 2012 John Wiley & Sons, Ltd. Published 2012 by John Wiley & Sons, Ltd.

384

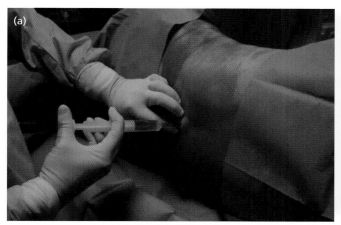
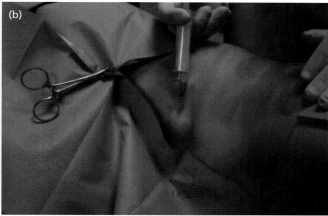

Figure 18.1 (a,b) Infiltrate the skin over the entry site and port pocket.

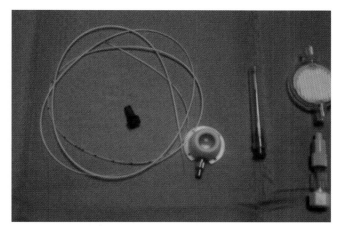

Figure 18.2 A set of access ports for epidural analgesia.

- access port or pump system devices;
- epidural or intrathecal catheter as planned.

Step 4. Mark the surface landmarks for needle entry
1. The targeted intervertebral space is identified by palpating the spinous processes of the adjacent vertebrae. To ensure that the needle entry site is exactly in the midline, the physician's middle and index fingers are placed on each side of the spinous processes. In obese patients it may be difficult to identify the midline, so place the C-arm in a lateral position to view the anteroposterior image of the vertebral column.
2. To identify the point of entry, view the following anatomical landmarks:
  ○ vertebral body of L1;
  ○ the line drawn on the posterior iliac crest is between the L4 and L5 intervertebral spaces.

Step 5. Technique of epidural port implantation
1. Infiltrate the skin and subcutaneous tissues, supraspinous and interspinous ligaments in the midline with local anesthetic. Then surgically make a 5 cm incision in the skin down to the lumbar fascia. Under hemostatic conditions, pack the incision wound (Figs 18.1 and 18.2).
2. Then prepare the pocket for the port or pump system. On the lower quadrant of the abdomen, make a 10 cm incision, down through the underlying subcutaneous fat layer. Prepare a subcutaneous pocket large enough to admit the particular port or pump system. Maintain meticulous hemostasis to avoid postoperative hematoma formation. Pack the pocket with an antibiotic sponge (Fig. 18.3).

Step 6. Direction of the needle
1. Move the C-arm to a posteroanterior position. As the patient lies in the lateral decubitus position, the image on the fluoroscopy will be the lateral view of the lumbar spine.
2. Identify the vertebral body, intervertebral space, and spinous process on the lateral view.

Step 2. Position and monitor the patient
1. Place the patient in the lateral decubitus position on the table with the head in hyperflexed position and the legs pulled and flexed towards the abdomen.
2. Support the abdomen and thorax with pillows, so the patient feels comfortable.
3. Obtain intravenous access. Administer oxygen by nasal cannula, monitor the vital signs noninvasively.
4. Prepare and drape the area in a sterile fashion.
The patient should not be over-sedated. The patient should remain sufficiently conscious to provide response to any questions.

Step 3. Drugs and equipment for implantation of drug delivery systems
- 10 ml syringe for skin infiltration with the local anesthetic;
- 10 cm, 25 gauge needle for local anesthesia;
- 10 ml syringe for contrast material;
- 5 ml loss of resistance syringe for entering epidural or intrathecal space;

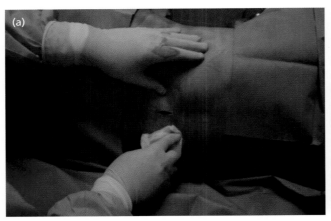

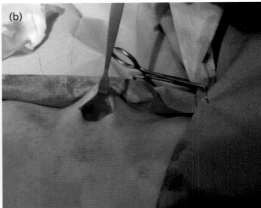

Figure 18.3 (a,b) Make an incision at the entry site and at the port pocket site.

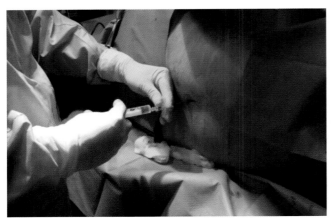

Figure 18.4 Loss of resistance technique.

3. The base of the spinal process appears as a virtual line on the lateral view. Anterior to this virtual line lies the ligamentum flavum. The target of the needle is the virtual line. Advance the needle through the supraspinous and interspinous ligament under fluoroscopy. Stop at the level of the "virtual line," the line drawn at the base of the spinous process. Entrance to the lumbar epidural space is possible either by "loss of resistance technique" or "hanging drop technique." We prefer the loss of resistance technique.

4. Remove the stylet of the needle. Attach a well-lubricated 5 ml syringe filled with saline.

5. Hold the hub of the epidural needle firmly with the left thumb and index finger.

6. Place the wrist of the left hand against the neck of the patient to prevent the advance of the needle due to unexpected movement of the patient.

7. Hold the syringe with the right hand; advance the needle under fluoroscopy with the thumb applying pressure on the plunger (Fig. 18.4).

8. As soon as the needle bevel passes through the ligamentum flavum, there will be a "loss of resistance" and the plunger slides freely (Fig. 18.5).

9. Gentle aspiration is required. If blood is aspirated, withdraw the needle outside the epidural space, redirect, and enter the epidural space again. If blood is aspirated, terminate the procedure.

10. For epidural catheter implantation one should be careful not to enter the intrathecal space. If the needle does enter the intrathecal space, cerebrospinal fluid (CSF) will be aspirated and the procedure should be aborted for another week.

Step 7. Confirm the position of the needle

1. Inject 2–5 ml of contrast solution; the "straight" view will appear in the lateral fluoroscopic view. One should wait about 30 seconds and be vigilant to visualize that the contrast solution stays in the epidural space. Rapid clearance of the contrast solution can signify that the needle is in the subarachnoid space. During the dural puncture, CSF may not have been aspirated (Fig. 18.6).

2. If the needle is within the subdural space, injection of a very small amount of contrast material will appear like a thin direct line at multiple levels. Unlike injection of the contrast solution in the subarachnoid space, contrast solution does not disappear in this situation.

3. Fill the epidural catheter with saline before inserting through the needle.

4. Insert and advance the catheter through the needle under fluoroscopy in the lateral view. The catheters have centimeter measurement marks on their surface. Measure the length of the needle and then introduce the catheter taking into consideration the desired depth of the catheter needed inside the epidural space (Fig. 18.7).

5. Aspirate. If blood is seen, advance the catheter several more millimeters, and aspirate again. If the aspiration test is

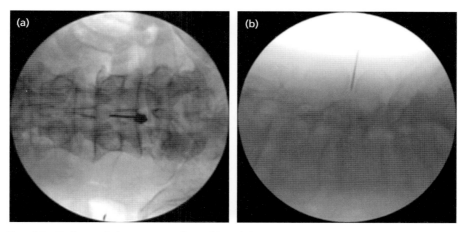

Figure 18.5 (a,b) Direction of the Tuohy needle in posteroanterior and lateral views.

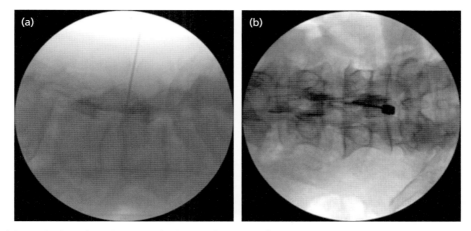

Figure 18.6 (a) Tip of the epidural needle within the epidural space. (b) Spread of the contrast material within the epidural space in lateral and posteroanterior views.

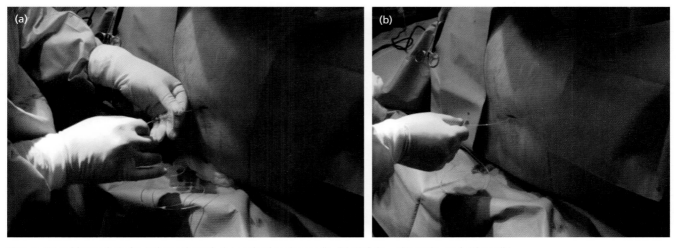

Figure 18.7 (a) Introduce the catheter through the epidural Tuohy needle. (b) Withdraw the Tuohy epidural needle.

still positive withdraw the catheter with the needle as a single unit and interrupt the procedure.

6. If the aspiration test is negative, inject contrast material through the catheter at this new location to verify the tip of the catheter in the epidural space both in posteroanterior and lateral views.

7. Next, tunnel the catheter subcutaneously. The distal end of the epidural catheter is connected (through the extension catheter) from the lumbar region to the port pocket.

8. Make the connection very secure between the catheter and the port.

9. Place the port into the subcutaneous pocket previously made. To prevent movement or rotation use at least two sutures. The clinician should follow the device guidelines for surgical procedure that are especially written for the device chosen (Fig. 18.8).

10. Then carefully close the incisions; a 2.0 absorbable suture is sufficient. Then close the skin edges with sterile strips (Fig. 18.9).

Technique of intrathecal pump implantation

• The steps for entering the epidural space are the same as described above. After entering the epidural space gently continue pushing the needle deeper and check if the needle is in the subarachnoid space. When the needle tip is within the intrathecal space, there should be free flow of the CSF (Fig. 18.10).

• Implant the catheter through the needle in the subarachnoid space. There should be a free flow of the CSF through the catheter (Fig. 18.11).

• Withdraw the needle meticulously and cautiously.

• Next clamp the intrathecal catheter to prevent CSF loss.

• Then, tunnel the catheter connecting the intrathecal catheter to the pump (the extension catheter) from the port pocket to the back with an incision using a tunneling device.

• Connect the catheter and the pump.

• Place the pump into the subcutaneous pocket. To prevent rotation use at least two sutures. It may be better to place the sutures into the pocket then enter through the pump suture loops (Figs 18.12–18.14).

• An ideal pocket is one that allows the pump to be placed in such a fashion that the refill port is clear of the incisional scar and easier to locate.

• Another aim is to have a pocket that allows placement of the pump without struggle but is tight enough to aid in preventing pump rotation.

• The depth of the pocket under the skin is critical for programmable pumps. A depth greater than 2.5 cm may not allow reliable telemetry.

• Carefully close the incisions with 2.0 absorbable sutures. Then close the skin edges with sterile strips.

Step 8. Postprocedure care

After implantation, patients should be kept in hospital for several days to arrange the drug delivery parameters. The patient and the family should be trained in the use of pump monitoring during this period. Periodic reprogramming then becomes essential. Migration of the catheter is much less likely, but it still can occur. By varying the programs from time to time, analgesia can be maintained.

After appropriate monitoring of the operative site and training of the patient and family in using the pump, the

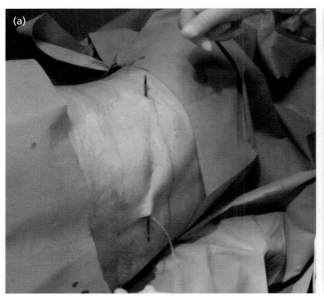
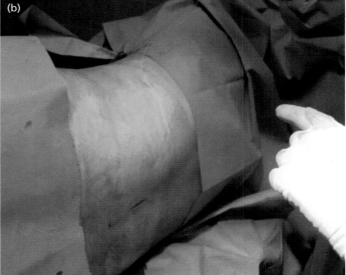

Figure 18.8 (a,b) Advance the catheter through the tunneling device toward the port pocket. Note that to advance the catheter toward the port pocket may need two steps through the tunneling device.

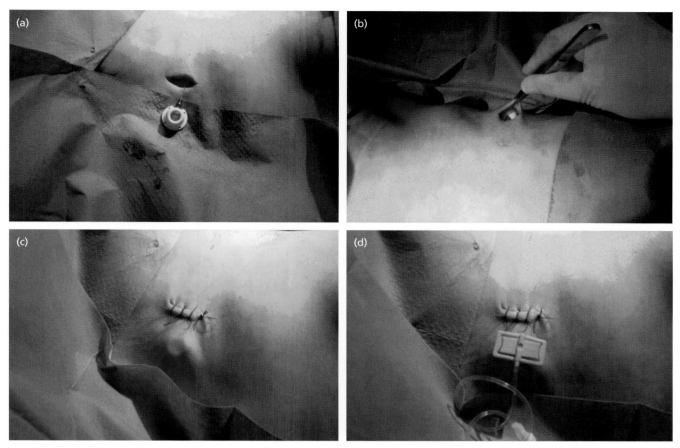

Figure 18.9 (a–d) Make the connection very secure between the catheter and the port. Place the port into the subcutaneous pocket previously made. To prevent movement or rotation use at least two sutures.

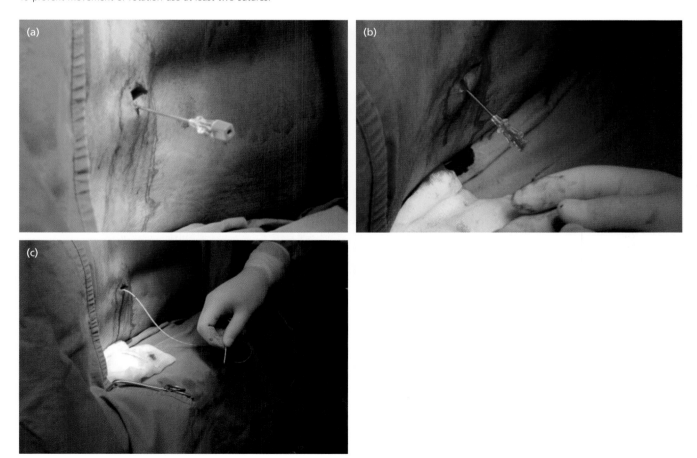

Figure 18.10 (a–c) Implant the catheter through the needle in the subarachnoid space. There should be a free flow of the CSF through the catheter.

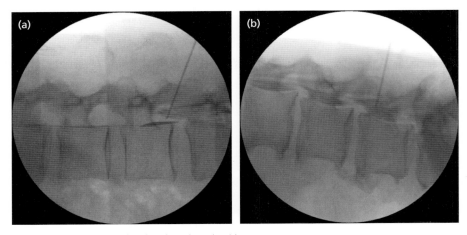

Figure 18.11 (a,b) Spread of the contrast material within the subarachnoid space.

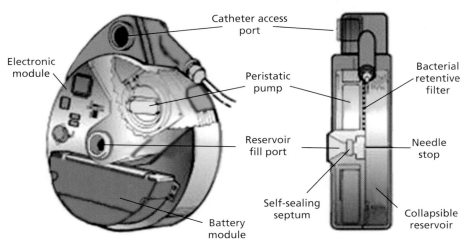

Figure 18.12 An intrathecal pump.

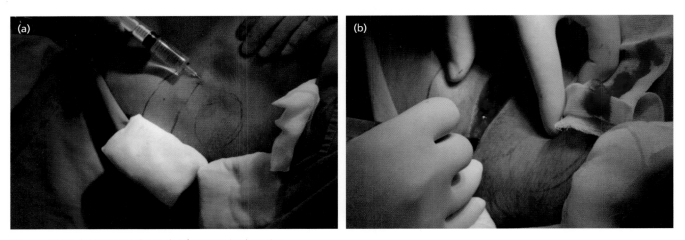

Figure 18.13 (a,b) Prepare the pocket for pump implantation.

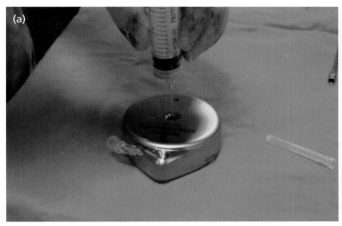
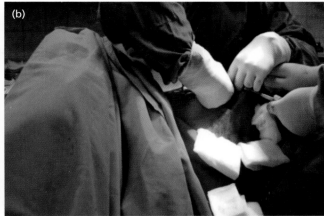

Figure 18.14 (a) Fill the pump. (b) Place the pump within the pump pocket.

Table 18.1 Spinal drug delivery systems

Type I. Percutaneous epidural or intrathecal catheter with or without subcutaneous tunneling.

Type II. Totally implanted epidural or intrathecal catheter with subcutaneous injection port.

Type III. Totally implanted epidural or intrathecal catheter with implanted infusion pump.

Type IV. Totally implanted epidural or intrathecal catheter with implanted programmable infusion pump.

Reproduced from Erdine and De Andres (2006) with permission from Editor-in-Chief of *Pain Practice*.

patient is discharged with instructions for further follow up and emergency action.

Classification of drug delivery systems

It is useful to review the classification of drug delivery systems, before the start of the above procedures.

There are various techniques to implant the drug delivery systems. They are classified in Table 18.1. The advantages and disadvantages of drug delivery systems are presented in Table 18.2. They should also be reviewed before performing the procedure. Inhibition of pain transmission by spinal analgesics is shown in Table 18.3.

The impact of drugs which are commonly introduced in drug delivery systems are described below in terms of pharmacology, pharmacodynamics, and their side effects.

Drugs used for intraspinal analgesia

Opioids

Morphine remains the current "gold standard" for spinally administered analgesic agents and is the only opioid approved by the Food and Drug Administration (FDA) for intrathecal delivery to treat chronic pain.

Because of its hydrophilic properties and potent receptor affinity, morphine is considered the "gold standard" for the treatment of chronic (mainly nociceptive and mixed) pain.

Morphine and hydromorphone are the two opioids recommended as initial medications for pump infusion. Fentanyl is considered a second-line opiate. Other opioids should be tried only when other opioids, nonopioids, and combinations have failed.

The onset, peak, and duration of action of each opioid are dependent on its ability to diffuse across the dura and into the dorsal horn. This ability is associated with the lipid solubility of the opioid, which is best defined by the oil–water coefficient. A higher coefficient corresponds to increased lipid solubility, thus a faster onset and peak action, as well as a more rapid clearance of the medication from the CSF.

Morphine has an oil–water coefficient of 1.4 and in comparison with other opioids a longer time of onset and peak and a prolonged clearance from the CSF. Delayed respiratory depression may be seen with intrathecal or epidural morphine because of prolonged clearance from the CSF, rostral migration, and its effect on opioid receptors of the ventral medulla.

Delayed respiratory depression may be seen within 6–12 hours, but has been reported up to 24 hours after a single bolus injection of intra-axial morphine.

Hydromorphone is a semi-synthetic hydrogenated ketone of morphine that has greater lipophilic properties than morphine, thus is faster acting and has greater potency. Intrathecal hydromorphone in a dose 20% that of morphine results in equal analgesia. Its increased lipophilicity compared with morphine also results in decreased distribution within the intrathecal space and rostral migration. Side effects, including nausea, vomiting, pruritus, and sedation, are less frequent than with intrathecal morphine. Both morphine and hydromorphone have been associated with catheter tip granuloma formation.

Table 18.2 Advantages and disadvantages of selected intraspinal drug-delivery devices

Device	Advantages	Disadvantages
Short-term epidural catheter	• No surgery • Can be done in any sterile environment • Easy replacement	• Catheter externalized (infection risk) • Catheter has external dressing • Restriction on bathing and clothing • Less precise tip placement • More likely to become disconnected (infection risk)
Permanent epidural or intrathecal catheter	• Internal fixation to avoid inadvertent catheter withdrawal • Physician can verify catheter and tip position with a normal spine film • No dressings on back • Catheter is larger and easier to clean and dress	• Catheter is externalized with some increased risk of infection • Restrictions on bathing and clothing • Commonly requires an ambulatory pump, but could be intermittent injections • Cost includes the mixture of drug and pump rental
Implantable epidural or intrathecal port	• Catheter and port are completely internal with (possibly) less infection risk • Physician can direct the catheter to the best possible catheter tip location • May be used for intermittent bolus dosing	• Port must be accessed through the skin for each administration or continuously during infusion with (possible) infection risk • The skin over the port must be monitored for infection • Needle-access discomfort
Implanted intrathecal catheter and pump	• Completely internalized system (decreased infection risk) • Less chance of catheter withdrawal • Greater patient satisfaction • Some pumps can be programmed to give boluses and infusions	• Requires surgical procedure for catheter fixation and pump insertion • Increased initial, implantation cost (possible long-term savings after 3 months over externalized systems)

Reproduced from Erdine and De Andres (2006) with permission from Editor-in-Chief of *Pain Practice*.

Table 18.3 Inhibition of pain transmission by spinal analgesics

Drug	Class	Mechanism of action
Morphine	Opioids	Inhibit C-fiber transmission by binding to presynaptic and postsynaptic opioid mu receptors in substantia gelatinosa and dorsal horn.
Hydromorphone		
Fentanyl		
Bupivacaine	Local anesthetic	Binds to plasma membrane of nerve cells causing distortion of the fast sodium channels, thus preventing the sodium influx that initiates the action potential.
Clonidine	Alpha-2-agonist	Binds to presynaptic and postsynaptic α-2 receptors in dorsal horn inhibiting neurotransmission and depresses release of C-fiber transmitters including substance P.
Gabapentin	Anticonvulsant	Uncertain – structural derivative of GABA; specific receptor identified on calcium channels.
Ziconotide	N-type voltage dependent calcium channel blocker	Thought to act on N-type channels in substantia gelatinosa to inhibit substance P release and glutamergic transmission.
Baclofen	Anticonvulsant	GABA-B receptor agonist which evokes hyperpolarization of the membrane, reducing terminal neurotransmitter release. The highest concentration of GABA-B receptors is in the substantia gelatinosa.

GABA (gamma-aminobutyric acid).
Reproduced from Erdine and De Andres (2006) with permission from Editor-in-Chief of *Pain Practice*.

Fentanyl and sufentanil are highly lipophilic and have a rapid time of onset and peak action, as well as rapid clearance from the intrathecal space. They are 100 and 1000 times more potent than morphine, respectively.

Given the rapid clearance from the intrathecal space, both fentanyl and sufentanil are thought to be associated with fewer supraspinal side effects and have a more segmental effect, but data on efficacy and safety with long-term intrathecal use of fentanyl and sufentanil are lacking. Fentanyl was recommended as a second-line drug for intrathecal therapy by the Polyanalgesic Consensus Conference of 2007 because it is a widely accepted and used drug, and is rarely associated with intrathecal granuloma formation.

Local anesthetics

Bupivacaine is the most commonly used local anesthetic and the only one currently supported by the published data for intrathecal infusion. However, it should be understood that currently the FDA does not approve any local anesthetic for use within a drug delivery system.

Although bupivacaine alone has not shown great promise for analgesia before producing intolerable side effects, a synergistic effect has been shown to occur when infused concurrently with opiates. Motor blockade is typically the limiting factor regarding the dose of bupivacaine infusion. It has been shown that infusions between 1 and 20 mg/day are safe to infuse; however, motor blockade has been noted as low as 10 mg/day.

Alpha-2 agonists

Clonidine is an alpha-2 agonist that also works presynaptically, binding to alpha-2 receptors and decreasing the release of neurotransmitters. It has also been shown to have an effect on postsynaptic G-coupled potassium channels resulting in hyperpolarization, and it has been found to activate spinal cholinergic receptors potentiating the analgesic effect. It is hydrophobic with an oil–water coefficient similar to that of fentanyl, resulting in a rapid onset and peak action as well as rapid clearance from the intrathecal space. Clonidine is approved by the FDA for intrathecal administration.

It has been shown to be an excellent adjuvant to opiate therapy as it may decrease the opiate requirement and prolong the development of tolerance to opiates.

The most common side effect is postural hypotension; however, it is also associated with sedation, dry mouth, dizziness, and constipation. A stability study showed that clonidine given in combination with hydromorphone is stable and may be used long term with an implantable drug delivery system. It may also cause hypotension and bradycardia.

Ziconotide

Ziconotide produces potent antinociceptive effects by selectively binding to N-type voltage-sensitive calcium channels on neuronal somata, dendrites, dendritic shafts, and axon terminals, thus blocking neurotransmission from primary nociceptive afferents.

Ziconotide was approved by the FDA in December 2004 for intrathecal use. It has been shown to aid in chronic nonmalignant pain, with greater efficacy noted in the treatment of neuropathic pain.

Possible side effects of ziconotide include allergic reaction, nausea, vomiting, seizures, fever, headache, change in mental status, asthenia, confusion, change in mood or perception, postural hypotension, abnormal gait, urinary retention, nystagmus/amblyopia, drowsiness/somnolence, dizziness or lightheadedness, weakness, or visual problems (e.g. double vision).

Baclofen

Baclofen is a gamma-aminobutyric acid-B (GABA-B) agonist that acts presynaptically by decreasing calcium conduction, which results in a decrease in the release of neurotransmitters. Postsynaptically it also increases potassium conductance and results in hyperpolarization of the second-order neurons. Use of intrathecal baclofen is approved by the FDA.

Evidence for its use in neuropathic pain and other pain conditions is limited. Adverse effects include drowsiness, sedation, weakness, headaches, confusion, hypotension, nausea, urinary retention, constipation, and sexual dysfunction. Overdose with baclofen may lead to respiratory depression and seizures, and may be fatal. Physostigmine may be beneficial in baclofen overdose. Baclofen withdrawal can also be life threatening and lead to hallucinations, anxiety, tachycardia, seizures, muscle rigidity, hypertension, and may even progress to disseminated intravascular coagulation, rhabdomyolysis, and death.

Intrathecal analgesic combinations

During the Polyanalgesic Consensus Conference of 2007, a panel of physicians and nonphysicians expert in the field of intrathecal analgesia reviewed relevant studies from 2000 to 2006 and updated an algorithm for the use of intrathecal opioid and nonopioids medications. It is now a widespread practice to try combinations of medications for intrathecal analgesia when the use of single agents fails. Common combinations are outlined in the recommendations of the Polyanalgesic Consensus Conference of 2007.

The stability of several intrathecal medications when used in combination has been studied. Combining morphine with clonidine, and morphine with hydromorphone and bupivacaine, has been shown to be stable. Morphine and hydromorphone by contrast have both been shown to destabilize ziconotide, especially at higher concentrations. Therefore, concentration limitations have been outlined. Ziconotide has been shown to remain stable when combined with clonidine at 2 g/ml and is less stable with bupivacaine (Table 18.4).

Table 18.4 2007 Polyanalgesic algorithm for intrathecal therapies

Line 1	(a) Morphine	↔	(b) Hydromorphone	↔	(c) Ziconotide
Line 2	(d) Fentanyl	↔	(e) Morphine/hydromorphone + ziconotide	↔	(f) Morphine/hydromorphone + bupivacaine/clonidine
Line 3	(g) Clonidine	↔	(h) Morphine/hydromorphone/fentanyl bupivacaine + /clonidine + ziconotide		
Line 4	(i) Sufentanil	↔	(j) Sufentanil + bupivacaine + /clonidine + ziconotide		
Line 5	(k) Ropivacaine, buprenophine, midazolam, meperidine, ketorolac				
Line 6	**Experimental drugs** Gabapentin, octreotide conpeptide, neostigmine, adenosine XEN2174, AM336, XEN, ZGX 160				

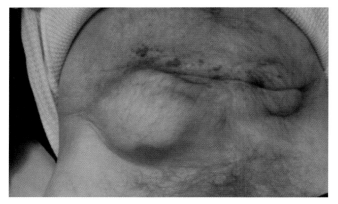

Figure 18.15 Infection at the pump pocket.

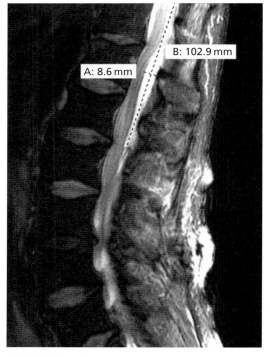

Figure 18.16 Epidural abscess.

Complications

The complications of intraspinal analgesia may be classified as follows.

1. Side effects related to the drugs used during intraspinal analgesia.

2. Complications related to the implantation technique and devices:

    (a) related to the procedure;

    (b) related to the catheter;

    (c) related to the implanted port or pump;

    (d) related to the administered agents.

Complications related to the procedure

(Figs 18.15–18.20)

Bleeding at the incision site and subcutaneous tunnel.

Epidural hematoma.

Infection, abscess formation.

CSF leakage.

Seroma at the implantation site.

Complications related to the catheter

Epidural:

- occlusion of the catheter;
- kinking of the catheter;
- curling up, knot formation;
- misplacement of the catheter;
- fibrosis in the epidural space;
- injection-related burning pain.

Intrathecal:

- neural damage;
- subarachnoid puncture headache;

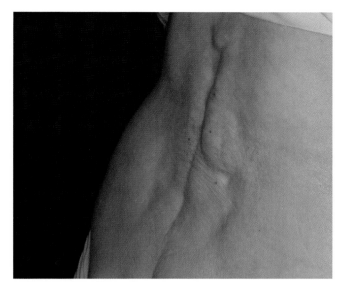

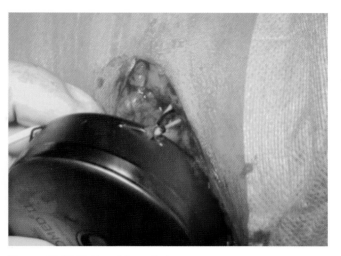

Figure 18.18 Kinking of the catheter.

Figure 18.17 Seroma formation.

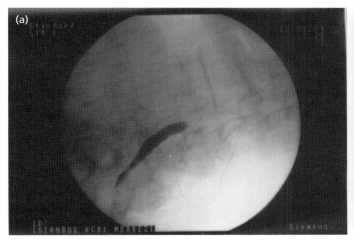

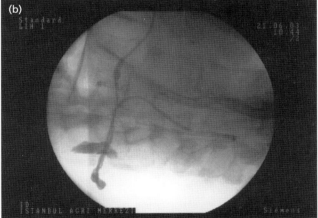

Figure 18.19 Fibrosis formation (a) within the epidural space and (b) along the catheter.

- subarachnoid fistula;
- granuloma formation;
- catheter migration.

Complications related to the implanted port or pump
Obstruction of the port or pump.
Leakage from the port membrane.
Disconnection of the catheter.
Seroma formation.
Skin necrosis.

Complications related to the administered agents
Pruritus.
Nausea and vomiting.

Urinary retention.
Constipation.
Respiratory depression.
Hormonal dysfunction.
Sedation and cognitive symptoms.

Complications related to the procedure

Bleeding
Some patients may have coagulation disorders, either because of the drugs administered orally (chemotherapeutic agents or nonsteroidal anti-inflammatory drugs used for pain relief) or because of tumor growth.

During the surgical procedure, the port or pump pocket should be examined meticulously. The patient should be

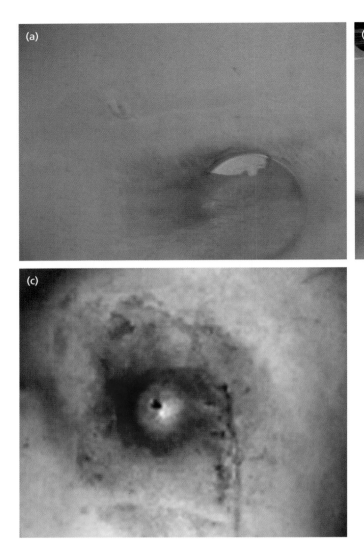

Figure 18.20 (a–c) Skin necrosis for port and pump.

kept in the hospital for observation for at least 48 hours after the procedure.

A hematoma may develop when the subcutaneous tunneling device is passed through the subcutaneous tissue. Ecchymosis may be observed along the route of the tunneling device.

Epidural hematoma

Epidural hematoma may develop owing to coagulation disorders or because of a traumatic epidural puncture or penetration of the blood vessels in the epidural space as the catheter is introduced. It may also occur spontaneously.

With large hematoma, there may be some neurological findings such as severe lumbar pain, bilateral lower extremity weakness; diffuse diminished pinprick sensation, paresthesia, and hypesthesia. To confirm the presence of an epidural hematoma, MRI is required.

Infection

Infection may be observed either immediately after implantation or later. Serious infection has not emerged as a common sequel to intraspinal analgesia.

The causes of infection are contamination from the injected solution, contamination by skin flora, and hematogenous spread. Possible sites for the infection are the exit site of the catheter, at the port and pump pocket, epidural space (epidural abscess), and in the intrathecal space (meningitis).

Diagnosis of epidural space infection includes acute loss of analgesia, fever, and elevations in white blood cells. In the immunosuppressed cancer population, fever and elevation in white blood cells may be delayed. Epidural space infection and catheter encapsulation present with three symptoms: (1) pain on injection; (2) retrograde flow of infusaide with pooling in the paravertebral tissues; and (3) loss of analgesia.

Epidural infection and abscess formation may be due to the hematogenous spread or extension of the superficial infection at the port site during injection. Untreated infections that progress and become epidural abscesses may subsequently cause neurological deficit due to the pressure on the spinal cord.

Development of pain due to an epidural abscess must be distinguished from injection-related burning pain. In both instances, there will be pain during injection, which was not felt in the earlier stages; pain increases during the injection and stops as soon as the injection is ceased.

With an epidural abscess, there will be a lack of analgesia despite an increased dose. At the beginning, there may be no fever, but the temperature will rise as the abscess develops. There will be a nonspecific low back pain and, if the abscess is large, there may be paresthesia due to the compression of the nerves in the region.

MRI is necessary to verify the extent of the problem. Should infection be confirmed, the drug delivery system should immediately be removed. A sample may be obtained by aspiration and the type of infection may be confirmed by culture and the appropriate antibiotic sensitivity determined. After 10 days of specific aggressive intravenous antibiotic treatment, MRI should be repeated to reevaluate the epidural space.

In cases of stubborn abscess, surgical intervention may be necessary.

Two factors may explain the incidence of meningitis for intrathecally inserted systems: injections performed through the skin into the reservoir are potentially septic, and the effect of the changes in the patient's reference mechanism due to the disease and anticancer treatment. One should consider prophylactic antibiotic coverage in all patients. Local skin infections can be treated with aggressive antibiotic coverage.

CSF leakage

CSF leakage occurs in two ways. First, during the epidural approach, the needle or catheter may rupture the dura accidentally. The second possibility is when the catheter is inserted intrathecally, the discrepancy between the size of the catheter and the needle may cause a short-duration CSF leak. To prevent leakage, a stylet or catheter should be inserted into the Tuohy needle immediately upon penetration of the intrathecal space. Despite these precautions, postdural puncture headache may develop.

Seroma formation

In some patients, after the implantation of the pump, a serosanguinous fluid collection (seroma) may develop and may last for up to 1 or 2 months. The size of the incision may play a role in the formation of the seroma. Although the seroma may be aspirated under aseptic conditions,

unless the fluid collection is excessive it is not advisable because of the risk of infection may increase. After aspiration, compression of the skin may be applied, which is sometimes helpful.

Complications related to the catheter

Epidural

Occlusion of the catheter
The catheter may be occluded owing to clot formation, development of fibrosis around the tip of the catheter, foreign particles in the injected solution, or kinking of the catheter. The solutions to be delivered should be carefully prepared. Filters should be used during the preparation. The risk of occlusion is higher in the epidural space.

Kinking of the catheter
The catheter can be kinked at several sites: inside the epidural space, in the subcutaneous tissue as it turns into the subcutaneous tunnel, and at the implantation site near the junction of the port or pump.

To prevent kinking of the catheter, several precautions should be taken. In every step of the implantation procedure, passage of fluid through the catheter should be maintained. If there is a difficulty of administration into the epidural space; the catheter may be withdrawn 1–2 cm. If there is still a difficulty, the catheter should be removed and then reinserted.

The other reason for kinking is the improper placement of the drug delivery system. The catheter should be externalized at the near edge of the pocket incision, to allow it to curve gradually. Before closing the incision, free flow of the drug to be delivered should be confirmed.

Curling up, knot formation
If excess catheter is inserted into the epidural or intrathecal space, curling or knotting may occur. Therefore the position of the tip of the catheter should be confirmed by injecting contrast material.

Misplacement of the catheter
The catheter should be placed very carefully into the target space. The possibilities for misplacement are the catheter entering: a vein, paravertebral space, subdural space, or intrathecal space while targeting the epidural space.

The catheter can enter a vein at the initial insertion, when blood appears during aspiration; the catheter may be advanced further or withdrawn until the aspiration of the blood ceases.

When the catheter is introduced epidurally with the loss of resistance technique, the same sensation may be felt if the needle is within the paravertebral space. Another possibility is that if the catheter is inserted too far within the epidural space, the tip may pass through the intervertebral foramen to a position outside the epidural space.

The subdural space is a potential space between the dural and the arachnoid membranes. If the catheter enters the subdural space, there is a potential hazard of serious side effects from the drugs delivered. If a local anesthetic is included in the mixture, there will be a sudden respiratory depression. The administration of opioids alone into the subdural space may also cause progressive respiratory depression which lasts longer than when observed after an intrathecal injection.

The catheter may enter the intrathecal space during the epidural approach. This may be due to the thickness of the dura and the catheter itself. Thus after epidural insertion of the catheter a test dose should always be given. Catheters initially placed within the epidural space can migrate to the intrathecal space.

To prevent misplacement of the catheter, it should be inserted under fluoroscopy, confirming in every step the correct position of the tip of the catheter.

Fibrosis in the epidural space

During chronic epidural delivery, nonspecific foreign body reactions develop in the epidural space. Epidural catheters may cause fibrous mass formation as a reaction within the epidural space. Dose escalation may develop due to the dural thickening and fibrotic reactions in the epidural space. During fibrous tissue formation, a resistance to the flow through the catheter develops initially. This resistance progresses and then the catheter may become blocked. In some patients, a fibrotic sheath develops around the catheter from the tip, through the tunneled area, toward the port system. In such instances, the concentration of the solution should be increased. If there is still a backflow, the system should be removed.

Injection-related burning pain

During long-term treatment, pain on epidural injection is observed in several patients. The reasons for such pain can only be speculated upon. Fibrous tissue developing in the epidural space, inflammation or infection may be the cause. The tip of the catheter may migrate to a position opposite to a nerve root and when a solution is injected, it may induce pain. This type of pain is sometimes so intractable that patients prefer the pain of the disease and desire the removal of the system.

Before deciding to remove the system, several steps can be taken. Depasteroid may be injected to relieve inflammation around the tip of the catheter.

Injection-related pain and fibrous tissue development are the main reasons for preferring the intrathecal route in patients in whom the pain responds to opioids.

Intrathecal

Neural damage

Spinal cord injury, nerve injury, and cauda equina injury have all occurred with placement of intrathecal catheters for implantable pumps. Use of fluoroscopy and insertion of the catheter below the level of the spinal cord may prevent neural damage. Inserting the needle at a gentle angle in a paramedian approach may minimize the risk of direct trauma to the spinal cord or nerve root. The use of general anesthesia is somewhat controversial. It may be better if the patient is awake enough to respond if the needle tip or catheter is on a neural tissue.

Subarachnoid fistula

If a system inserted intrathecally has to be removed for any reason, a cerebrospinal fistula may develop. The CSF flow through this fistula collects in the subcutaneous tissue. In such patients, fistulectomy should be performed. Despite fistulectomy the flow of CSF may continue. In such patients, a catheter should be inserted intrathecally just above the level of the fistula, and CSF flow maintained through this catheter for a period, thus enhancing the healing of the dura around the fistula.

Granuloma formation

An intrathecal granuloma is an inflammatory mass forming at the tip of an intrathecal catheter in response to the administration of medications. Intrathecal granulomas develop as a result of an inflammatory process. Granulomas are unrelated to infection and are sterile masses. High concentrations of morphine or hydromorphone are accused of being responsible for granulomas.

Patients may complain of increased pain and neurological deficit. They may present with subtle changes in history and physical examination or they may present with obvious changes. MRI is the "gold standard" diagnostic tool. The best study is a T1-weighted gadolinium enhanced study.

Another more affordable method is the side-port contrast study. Contrast is injected through the side port of the pump under fluoroscopy to determine whether there is a mass or obstruction. This can also be done under computed tomography (CT) without risk to the pump or its mechanism. Before infusing dye into the side port, the catheter must be aspirated to clear any drug from the infusion tubing.

If the granuloma becomes large enough, it can compress the spinal cord resulting in neurological injury. With the catheter in the high thoracic or cervical canal, should the patient suffer a compressive lesion, the damage is more serious. In addition, for catheter placement with a needle, entering the dura in a region where the dura is close to the spinal cord carries the increased risk of spinal cord injury.

Subarachnoid puncture headache

Spinal headaches occur frequently after insertion of intrathecal catheters. Risk for headache appears to be related to the size of the needle, age and sex of the patient, number of dural punctures (attempts), previous spine surgery, and direction of the bevel. Patients with a previous laminectomy and scar tissue formation at the site of the needle insertion may be at increased risk of CSF leak. In these situations it is reasonable to place the spinal catheter above the level of the fusion, again using a gentle angled approach.

Enter the dura using an oblique angle. The bevel should be placed vertically, separating as opposed to cutting the dural fibers. A purse string suture placed around the Tuohy needle seems to decrease distal CSF leak as well. Whenever possible, do not enter the thecal sac at the site of a previous laminectomy.

Catheter migration

Migration of the catheter may also be the cause for decreased efficiency, depending on the location of the tip of the catheter. Changes in symptoms can be sudden and abrupt or may slowly develop over a long period. A differential diagnosis is necessary for the disease progression. CT, MRI, or side-port myelography may help to decide.

Complications related to the implanted port or pump

Obstruction of the port or pump

Obstruction of the port or pump may be due to catheter occlusion or kinking. Besides that, the solutions to be delivered should be carefully prepared. Filters should be used during preparation. Some access ports and pumps have internal filters; if a contrast material is injected, the contrast solution may form a layer over the filter, thereby making the injection difficult. Dilution of the contrast material is necessary if it is to be injected.

Occlusion due to the pump may occur because of valve failure or malfunction of the pump.

Leakage from the port membrane

If a needle other than a Huber type is used, there is a risk of leakage from the port membrane.

Disconnection of the catheter

The satisfactory connection of the catheter with the drug delivery system may still be a problem. If there is a disconnection, the efficacy of the intraspinal administered analgesics will suddenly drop. The leak can be visualized by injecting contrast material through the port or pump system.

Skin necrosis

In debilitated cancer patients, skin necrosis may develop at the edges of the port or pump pocket. If the necrosis is over a small area, instead of removing the system, one should try to reopen, clean and resuture the incision. If one cannot succeed, then the drug delivery system has to be removed.

Complications related to the administered agents

Pruritus

Pruritus is one of the most frequent side effects after intraspinal opioid delivery. It occurs after several hours of intraspinal opioid delivery. It decreases with time.

The mechanism of pruritus is not well described. It is probably not related to histamine release but the interaction of the opioids with the trigeminal nucleus located on the surface of the medulla.

Antihistamines or opioid antagonists may be administered if the symptoms are severe.

Nausea and vomiting

Nausea may start 4 hours after intraspinal delivery and vomiting may follow. Generally antiemetic agents may help. Nausea and vomiting may be due to the interaction of the opioid with the opioid receptors in the area postrema.

Urinary retention

The incidence of urinary retention is between 42 and 80% after intraspinal opioid delivery. It is more frequent in patients with prostate hypertrophy. Inhibition of the parasympathetic fibers causes atony in the detrusor muscle. A temporary urinary catheter may be necessary in some patients. Generally it lasts for several days.

Constipation

Opioids may decrease gastrointestinal motility and cause constipation. Dietary changes may be helpful.

Respiratory depression

The risk of respiratory depression is rare in patients who have been administered opioids by oral or other routes before intraspinal delivery. In elderly patients, the risk is higher. Late respiratory depression develops within 6–12 hours after the first intraspinal opioid delivery.

Naloxone should be considered if the respiratory distress is severe and the respiratory rate decreases. Naloxone, 0.4 mg in 10 ml of saline, should be given every 1–2 minutes at a dose of 40–80 µg. The effect of naloxone is short and lasts for 20–40 minutes.

Hormonal dysfunction

A decrease in testosterone production in patients receiving chronic intrathecal opiate therapy was demonstrated in a randomized controlled trial. It was associated with a decrease in libido and potency.

Sedation and cognitive symptoms

Sedation and somnolence may occur with all opioids. In very rare cases euphoria, anxiety, or catatonia may develop.

Helpful hints

Successful use of intraspinal analgesia begins with proper patient selection. In selection of patients for intraspinal therapy a careful evaluation and analysis of the pain is necessary before selecting the route and the drug delivery system. The physician should have a thorough understanding of the patient's characteristics such as life expectancy, source of pain, age, weight, spinal canal assessment, and the environment of the patient. This is also important in the development of complications, several of which can arise owing to the wrong choice of route or system.

The general and mental status of the patient must be evaluated carefully in the preoperative period. If physiological and psychological abnormalities are underestimated, the risk of complications associated with these systems increase.

Preexisting structural abnormalities, such as a cerebral infarct, hemorrhage, or abscess, or neurodegenerative disorders such as multiple sclerosis or Alzheimer's disease, must be considered.

Life expectancy of the patient is an important factor in selecting the drug delivery system. A percutaneous catheter or subcutaneously inserted catheter may be preferred if a patient has a life expectancy of days to weeks, whereas access ports with epidural or intrathecal catheters for several weeks to months, and implantable intrathecal pumps, should be considered for a life expectancy of months to years, especially in noncancer patients.

Not all pain responds to spinal opioids. The route of administration, whether epidural or intrathecal, will differ according to opioid responsiveness. Thus a preimplantation trial is necessary before implanting the drug delivery system. The decision to implant should be made only after a positive response to this trial is obtained. During the trial, the response to opioids, the need for the adjuvant drugs such as clonidine or local anesthetics, and the route of administration (epidural or intrathecal) can be assessed. The preimplantation trial should last from at least three days to a week.

Guidelines for appropriate selection of the route are as follows:

• For patients with short life expectancy, the epidural route may be preferred; percutaneously or subcutaneously implanted catheters/ports are most cost effective.

• Drugs other than morphine, like local anaesthetic, may effectively be used by the epidural route, and the intrathecal route to some extent.

• The epidural route may be confined to cancer patients with life expectancy of weeks to 2 or 3 months. Fibrosis, occlusion of the catheter, or burning pain in the injection site develop with longer duration.

• In noncancer patients, the intrathecal route is the only choice. Also in cancer patients with long life expectancy, the intrathecal route should be preferred.

• The intrathecal route is the only choice if a pump implantation is planned.

The patient's environment is also an important factor. The caregiver should be trained in using the drug delivery system, and about the drugs to be delivered.

As a conclusion, intraspinal analgesia using drug delivery systems is an important advance. However, only experienced, skillful pain physicians should perform it in an environment where the patient can be followed up for many months and even years.

The physician should be aware of the complications as well as how to cope with them. Implantation of a drug delivery system is perhaps the easiest first step of intraspinal analgesia.

The 2003 Polyanalgesic Conference noted that of the 18 agents for which clinical or preclinical data for intrathecal infusion were found, only one (ziconotide) had extensive data as a result of a formal development program for intrathecal administration. The mechanisms by which the agents most commonly used for intraspinal analgesia are thought to inhibit pain transmission are summarized in Table 18.3.

Table 18.4 shows the recommendation of the Polyanalgesic Algorithm for intrathecal therapies. According to the consensus meeting in 2007:

• If side effects occur, switch to another opioid.

• If maximum dosage is reached without adequate analgesia, add adjuvant medication (line 2).

• If the patient has neuropathic pain, consider starting with opioid monotherapy (morphine or hydromorphone) or, in selected patients with pure or predominant neuropathic pain, consider opioid plus adjuvant medication (bupivacaine or clonidine) (line 3).

• Some of the panel advocated the use of bupivacaine first because of concern about clonidine-induced hypotension.

• If side effects or lack of analgesia on second first-line opioid occur, you may switch to fentanyl (line 4).

• There are limited preclinical data and limited clinical experience; therefore, caution in the use of these agents should be considered.

Following that recommendation meant changes in clinical guidelines (the algorithm) for intraspinal drug infusion in pain management. They are as follows:

• addition of hydromorphone to first line;

• second-line change to morphine or hydromorphone with bupivacaine or clonidine;

• third-line change to all tri-mixtures;

• position of ziconotide within the algorithm dependent upon FDA approved indications;

• expansion to the application of the algorithm during the trialing period (pre-pump implant).

Table 18.5 Concentrations and doses of intrathecal agents recommended by the Polyanalgesic Consensus panelists, 2007

Drug	Maximum concentration	Maximum dose/day
Morphine	20 mg/ml	15 mg
Hydromorphone	10 mg/ml	4 mg
Fentanyl	2 mg/ml	No known upper limit
Sufentanil	50 μg/ml	No known upper limit
Bupivacaine	40 mg/ml	30 mg
Clonidine	2 mg/ml	1.0 mg
Ziconotide	100 μg/ml	19.2 μg (company recommendations)

Source: Deer et al. (2007).

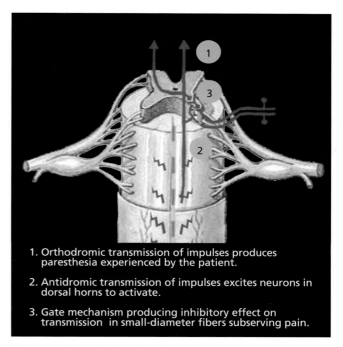

1. Orthodromic transmission of impulses produces paresthesia experienced by the patient.

2. Antidromic transmission of impulses excites neurons in dorsal horns to activate.

3. Gate mechanism producing inhibitory effect on transmission in small-diameter fibers subserving pain.

Figure 18.22 Mechanism of spinal cord stimulation.

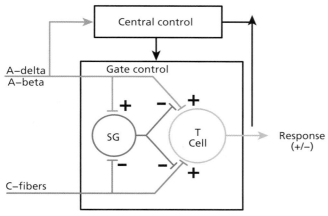

Figure 18.21 Gate control theory.

The concentrations and doses/days are provided in Table 18.5.

Technique of spinal cord stimulation

History

Many attempts to use electrical central nervous system stimulation for the treatment of pain emerged in the 1950s and 1960s based on the gate control theory of pain proposed by Melzack and Wall in 1965. In 1967, Shealy and associates introduced spinal cord stimulation. Initial spinal cord stimulation procedures involved open intrathecal implantation of electrodes through laminotomy. Development of percutaneous electrodes in 1975 has facilitated a wider application of spinal cord stimulation. The first pulse generators using a lithium battery were developed in the 1970s. Although unipolar electrodes were used in the initial stages, bipolar and quadripolar electrodes have been developed since the 1980s.

Shealy and colleagues used the term "dorsal column stimulation" initially, rationalizing that stimulation was effective on the dorsal column. Later, as electrical stimulation was proven to be effective in other regions of the spinal cord, newer spinal cord stimulation modalities were introduced.

The anatomy of spinal cord stimulation is similar to that described in other chapters (vide supra) and will not be described here.

Mechanism of action of spinal cord stimulation

Initially the basic explanation was the gate control theory by Melzack and Wall. Their proposition was based on the theory that stimulation of A-beta fibers modulates the dorsal horn "gate," reducing the nociceptive input from the periphery to the central nervous system, and modulating the transmission in the spinothalamic tract (Figs 18.21 and 18.22).

Activation of the central inhibitory mechanisms, influencing the sympathetic efferent neurons, and activation of putative neurotransmitters or neuromodulators may also play a role.

However, other mechanisms may play a more significant role in mechanisms of action of spinal cord stimulation. One of these is increased dorsal horn inhibitory action of GABA. There may also be a potential role for adenosine in stimulation.

Indications
- Radicular neuropathic pain.
- Failed back surgery syndrome.

- Ischemic pain due to peripheral vascular disease.
- Complex regional pain syndromes type I, type II.
- Phantom pain.
- Postherpetic neuralgia.
- Deafferentation pain.
- Angina pectoris.
- Cerebral palsy.
- Multiple sclerosis.

Contraindications
- Systemic or local infection.
- Coagulopathy.
- Anomalies of spinal canal.
- Spina bifida.
- Drug dependence, with behavioral abnormalities.
- Psychopathologies.

Technique of spinal cord stimulation

Step 1. Prepare the patient for the procedure
1. Physical examination (including examination of the entry site for local infection and distorted anatomy), lumbosacral MRI, urology evaluation (if necessary), and laboratory studies, including complete blood count with platelets, prothrombin time, partial thromboplastin time, platelet function studies and bleeding time, and urine analysis, are required.
2. For preoperative medication, use the standard recommendations for conscious sedation from the American Society of Anesthesiologists. Preprocedure sedatives, analgesics, and ancillary drugs are administered as needed in the surgical holding area. The patient is given 1 g of ceftriaxone (Rocephin) intravenously before the start of the procedure. Ciprofloxin (Cipro), 400 mg, is also given 1 hour before it.
3. Before the implantation, one should decide on the side and the location of the generator. The most appropriate location for the implantation of the generator is the right or left lower quadrant of the abdomen. The generator should not touch the iliac crest, the symphysis pubis, the ilioinguinal ligament, or the costal margin when seated.
4. The anatomic constraints tend to be the iliac crest, the symphysis pubis, the ilioinguinal ligament, and the costal margin. One should not be close to these structures during implantation.
5. For all patients, the medical evaluation must include a review of the patient's medical history, a physical examination, and an accurate description of the pain characteristics to allow a diagnosis and establish a treatment algorithm. A psychological/behavioral evaluation is also essential and should include a review of the patient's history and medical records, a clinical interview, a mental status examination, psychological testing, and determination of suitability for

implantation. Appropriate education should be given about the expectations and goals of spinal cord stimulation, the trial, and possible complications (patient dissatisfaction often is related to the difference between expectations and outcomes). An understanding is that the purpose of spinal cord stimulation will enable patients to take more responsibility for their own care. Finally, patients should recognize that their needs and response may change during the course of long-term spinal cord stimulation.
6. Following patient selection, a trial period is required to test the efficacy of analgesics. Thus, the screening period also allows assessment of analgesic effect and helps to ensure that patients have realistic expectations of treatment. This screening period may vary from several weeks to a month.

Implantation of the trial electrode

Step 2. Position and monitor the patient
1. Place the patient prone on the table. Place a pillow under the abdomen to flatten the lumbar lordosis.
2. Obtain an intravenous access.
3. Administer oxygen by nasal cannula, monitor the vital signs noninvasively.
4. Prepare and drape the area in a sterile fashion.
5. The patient should not be over-sedated. The patient should remain sufficiently conscious to provide responses to any questions.

Step 3. Drugs and equipment for trial electrode implantation
- trial electrode;
- 25 gauge infiltration needle;
- 15–17 gauge needle;
- 5 ml syringe;
- 10 ml syringe;
- loss-of-resistance syringe;
- 2–0 nylon suture;
- needle driver;
- connecting cables to stimulator box;
- device-specific power source (stimulator box);
- 1% lidocaine.

Step 4. Mark the surface landmarks for needle entry
1. The target intervertebral space is identified by palpating the spinous processes above and below. To ensure that the needle entry site is exactly in the midline, the physician's middle and index fingers are placed on each side of the spinous processes.
2. The anatomical landmarks are as follows.
  ○ The vertebral body of L1 is just below the vertebral body of T12 where the ribs appear bilaterally (Fig. 18.23).
  ○ The line drawn on the posterior iliac crest is between the L4–L5 intervertebral space.

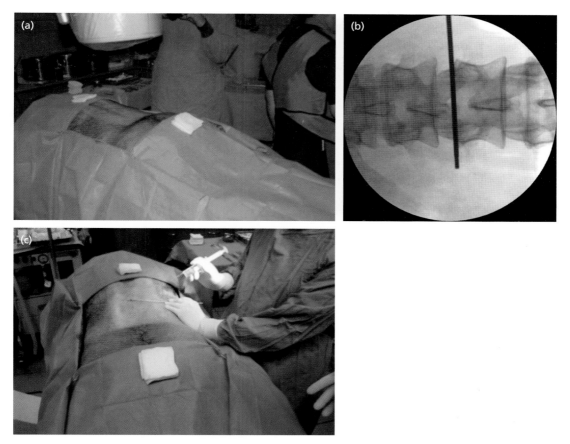

Figure 18.23 (a–c) Identify the entry point at the T12–L1 level for lower extremities and infiltrate the skin.

3. The point entry for lower extremity pain is the L1–T12 level. Infiltrate the skin, subcutaneous tissues, and supraspinous and interspinous ligaments at the midline with local anesthetic.

Step 5. Direction of the needle
1. Place the C-arm in a posteroanterior position. Identify the midpoint of the intervertebral space at the target level. Infiltrate the skin with local anesthetic solution using a short 25 gauge needle down to the lamina. Introduce the needle about 1 cm paramedially at the level of the tip of the spinous process. The needle is then angled slightly medially and advanced to make contact with the lamina. Once the bony contact is made, redirect the needle at an angle of 45° to the parasagittal and 15° to the axial plane medial and cephalad (Fig. 18.24).
2. Then position the C-arm laterally and advance the needle with the loss of resistance technique. Instead of saline, use sterile distilled water during the loss of resistance technique. Do not inject contrast material into the epidural space as it will change the medium of the epidural space and the patient cannot respond efficiently during the stimulation phase (Fig. 18.25).

3. Then insert the guidewire through the epidural needle into the epidural space. If there is difficulty while advancing the guidewire, do not force it. The guidewire should stay in the posterior epidural space. If it is directed toward the anterior epidural space, the needle has to be repositioned within the epidural space. The aim of inserting the guidewire is to open a space within the epidural space for the electrode (Fig. 18.26).

Step 6. Confirm the position of the electrode
1. Withdraw the guidewire; insert the electrode into the needle toward the epidural space. The electrode should stay in the posterior epidural space, not course towards the anterior epidural space (Figs 18.27 and 18.28).
2. Place the C-arm in a posteroanterior position again; advance the electrode under posteroanterior view (Fig. 18.29).
3. The electrode should be at least 7 or 8 cm within the epidural space to prevent the risk of coming out it.
4. Depending on the patient's pathology, one electrode is placed at the midline or laterally. One or more electrodes can be placed.
Note: in some cases the electrode may enter the subarachnoid space. The aspiration test is mandatory as soon

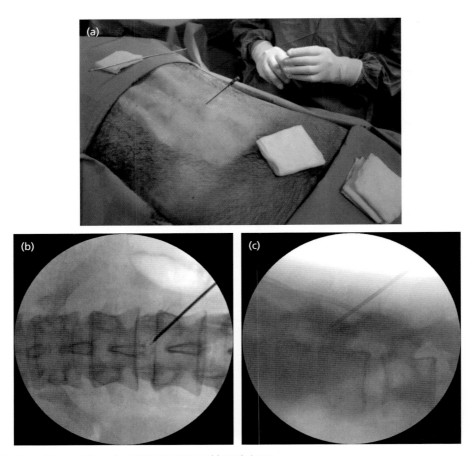

Figure 18.24 (a–c) Direction of the needle under posteroanterior and lateral views.

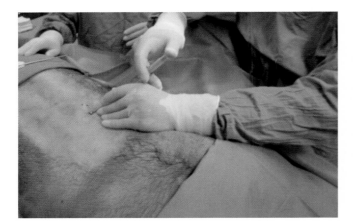

Figure 18.25 Loss of resistance technique.

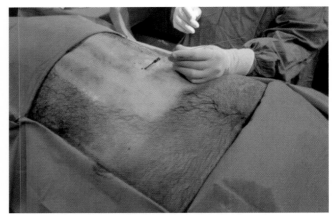

Figure 18.26 Introduce the guidewire.

as the needle enters the epidural space. Despite a negative aspiration test, the electrode may enter the subarachnoid space. The electrode will suddenly move freely within the subarachnoid space. Another way of verifying that the electrode is within the subarachnoid space is the stimulation test. The patient will respond to both the motor and sensory testing at very low stimulation settings.

5. After confirming the correct position of the electrode, it is connected to the "pulse generator" for the stimulation test. The device should be totally dry and there should be no blood at the connection point.

Step 7. Stimulation
The patient should not be over-sedated. They should remain sufficiently conscious to provide responses to the physician's

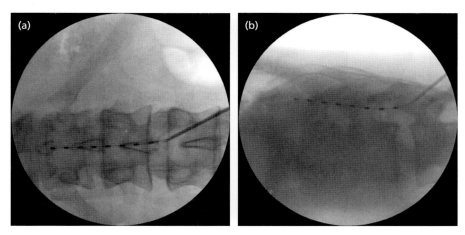

Figure 18.27 The electrode in (a) posteroanterior and (b) lateral views.

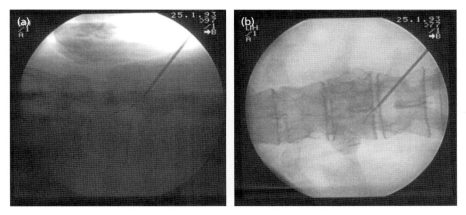

Figure 18.28 The electrode within the anterior epidural space, (a) lateral and (b) posteroanterior views.

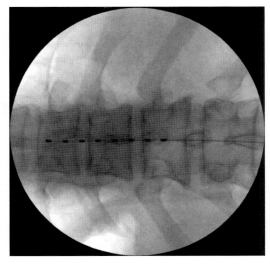

Figure 18.29 The electrode in position in posteroanterior view.

questions. Stimulation is planned methodically, setting the amplitude, rate, and pulse width. The amplitude is gradually increased by 0.05–0.1 V increments. The range of rate is optimally either as low as 10 or as high as 120 Hz. At lower rates less energy is used. At higher rates the amplitude of stimulation increases and tetanus may develop. Lower rates are preferred for peripheral stimulation. The pulse width is between 0 and 450 μs. The narrower pulse width covers less area. Sometimes when the pulse width is increased, stimulation felt by the patient may increase (Fig. 18.30).

The stimulation test should start with stimulating the region at 2 Hz, with 0.1–1.5 V settings. Contraction of the lower extremity does not always mean that the electrode is in the correct position. Next, seek paresthesia at the desired region. One should stimulate at 50–100 Hz with a 0.1–1.5 V setting. Generally, the patient feels paresthesia at the 0.5 V setting. The sensory test has to be repeated on the next day.

After the position of the electrode is confirmed, slightly withdraw the epidural needle to the fascia. Make a 5 cm incision, dissect down to the supraspinous ligament, withdraw the needle, and check the position of the electrode under fluoroscopy (Fig. 18.31).

Step 8. Placement of the electrode

1. Prepare a large pocket, because the extra lead or extension may be required to be coiled behind it. Push the protective boot over the proximal portion of the lead while stabilizing the lead body.

2. Wipe off any remaining body fluids from the surfaces of the lead contacts and extension setscrew connector.

3. Insert the lead fully into the extension setscrew connector. The four metal bands on the proximal end of the lead should be aligned under the four setscrews. Sterile water may be used as a lubricant to facilitate the insertion of the lead. Do not use saline.

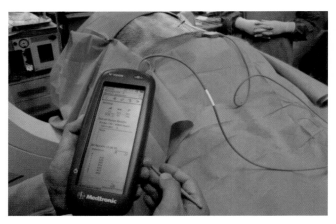

Figure 18.30 Test stimulation.

4. Tighten each of the four screws by turning them clockwise in the setscrew socket with the hex wrench. Tighten the setscrews only until they touch the contacts. Do not over-tighten setscrews: excessive torque may damage the lead contacts. Push the protective boot completely over the lead-extension connection. Secure the connection with nonabsorbable sutures around both the grooved ends of the boot. Do not tie a suture directly to the extension or the lead (Figs 18.32–18.34).

5. Suture the anchors securely to the ligament. Using a tunneling device, pull the extension at a distant point where the permanent generator will be placed in the next step.

6. Then carefully close the incisions. A 2.0 absorbable suture is sufficient. Then oppose the skin edges with sterile strips.

Cervical electrode placement

All steps are as explained above (vida supra) (Figs 18.35–18.37).

Trial period

Considering the placebo effect of a procedure, it is essential to prolong the trial period up to one month. For the cervical region, the patient should wear a collar and should be advised to rotate the head carefully.

Permanent electrode placement

Step 1. Preparation of the pocket

1. Before the implantation, one should decide on the side and the location of the pulse generator. The most appropriate location for the implantation of large devices is the right or left lower quadrant of the abdomen. The generator should not touch the iliac crest, the symphysis pubis, the ilioinguinal ligament, or the costal margin when seated. The

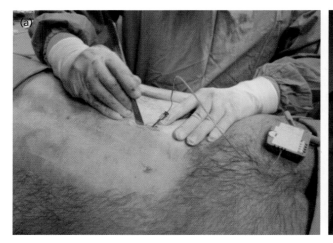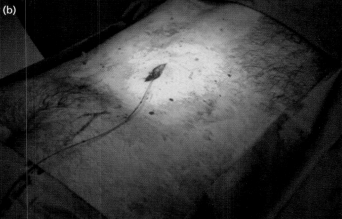

Figure 18.31 (a) Make an incision around the needle. (b) Withdraw the needle meticulously.

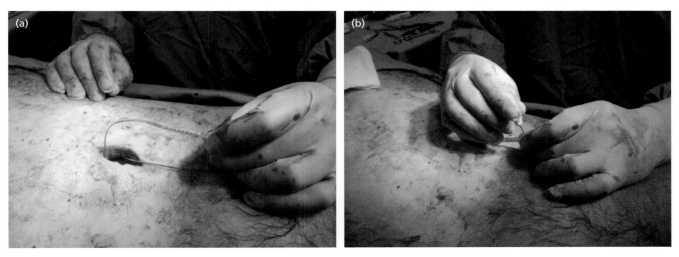

Figure 18.32 (a,b) Connect the electrode to the extension.

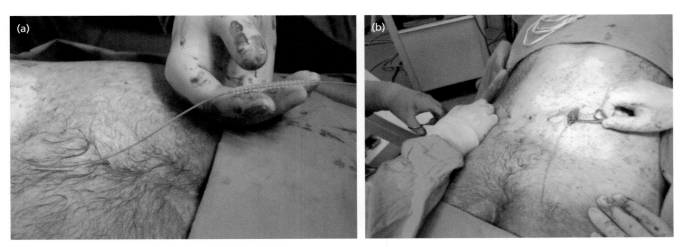

Figure 18.33 (a,b) Advance the extension through the subcutaneous tunneling device.

anatomic constraints tend to be the iliac crest, the symphysis pubis, the ilioinguinal ligament, and the costal margin.

2. Then prepare the pocket for the pulse generator on the lower quadrant of the abdomen.

3. Make a 10 cm incision, down through the underlying subcutaneous fat layer. Prepare a subcutaneous pocket large enough to admit the particular pulse generator. Maintain meticulous hemostasis to avoid postoperative hematoma formation.

Step 2. Lead tunneling

1. Attach the metal tunneling tip to the tunneling tool. Remove the tunneling tip and tunneling tool, leaving the tube in place in the tunnel.

2. Gently feed the lead through the tube.

3. Pull the tube out to remove it from the tunnel, leaving the lead in position.

Step 3. Making the lead-extension connection

1. Push the protective boot over the proximal portion of the lead while stabilizing the lead body.

2. Wipe off any remaining body fluids from the surfaces of the lead contacts and extension setscrew connector.

3. Insert the lead fully into the extension setscrew connector. The four metal bands on the proximal end of the lead should be aligned under the four setscrews. Sterile water may be used as a lubricant to facilitate the insertion of the lead. Do not use saline.

4. Tighten each of the four screws by turning them clockwise in the setscrew socket with the hex wrench. Tighten the setscrews only until they touch the contacts. Do not over-tighten setscrews: excessive torque may damage the lead contacts. Push the protective boot completely over the lead-extension connection. Secure the connection with

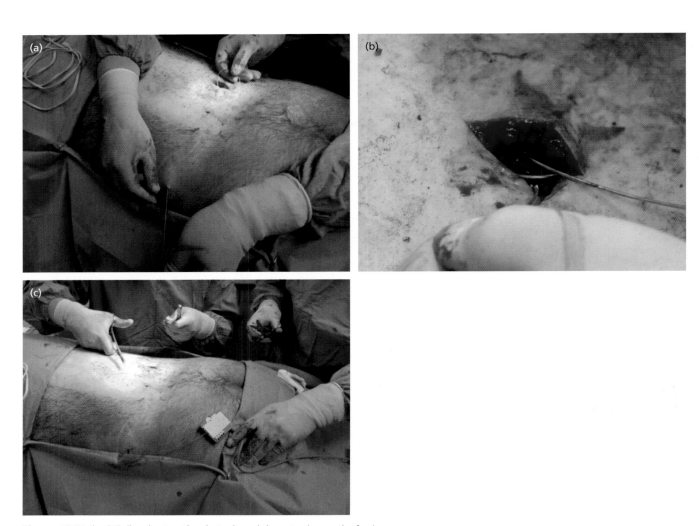

Figure 18.34 (a–c) Coil and suture the electrode and the extension on the fascia.

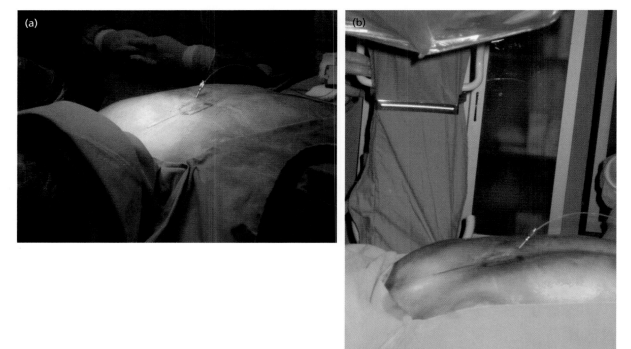

Figure 18.35 (a,b) Position of the needle for cervical electrode placement.

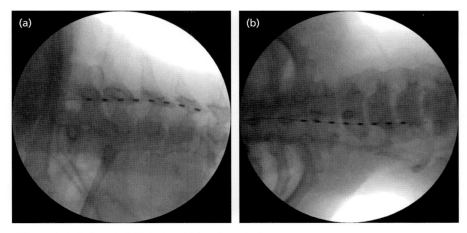

Figure 18.36 Position of the cervical electrode in (a) lateral and (b) posteroanterior views.

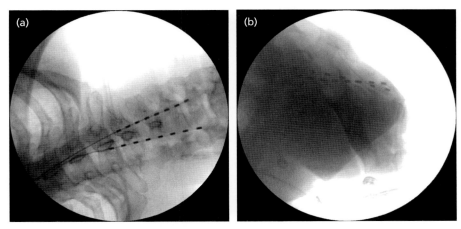

Figure 18.37 Position of double electrodes in (a) lateral and (b) posteroanterior views in the cervical region.

nonabsorbable sutures around both the grooved ends of the boot. Do not tie a suture directly to the extension or the lead.

Step 4. Making the extension–neurostimulator connection
1. Check the neurostimulator sockets by obstructing setscrews if necessary, partially back out the setscrews.
2. To back out a setscrew, insert the hex wrench through the pre-pierced hole in the rubber grommet and turn the setscrew counterclockwise only until the neurostimulator socket is unobstructed.
3. Wipe off any body fluids from the extension connector pins and connector block.
4. Check that the encapsulated diagram on the extension matches the diagram on the neurostimulator.
5. Insert the extensor connector pins.
6. Once the extensor connector pins are fully inserted in the neurostimulator sockets, do the following for each setscrew.

7. Insert the hex wrench through each rubber grommet to engage setscrews. Tighten each setscrew by turning clockwise with the hex wrench. Tighten the setscrews only until they touch the contacts. Continue tightening for a maximum of a quarter of a turn only.
8. Place the neurostimulator in the pocket, do not loop or coil the extension on the top of the neurostimulator etched identification side. Wrap any excess around the perimeter of the neurostimulator.
9. The neurostimulator has two suture holes in the connector block to secure it in the subcutaneous pocket.
10. The neurostimulator should be located no more than 3.8 cm beneath the surface of the skin to ensure proper programming. The device must be placed parallel to the skin surface.
11. The neurostimulator should be placed away from bony structures and with the etched identification side facing away from the muscle tissue to minimize pain at the neurostimulator site, and to minimize the possibility of skeletal

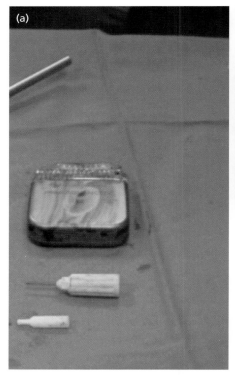

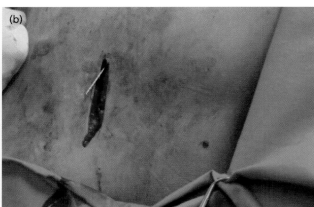

Figure 18.38 (a,b) Prepare the pocket for the lesion generator.

muscle stimulation, which may be perceived by the patient as twitching and burning.

12. Then carefully close the incisions. A 2.0 absorbable suture is sufficient. Then oppose the skin edges with sterile strips.

13. Check the neurostimulator function using the physician programmer (Figs 18.38 and 18.39).

Step 5. Postprocedure care

After the implantation, the patient should be kept in hospital for several days to arrange the stimulation parameters. The patient and their family should be trained in the use of the pulse generator during this period. The ideal stimulation pattern – and resulting pain relief – are often lost within the first few weeks after implantation. Periodic reprogramming then becomes essential. As the fibrous tissue invests the lead electrodes, resistance to delivery of the electrical impulses can increase. The result is the need to increase the amplitude substantially over time. This should be expected, and the patient made aware that it is a normal occurrence. This maturation process can often require reprogramming of the electrode array, pulse width, and frequency. The three-dimensional space surrounding the lead can be altered by the natural process of healing in a manner that renders the stimulator system ineffective, despite a successful trial.

Migration of the lead after maturation is much less likely, but it still can occur. "Electrical repositioning" of the elec-trode array recovers the optimal stimulation pattern. By varying the programs from time to time, accommodation can be avoided. Accommodation describes the phenomenon by which the body comes to "ignore" a steady, unvarying electrical stimulus over time. Patients who leave their stimulator systems on continuously may accommodate much more rapidly, causing the stimulation to become ineffective.

Complications
Early complications:
- Bleeding.
  - Bleeding at the surgery site.
  - Bleeding at the subcutaneous tunnel.
  - Epidural hematoma.
- Nerve injury, spinal cord injury.
- Inadvertent dural puncture, postdural puncture headache.
- Early infection: infection at the epidural space, epidural abscess, meningitis, discitis.
- Edema and seroma formation at the generator site.
Late complications:
- Epidural fibrosis.
- Spinal stenosis due to the narrowing of the spinal canal.
- Infection at the generator pocket or around the leads at the paraspinous region.
- Skin necrosis around the generator or leads.

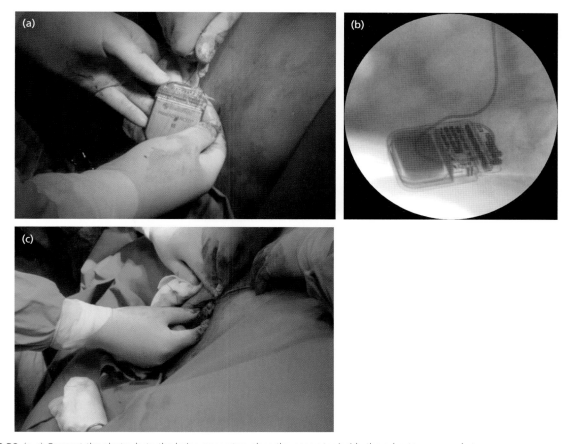

Figure 18.39 (a–c) Connect the electrode to the lesion generator; place the generator inside the subcutaneous pocket.

Complications related to the device:
- Migration of electrode.
- Lead breakage.
- Hardware malfunction.
- Unwanted stimulation.
- Burning of the skin due to overheating.

Early complications

Bleeding
Bleeding at the site of surgery during the procedure or in the early period is not a frequent complication.

Before the procedure, laboratory studies, including complete blood count with platelets, prothrombin time, partial thromboplastin time, platelet function studies and bleeding time, are required.

During the surgical procedure, the port or pump pocket should be examined meticulously. The patient should be kept in the hospital for observation for at least 48 hours after the procedure.

A hematoma may develop when the subcutaneous tunneling device is passed through the subcutaneous tissue. Ecchymosis may be observed along the route of the tunneling device.

Controlling the bleeding at the surgery site is not a problem. However, epidural hematoma developing during the insertion of the electrode may cause serious problems.

Epidural hematoma may develop owing to coagulation disorders, coexisting liver disease, difficult lead placement with multiple passes, or surgical lead placement.

With large hematoma, there may be some neurological findings such as severe lumbar pain, bilateral lower extremity weakness, diffuse diminished pinprick sensation, paresthesia and hypesthesia. To confirm the presence of an epidural hematoma, CT is required. MRI is contraindicated with an indwelling lead. In the case of epidural hematoma, the leads should immediately be removed and an MRI obtained. When epidural hematoma is confirmed, surgical evacuation should be done as soon as possible within 24 hours.

Spinal cord or nerve injury
Direct trauma to the spinal cord or nerve roots may occur owing to the needle or electrode placement.

One should be more careful in the cervical region while placing the electrode as the epidural space in the cervical region is already 1–2 mm and the electrode may compress the nerve root or the spinal cord.

If the electrode is in very close proximity with the neural foramen, it may compress the nerve roots. Paresthesia will develop without stimulation. The electrode should immediately be removed.

Inadvertent dural puncture

Inadvertent dural puncture may occur while advancing the needle or electrode. If dural puncture occurs while advancing the needle into the epidural space, CSF may be aspirated. However, in some cases the aspiration test may be negative.

If dural puncture occurs while advancing the electrode, the electrode will immediately move in a more free fashion.

Previous surgery at the site of the needle placement, obesity, spinal stenosis, calcified ligaments, and movement of the patient are the risk factors.

A midline approach at an angle of entry greater than 60° increases the risk of dural puncture.

In the case of dural puncture, postdural puncture headache may develop with signs of positional headache, nausea, nystagmus, and tinnitus. If hydration, caffeine, or bed rest do not relieve the symptoms, a blood patch may be considered.

Infection

The risk of infection during the procedure is not as great as anticipated. Infection may develop at the generator pocket or lead tunnel. Risk factors include immunocompromised state, uncontrolled diabetes mellitus, history of chronic skin infections, history of methicillin-resistant infection or colonization with *Staphylococcus aureus*, and wound breakdown at the surgery site.

Epidural abscess

If infection is not treated, an epidural abscess may develop. At the early stages, fever may not develop. Epidural abscess should be suspected when there is severe pain at the lead implant site.

A diagnosis of abscess or disc infection requires a CT scan or surgical tissue sampling. A diagnosis of meningitis requires cerebrospinal fluid analysis. In the case of epidural abscess, the generator should immediately be removed.

Seroma formation

A seroma is a noninfectious process that involves the seepage of serum from the tissues of the pocket into the area surrounding the generator. This may be caused by excessive tissue trauma, such as aggressive sharp dissection, excessive use of cautery, or forceful blunt retraction. Diagnosis can be confirmed by aspiration of a straw-colored fluid that is negative on microscopic exam for bacteria and subsequent culture. Pressure may be applied to the tissue or careful aspiration may be helpful.

Treatment can be by pressure applied to the tissue, needle aspiration, or by surgical incision.

Late complications

Epidural fibrosis

Epidural fibrosis can occur around the electrode. In some settings, the amount of fibrosis does not appear to cause any change in the patient's condition and does not require treatment. However, in some patients, epidural fibrosis may affect the programming of the system. In widely spaced dual-lead octapolar systems, the leads may be reprogrammed to capture other fibers and to salvage a good outcome. Painful stimulation may also occur with fibrosis, causing current transfer to the lateral nerve roots and spinal structures. In such cases the electrode has to be removed.

Spinal stenosis

The lead volume itself may create further narrowing of the spinal canal and create a spinal stenosis. If epidural fibrosis develops in those cases, the symptoms become more severe.

Erosion of the skin around the generator

Erosion of the skin may occur due to weight loss so that the connectors or generators become excessively superficial, causing pain and possible tissue breakdown. In thin patients or in those with weight loss, the generator may require revision to a different location or to a tissue plane below the fascia.

Complications related to the device

Lead migration

Lead migration can occur due to poor anchoring, or excessive movement of the patient. Diagnosis can be made by plain radiography, comparing the initial placement of the electrode. In the case of lead migration, reprogramming may be helpful in some cases. If appropriate paresthesia cannot be captured, repositioning of the electrode is necessary.

Lead fracture

In the case of lead fracture, painful stimulation will occur. Diagnosis is made by computer analysis or plain radiography. To reverse lead fracture, the leads should be placed to relieve stress on the materials. Trauma may also cause lead fracture. Surgical revision is necessary.

Loss of stimulation

Loss of stimulation may be due to epidural fibrosis, lead migration, disease progression, or malfunction of the device.

Burning of the skin due to overheating

In the past few years, a new complication has developed owing to recharging of generators. In rare cases, burning of the skin can occur due to overheating. Treatment includes immediate treatment of the burn, consultation with a plastic surgeon, and eventual revision of the device.

Helpful hints

Before the procedure, detailed information about the procedure, expectations of the therapy, outcomes, risks, and complications should be given to the patient and their family.

Consultation with other disciplines such as neurosurgery, psychiatry, physical therapy and rehabilitation, and internal medicine if necessary, should be warranted. The physician should be aware that the procedure for spinal cord stimulation is just the first step of a long journey with the patient and the family. The center performing spinal cord stimulation should have all facilities for a long-term follow up of the patient.

At the beginning of the surgery, the patient should be assessed for skin disorders or infection, not only at the site of the needle entry or incision but also on other parts of the body. Preventive intravenous third-generation cephalosporin is recommended.

The area of the needle entry and incision, both for the trial and permanent implantation, should be very carefully prepared and draped. The patient may be sedated, but they should be conscious enough to respond to questions during the stimulation as well as any complications that may arise during the needle entry or while advancing the electrode. For implanting the permanent generation, general anesthesia may also be considered.

Wipe body fluids off the lead contacts before connecting, as a contamination of connections can affect stimulation.

Do not loop or coil the extension on top of the neurostimulator. Wrap the excess extension around the perimeter of the neurostimulator. This avoids any increase in the subcutaneous pocket depth, helps to minimize potential damage during neurostimulator replacement surgery, and helps to minimize potential kinking of the extension.

Handle the implanted components of the neurostimulation system with extreme care. These components may be damaged by excessive traction or sharp instruments. Do not bend, kink, or stretch the lead, whether or not the stylet is in place. Do not bend or kink the stylet. Be careful when using sharp instruments around the lead to avoid nicking or damaging the lead.

Place the neurostimulator with the marked identification side facing away from the muscle. This helps to minimize the possibility of skeletal muscle stimulation that may be perceived as twitching or burning.

While removing the percutaneous extension suture, use caution to avoid cutting the lead's insulation, which can result in loss of stimulation and lead failure.

If resistance is felt when removing the lead from the percutaneous extension setscrew connector, loosen the setscrews slightly to ensure that they clear the lead contacts.

Avoid disengaging the setscrews. Inspect the lead contacts for damage (flattening or stretching the lead) if resistance was felt before removal.

The wound should be closed in the usual fashion using either interrupted or running absorbable sutures or multiple layers to assure that all dead space is obliterated and there is no tension on the skin.

A sterile nonocclusive dressing should be applied over the wound and should remain undisturbed for 48–72 hours. Removal of the sutures should take place 7 to 10 days later, depending on the general health of the patient.

The patient should be followed up for at least 24 hours for possible neurological complications. Stimulation patterns should be checked in the next day as well as for the 6 weeks after implantation if necessary.

Typically, good stimulation can be achieved using the following upper cervical placements for specific nerve involvement: C1–C3, facial pain; C2–C3, upper neck; C4–C5, radial nerve; just below C5, median nerve; C6–C7, ulnar nerve.

A percutaneous lead with a broad area of coverage can provide good stimulation for these areas with four- or eight-contact electrodes. When pain is bilateral, the lead can be placed at the midline, or two separate electrode arrays (placed bilaterally on the spinal cord) can be used (Table 18.6).

Technique of sacral nerve root stimulation (contributed by S. Ozyalcin)

History

Applying electrical stimulation to the vagina, perineum, and anal regions has been used for the treatment of incontinence. In 1963 Caldwell placed an electrode at the base of the pelvis, which started the use of this technique in clinical practice. Since 1988 technical improvement by Schmidt and Tanagho and a proposed mechanism by Craggs and Fowler in 1996 have popularized this technique for pelvic pain.

Mechanism of action of sacral nerve stimulation

Although the exact mechanism of sacral stimulation remains unclear, it is assumed that the sacral nerve roots or sacral nerves mediate various types of sacral and pelvic pain

Table 18.6 Mechanisms of spinal cord stimulation

Orthodromic transmission of impulses produces paresthesia experienced by the patient.
Antidromic transmission of impulses excites neurons in dorsal horns to active.
Gate mechanism producing inhibitory effect on transmission in small-diameter fibers subserving pain.

fiber. There is a rational basis for stimulation. The stimulation of the S3 nerve root influences the sensory threshold of the bladder to function. It has been hypothesized that the effects of sacral neuromodulation depend on electrical stimulation of afferent axons in the spinal roots, which in turn modulate voiding and continence reflex pathways in the central nervous system. Sacral neuromodulation activates somatic afferent axons that modulate sensory processing and micturition reflex pathways in the spinal cord.

Anatomy

The sacrum is a large, triangular bone at the base of the spine and at the superior and posterior aspect of the pelvic cavity; there the sacrum is inserted like a wedge between the two iliac crests. Its upper part connects with the last lumbar vertebra and the inferior part articulates with the coccyx.

Although the vertebral components of the sacrum are fused into a single bone, the sacral vertebrae are still numbered as if they are separate vertebrae for counting the sacral foramen and sacral nerves. There are four anterior sacral foramina through which the sacral nerves exit and the lateral sacral arteries enter. The posterior surface of the sacrum is convex. One can identify four dorsal sacral foramina. The dorsal S1 foramen is located approximately 1 cm medial to the posterior superior iliac spine, whereas the S2 foramen is 1 cm medial and 1 cm inferior to the posterior superior iliac spine. The S4 foramen is immediately lateral and just superior to the sacral cornua. The S3 foramen is located midway between the S2 and S4 foramina. The sacral foramina are somewhat rounded in form and diminish in size from superior to inferior position.

Course of sacral nerves

Sacral nerves initially course through soft retroperitoneal spaces and then traverse within the bony sacrum. Sacral nerve roots divide into anterior and posterior divisions that exit the sacrum through their respective aspects of sacral foramina (S1–S4); the fifth sacral nerve and the coccygeal nerve exit inferiorly through the sacral hiatus. Posteriorly, they emerge from the sacral foramina; they divide as the posterior branches of sacral nerves (including the medial cluneal nerves). Anteriorly, they emerge from the anterior sacral foramina, and contribute to the sacral plexus (S1–S4) and coccygeal plexus.

Innervation

Posterior divisions supply the skin and musculature of the gluteal region. Anterior divisions, of L4 and L5, form the sacral plexus, which innervates the pelvic structures, perineum, and much of the lower extremity, mostly through its large sciatic nerve (L4–S3) (Fig. 18.40).

Indications

- Voiding disorders.
  - Urinary incontinence.
  - Urinary retention.
  - Voiding dysfunction.
- Chronic pelvic pain.
  - Interstitial cystitis.
  - Pudendal neuralgia.
  - Vulvodynia.

Contraindications

- Local or systemic infection.
- Coagulopathy.
- Inflammatory process within the bowel.
- Rectal prolapse or prosidynia.
- Pregnancy.

Technique of sacral nerve stimulation

Sacral stimulation has historically been achieved with the percutaneous placement of a catheter-type electrode through the skin and into the actual sacral foramen. The goal is stimulation of sacral nerve roots responsible for various types of sacral and/or pelvic pain.

There are two approaches now available to place the electrodes close to these sacral nerve roots: (1) posterior sacral foraminal approach; (2) retrograde lumbar approach.

The common technique of placement of electrodes is by the posterior sacral foraminal approach.

Step 1. Prepare the patient before the procedure
For all patients, the evaluation must include a review of the medical history, a physical examination, and an accurate description of the pain characteristics to allow a diagnosis and establish a treatment algorithm. A psychological/behavioral evaluation also is essential. Appropriate instructions should be given to the patient about the expectations and goals of sacral stimulation, the trial, and possible complications.

Physical examination
Physical examination includes examination of the entry site for local infection and distorted anatomy. Further lumbosacral MRI, urology evaluation and laboratory studies, complete blood count with platelets, prothrombin time, partial thromboplastin time, platelet function studies and bleeding time, and urine analysis are required.

For preoperative medication, use the standard recommendations for conscious sedation by the American Society of Anesthesiologists. Preprocedure sedatives, analgesics, and ancillary drugs are administered as needed in the surgical holding area. The patient is given 1 g of ceftriaxone (Rocephin) intravenously before the start of the procedure. Ciprofloxin (Cipro), 400 mg, can also be given 1 hour before the procedure.

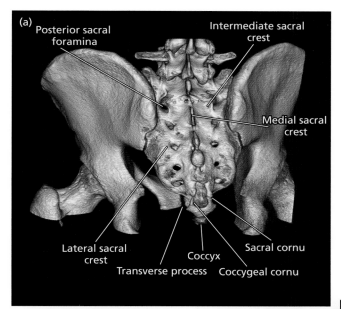

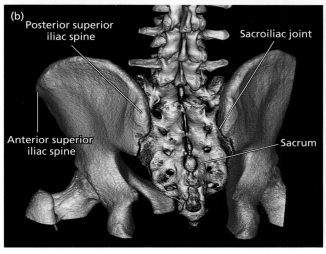

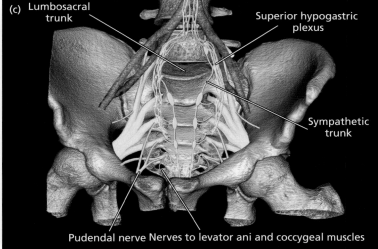

Figure 18.40 (a–c) Anatomy and innervation of sacrum.

Before the implantation, one should decide on the side and the location of the generator if required. The most appropriate location for the implantation of the generator is the right or left lower quadrant of the abdomen. The generator should not touch the iliac crest, the symphysis pubis, the ilioinguinal ligament, or the costal margin when seated.

Step 2. Position and monitor the patient (Fig. 18.41)
1. Place the patient in the prone position, which allows a 30° flexion at the hips and knees.
2. Obtain an intravenous access.
3. Administer oxygen by nasal cannula.
4. Monitor the vital signs noninvasively.

5. Prepare the sacrum and perineum for sterile surgery.
6. Drape to allow observation of the pelvic floor for muscle response to stimulation.
7. Provide visual access to soles of the feet to confirm muscle responses to stimulation.
8. The patient should not be over-sedated. The patient should remain sufficiently conscious to provide responses to any questions.

Step 3. Drugs and equipment for trial electrode implantation
• 20 ml syringe for skin infiltration;
• 1½ inch, 20 gauge needle for skin infiltration;
• no. 11 blade scalpel;
• a 2/0 or 3/0 nonabsorbable suture;

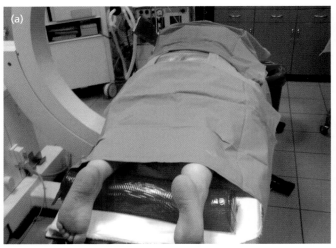 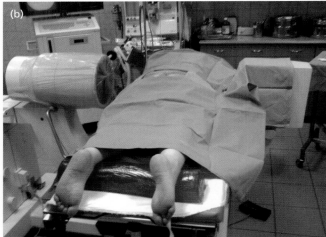

Figure 18.41 Position of (a) the patient and (b) the C-arm for sacral stimulation.

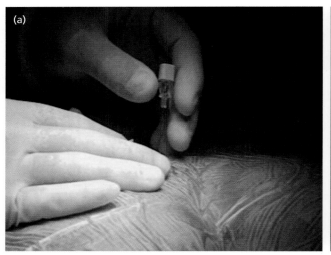 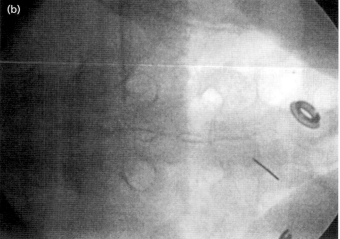

Figure 18.42 (a,b) Position of the needle in posteroanterior view on the sacral foramina.

- introducer kit for the trial period;
- trial electrode;
- sacral nerve stimulator;
- patient programmer;
- 1% lidocaine for skin infiltration.

Step 4. Visualization (posterior sacral foraminal approach)
1. Place the C-arm in a posteroanterior position. Try to visualize the S1 and S2 foramen (Fig. 18.42).
2. To verify the position of S1, measure the distance from the posterior iliac crest: it should be approximately 1–2 cm towards the medial direction. If the distance is longer, then it is usually the S2 foramen.
3. The site of entry is visualized by adjusting the fluoroscopic beam to align the chosen posterior sacral aspect of foramen with the anterior aspect of the foramen.

Note: generally the S3 foramen is preferred for sacral stimulation.

Step 5. Direction of the needle
1. Infiltrate the skin with 1% lidocaine. Insert a 20 gauge insulated foramen needle with an angle of 60° with the skin and 90° with the sacrum into the selected sacral foramen.
2. Position the C-arm laterally, advance the stimulation needle.
3. Cease insertion at the point when desired response is obtained. The insertion depth is usually 2.5–4 cm.

Step 6. Stimulation
1. Connect the mini-hook from the patient cable to the noninsulated section of the foramen needle (Fig. 18.43).

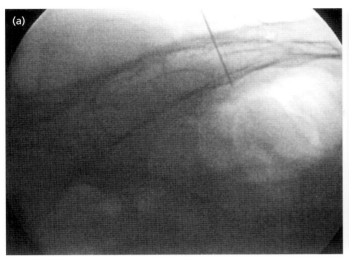

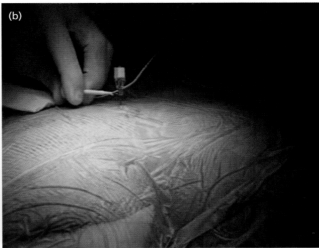

Figure 18.43 (a) Needle in lateral view. (b) Stimulate the needle using the alligator.

Trial sacral stimulation (posterior approach)
2. Patients must undergo acute percutaneous electrical stimulation of the ventral ramus at the level of the third S3, and possibly S2 and S4 sacral foramina, to establish functional integrity of the sacral nerves, to locate the nerves that can elicit beneficial responses, and to confirm that nerve stimulation elicits contractions of the appropriate muscle groups. The search for the S3 foramen can be done either with anatomic palpation or fluoroscopy.
3. If adequate responses are obtained during the acute testing, then test stimulation needs to be conducted for several days (not to exceed 7 days). Stimulation is achieved by replacing the stimulation needle with a temporary screening lead placed through the needle and connected to the same external screener that is used during the test phase. The amplitude of stimulation and "on/off" is controlled by the patient.

The patient controls the amplitude of the stimulation so that it is sensed but painless. Patients are informed that the sensation can change according to their positioning (sitting, standing, lying) and movements. Continuous stimulation is used (day and night, 10 Hz, 210 ms), and patients must be educated to manage power according to the severity of symptoms and feelings. They have to report all modifications of stimulation parameters on the voiding diary.
4. Urinary retention and dysfunctional voiding can be resolved by inhibition of the guarding reflexes. Detrusor overactivity can be suppressed by direct inhibition of bladder preganglionic neurons. Inhibition of interneuronal transmission in the afferent limb of the micturition reflex can also block detrusor overactivity.

In all patients, criteria for a successful trial includes a greater than 50% reduction in pain level, a reduced consumption of pain medications, and an increase in activities

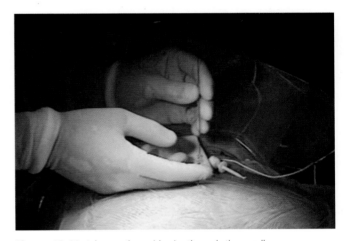

Figure 18.44 Advance the guidewire through the needle.

of daily living. If the patient had a successful trial, then permanent sacral electrodes are implanted. After trial stimulation, permanent stimulation can be done by implanting the permanent electrodes similarly to the trial stimulation.

Step 7. Permanent sacral stimulation
1. Remove the foramen needle stylet and replace with a directional guide, aligning the bottom of the appropriate depth marker on the directional guide with the top of the needle hub. Arrange the depth with the depth marker.
2. Holding the proximal portion of the directional guide in place, gently remove the foramen needle from the patient and from the directional guide (Fig. 18.44).
3. Make a small incision on either side of the directional guide.

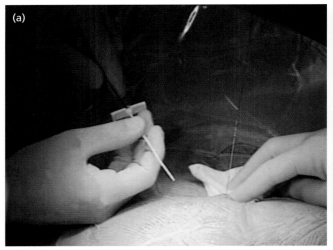

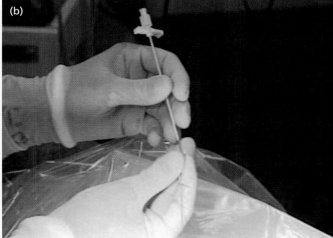

Figure 18.45 (a,b) Advance the dilator through the guidewire.

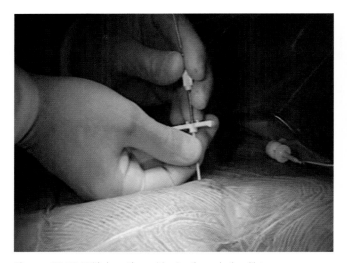

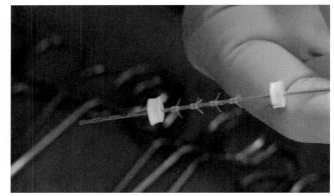

Figure 18.47 The hooves on the electrode fixing the electrode to the sacrum.

Figure 18.46 Withdraw the guidewire through the dilator.

4. Holding the directional guide in place near the skin, fit the dilator and introducer sheath over the directional guide and advance into the foramen. Align the bottom of the third most proximal depth marker on the directional guide with the top of the dilator (Fig. 18.45).

5. Unlock the dilator from the introducer sheath; remove the directional guide and dilator, leaving the introducer sheath in place (Fig. 18.46).

6. Insert the lead into the introducer sheath and advance the lead until visual marker band C on the lead lines up with the top of the introducer sheath handle. Using fluoroscopy, confirm that electrode 0 of the lead is proximal to the radiopaque marker band at the distal tip of the sheath (Fig. 18.47).

7. While holding the lead in place, retract the introducer sheath until visual marker band D on the lead lines up with the introducer sheath handle. Optimal motor responses

should be observed intraoperatively at 1–2 V amplitude during test stimulation. If strong motor responses are obtained at amplitude levels less than 1 V intraoperatively, the lead may be placed too close to the intended sacral nerve and should be repositioned farther away.

8. When satisfied with lead position, hold the lead in place and carefully withdraw the introducer sheath and lead stylet. Use care not to dislodge the lead from its position (Fig. 18.48).

Permanent sacral stimulation: lumbar retrograde approach

Step 1. Position of the patient
The patient is positioned prone on a radiolucent table.

Step 2. Placement of electrodes
Electrodes are placed percutaneously in the epidural space under fluoroscopic guidance at the appropriate level as

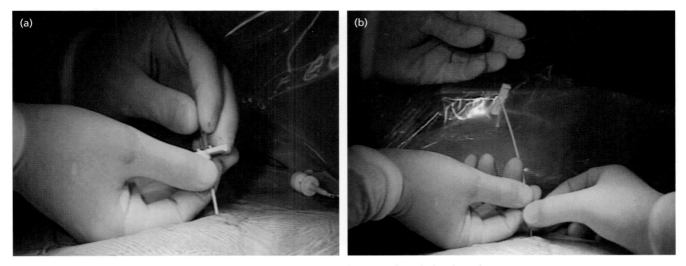

Figure 18.48 (a) Advance the electrode through the needle. (b) Withdraw the dilator through the electrode.

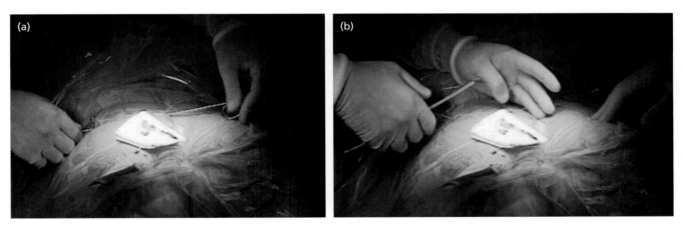

Figure 18.49 (a,b) Prepare the subcutaneous pocket.

determined by patient paresthesia, usually at the L4–L5 disc space (Fig. 18.49).

Step 3. Direction of the electrodes

The lumbar and sacral nerve roots are approached in a caudal direction (retrograde approach). In this approach, a Tuohy-type needle is inserted into the skin at a level superior rather than inferior to the interlaminar space and advanced in a caudal rather than a cranial direction. To reach sacral nerve roots, it is imperative to insert the needle in the same direction that the nerve root travels within the epidural nerve root sleeve. Therefore, the needle has to be placed in a paramedial fashion and advanced caudally into the epidural space. Once the epidural space is reached, the electrode should follow the path of the needle and continue to advance toward the targeted nerve root. Quattrode or Octrode multielectrode systems are recommended.

Step 4. Confirm the target site

Initial positioning is according to the anatomically predicted locations appropriate for the patient's pain. The exact position of the physiologic target varies and can be determined only intraoperatively by communicating with the patient about the location of the perceived paresthesias as different neural targets are stimulated. The perceptual threshold is defined as the stimulation amplitude at which level the patient first perceives the paresthesia. The discomfort threshold is the amplitude at which the paresthesias become uncomfortable.

Step 5. Creating the neurostimulator pocket

1. The neurostimulator is placed in the upper buttock area. Create a subcutaneous pocket by blunt dissection to the anterior surface of the muscle.
2. The neurostimulator should be located no more than 3.8 cm beneath the surface of the skin to ensure proper

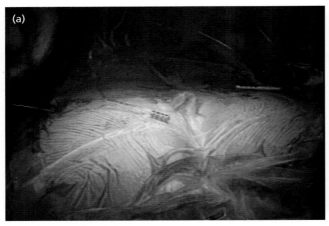 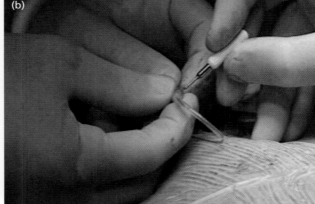

Figure 18.50 (a,b) Connect the extension with the electrode.

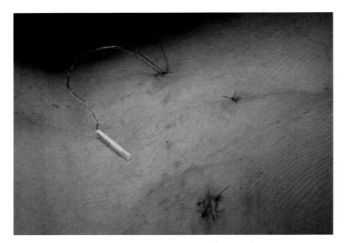

Figure 18.51 Distal end of the extension.

programming. The device must be placed parallel to the skin surface. The neurostimulator should be placed away from bony structures and with the etched identification side facing away from the muscle tissue to minimize pain at the neurostimulator site, and to minimize the possibility of skeletal muscle stimulation which may be perceived by the patient as twitching and burning.

Step 6. Lead tunneling
1. Attach the metal tunneling tip to the tunneling tool. Remove the tunneling tip and tunneling tool, leaving the tube in place in the tunnel.
2. Gently feed the lead through the tube.
3. Pull the tube out to remove it from the tunnel, leaving the lead in position.

Step 7. Making the lead–extension connection
1. Push the protective boot over the proximal portion of the lead while stabilizing the lead body.

2. Wipe off any remaining body fluids from the surfaces of the lead contacts and extension setscrew connector.
3. Insert the lead fully into the extension setscrew connector. The four metal bands on the proximal end of the lead should be aligned under the four setscrews. Sterile water may be used as a lubricant to facilitate the insertion of the lead. Do not use saline.
4. Tighten each of the four screws by turning them clockwise in the setscrew socket with the hex wrench. Tighten the setscrews only until they touch the contacts. Do not over-tighten setscrews: excessive torque may damage the lead contacts. Push the protective boot completely over the lead–extension connection. Secure the connection with nonabsorbable sutures around both the grooved ends of the boot. Do not tie a suture directly to the extension or the lead.

Step 8. Making the extension–neurostimulator connection (Figs 18.50–18.54)
1. Check the neurostimulator sockets by obstructing setscrews if necessary, partially back out the setscrews.
2. To back out the setscrew, insert the hex wrench through the pre-pierced hole in the rubber grommet and turn the setscrew counterclockwise only until the neurostimulator socket is unobstructed.
3. Wipe off any body fluids from the extension connector pins and connector block.
4. Check that the encapsulated diagram on the extension matches the diagram on the neurostimulator.
5. Insert the extensor connector pins.
6. Once the extensor connector pins are fully insert in the neurostimulator sockets, do the following for each setscrew.
7. Insert the hex wrench through each rubber grommet to engage setscrews. Tighten each setscrew by turning clockwise with the hex wrench. Tighten the setscrews only until they touch the contacts. Continue tightening for a maximum of a quarter of a turn only.

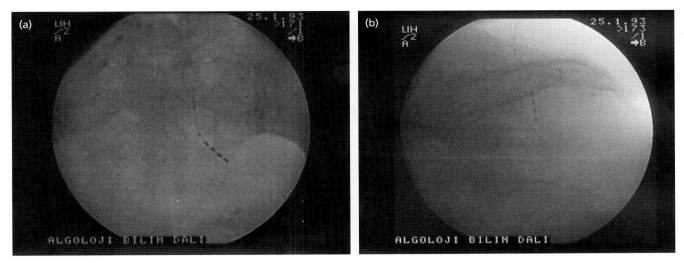

Figure 18.52 Position of the electrode in (a) lateral and (b) posteroanterior views.

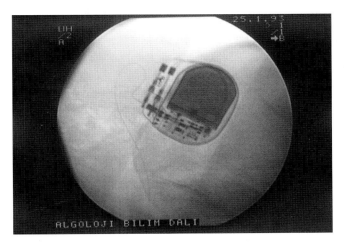

Figure 18.53 The lesion generator in place.

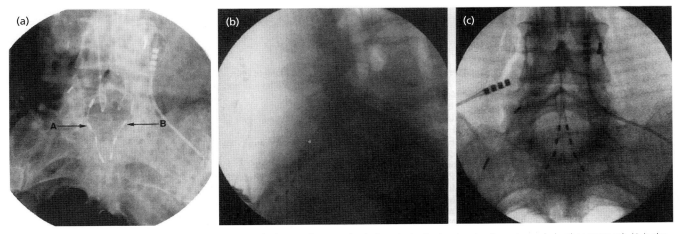

Figure 18.54 (a) Anteroposterior view of the sacrum with the sacral nerve stimulating electrodes in place by the retrograde lumbar approach (A is the left-side electrode, B is the right-side electrode). (b) Lateral view of the same in the caudal canal. (c) Electrodes in final position.

8. Place the neurostimulator in the pocket; do not loop or coil the extension on the top of the neurostimulator etched identification side. Wrap any excess around the perimeter of the neurostimulator.

9. The neurostimulator has two suture holes in the connector block to secure it in the subcutaneous pocket.

10. Check the neurostimulation function using the physician programmer.

Step 9. Postprocedure care

After the implantation, the patient should be kept in hospital for several days to arrange the stimulation parameters. The patient and their family should be trained in the use of the pulse generator during this period. The ideal stimulation pattern and resulting pain relief are often lost within the first few weeks after implantation. Periodic reprogramming then becomes essential. As the fibrous tissue invests the lead electrodes, resistance to delivery of the electrical impulses can increase. The result is the need to increase the amplitude substantially over time. This should be expected, and the patient made aware that it is a normal occurrence. This maturation process can often require reprogramming of the electrode array, pulse width, and frequency. The three-dimensional space surrounding the lead can be altered by the natural process of healing in a manner that renders the stimulator system ineffective, despite a successful trial.

Migration of the lead after maturation is much less likely, but it still can occur. "Electrical repositioning" of the electrode array recovers the optimal stimulation pattern. By varying the programs from time to time, accommodation can be avoided. Accommodation describes the phenomenon by which the body comes to "ignore" a steady, unvarying electrical stimulus over time. Patients who leave their stimulator systems on continuously may accommodate much more rapidly, causing the stimulation to become ineffective.

Complications

Hemorrhage, hematoma.
Nerve injury.
Paralysis.
Seroma at the neurostimulator site.
Allergic or immune system response to the implanted materials.
Infection.
Lead or neurostimulator erosion or migration.
Undesirable change in stimulation.
Change in bowel and/or bladder function.
Change in erectile and/or ejaculatory behavior.

• Hemorrhage, hematoma

Bleeding at the site of surgery during the procedure or in the early period is not a frequent complication.

Before the procedure, laboratory studies, including complete blood count with platelets, prothrombin time, partial thromboplastin time, platelet function studies, and bleeding time are required.

During the surgical procedure, the port or pump pocket should be examined meticulously. The patient should be kept in hospital for observation for at least 48 hours after the procedure.

A hematoma may develop when the subcutaneous tunneling device is passed through the subcutaneous tissue. Ecchymosis may be observed along the route of the tunneling device.

Controlling the bleeding at the surgery site is not a problem. However, epidural hematoma developing during the insertion of the electrode may cause serious problems.

Epidural hematoma may develop owing to coagulation disorders, coexisting liver disease, difficult lead placement with multiple passes, or surgical lead placement.

With large hematoma, there may be some neurological findings such as severe lumbar pain, bilateral lower extremity weakness, diffuse diminished pinprick sensation, paresthesia, and hypesthesia. To confirm the presence of an epidural hematoma, CT is required. MRI is contraindicated with an indwelling lead. In the case of epidural hematoma, the leads should immediately be removed and an MRI obtained. When epidural hematoma is confirmed, treatment is surgical evacuation as soon as possible within 24 hours.

• Nerve injury

Direct trauma to the nerve roots may occur due to the needle or electrode placement. If the electrode is in very close proximity with the neural foramen, it may compress the nerve roots. Paresthesia will develop without stimulation. The electrode should immediately be removed.

• Paralysis

This is a very rare complication under fluoroscopic guidance.

• Seroma at the neurostimulator site

A seroma is a noninfectious process that involves the seepage of serum from the tissues of the pocket into the area surrounding the generator. This may be caused by excessive tissue trauma, such as aggressive sharp dissection, excessive use of cautery, or forceful blunt retraction. Diagnosis can be confirmed by aspiration of a straw-colored fluid that is negative on microscopic exam for bacteria and subsequent culture. Pressure may be applied to the tissue or careful aspiration may be helpful. Treatment can be by pressure applied to the tissue, or needle aspiration.

• Allergic or immune system response to the implanted materials

This is also a very rare complication.

• Infection

The risk of infection during the procedure is not as great as anticipated. Infection may develop at the generator pocket or lead tunnel. Risk factors include immunocompromised state, uncontrolled diabetes mellitus, history of chronic skin infections, history of methicillin-resistant infection or colonization by *Staphylococcus aureus*, and wound breakdown at the surgery site.

- **Lead or neurostimulator erosion or migration**

Lead migration can occur owing to poor anchoring or excessive movement of the patient. Diagnosis can be made by plain radiography, comparing the initial placement of the electrode. In the case of lead migration, reprogramming may be helpful in some cases. If appropriate paresthesia cannot be captured, repositioning of the electrode is necessary.

- **Undesirable change in stimulation**

This is possibly related to cellular changes around the electrode. Shifts in electrode position, loose electrical connections, or lead/extension fractures have been described as uncomfortable by some patients.

- **Change in bowel and or bladder function**

Owing to stimulation parameters, change in bowel or bladder function may occur. It may take some time for the patient to accommodate to stimulation parameters.

- **Change in erectile and/or ejaculatory behavior**

Owing to stimulation parameters, change in erectile and/or ejaculatory behavior may occur. It may take some time for the patient to accommodate to stimulation parameters.

Helpful hints

Please review the helpful hints described in the previous section (spinal cord stimulation).

Vertebroplasty

History

Percutaneous vertebroplasty is a percutaneous procedure used to treat vertebral compression fractures by injecting bone cement (usually methylmethacrylate) directly into the vertebral body. Polymethylmethacrylate (PMMA) was used by Charnley in 1970 during hip prosthesis. The first percutaneous vertebroplasty was performed in France in 1984 for the treatment of painful cervical hemangiomas, reported by Galibert, Deramond, Rosat and LeGars in 1989. In 1988, Duquesnel used vertebroplasty in vertebral compression fractures due to osteoporosis and metastatic tumors.

Anatomy

The lumbar vertebrae are the largest segments of the functioning part of the vertebral column. They are characterized by the absence of the foramen transversorium within the transverse process, and by the absence of facets on the sides of the body.

As with other vertebrae, each lumbar vertebra consists of a vertebral body and a vertebral arch. The vertebral arch, consisting of a pair of pedicles and a pair of laminae, encloses the vertebral foramen.

The vertebral body of each lumbar vertebra is large, wider from side to side than from front to back, and a little thicker in front than in back. It is flattened or slightly concave above and below, concave behind, and deeply constricted in front and at the sides.

The pedicles are very strong, directed backward from the upper part of the vertebral body; consequently, the inferior vertebral notches are of considerable depth. The pedicles change in morphology from the upper lumbar to the lower lumbar. They increase in sagittal width from 9 to 18 mm at L5. They increase in angulation in the axial plane from 10 to 20° by L5. The pedicle is sometimes used as a portal of entrance into the vertebral body for fixation with pedicle screws or for placement of bone cement as with kyphoplasty or vertebroplasty.

The laminae are broad, short, and strong. They form the posterior portion of the vertebral arch. In the upper lumbar region the lamina are taller than wide but in the lower lumbar vertebra the lamina are wider than tall. The lamina connect the spinous process to the pedicles.

The vertebral foramen within the arch is triangular, larger than in the thoracic vertebrae, but smaller than in the cervical vertebrae.

The spinous process is thick, broad, and somewhat quadrilateral; it projects backward and ends in a rough, uneven border, thickest below where it is occasionally notched.

The superior and inferior articular processes are well defined, projecting respectively upward and downward from the junctions of pedicles and laminae. The facets on the superior processes are concave, and look backward and medial-ward; those on the inferior are convex, and are directed forward and lateral-ward. The former are wider apart than the latter, because in the articulated column the inferior articular processes are embraced by the superior processes of the subjacent vertebra.

The transverse processes are long and slender. They are horizontal in the upper three lumbar vertebrae and incline a little upward in the lower two. In the upper three vertebrae they arise from the junctions of the pedicles and laminae, but in the lower two they are set farther forward and spring from the pedicles and posterior parts of the vertebral bodies. They are situated in front of the articular processes instead of behind them as in the thoracic vertebrae, and are homologous with the ribs.

Of the three tubercles noticed in connection with the transverse processes of the lower lumbar vertebrae, the superior one is connected in the lumbar region with the back part of the superior articular process, and is named the mammillary process. The inferior is situated at the back part of the base of the transverse process, and is called the accessory process.

The fifth lumbar vertebra has certain peculiarities. Some individuals have four lumbar vertebrae, whereas others have six. Lumbar disorders that normally affect L5 will affect L4 or L6 in these individuals.

The first lumbar vertebra is level with the anterior end of the ninth rib. This level is also called the transpyloric plane, because the pylorus of the stomach is at this level.

The fifth lumbar vertebra is characterized by its body being much deeper in front than behind, which accords with the prominence of the sacrovertebral articulation, by the smaller size of its spinous process, by the wide interval between the inferior articular processes, and by the thickness of its transverse processes, which spring from the body as well as from the pedicles.

Indications

- Osteoporotic or osteolytic compression fractures of the thoracic or lumbar vertebrae, nonresponsive to medical treatment.
- Osteolytic metastasis related to a destruction of the vertebral body.
- Multiple myeloma.
- Aggressive vertebral hemangiomas (or eosinophilia granulomas of the spine).
- Painful vertebral fracture associated with osteonecrosis (Kummell disease).
- Reinforcement, or stabilization, of vertebral body before surgery.

Contraindications

- Coagulopathy.
- Local or systemic infection.

- Allergy to any materials used, such as contrast solution or cement.
- Retropulsed bone fragment resulting in myelopathy.
- Significant vertebral collapse with vertebral height reduced by two-thirds.
- Neurologic symptoms related to vertebral compression.
- Radiculopathy in excess of vertebral pain caused by a compressive syndrome unrelated to vertebral collapse.
- Asymptomatic retropulsion of a fracture fragment.
- Complete vertebral collapse.
- Epidural tumor.
- The presence of cortical destruction or epidural or foraminal stenosis.
- Patient unable or unwilling to give informed consent.
- Patient unable to lie down in prone position.
- Vertebroplasty may be performed by (1) a transpedicular approach (Fig. 18.55) or (2) an extrapedicular approach (Fig. 18.56).

Technique of vertebroplasty by transpedicular approach

Step 1. Prepare the patient before the procedure
1. The patient should be aware of why this procedure is being done and what to expect from it. All complications and side effects related to the procedure should be explained in detail, before it is started. Valid written consent should be obtained.
2. The type of analgesia or sedation needs to be ascertained before performance of the invasive procedure. Intravenous

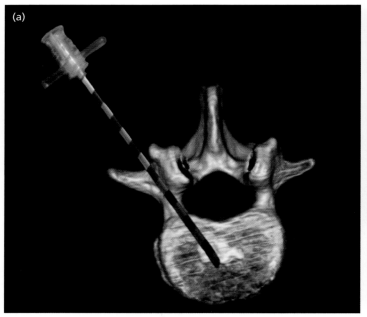
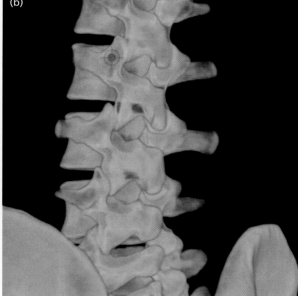

Figure 18.55 (a,b) Three-dimensional CT scans showing the entry point and direction of the needle for transpedicular vertebroplasty.

fentanyl, midazolam, and/or propofol may be used judiciously for the patient's comfort. CT imaging for the diameter of the pedicles to be entered is helpful. Recent plain radiographs should be examined. Recent MRI should be available, particularly a T2-weighted sagittal image and axial views through the levels of pathology to be treated. Prothrombin time, partial thromboplastin time, and platelet function studies should be done.

Step 2. Position and monitor the patient
1. Place the patient prone on the table. Place a pillow under the abdomen to flatten the lumbar lordosis.
2. Obtain an intravenous access.
3. Administer oxygen by nasal cannula, monitor the vital signs noninvasively.

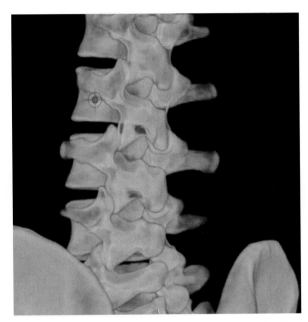

Figure 18.56 Position of the needle for extrapedicular vertebroplasty.

4. Prepare and drape the area in a sterile fashion.
5. The patient should not be over-sedated. The patient should remain sufficiently conscious to provide responses to any questions.

Step 3. Drugs and equipment for vertebroplasty
• 5 ml syringe for skin infiltration;
• 5 ml syringe for contrast solution;
• 25 gauge 1½ inch needle for skin infiltration;
• no. 11 blade scalpel;
• 11 or 13 gauge bone biopsy needle;
• sterile hammer;
• disposable mixing bowl and ladle;
• disposable PMMA injection syringe;
• 1% lidocaine for local anesthesia;
• nonionic contrast material;
• powder methylmethacrylate polymer;
• 10 ml of liquid methylmethacrylate monomer;
• 12 g barium sulfate.

Step 4. Visualization
1. Place the C-arm in a posteroanterior position. Identify the midpoint of the intervertebral space at the target level. Adjust the lower endplate of the target vertebral body to be aligned by moving the C-arm in a cephalocaudal direction (Fig. 18.57).
2. Oblique the C-arm in the coronal plane approximately 45° for L4–L5 and L5–S1 levels and 30° for upper levels until the facet joint is delineated and the "Scottie dog" view appears (Fig. 18.58).
3. It is important to oblique the fluoroscopic view enough to place the facet joint in the middle of the vertebral body and the spinous processes to the contralateral side. This facilitates a central placement of the needle. The target for entry is the superior lateral quadrant of the pedicle in the fluoroscopic view.

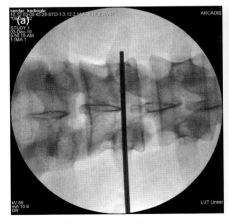
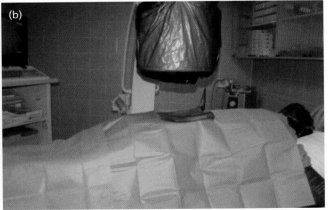

Figure 18.57 (a,b) Identify the entry level in posteroanterior view.

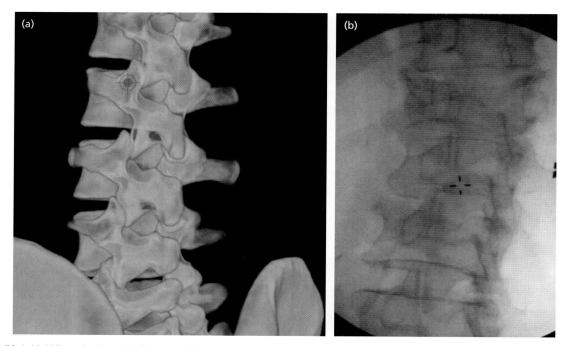

Figure 18.58 (a,b) Oblique the C-arm in the coronal plane approximately 45° for L4–L5 and L5–S1 levels and 30° for upper levels. (Courtesy of R. Benyamin.)

Step 5. Mark the surface landmarks for the needle entry
1. Infiltrate the skin and subcutaneous tissue over the center of the pedicle using 1 ml of 1% lidocaine and a 25 gauge needle (Fig. 18.59).
2. A small skin incision is made with a no. 11 blade scalpel to allow insertion of a large-bore biopsy needle.

Step 6. Direction of the needle
1. An 11 gauge bone biopsy needle or a 13 gauge needle is inserted under tunnel vision to the upper outer quadrant of the face of pedicle (Fig. 18.60).
2. The needle shaft should contact the center of the pedicle. Once contact has been made with bone, advance the needle through the cortex of the bone; this should be accomplished with a twisting motion of the needle or gentle tapping of the needle with a sterile hammer (Fig. 18.61).

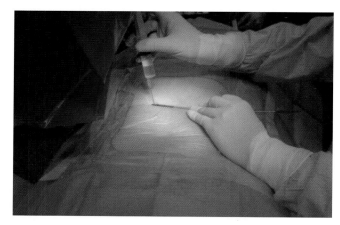

Figure 18.59 Infiltrate the skin over the entry point.

Step 7. Confirm the position of the needle
1. Rotate the C-arm laterally. In the lateral view, the needle needs to be at the upper midpoint of the pedicle so that the needle advances in the midpoint of the pedicle (Fig. 18.62).
2. The target point is at the junction of the anterior and middle third of the vertebral body. One should hold the needle with one hand and use the hammer with the other.
3. Rotate the C-arm to a posteroanterior position. The direction of the needle should be parallel to the endplates of the vertebral body.
4. Repeat the procedure from the contralateral side.

Step 8. Vertebroplasty
1. After confirming the final position of the needle, the cement is prepared for injection (Fig. 18.63).
2. There are several manufacturers producing the vertebroplasty kit. One should follow their guidelines. The powder is mixed with the liquid monomer (approximately 7.5 ml). The liquid monomer is titrated until it takes on a "toothpaste" or "cake-glaze" consistency. There are several delivery systems available that may be used to simplify the mixing and delivery in addition to decreasing fumes.

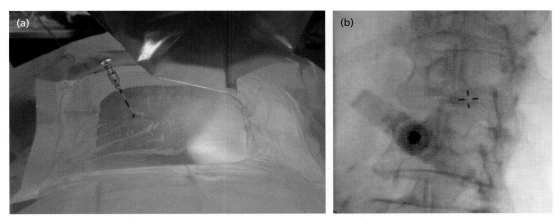

Figure 18.60 (a,b) Introduce the needle in "tunneled vision."

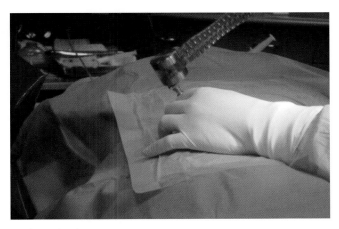

Figure 18.61 Advance the needle by gently tapping it.

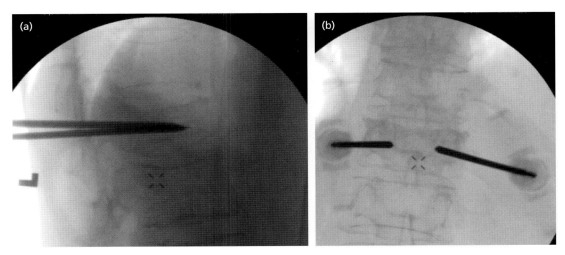

Figure 18.62 (a,b) Position of the needles in lateral and posteroanterior views.

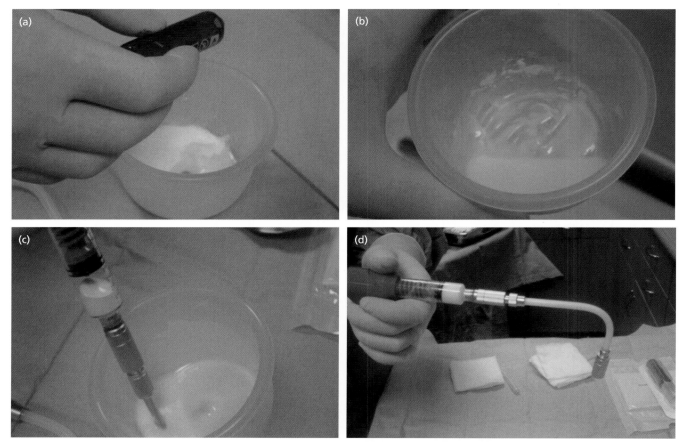

Figure 18.63 (a–d) Preparation of the cement.

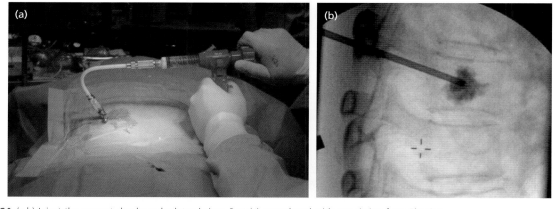

Figure 18.64 (a,b) Inject the cement slowly under lateral view. Part (a) reproduced with permission from Elsevier.

3. Then, the stylet is removed from the needle and the cement is slowly injected under continuous fluoroscopic imaging under a lateral view (Fig. 18.64).

4. Total amount to be injected varies according to the area. In the lumbar region, a total of 3–6 ml is usually enough, whereas 2–3 ml is sufficient in the thoracic area. If there is any sign of cement extrusion or if it moves toward the intervertebral foramen, the injection should immediately stop (Figs 18.65 and Fig. 18.66).

Step 9. Postprocedure care

After the procedure, the patient should be followed for 3 hours before discharge from the recovery room. The patient should lie down supine for 2 hours and then be allowed to sit. Vital signs, especially neurological monitoring, should be evaluated every 15 minutes for 1 hour, then every 30 minutes for the rest of patient's stay in the clinic. At discharge, the patient and their family should be warned to call the physician if the back pain returns, and if weakness in the lower extremities and fever over 100 °F occurs.

Technique of vertebroplasty by extrapedicular approach

Above the T8 level, the relationship between the vertebral body and the pedicle is different than below the T8 level. The pedicle is perpendicular to the vertebral body, thus a transpedicular approach is difficult and may result in the needle entering the spinal canal. An extrapedicular approach may be safer. Mark the spinous processes of upper and lower levels. Draw a second line perpendicular to the first line just below the transverse process and the pedicles.

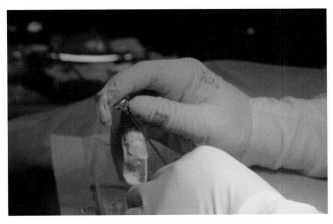

Figure 18.65 Insert the stylet inside the needle before withdrawing the needle.

Visualization of landmarks

1. Rotate the C-arm oblique 20–30° for thoracic levels, 45–50° for L1–L3 levels, 50–55⁰ for L4, and 55–60° for L5 levels.
2. The entry point is just below the pedicle. Infiltrate the skin toward the pedicle with 1% lidocaine.
3. Advance an 11 gauge needle for lumbar and 13 gauge needle for thoracic levels in a tunneled vision until a bony contact is made below the pedicle (Fig. 18.67).
4. Advancing the needle through the cortex of the bone may be accomplished with a twisting motion or gentle tapping of it with a sterile hammer under a lateral view (Fig. 18.68).
5. The depth of the needle is 70% of the vertebral body in a lateral view and in the middle of the vertebral body in a posteroanterior view (Figs 18.69 and 18.70).
6. The remaining steps are as described above.

Complications

• **Hemorrhage**

To prevent hemorrhage in the region, applying pressure and cold packs after the procedure may be helpful.

• **Infection**

The risk of infection should be kept in mind and, similar to all spinal procedures, prophylactic antibiotics should be administered.

• **Cement extrusion, leakage**

Leakage may occur due to the lower viscosity of the cement or due to technical failure.

  ○ Paravertebral leakage

  Cement extrusion into the paravertebral muscles can cause severe localized pain due to the exothermic reaction during PMMA cement curing and the effect of the mass of cement on muscle motion (Fig. 18.71).

  ○ Intravenous leakage

  Leakage of cement into the venous circulation can produce generalized toxic reactions and, when entering the

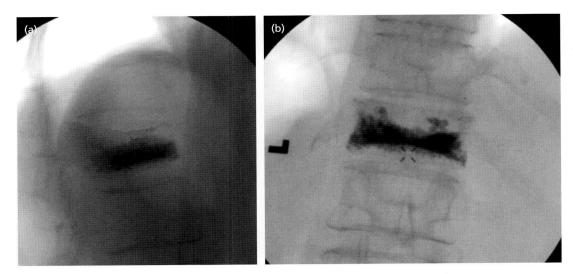

Figure 18.66 View of the cement in (a) lateral and (b) posteroanterior views.

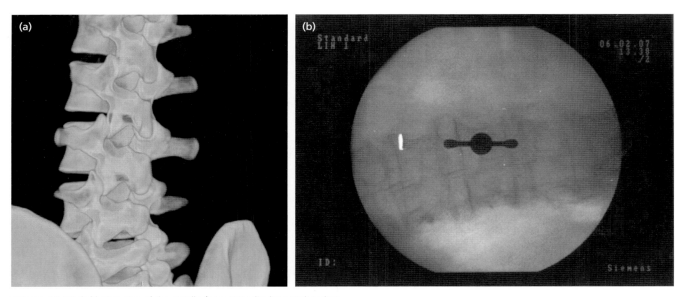

Figure 18.67 (a,b) Direction of the needle for extrapedicular vertebroplasty.

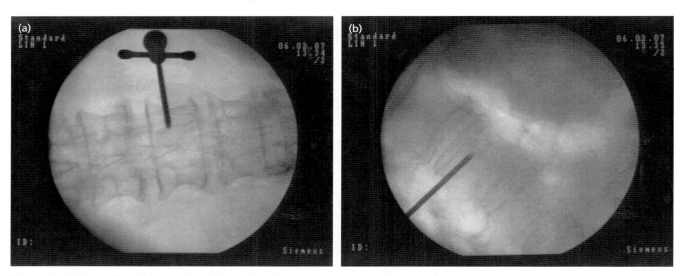

Figure 18.68 The position of the needles in (a) lateral and (b) posteroanterior views for extrapedicular approach.

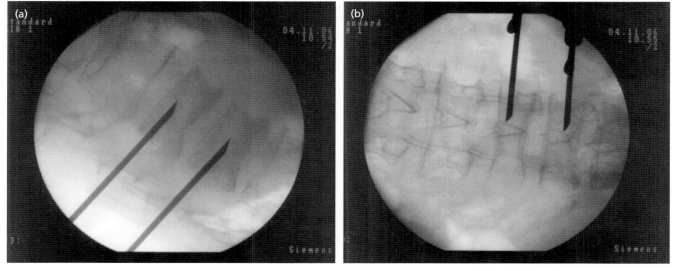

Figure 18.69 (a,b) Position of double needles for extrapedicular approach.

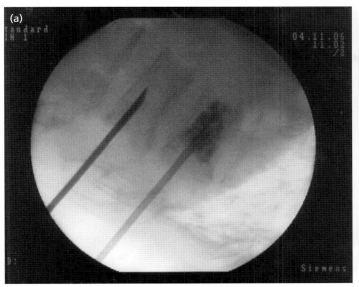

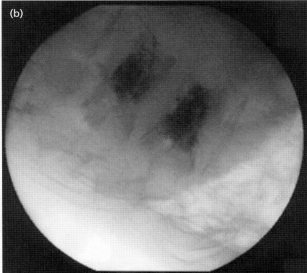

Figure 18.70 (a,b) View of cement for extrapedicular approach.

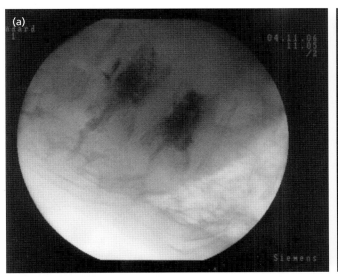

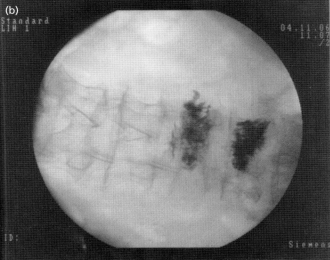

Figure 18.71 (a,b) Paravertebral leakage of the cement.

inferior vena cava, possibly life-threatening pulmonary embolization.

○ Leakage into the spinal canal

Leakage of cement into the epidural space may compress the spinal cord and/or nerve roots. Extravertebral PMMA is frequently seen anterior to the vertebral body adjacent to the periosteum but rarely causes any clinical symptoms. A more problematic complication is foraminal PMMA that occurs due to leakage through the fractured posterior vertebral body wall or through the pedicle wall fractured by the cannula. Such complications result in neuritis along the affected intercostal or segmental nerve.

The spinal canal may be compromised through retropulsion of bone fragments during filling of the vertebral body or PMMA transfer through the posterior fracture site itself into the spinal canal. If symptoms are significant in either case, urgent neurosurgical consultation is required for possible surgical decompression. Neurological deficits, when they occur, usually occur within 24 hours after vertebroplasty, although in more than half of patients post-PMMA, neurological deficits did not occur until an average of 37 days later.

Transient radiculopathy has been reported in 3–6% of patients and has been successfully treated in most cases with steroids and anti-inflammatory medications.

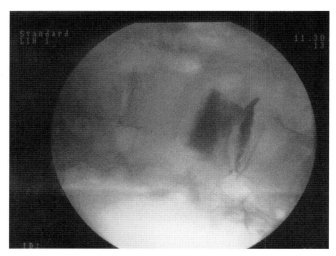

Figure 18.72 Intradiscal leakage of the cement.

○ Leakage to the intervertebral disc.
Leakage to the intervertebral disc is possible owing to fractures of the upper and lower endplates (Fig. 18.72).

• **Pulmonary emboli**
Pulmonary embolism through the azygous system anterior to the spine has an incidence of 0.1–0.6%, although only rarely is such embolism clinically significant. If there is significant dyspnea immediately after vertebroplasty, a CT should be obtained if the X-ray is negative.

• **Fracture of lamina, pedicle**
Cannula placement complications include fracture of the medial wall of the pedicle, cannula placement through the endplate into the intervertebral disc, and nerve injury if the cannula is placed inferiorly in the pedicle fracturing the inferior cortex.

• **Rib fracture**
Rib fracture is related to the positioning of the patient.

Helpful hints

Although it is probably one of the most rewarding interventional procedures, vertebroplasty should only be performed by an experienced physician. Complete pain relief can occur very early after vertebroplasty and the patient may be discharged on the same day.

Careful attention to the technique guidelines, adequate training, and possible proctoring the early cases will ensure the safety of the procedure. Although the complication rate is very low, those performing vertebroplasty should be ready to manage life-threatening complications, such as anaphylactic reactions or potentially devastating neurological sequelae.

Physical and neurological assessment of the patient before the procedure is mandatory. The dimension of the pedicles should be measured by a recent CT.

The possible complications of vertebroplasty should be explained in detail before the procedure and the written consent of the patient should be obtained.

Kyphoplasty

Definition

This technique was first performed in 1998. It may be defined as inserting an inflatable balloon within the vertebral body through a trocar. The cavity formed in the vertebral body is filled with bone cement.

Kyphoplasty was developed to cope with high rates of cement leakage by vertebroplasty and the inability of vertebroplasty to correct fracture deformity. Creation of a cavity within the vertebral body decreases the potential for cement leakage as well as creating a high density zone in the vertebral body.

Indications

• Painful or progressive osteoporotic or osteolytic compression fractures.

Contraindications

• Local or systemic infection.
• Coagulopathy.
• Cardiopulmonary insufficiency.
• Height loss of the vertebral body greater than 80% of the pre-fracture height.
• True burst fractures.
• Fractures associated with neurological findings.

Technique of kyphoplasty

Step 1. Prepare the patient before the procedure
1. The patient should be aware of why this procedure is being done and what to expect from it. All complications and side effects related to the procedure should be explained in detail, before it is started. Valid written consent should be obtained.
2. The type of analgesia or sedation needs to be ascertained before performance of the invasive procedure. Intravenous fentanyl, midazolam, and/or propofol may be used judiciously for the patient's comfort. If radiofrequency thermocoagulation or pulsed radiofrequency is planned, the patient needs to be awake to respond to the stimulation test.
3. CT imaging for the diameter of the pedicles to be entered is helpful. Recent plain radiographs should be examined. Recent MRI should be available, particularly a T2-weighted sagittal image and axial views through the levels of pathology to be treated. Prothrombin time, partial thromboplastin time, and platelet function studies should be done.

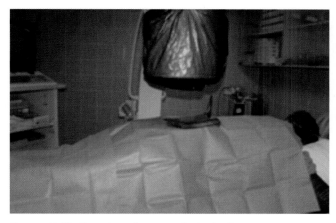

Figure 18.73 Place the patient prone for kyphoplasty.

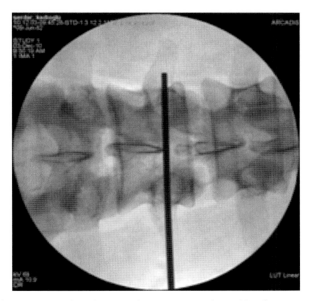

Figure 18.74 Place the C-arm in a posteroanterior position first. Identify the midpoint of the intervertebral space at the target level.

Step 2. Position and monitor the patient
1. Place the patient prone on the table. Place a pillow under the abdomen to flatten the lumbar lordosis (Fig. 18.73).
2. Obtain an intravenous access.
3. Administer oxygen by nasal cannula, monitor the vital signs noninvasively.
4. Prepare and drape the area in a sterile fashion.
The patient should not be over-sedated. The patient should remain sufficiently conscious to provide responses to any questions.

Step 3. Drugs and equipment
• 5 ml syringe for skin infiltration;
• 5 ml syringe for contrast material;
• 25 gauge, 1½ inch needle for skin infiltration;
• no. 11 blade scalpel;

• 11 and 13 gauge bone biopsy needle;
• catheter with inflatable balloon;
• sterile hammer;
• disposable mixing bowl and ladle;
• disposable PMMA injection syringe;
• 1% lidocaine for local anesthesia;
• nonionic contrast material;
• powder methylmethacrylate polymer;
• 10 ml of liquid methylmethacrylate monomer.

Step 4. Visualization
1. Place the C-arm in a posteroanterior position first. Identify the midpoint of the intervertebral space at the target level. Adjust the lower endplate of the target vertebral body to be aligned by moving the C-arm in a cephalocaudal direction (Fig. 18.74).
2. Oblique the C-arm in the coronal plane approximately 45° for L4–L5 and L5–S1 levels and 30° for upper levels until the facet joint is delineated and the "Scottie dog" view appears (Fig. 18.75).
3. It is important to oblique the fluoroscopic view enough to place the facet joint in the middle of the vertebral body and the spinous processes to the contralateral side. This facilitates a central placement of the needle. The target for entry is the superior lateral quadrant of the pedicle in the fluoroscopic view.

Step 5. Mark the surface landmarks for the needle entry
1. Infiltrate the skin over the center of the pedicle toward the pedicle using 1 ml of 1% lidocaine and a 25 gauge needle (Fig. 18.76).
2. A small skin incision is made with a no. 11 blade scalpel to allow insertion of a large-bore biopsy needle.

Step 6. Direction of the needle
1. An 11 gauge bone biopsy needle for lumbar or a 13 gauge needle for thoracic vertebrae is inserted under tunneled vision to the upper outer half of the face of pedicle, which appears as the "Scottie dog." In the higher thoracic region an extrapedicular route lateral to the pedicle is recommended. This approach allows the needle tip to be angled more toward the center of the vertebra and thus allows easy filling of the vertebra with a single needle.
2. The needle shaft should contact the center of the pedicle. Once contact has been made with bone, advance the needle through the cortex.
3. Advancing the needle through the cortex of the bone may be accomplished with a twisting motion or gentle tapping of the needle with a sterile hammer.

Step 7. Confirm the position of the needle
1. Rotate the C-arm laterally. In the lateral view, the needle needs to be at the upper midpoint of the pedicle so that the needle advances in the midpoint of the pedicle.

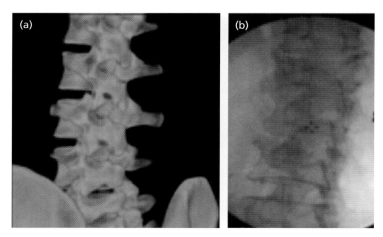

Figure 18.75 (a,b) Oblique the C-arm in the coronal plane approximately 45° for L4–L5 and L5–S1 levels and 30°, for upper levels.

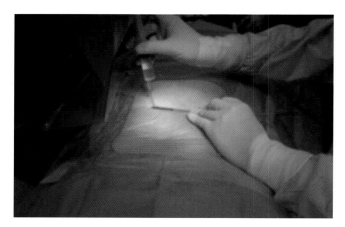

Figure 18.76 Infiltration at the entry point.

2. The target point is at the junction of the anterior and middle third of the vertebral body.
3. Rotate the C-arm to a posteroanterior position. The direction of the needle should be parallel to the endplates of the vertebral body.

Step 8. Kyphoplasty (Figs 18.77–18.79)
1. When the tips of the cannulas have passed the plane of the posterior wall of the vertebral body, the trocar is removed and a drill is introduced to make a channel in the vertebral body (diameter 3.3 mm) for insertion of the catheter with the deflated balloon.
2. The size of the balloon is selected on the basis of the vertebral body to be treated: 6 mm balloons for lumbar and 4 mm balloons for thoracic vertebral bodies are preferred.
3. After placing the needles bilaterally, the balloons are inflated with contrast material in 0.5 ml increments under fluoroscopy with a continuous control of pressure and volume until vertebral body height is restored.
4. After restoration of the vertebral body height, the balloons are retracted and bone cement is injected under fluoroscopy with visualization in two planes.

Step 9. Postprocedure care
After the procedure, the patient should be followed up for 3 hours before discharge. They should lie down supine for 2 hours and then may sit. Vital signs, especially neurological monitoring, should be evaluated every 15 minutes for 1 hour, then every 30 minutes for the rest of the patient's stay.

Complications
The complications of kyphoplasty are as described above for vertebroplasty.

Helpful hints
Patient selection is an important issue for kyphoplasty. The existence of multiple fractures may complicate the diagnosis. Thus a recent MRI or CT are required to identify recent fractures. Sagittal T1-weighted MR sequences can distinguish acute or nonhealed fractures from healed fractures.

If one compares vertebroplasty with kyphoplasty, vertebroplasty is less expensive, faster for the physician and the patient, and may be indicated to treat even older fractures. With kyphoplasty, more anatomic correction of spinal deformity than vertebroplasty is possible. In recent fractures, less than 3 months old, greater height restoration is possible. It is indicated for patients with extensive kyphosis due to multiple recent vertebral compression fractures. The risk of PMMA extravasation is much less than with vertebroplasty.

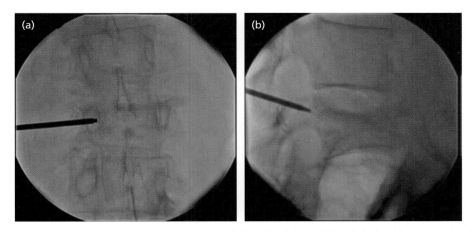

Figure 18.77 (a) In the anteroposterior view the trocar is now at the medial border of the pedicle, which should correspond to the posterior vertebral body cortex. (b) At this point the spinal canal is now cleared and the trocar may be advanced in the lateral projection. (Courtesy of R. Justiz.)

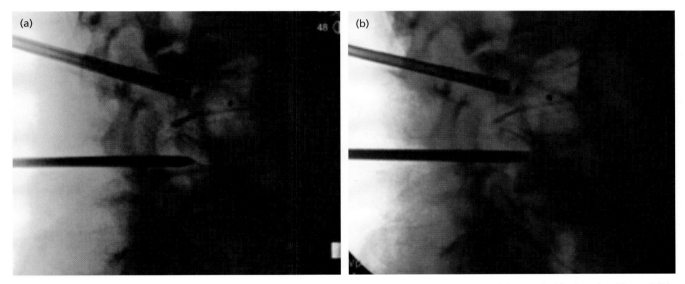

Figure 18.78 (a,b) The trocar may now be advanced in the lateral view 2 cm anterior to the posterior cortex of the vertebral body. A hand bone drill is then inserted and advanced 2–3 cm short of the anterior cortex of the vertebral body. (Courtesy of R. Justiz.)

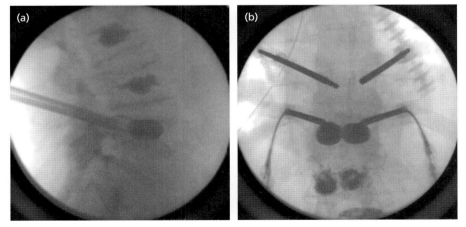

Figure 18.79 (a,b) After placing the needles bilaterally, the balloons are inflated with contrast material in 0.5 ml increments under fluoroscopy. The balloons are retracted and bone cement is injected under fluoroscopy with visualization in two planes. (Courtesy of A. Burton.)

Further reading

Allen, J.W., Horias, K.A., Tozier, N.A. & Yaksh, T.L. (2006) Opiate pharmacology of intrathecal granulomas. *Anesthesiology* **105**(3), 590–598.

Benyamin, R. & Vallejo, R. (2005) Vertebroplasty. *Techniques in Regional Anesthesia and Pain Management* **9**, 62–67.

Boswell, M.V., Trescot, A.M., Datta, S., et al. (2004) Safety and efficacy of spinal cord stimulation for the treatment of chronic pain: a 20-year literature review. *Journal of Neurosurgery: Spine* **100** (3 Suppl.), 254–267.

Burton, A. & Mendel, E. (2003) Vertebroplasty and kyphoplasty. *Pain Physician* **6**, 335–343.

Deer, T., Krames, E.S., Hassenbusch, S.J., et al. (2007) Polyanalgesic consensus conference 2007: recommendations for the management of pain by intrathecal (intraspinal) drug delivery: report of an interdisciplinary expert panel. *Neuromodulation* **10**, 300–328.

Deer, T.R. & Stewart, C.D. (2008) Complications of spinal cord stimulation: identification, treatment, and prevention. *Pain Medicine* **9**(1 Suppl.), S93–S101.

Deer, T., Winkenmüller, W., Erdine, S., Bedder, M. & Burchiel, K. (1999) Intrathecal therapy for cancer and non malignant pain: patient selection and patient management. *Neuromodulation* **2**(2), 55–66.

DuPen, S.L. (1998) Implantable spinal catheter and drug systems complications. *Techniques in Regional Anesthesia and Pain Management* **2**(3), 152–160.

Erdine, S. & De Andres, J. (2006) Drug delivery systems. *Pain Practice* **6**(1), 51–57.

Follett, K.A., Boortz-Marx, R.L., Drake, J.M., et al. (2004) Prevention and management of intrathecal drug delivery and spinal cord stimulation system infections. *Anesthesiology* **100**(6), 1582–1594.

Forouzanfar, T., Kemler, M.A., Weber, W.E., Kessels, A.G. & Van Kleef, M. (2004) Spinal cord stimulation in complex regional pain syndrome: cervical and lumbar devices are comparably effective. *British Journal of Anaesthesia* **92**(3), 348–353.

Gybels, J., Erdine, S., Maeyaert, J., et al. (1998) Neuromodulation of pain. A consensus statement prepared in Brussels 16–18 January 1998 by the following task force of the European Federation of IASP Chapters (EFIC). *European Journal of Pain* **2**(3), 203–209.

Hassenbusch, S.J., Portenoy, R.K., Cousins, M., et al. (2004) Polyanalgesic Consensus Conference 2003: an update on the management of pain by intraspinal drug delivery – report of an expert panel. *Journal of Pain and Symptom Management* **27**(6), 540–563.

Hu, Y.C. & Hart, D.J. (2007) Complications of vertebroplasty and kyphoplasty. *Techniques in Regional Anesthesia and Pain Management* **11**(3), 164–170.

Jones, R.L. & Rawlins, P.K. (2005) The diagnosis of intrathecal infusion pump system failure. *Pain Physician* **8**(3), 291–296.

Kumar, K., Buchser, E., Linderoth, B., Meglio, M. & Van Buyten, J.-P. (2007) Avoiding complications from spinal cord stimulation: practical recommendations from an international panel of experts. *Neuromodulation* **10**(1), 24–33.

Mailis-Gagnon, A., Furlan, A.D., Sandoval, J.A. & Taylor, R. (2004) Spinal cord stimulation for chronic pain. *Cochrane Database of Systematic Reviews* **3**, CD003783.

McIntyre, P.J., Deer, T.R. & Hayek, S.M. (2007) Complications of spinal infusion therapies. *Techniques in Regional Anesthesia and Pain Management* **11**, 183–192.

Perez, M.R. & Pulley, S.C. (2010) Intrathecal analgesia in cancer pain. *Techniques in Regional Anesthesia and Pain Management* **14**(1), 10–18.

Raffaeli, W., Andruccioli, J., Righetti, D., Caminiti, A. & Balestri, M. (2006) Intraspinal therapy for the treatment of chronic pain: a review of the literature between 1990 and 2005 and suggested protocol for its rational and safe use. *Neuromodulation* **9**(4), 290–308.

Rosenow, J.M., Stanton-Hicks, M., Rezai, A.R. & Henderson, J.M. (2006) Failure modes of spinal cord stimulator hardware. *Journal of Neurosurgery: Spine* **5**(3), 183–190.

Ruan, X. (2007) Drug-related side effects of long-term intrathecal morphine therapy: a focused review. *Pain Physician* **10**, 357–366.

Smith, H.S., Deer, T.R., Staats, P.S., Singh, V., Sehgal, N. & Cordner, H. (2008) Intrathecal drug delivery. *Pain Physician* **11**(2 Suppl.), S89–S104.

Soin, A., Kapural, L. & Mekhail, N. (2007) Imaging for percutaneous vertebral augmentation. *Techniques in Regional Anesthesia and Pain Management* **11**, 90–94.

Taylor, R.S., Van Buyten, J.P. & Buchser, E. (2005) Spinal cord stimulation for chronic back and leg pain and failed back surgery syndrome: a systematic review and analysis of prognostic factors. *Spine* **30**(1), 152–160.

Taylor, R.S., Van Buyten, J.-P. & Buchser, E. (2006) Spinal cord stimulation for complex regional pain syndrome: a systematic review of the clinical and cost-effectiveness literature and assessment of prognostic factors. *European Journal of Pain* **10**(2), 91–101.

Turner, J.A., Loeser, J.D., Deyo, R.A. & Sanders, S.B. (2004) Spinal cord stimulation for patients with failed back surgery syndrome or complex regional pain syndrome: a systematic review of effectiveness and complications. *Pain* **108**(1–2), 137–147.

Turner, J.A., Sears, J.M. & Loeser, J.D. (2007) Programmable intrathecal opioid delivery systems for chronic nonmalignant pain: a systematic review of effectiveness and complications. *Clinical Journal of Pain* **23**(2), 180–195.

Vallejo, R., Benyamin, R., Yousuf, N. & Kramer, J. (2006) Vertebroplasty. *Pain Practice* **6**(3), 203–205.

Waara-Wolleat, K.L., Hildebrand, K.R. & Stewart, G.R. (2006) A review of intrathecal fentanyl and sufentanil for the treatment of chronic pain. *Pain Medicine* **7**(3), 251–259.

Wallace, M.S., Charapata, S.G., Fisher, R., et al. (2006) Intrathecal ziconotide treatment of chronic non-malignant pain: a randomized double blind placebo controlled clinical trial. *Neuromodulation* **9**(2), 75–86.

Woods, D.M., Hayek, S.M. & Bedder, M. (2007) Complications of neurostimulation. *Techniques in Regional Anesthesia and Pain Management* **11**(3), 178–182.

Index

Pain-Relieving Procedures: The Illustrated Guide, First Edition. P. Prithvi Raj and Serdar Erdine.
© 2012 John Wiley & Sons, Ltd. Published 2012 by John Wiley & Sons, Ltd.

Index

Index

Index